Brain Imaging in Clinical Psychiatry

Brain Imaging in Clinical Psychiatry

edited by

**K. Ranga Rama Krishnan
and P. Murali Doraiswamy**

*Duke University Medical Center
Durham, North Carolina*

MARCEL DEKKER, INC.   NEW YORK · BASEL · HONG KONG

ISBN: 0-8247-9859-7

The publisher offers discounts on this book when ordered in bulk quantities. For more information, write to Special Sales/Professional Marketing at the address below.

This book is printed on acid-free paper.

Marcel Dekker, Inc.
270 Madison Avenue, New York, New York 10016

Current printing (last digit):
10 9 8 7 6 5 4 3 2 1

PRINTED IN THE UNITED STATES OF AMERICA

This book is dedicated to our families.

Preface

The search for brain pathology as an underlying cause of psychiatric disorders continues to be the driving force behind biological psychiatry. Until about a decade ago, the only way to evaluate abnormalities in brain structure was by postmortem neuropathological studies. These studies were limited by several confounding factors, such as postmortem changes in the brain, problems with fixation, heterogeneous samples, agonal factors, and comorbid medical conditions including cardiovascular and cerebrovascular disease. Thus the results of the early postmortem studies were often contradictory and difficult to interpret. Early imaging techniques such as skull x-rays and ventriculograms were insensitive and provided limited information.

The advent of computed tomography (CT) enabled observation of living brain tissue for the first time. In the years since CT began providing in vivo evidence of cerebral atrophy, for example, enlarged ventricles and sulcal dilation in schizophrenia, there have been numerous reports of CT showing gross morphological changes in patients with psychotic disorders.

Magnetic resonance imaging (MRI)—with its greater tissue differentiation, three-dimensional acquisition capability, and increased flexibility in acquiring and reslicing the brain in orientations that facilitate rendering, visualizing, and quantifying specific structures in the brain—has led to a veritable explosion of studies documenting regional changes in the brain in psychiatric disorders. Patients with psychiatric disorders generally manifest subtle brain abnormalities that are best characterized by quantitative measures.

Magnetic resonance spectroscopy (MRS) is a unique, noninvasive tool that is useful for probing metabolic function in the living brain without using any radioactive compounds. MRS has been successfully applied in investigating neuropsychiatric disorders including schizophrenia, Alzheimer's disease, and depression. Some MRS measured neurochemicals may also have clinical utility as adjuncts in following progression of a disease.

Positron emission tomography (PET) and single photon emission computed tomography (SPECT) now afford unprecedented opportunities for studying in vivo neurochemistry, cerebral blood flow, and receptor binding. A number of studies using these technologies have begun to elucidate the pathophysiology of neuropsychiatric disorders and have led to increased clinical use of these methods in neuropsychiatry (e.g., for Alzheimer's disease and temporal lobe epilepsy). Functional MRI has begun to complement and extend both the time and spatial resolution of neuronal and activation studies and has the potential to revolutionize our understanding of human brain function in neuropsychiatric disorders.

This book provides clinicians and researchers with a background and comprehensive introduction for imaging neuropsychiatric disorders. It addresses relevant questions regarding the current state of imaging in different neuropsychiatric disorders and indicates the potential clinical value of the various neuroimaging techniques.

The general format is organized by specific disorder categories and by imaging modalities. The contributors are primarily clinical scientists who utilize neuroimaging in their research. Chapters 1A, 1B, and 2 are designed to provide a basic understanding of the general principles of MRI, MRS, SPECT and PET. For a more detailed discussion on instrumentation and technical aspects of these modalities, readers are referred to the references in these chapters. Chapter 4, on normal functional neuroanatomy, is restricted to a discussion of the limbic system and planum temporale. We selected this region given its obvious relevance to neuropsychiatry and its significance in contemporary neuropsychiatric imaging studies. The normal functional anatomy of other cortical and subcortical areas, as well as more theoretical discussions of brain circuitry, are not elaborated separately in order to limit the length of this book. Chapter 5 summarizes imaging studies of normal brain development and is restricted to issues relevant to interpreting imaging studies of child and adolescent psychiatric disorders. It does not address other aspects of brain maturation, such as changes during birth and infancy, that were felt to be more relevant to a neuroradiologist or pediatric neurologist.

The subsequent chapters discuss specific structural and functional imaging findings in selected childhood and adult psychiatric disorders, including developmental disorders (Chapter 6), mood disorders (Chapters 7–10), eating disorders (Chapter 12), schizophrenia and psychotic disorders (Chapters 12–15), anxiety disorders (Chapters 16 and 17), and personality disorders (Chapter 18). Chapters 19–23 review imaging progress in selected neuropsychiatric conditions such as dementia, adult aging, HIV dementia, and in chronic fatigue syndrome. The disorders selected in each case represent, in our opinion, the areas of greatest current interest to psychiatrists and clinical neuropsychiatric researchers. Chapters on imaging findings in alcoholism and substance abuse and fMRI studies in psychiatry may be included in future editions of this book, as new information on these topics becomes available. Each chapter was written to provide a comprehensive yet concise update useful for both clinicians and researchers. The chapters emphasize the utility of imaging in unraveling pathophysiologic mechanisms rather than as a diagnostic tool. In routine psychiatric practice, neuroimaging is not essential in most typical clinical presentations, for either diagnosis or treatment.

We are grateful to our many contributors for their substantial time commitments in the preparation of their chapters. Finally, we are grateful to our colleagues and families for their support and patience during the production of this book.

K. Ranga Rama Krishnan
P. Murali Doraiswamy

Contents

Contents

Contributors

Eileen Ahearn, M.D., Ph.D. Department of Psychiatry and Behavioral Sciences, Duke University Medical Center, Durham, North Carolina

Kevin John Black, M.D. Departments of Psychiatry, Neurology, and Radiology, Washington University School of Medicine, St. Louis, Missouri

Sarah W. Book, M.D. Department of Psychiatry and Behavioral Sciences, Clinical Psychopharmacology Research Division, Medical University of South Carolina, Charleston, South Carolina

Kelly N. Botteron, M.D. Departments of Psychiatry and Radiology, Mallinckrodt Institute of Radiology, Washington University School of Medicine, St. Louis, Missouri

Olga Brawman-Mintzer, M.D. Department of Psychiatry and Behavioral Sciences, Clinical Psychopharmacology Research Division, Medical University of South Carolina, Charleston, South Carolina

Christopher E. Byrum, M.D., Ph.D. Department of Psychiatry and Behavioral Sciences, Duke University Medical Center, Durham, North Carolina

F. Xavier Castellanos, M.D. Child Psychiatry Branch, National Institute of Mental Health, Bethesda, Maryland

H. Cecil Charles, Ph.D. Department of Radiology, Duke University Medical Center, Durham, North Carolina

Jennifer Cousins   Department of Psychiatry, Duke University Medical Center, Durham, North Carolina

Jonathan R. T. Davidson, M.D.   Department of Psychiatry and Behavioral Sciences, Duke University Medical Center, Durham, North Carolina

Michael Devous, Sr.   Department of Psychiatry, University of Texas Southwestern Medical Center, Dallas, Texas

Gary S. Figiel, M.D.   Department of Psychiatry and Behavioral Sciences, Emory University, Atlanta, Georgia

Mark S. George, M.D.   Functional Neuroimaging Division, Department of Psychiatry and Behavioral Sciences, Medical University of South Carolina, Charleston, South Carolina

Jay N. Giedd, M.D.   Child Psychiatry Branch, National Institute of Mental Health, Bethesda, Maryland

Michael Gonzalez   Department of Psychiatry, Duke University Medical Center, Durham, North Carolina

Raquel E. Gur, M.D., Ph.D.   Department of Psychiatry, Mental Health Clinical Research Center, University of Pennsylvania, Philadelphia, Pennsylvania

John M. Hoffman, M.D.   Departments of Neurology and Radiology, Center for Positron Emission Tomography, Emory University School of Medicine, Atlanta, Georgia

Mustafa M. Husain, M.D.   Department of Psychiatry, University of Texas Southwestern Medical Center, Dallas, Texas

Dilip V. Jeste, M.D.   Department of Psychiatry, University of California—San Diego, and VA Medical Center, San Diego, California

Ingrid Kemperman, M.D.   Department of Psychiatry, The New York Hospital—Cornell Medical Center, New York, New York

Matcheri S. Keshavan, M.D.   Department of Psychiatry, University of Pittsburgh, Western Psychiatric Institute and Clinic, Pittsburgh, Pennsylvania

K. Ranga Rama Krishnan, M.D.   Department of Psychiatry and Behavioral Sciences, Duke University Medical Center, Durham, North Carolina

Anand Kumar, M.D. Director, Mood and Memory Disorders Clinic, Section of Geriatric Psychiatry, University of Pennsylvania School of Medicine, Philadelphia, Pennsylvania

R. Bruce Lydiard, M.D. Department of Psychiatry and Behavioral Science, Clinical Psychopharmacology Research Division, Medical University of South Carolina, Charleston, South Carolina

James R. MacFall, Ph.D. Department of Radiology, Duke University Medical Center, Durham, North Carolina

David J. Madden, Ph.D. Center for the Study of Aging and Human Development of Department of Psychiatry and Behavioral Science, Duke University Medical Center, Durham, North Carolina

Robert W. McCarley, M.D. Department of Psychiatry, Harvard Medical School, Boston; Brockton Veterans Affairs Medical Center, Brockton; Massachusetts Mental Health Center, Boston; and McLean Hospital, Belmont, Massachusetts

Constance M. Moore, M.Sc., Ph.D. Brain Imaging Center, McLean Hospital, Belmont, and Harvard Medical School, Boston, Massachusetts

Lyn M. Harper Mozley, Ph.D. Department of Psychiatry, Mental Health Clinical Research Center, University of Pennsylvania, Philadelphia, Pennsylvania

Jay W. Pettegrew, M.D., Ph.D. Department of Psychiatry and Neurology, University of Pittsburgh, Western Psychiatric Institute and Clinic, Pittsburgh, Pennsylvania

Nicholas L. S. Potts, M.D. Department of Psychiatry and Behavioral Sciences, Duke University Medical Center, Durham, North Carolina

Perry F. Renshaw, M.D., Ph.D. Brain Imaging Center, McLean Hospital, Belmont, and Harvard Medical School, Boston, Massachusetts

Mark J. Russ, M.D. Director of Critical Care Psychiatry, Hillside Hospital, Long Island Jewish Medical Center, Glen Oaks, New York

Martha E. Shenton, Ph.D. Department of Psychiatry, Harvard Medical School, Boston; Brockton Veterans Affairs Medical Center, Brockton; Massachusetts Mental Health Center, Boston; and McLean Hospital, Belmont, Massachusetts

David Silbersweig, M.D.   Functional Neuroimaging Laboratory, Departments of Psychiatry, Neurology, and Neuroscience, The New York Hospital—Cornell Medical Center, New York, New York

Theodore B. Snyderman   Department of Psychiatry and Behavioral Sciences, Duke University Medical Center, Durham, North Carolina

David C. Steffens, M.D.   Geriatric Depression Clinic, Duke University Medical Center, Durham, North Carolina

Emily Stern, M.D.   Functional Neuroimaging Laboratory, Departments of Psychiatry and Radiology, The New York Hospital—Cornell Medical Center, New York, New York

Charlie L. Swanson, Jr., M.D.   Department of Psychiatry, Mental Health Clinical Research Center, University of Pennsylvania, Philadelphia, Pennsylvania

Laura L. Symonds, Ph.D.   Department of Psychiatry, University of California—San Diego, San Diego, California

Jill E. Thompson, M.D.   Department of Radiology, University of North Carolina Hospitals, Chapel Hill, North Carolina

John Travers, M.D.   Department of Psychiatry and Behavioral Sciences, Duke University Medical Center, Durham, North Carolina

Madhukar H. Trivedi, M.D.   Department of Psychiatry, University of Texas Southwestern Medical Center, Dallas, Texas

Gerardo Villarreal, M.D.*   Department of Psychiatry and Behavioral Sciences, Clinical Psychopharmacology Research Division, Medical University of South Carolina, Charleston, South Carolina

Cynthia G. Wible, Ph.D.   Department of Psychiatry, Harvard Medical School, Boston; Brockton Veterans Affairs Medical Center, Brockton; Massachusetts Mental Health Center, Boston; and McLean Hospital, Belmont, Massachusetts

---

* *Current affiliation*: Department of Psychiatry, Appalachian Regional Healthcare, Harlan, Kentucky

1A

Basic Principles of Magnetic Resonance Imaging

K. Ranga Rama Krishnan and James R. MacFall
Duke University Medical Center, Durham, North Carolina

This chapter will provide a brief introduction to the principles underlying magnetic resonance imaging (MRI). The focus and intent of this chapter is to educate the reader about some of the basic concepts underlying magnetic resonance imaging. Mathematical details will not be provided. Additional information regarding the principles of magnetic resonance imaging are available from a variety of sources for the interested reader [1–8].

I. INTRODUCTION

Magnetic resonance is a primary interaction between a magnetically active nucleus (such as hydrodgen in water, phosphorus in cellular metabolism, or fluorine in many medicinal preparations) and a magnetic field. When such a nuclear magnet is placed in a magnetic field, it tries to align itself with the field. In this process it oscillates like a spinning top at a frequency called the Larmor frequency, which is faster with stronger magnetic fields. If the magnetic field is graded, i.e., varied, then this frequency of oscillation will also vary. The frequency of oscillation depends upon the properties of the nuclear magnet and the magnetic field.

In order to simplify and present the principles underlying magnetic resonance imaging and spectroscopy, we present the principles in the form of concepts. The concepts are built in a sequential fashion to help the reader grasp the basic principles.

II. MAGNETIC NUCLEI

Atomic elements are made up of many particles. The following particles are important for understanding magnetic resonance: protons (positively charged), neutrons (not charged), and electrons (negatively charged). Protons and neutrons are present in the nucleus, and electrons orbit around the nucleus.

When the nucleus contains an odd number of either protons or neutrons, it is magnetic. Examples of common elements include hydrogen (one proton), C^{13} (13 protons, whereas the usual carbon has 12 protons), and P^{31} (31 protons). Of the many elements, the most abundant in living tissue is hydrogen. Hydrogen also has the strongest magnetic interaction of the biologically interesting nuclei. Hydrogen is therefore the element of most interest to magnetic resonance imaging.

Why is hydrogen magnetic? The simplest explanation is based on the fundamental properties of atoms. First, protons and neutrons, in addition to having a defined mass, spin about their axes. The main component of spin is called *angular momentum*, which is related to spin number. Just like a dynamo in a power plant, the spinning nuclear charge of a proton produces a magnetic field, called the *magnetic moment*. Since a neutron can be thought of as a proton and an electron bound together by a neutrino, the spinning charges in the neutron also produce a (different) magnetic field.

The number of protons determines the electrical charge of the nucleus. Both protons and neutrons have a spin value of h/2, where h is Planck's constant. (Note that the spin value can be plus or minus.) Inside the nucleus, protons and neutrons tend to pair off oppositely in terms of spin to each other. Thus, paired neutrons and paired protons (with opposite spin values) produce no significant magnetic field. The single unpaired proton or neutron, however, does produce magnetic effects. Since protons and neutrons are distinct particles and have very different magnetic moments, they are not usually simultaneously observable.

III. NUCLEAR MAGNETIC RESONANCE

When a hydrogen atom is placed in a magnetic field, it behaves like a magnet, i.e., it aligns itself with the direction of the magnetic field. Because it has an inherent spin, it does not just align itself in the direction of the field, but oscillates (like a top) around the magnetic field. The frequency (also called the Larmor frequency) of oscillation is proportional to the strength of the magnetic field and the strength of the magnetic moment. The proportionality constant is called the *nuclear gyromagnetic ratio*, which is the ratio of the magnetic moment to its angular momentum.

The meaning of the word resonance as used in nuclear magnetic resonance (NMR) is similar to that used when describing the resonance of a tuning fork. Resonance is when the applied frequency (sound in the case of a tuning fork or magnetic in the case of NMR) is of the identical frequency as the object. In the case of atomic nuclei, the resonance frequency is the Larmor frequency.

When the magnetic field strength is varied, the Larmor frequency changes. Thus, if the magnetic field is established as a gradient, the Larmor frequency will vary depending on where the magnetic nuclei are located on the gradient. Magnetic nuclei have the following characteristics:

1. They have unpaired protons or neutrons.
2. They oscillate in the direction of the magnetic field.
3. The frequency of oscillation is proportional to the strength of the field.

IV. RADIOFREQUENCY STIMULATION AND RELEASE OF ENERGY

Magnetic nuclei in a magnetic field can be stimulated by other magnetic fields. These fields can be created by magnets or, if the magnetic field is strong enough, by radiofrequency waves tuned to the Larmor frequency of the atomic nuclei in that particular magnetic field. This is true for magnets with a field strength of from approximately 600–4000 G (the earth's magnetic field is 1/2 G, and a typical refrigerator magnet measures about 100 G). When the magnetic field created by the radiofrequency field is turned on, a remarkable thing happens: the atom oscillates in the direction of this new field, causing the nuclei to move in and out of alignment with the main (non–radiofrequency-created) field. When the field is turned off, the nuclei relax, emit the absorbed energy, and return to the prestimulated state (aligned again with the main field). This process can be repeated over and over as long as enough time is allowed for the nuclear "relaxation."

V. MAGNETIZATION VECTORS

So far we have discussed the behavior of single atoms, whereas of concern to NMR applications in medicine is the behavior of billions of atoms. When hydrogen atoms are placed in a magnetic field, a preponderance of magnetic moments will point in the direction of the field (parallel to the field). The preponderance is actually quite small in the fields used in clinical scanners. The direction of this preponderance of magnetic moments is described in the form of a magnetization vector (a mathematical construct used to describe strength and direction).

The realignment of magnetization induced by a radiofrequency pulse changes the direction of the magnetization vector. Pulses are defined by the angle to which they change the direction of the magnetization vector, i.e., a 90° pulse changes the direction by 90°. The greater the change, the greater the strength of the pulse.

VI. NMR SIGNAL OR FREE INDUCTION DECAY

When the hydrogen atoms in a magnetic field are stimulated by radiofrequency, they realign themselves (actually oscillate) in the direction of the new magnetic field. When the field is turned off, the rotating magnetization vector will produce an electromagnetic field at the Larmor frequency. For strong enough magnetic fields, the electromagnetic field is at radiofrequency and the collection of nuclei act briefly like a small radio transmitter. This field can be detected by tuning a radiofrequency antenna (receiving coil) to the Larmor frequency. This detected signal is the NMR signal. The signal will decay as the magnetization returns to equilibrium. The decay of this signal is called *free induction decay* (FID).

VII. RELAXATION

After the radiofrequency (RF) magnetic field is turned off, the nuclei return to their prestimulation condition (aligned with the main magnetic field). The term *relaxation* is used to describe this return of magnetization to equilibrium. The time to recover 63% of the magnetization is called the T_1 relaxation time.

The magnetization vector is described in terms of two component vectors. One, the *longitudinal vector*, is along the z axis (the magnetic field direction), and the other, at right angles to the z axis, is called the *transverse vector*. In the case of clinical MRI, the z axis or longitudinal axis is along the length of the base of the magnet. If the individual is lying on his back inside the scanner, the z axis is the head-foot direction. By convention, the y axis refers to the front-back and the x axis is right-left. Before the RF pulse is applied, the magnetization vector is described entirely by the longitudinal component. After the RF pulse is applied, the vector is described by both the longitudinal and transverse component. The length of the magnetization vector is the same before and after the stimulation, and it depends on the number of hydrogen atoms. The stronger the RF pulse, i.e., the greater the deflection of the vector, the greater the length of the transverse vector (maximum at 90°) and the shorter the longitudinal vector. Two components are used because the receiver only measures the transverse component. When the pulse is turned off, the transverse component shortens and the longitudinal component returns to its original position.

A. T₁ Relaxation

T_1 relaxation is exponential and is the time taken to recover 63% of the longitudinal vector. Thus, it represents the time to regain the ability to make a signal. This is also called spin-lattice relaxation time. T_1 for pure water is about 3000 ms (or 3 s) in most clinical scanners. This relaxation time is influenced by the microenvironment of the hydrogen atoms and in tissues can vary between 150 (fat) 900 (gray matter), 750 (white matter), and 2000 ms (cerebrospinal fluid). These values are for 1.5 Tesla (15000 Gauss) magnets. The values are smaller at lower fields—almost 20% lower at 0.5 Tesla.

B. T_2 Relaxation

T_2 relaxation refers to the relaxation of the transverse component. This is also approximately exponential. In contrast to T_1, however, it represents the time over which the signal disappears. In pure water T_1 and T_2 are approximately equal. In tissues, however, T_2 is usually much shorter (factors of 1/5 to 1/10) than T_1. For example, in brain, the T_2 value is about 70 ms and in cerebrospinal fluid it is 300 ms.

The mechanism for transverse relaxation involves dephasing. The many billions of hydrogen atoms in the magnetic field experience local magnetic field effects from neighboring atoms. These local magnetic fields can be very different (especially if it is not made up of the same molecules in the same environment). This causes the hydrogen atoms to oscillate at slightly different frequencies. Thus, although immediately after the pulse they oscillate about the same frequency, when the pulse is turned off, the different atoms can oscillate at different frequencies depending on the local environment. This causes the hydrogen atoms to dephase. Thus T_2 is always shorter than T_1.

C. T_2^*

There are two sources of dephasing. The first is random, thermal motion of neighboring atoms in tissues, and the second is nonuniformity of the magnetic field due to local variations in the main field due to shielding of the main field by tissue structure variations (such as air tissue or bone tissue interfaces) T_2 refers to the random effects, while T_2' refers to the dephasing due to nonuniformity of the magnetic field. In tissues in such nonuniform regions, T_2' can be very short (1–10 ms). These two numbers are combined into a single number called T_2^*. When random effects predominate, T_2^* is close to (but less than) T_2, while when nonuniformity effects predominate, T_2^* is close to (but less than) T_2'. T_2^* always describes the decay time of the free induction signal.

VIII. APPLICATION TO NMR IMAGING

In NMR imaging the subject is placed in a magnetic field (magnet bore), after which the area of interest is stimulated by a radiofrequency coil. The

NMR signal is picked up by a receiver coil, and is then used to localize and characterize the area of interest.

Nuclear magnetic resonance was originally used as an analytical technique in physics and later in chemistry. In the last decade, principles of magnetic resonance have been applied to examining animals and humans. In magnetic resonance imaging the living object is essentially placed inside a large magnet and stimulated by radiofrequency using the transmitting coil. The signal from the object is picked up in a receiving coil and the information is used to construct the image. Thus, a magnetic resonance image is a representation of the NMR signal from hydrogen atoms in the living subject. When NMR imaging was first developed, NMR signals were collected from a whole line or column of elements and/or from individual elements. With more advanced technology signals are collected either in two dimensions, that is, from a whole plane of elements, and the data is processed so that an image of the plane is obtained and/or the NMR signal is obtained from the whole three-dimensional object at the same time and the data is processed to characterize all the volume elements. At the current time, most NMR images used are either planar imaging or three-dimensional imaging. Planar imaging is primarily used for clinical purposes, and three-dimensional imaging is becoming more popular for morphometric methods because it allows thinner slices do planar methods.

A. Slice Selection

In planar imaging the first step is to isolate the slice to be imaged. In all of the imaging methods available, the object is placed in a field gradient whose direction is perpendicular to the plane of the slice. For example, for an axial slice the gradient would be in the z direction along the head-to-foot axis of the subject. The object is then irradiated with a pulse whose frequency spectrum corresponds to a small range of frequency values. Only those nuclei in the slice in which these range of frequencies are available will be excited. In the presence of the gradient field the hydrogens in the body are spatially encoded, that is, there is a relationship between the resonant frequency and their position in the gradient. In this way, through the application of a gradient to the body and exposure of the tissue to the radio signal of a narrow frequency range, only in the slice are hydrogen nuclei stimulated and the plane is isolated from neighboring regions. Although in theory it is possible to produce a stimulating pulse of a single frequency, such a pulse would be too long in duration (several seconds) to be practical. Thus, in practice the frequencies are restricted to a range sufficient to produce a signal that can be easily detected, resulting in slice thicknesses of 5–20 mm. The slice can be selected with equal ease in the transverse sagittal coronal or in any other direction.

B. Observe Gradient

The above-described slice selection provides spatial resolution in one direction. The slice must then be imaged in two dimensions. To accomplish this a second gradient is turned on immediately following the excitation pulse. A result of applying the second gradient is that the nuclei resonate at different frequencies along the gradient, i.e., they are spatially encoded in a second dimension. The Fourier transform of the signal analyzes both frequencies and gives a profile of the object along the direction of the gradient. These two techniques provide spatial resolution along two axes.

C. Gradient Echo

Application of a gradient causes protons to oscillate at different positions at different frequencies. This causes dephasing and loss of signal. If the gradient is reversed, the dephasing is reversed and the signal returns to maximum. This is called a *gradient echo*. Its use in these sequences allows the acquisition of a smoothly varying signal that minimizes certain image anomalies or artifacts.

D. Phase Encoding

The above methods provide resolution in two dimensions. To obtain the third dimension, phase encoding is used. Phase encoding depends on the detection of the two components of the transverse vector, i.e., in the x and y plane. The x component is proportional to the cosine and the y component to the sine of the phase of magnetization in the xy plane.

Following the radiofrequency pulse, the signals are in phase in the xy plane for a brief time ($t \sim 1$ ms). A phase-encoding gradient is now applied. When the gradient is on, depending on the position, the precession frequency is changed. This change in frequency changes the phase of the signal relative to the signals from the other positions. Repeated phase-encoding gradients can thus be used to determine the location of the precessing magnetic moments that create the signals. Phase encoding can be applied along three dimensions to give three-dimensional spatial resolution.

E. Spatial Resolution and Temporal Resolution

As spatial resolution is increased, i.e., by decreasing the volume of each element, the signal-to-noise ratio also decreases. The signal-to-noise ratio is often improved by signal averaging, which is accomplished by obtaining the signal repeatedly and averaging the results. The signal-to-noise ratio increases linearly with the square root of the number of signal acquisitions averaged. Increased temporal resolution also causes loss of signal-to-noise ratio, because the time available for signal averaging is decreased.

IX. SPIN ECHO

After a 90° pulse is applied, the precessing nuclei go out of phase. This is complete at about $2T_2$. When a 180° pulse is applied after a specified time interval, the phase of the nuclear magnetic moments is reversed. Thus, a moment that had a large phase accumulation now has a large negative phase. Since the nuclei are still oscillating at the same rate as the original decay, they begin to catch up with each other. At a time twice the interval between the 90° and 180° pulse, the oscillating nuclei get back into phase. This reoccurrence of the signal is called an echo, and the sequence is called a spin echo sequence. The time between the 90° pulse and the echo is called the echo time, or TE. When the two pulses are repeated several times, there is a decline in the height of the echo. This decrease is related to T_2. In regions of short T_2 there is rapid degradation compared to regions of larger T_2. This phenomenon is used to produce tissue contrast between tissues with different T_2 values.

A. T_1-Weighted Images

T_1 is much longer than T_2. Encoding T_1 information depends on the intervals between repetitions of spin echo sequences. This interval is called the repetition time, or TR. The length of the repetition time affects the amplitude of the free induction decay because the shorter the repetition time, the less time there is for the longitudinal vector to return to equilibrium. Thus, at times shorter than T_1 the longitudinal vector still has not fully returned to its equilibrium magnitude. When a subsequent repetition of the pulse sequence is applied, the signal create from this longitudinal magnetization is smaller. This essentially leads to a lower amplitude of free induction decay. Since different tissues have different T_1, this provides the T_1 contrast. When T_1 is long, the voxels appear dark and when T_1 is short, they appear bright.

B. T_2-Weighted Images

T_2-weighted images are obtained from a pulse sequence that uses a long TE value so that T_2 is an important factor in controlling image intensity. One of the popular methods of producing T_2-weighted images uses a spin echo sequence with a repetition time longer than T_1. This reduces the effect of T_1 on the free induction decay. In T_2-weighted images, long T_2 voxels appear bright and short T_2 appear dark. By varying the echo time, T_2 contrast is altered.

X. TISSUE CONTRAST

Tissue contrast is provided by hydrogen distribution (also known as proton density), T_1, and T_2. Scanning pulse sequences are optimized for emphasizing one contrast versus another. In MR morphometry attempts are made to estimate volumes of structure based on these scanning sequences. It must be remembered that NMR characteristics of tissue rather than the tissue itself are assessed. Magnetic resonance images are essentially physicochemical maps.

In the brain, every voxel contains extracellular fluid and millions of cells of different types (e.g., glial, neurons), and the cells themselves vary in the composition of their membranes (e.g., mitochondrial, endoplasmic reticulum). Thus, the microenvironment can vary substantially from site to site. In the white matter, myelin, which is essentially lipid, alters the signal. In addition, water content is lower in gray matter than white matter.

XI. ECHO PLANAR IMAGING

Manfield devised a method to rapidly (≥ 0.5 s) record the entire image using just the free induction decay. This is done using rapid gradient reversal to impose periodicity in one direction while another (perpendicular) gradient is applied to enable the voxels to be read without overlaps. This is used for functional MRI studies.

XII. MR MORPHOMETRY

MR morphometry basically requires segmentation of tissue and definition of boundaries of structures. Volumes are estimated from slices of a structure, i.e., two-dimensional probes of the structure. Segmentation is accomplished manually and/or semiautomatically. There are numerous semiautomatic segmentation methods. Most of the methods use either Bayesian classification neural networks or k-nearest-neighbor methods.

Factors that affect the sensitivity and accuracy of volume assessment include:

1. The number of slices that intersect the tissue
2. The orientation of slices relative to the tissue
3. Partial volume effects (i.e., voxels which at the edges seem to have an admixture of tissues)
4. Magnetic field inhomogeneities
5. Contrast as produced by the MR sequences

MR morphometry methods have improved greatly over the last few years and, at least for well-defined structures, have become extremely reliable. In the following chapters the application of MR morphometry to assess neuroanatomical changes in different brain regions will be described.

XIII.   CLINICAL APPLICATIONS OF MRI IN PSYCHIATRY

MRI is widely used in the assessment of neurological disorders such as stroke, tumors, demyelinating disease, etc. Its use in the diagnosis and follow-up of dementia is also relatively well established (see Chapter 19). However, its use in other psychiatric disorders is less well established. Although many consistent imaging findings have begun to emerge in neuropsychiatric disorders, they are by themselves insufficient to alter treatment. They are therefore used only when the clinical evaluation of an individual raises the possibility of another neurological disorder. In this context MRI becomes useful in clinical differential diagnosis. It is likely that, as this technology advances and our knowledge of the pathophysiology of neuropsychiatric diseases evolves, MRI will become integral in the evaluation of patients.

REFERENCES

1.   E. R. Andrew, G. Bydder, J. Griffiths, R. Iles, and P. Styles, *Clinical Magnetic Resonance: Imaging and Spectroscopy*, Wiley, New York, 1990.
2.   W. G. Bradley, W. R. Adey, and A. N. Hasso, *Magnetic Resonance Imaging of the Brain, Head, and Neck*, Aspen Systems, Rockville, MD, 1985.
3.   R. R. Ernst, G. Bodenhausen, and A. Wokaun, *Principles of Nuclear Magnetic Resonance in One and Two Dimensions*, Oxford University Press, Oxford, 1987.
4.   L. Kaufman, L. Crooks, and A. Margulis, eds., *Nuclear Magnetic Resonance Imaging in Medicine*, Igaku-Shoin, New York, 1981.
5.   P. C. Lauterbur, Image formation by induced local interactions: Examples employing nuclear magnetic resonance, *Nature (London) 242*:190 (1973).
6.   P. Mansfield and P. G. Morris, *NMR Imaging in Biomedicine*, Academic Press, New York, 1982.
7.   C. P. Slichter, *Principles of Magnetic Resonance*, Springer-Verlag, Berlin, 1990.
8.   S. W. Young, *Nuclear Magnetic Resonance Imaging: Basic Principles*, Raven Press, New York, 1984.

1B

Magnetic Resonance Spectroscopy

H. Cecil Charles, Theodore B. Snyderman, and Eileen Ahearn
Duke University Medical Center, Durham, North Carolina

I. INTRODUCTION

Magnetic resonance spectroscopy (MRS) utilizes the same general hardware as that of magnetic resonance imaging (MRI). MRS allows one to measure tissue metabolites and examine steady-state metabolic processes. Because it is non-invasive, MRS facilitates examination of multiple subjects, and provides access to information regarding drug effects on metabolic processes in individual subjects over time. This chapter will provide background information for understanding the use of MRS in neuropsychiatry.

II. MAGNETIC RESONANCE SPECTROSCOPY PHYSICS

In MRS, the physical processes are the same as in magnetic resonance imaging. However, MRS generally requires a scanning system with far greater magnetic field homogeneity and better system stability than is essential for routine MRI. The enhanced magnetic field homogeneity allows detection of structural moieties of different metabolic species which resonate at slightly different frequencies (or chemical shifts). These chemical shifts result from variations in the local magnetic field at the molecular level due to shielding of the nuclei by the electron fields of the molecule. An example of a proton (1H) spectrum spectrum is given in Fig. 1. For magnetic resonance spectros-

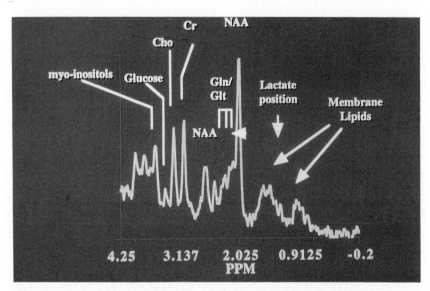

Fig. 1 Assignment of 1H-MR spectrum from human brain. Abbreviations: NAA = N-acetyl aspartate; Cho = choline; Cr = creatinine; Gln = glutatmine.

copy, the static magnetic field strength must be strong enough to provide adequate dispersion of the chemical shifts; thus, the greater the strength of the field, in general, the greater the dispersion. In addition to the field strength, magnetic field homogeneity should be maximized. Increasing field homogeneity yields improved signal-to-noise ratio, thus the detectability of metabolite signals. Homogeneity of the magnetic field is often improved by adjustments called shimming. Automatic shimming programs are available on many scanners, and these have enhanced the quality of acquisition across the spectrum.

A. Single Frequency and Multinuclear Capabilities

Most MRI systems are designed to operate only at hydrogen frequencies allowing imaging and 1H MRS data to be acquired. Additional capabilities in hardware in the radiofrequency section (amplifiers, frequency generation, receivers, coil arrays) are required for multinuclear (e.g. 19F, 31P) applications. These capabilities are generally optional on scanners and must be specified at the time of purchase or added later to allow MRS and MRI of nuclei other than hydrogen. In the area of neuropsychiatry, phosphorus and fluorine are the dominant other nuclei studies with lithium, sodium, and xenon as other possibilities.

III. LOCALIZATION OF THE SPECTRUM

There are several methods which are available for localization in NMR spectroscopy. The earliest methods utilized a radiofrequency coil placed against the surface of the object of interest, recording the "nominal" hemispherical volume, defined predominantly by the geometry of the coil. While this technique is useful for examining cortical regions of the brain with poor regional localization, its application in psychiatry appears to be limited to very general studies, e.g., simple detection of lithium or fluorinated drugs in the brain. For deeper structures inside the brain and for image-guided localization, other techniques have been developed. The desire to acquire either single volume elements (voxel) or simultaneous multiple volume elements has resulted in a handful of robust techniques.

A. Single or Multivoxel

These localization methods are classified as either single voxel or multivoxel methods. Single voxel methods obtain a single NMR spectrum from a single volume of tissue. This may be useful if the spectrum is to be obtained from a known region, e.g., a tumor, but otherwise it is too time consuming to query multiple regions of the brain as is often required in neuropsychiatric conditions. Multiple voxel spectroscopy or chemical shift imaging (CSI) allows examination of a larger spatial region with spatial encoding of many volume elements. In one type of multiple voxel spectroscopy, the data can be reformatted to produce an image demonstrating the spatial dimension of a particular metabolite. This is referred to as spectroscopic imaging or chemical shift imaging.

Simply put, for a given volume element size (e.g., 1 cc) either CSI or SVS will give the same signal-to-noise for a constant scan time but CSI provides multiple volume elements. The advantage of CSI has a price, the voxel definition is more complicated (although chemical shift effects cause the SVS to be more complicated than a cube) and the data processing is a bit more involved due to the large number of spectra obtained as opposed to the SVS technique. CSI uses scan techniques similar to those of conventional imaging, and with appropriate processing, one obtains localized spectra, spectrally resolved images, or both.

Clinical application of single voxel methods in the brain across subjects, and even across different sessions with the same subject, requires careful positioning of the patient and the volume element. However, the methods themselves are easier to undertake and data analysis is relatively straightforward compared to multivoxel techniques.

B. Specific Techniques of Localized MRS

1. STEAM, PRESS, and ISIS

These techniques (STEAM, PRESS, and ISIS) represent the three generally used single voxel methods. All three techniques use three sequential and mutually orthogonal slice selections to localize the signal to the "cube" at the intersection of the slices. The STEAM uses three 90° RF pulses in sequence to form a stimulated echo arising from the "cube". The PRESS technique is similar but uses a 90°–180°–180° double spin echo approach with the second echo arising from the "cube". The ISIS technique uses a series of three 180° inversion pulses followed by an excitation pulse. The inversion pulses are asserted in an eight step encoding pattern such that the sum of the eight acquisitions yields a spectrum from the "cube". In contrast to the STEAM and PRESS techniques which localize in a single pass, the ISIS requires the 8 cycles and is thus more sensitive to motion artifacts.

C. Phase Encoding

In addition to slice selection with above methods, phase encoding can be added to accomplish chemical shift imaging. With hydrogen usually the STEAM or PRESS technique is used to select a large voxel and then phase encoding is done in one, two or three directions. An example of a two dimen-

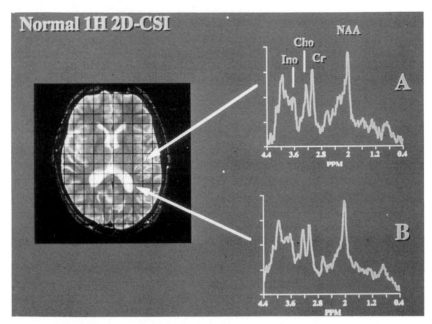

Fig. 2 Schematic of 2DCSI MRS method with spectra from two voxels. Ino = myoinositol. Other abbreviations as in Fig. 1.

sionally encoded slice is shown in Fig. 2 with extracted spectra from the chemical shift dimension.

D. Spectrum Referencing by Chemical Shift

For most MRS studies, peak assignment is based on the chemical shift relative to an internal standard, e.g., the water resonance in 1H MRS and creatine phosphate in 31P MRS. Often an additional scan is taken with the water unsuppressed to obtain a good reference for the water suppressed hydrogen spectra.

IV. QUANTIFICATION

Quantification in spectroscopy imaging is primarily based on the assumption that the area of a particular spectroscopic peak is proportional to the concentration of the metabolite represented by that peak. Usually, the spectra are obtained under conditions where this assumption has to be modified by a number of issues: 1) the repetition time is usually on the order of T1 of the metabolites, thus the signals are weaker than they would be in a fully relaxed state; 2) the echo times in 1H spectra are either of minimal influence (short echo $\leq$ 40 ms) or major influence (long echo $>$ 40 ms) as both T2 relaxation is occurring in the echo time, and modulation of complex spin patterns (e.g., glutamate/glutamine) attenuate the observed signal; 3) the peak results from more than one metabolite, each with different relaxation parameters (e.g., the choline pool and the creatine/creatine phosphate peak); 4) in pools such as these, the metabolites may be in physiologic exchange and this exchange is affected by disease; and 5) hardware conditions may vary from subject to subject or within a subject (e.g., non-uniform radiofrequency coil profiles). Several alternatives have been suggested and pursued, such as referencing the signal to the water signal in the same volume element, referencing the signal to an external standard sample, referencing the signal to contralateral "normal" tissue in the case of lesions, and even referencing the signal to an electrical standard signal injected in the receiver path. Each tactic has advantages and disadvantages that will not be discussed here. It suffices to point out that the terms absolute quantification, quantification, and others applied to this field in general reflect some type of reference normalization of the signal to allow better comparisons among subjects and sites.

V. PROTON SPECTRA OF THE HUMAN BRAIN

Proton NMR spectra of a normal human brain usually reveal four major resonances in addition to water. In proton spectroscopic imaging, a particularly important problem to address is the fact that the water signal (nominally 40–50 molar concentration) swamps the metabolite signals (1–10 mMolar concentration) and water suppression techniques are used to reduce the water signal and minimize the dynamic range problem for the receiver system. The major metabolites in the hydrogen spectra are discussed in the following.

A. *N*-Acetyl Aspartate

N-acetyl aspartate is only present within neurons, and is rarely present in glial cells. *N*-acetyl aspartate is generally considered to be a marker of viable or functional neurons. Therefore, when there is neuronal loss or reduction in neuronal function, *N*-acetyl aspartate concentrations are usually reduced. In stroke patients, at the region of the stroke, following death of the tissue, *N*-acetyl aspartate is depleted. It is also reduced in degenerative disorders such as Alzheimer's Disease and absent in tumors which do not contain neurons. In addition to irreversible alterations of *N*-acetyl aspartate, reversible alterations have been noted in conditions where there is transient neuronal dysfunction. The concentration of NAA is about 8–10 mM in a normal brain.

B. Choline

The choline peak results primarily from a pool of compounds composed of phosphocholine and glycerophosphocholine, with smaller contributions from choline and acetylcholine and CDP-choline, yielding a total concentration of about 2 mM. These are important constituents in membrane synthesis and breakdown. The choline signal is altered in a variety of conditions which involve membrane metabolism; thus in multiple sclerosis, in the regions of acute demyelination, choline is increased. It is also increased in depression where it may be reversible. Similar changes have been reported in Alzheimer's disease.

C. Creatine

Creatine readings generally reflect creatine and creatine phosphate. Creatine concentrations tend to be relatively stable in some neuropsychiatric disorders and are therefore often used as an internal concentration reference with other signals reported as normalized ratios to the creatine/creatine phosphate signal. While this needs to be done with some care, it is a simple and effective way of analyzing the spectral data. Creatine changes do occur in disorders (e.g., tumors) and this possibility must be considered when using it as a reference.

D. Inositol

The inositol peak reflects a pool of compounds including myoinositol, and other inositol compounds. It probably also reflects membrane stabilization and turnover. Inositol concentrations are reported to be increased in patients with Alzheimer's disease. Inositol is usually not detected on long echo proton spectroscopy, it is usually seen better when the spectra are obtained with shorter echo times, as the spectrum is observed at 1.5 Tesla as a deceptively simple single peak although the pattern is far more complicated. At long echo times, the signal is modulated and thus attenuated.

VI. ^{31}P SPECTROSCOPY

^{31}P spectroscopy of the human brain measures several major resonances. One resonance for each of the phosphates of ATP, Phospho-creatinine, and inorganic phosphate is present and the frequency difference between them reflects intracellular pH. In addition, two relatively broad spectra are seen for phosphor-monoesters and phospho-diesters, which are also membrane phospho-lipid constituents. Since the spectra primarily examine the mobile molecules containing ^{31}P, rather than those which are immobilized, they primarily reflect smaller membranes at the phospho-choline phosphate ethanolamine rather than phospholipids which are rigid constituents of the membrane. In psychiatric disorders, phospho-monoester and phospho-diester alterations have been reported in schizophrenia and Alzheimer's disease. This will be discussed in later chapters. Because brain phosphate concentrations are relatively small and the T_2 of brain phosphates is short, the voxels of interest have tended to be large, usually between 8 to 20 ml or more. This usually means that the voxels contain multiple tissues which has been a considerable challenge to their application in psychiatric disorders.

VII. ^{19}F SPECTROSCOPY

Fluorinated compounds are not usually present in the body, but many of the psychotropic drugs which are utilized, such as fluoxetine, contain fluorine. With fluorine ^{19}F spectroscopy it is possible to examine the concentration of these drugs in the brain and these techniques have been applied to assess fluoxetine concentration as well as fluphenazine concentration in the brain.

VIII. CLINICAL APPLICATION OF MRS

MRS is still a research tool. Its clinical utility is slowly being established for tumors, strokes and possibly dementia (see Chapter 19). Its current clinical utility is related to drug development and examining the course of disease. In the future, it is likely to be important for diagnostic purposes.

REFERENCES

1. P. A. Bottomley, Spatial localization in NMR spectroscopy in vivo, *Ann. N.Y. Acad. Sci. 508*:333–348 (1987).
2. P. A. Bottomley, H. C. Charles, P. B. Roemer, D. Flamig, H. Engeseth, W. A. Edelstein, and O. M. Mueller, Human in vivo phosphate metabolite imaging with ^{31}P NMR, *Magn. Reson. Med. 7*:319–336 (1988).
3. T. R. Brown, B. M. Kincaid, and K. Ugurbil, NMR chemical shift imaging in three dimensions, *Proc. Natl. Acad. Sci. U.S.A. 79*, 1982, 3523–3526.
4. J. Frahm, T. Michaelis, K. D. Merboldt, W. Haenicke, M. L. Gyngell, Chien, and H. Bruhn, Localized NMR spectroscopy in vivo: Progress and problems, *NMR Biomed. 2*:188–195 (1989).
5. J. Frahm, H. Bruhn, M. L. Gyngell, K. D. Merboldt, W. Haenicke, and R. Sauter, Localized high resolution proton spectroscopy using stimulated echoes: Initial application to human brain, *Magn. Reson. Med. 9*, 79–91 (1989).

6. K. K. Kwong, A. L. Hopkins, J. W. Belliveau, D. A. Chesler, L. M Porkka, R. C. McKinstry, D. A. Finelli, G. J. Hunter, J. B. Moore, R. G. Barr, and B. R. Rosen, Proton NMR imaging of cerebral blood flow using $H_2{}^{17}O$, *Magn. Reson. Med. 22*, 154–158 (1991).

7. K. K. Kwong, J. W. Belliveau, D. A. Chesler, I. E. Goldberg, R. M. Weisskoff, B. P. Poncelet, D. N. Kennedy, B. E. Hoppel, M. S. Cohen, R. Turner, H. M. Cheng, T. J. Brady, and B. R. Rosen, Dynamic magnetic resonance imaging of human brain activity during primary sensory stimulation, *Proc. Natl. Acad. Sci. U.S.A. 89*, 5675–5679 (1992).

8. S. Ogawa, T. M. Lee, A. S. Nayak and P. Glynn, Oxygenation-sensitive contrast in magnetic resonance image of rodent brain at high magnetic fields, *Magn. Reson. Med. 14*, 68–78 (1990).

9. S. Ogawa, D. Tank, R. Menon, J. M. Ellerman, S. G. Kim, H. Merkle, and K. Ugurbil, Intrinsic signal changes accompanying sensory stimulation: Functional brain mapping with magnetic resonance imaging, *Proc. Natl. Acad. Sci. U.S.A. 89*, 5951–5955 (1992).

10. L. Pauling and C. D. Coryell, The magnetic properties and structure of hemoglobin, oxyhemoglobin and carbonmonoxyhemoglobin, *Proc. Natl. Acad. Sci. U.S.A. 22*, 210–216 (1936).

11. S. Posse, B. Schuknecht, M. E. Smith, P. C. M. Van Zijl, N. Herschkowitz, and C. T. W. Moonen, Short echo time spectroscopic imaging, *J. Comput. Assist. Tomogr. 17*, 1–14 (1993).

12. K. R. Thulborn, J. C. Waterton, P. M. Matthews, and G. K. Radda, Oxygenation dependence of the transverse relaxation time of water protons in whole blood at high field, *Biochim. Biophys. Acta 714*, 265–270 (1982).

13. F. Turner, D. Le Bihan, J. Maier, R. Vavrek, L. K. Hedge and J. Pekar, Echoplanar imaging of intravoxel incoherent motions, *Radiology 177*, 407–414 (1990).

14. R. Turner, D. Le Biham, C. T. W. Moonen, D. Despres, and J. Frank, Echoplanar time course MRI of cat brain deoxygenation changes, *Magn. Reson. Med. 2*, 159–166 (1991).

15. F. Turner, P Jezzard, H. Wjn, K. K. Kwong, D. Le Bihan, T. Zeffiro, and R. S. Balaban, Functional mapping of the human visual cortex at 4 tesla and 1.5 tesla using deoxygenation contrast EPI, *Magn. Reson. Med. 29*, 277–279 (1993).

2

Positron Emission Tomography: Basic Principles

John M. Hoffman
Emory University School of Medicine, Atlanta, Georgia

Positron emission tomography (PET) and single photon emission computed tomography (SPECT) are modern imaging techniques that allow for in vivo qualitative, semi-quantitative, and quantitative assessment of cerebral physiology and biochemistry including cerebral blood flow (CBF), cerebral glucose metabolism (LCMRGlc), cerebral oxygen metabolism ($CMRO_2$), cerebral oxygen extraction, and blood-brain barrier permeability [1–3]. During the past decade there has been increasing interest in using these cross-sectional physiological imaging techniques in research and clinical practice [4].

The scientific foundation for PET methodology is the fact that the blood supply and glucose metabolism within a brain region varies in relation to the chemical changes underlying the functional activity of that brain region [5–8]. Kety and Schmidt were the first to describe techniques to measure whole brain blood flow using arterial venous differences and an inert gas (nitrous oxide) [9,10]. Since the development of the Kety-Schmidt technique, new and improved methodologies have been developed for measuring cerebral glucose metabolic activity [11,12] and cerebral blood flow [13–18] within specified brain regions. The basic principle for these methodologies rests on the assumption that neural activity, energy metabolism, and cerebral blood flow are tightly linked [8,19,20]. As neuronal activity increases, there is an associated increase in blood flow, which supports the oxygen and glucose consumption required. This particular physiological finding is present in most conditions. However, in certain situations such as intense sensory stimulation, cerebral blood flow and metabolic response can become uncoupled [21]. Physiological variables such as CBF, LCMRGlc, $CMRO_2$, oxygen extraction [13,16,17], and blood-brain barrier permeability [22] are measured by the PET tomograph from the tissue build-up and clearance of positron-emitting radionuclides that are either injected or inhaled.

PET is assuming increasing importance in the management of patients with various neurological and psychiatric disorders [1,4]. Presently more than 60 PET centers in the United States provide clinical PET services [1,4]. PET is being used clinically [1,2] in the evaluation of patients with dementia [23], brain tumors [24,25], medically refractory partial complex seizures [26–28], cerebrovascular disease [29], and various psychiatric disorders [30,31]. As its application becomes more widespread, it may be possible to use the results to physiologically characterize, classify, and diagnose various neurological and psychiatric disorders. Initially, the research and clinical PET studies conducted were primarily of the brain, typical of the evolution of any imaging modality. Recently, PET techniques have been applied to other relevant disorders, including oncology and cardiac disease [1]. This chapter provides an historical overview of the development of PET and reviews the physics, chemistry, methodology, and instrumentation as it relates to psychiatric illness.

Positron imaging was suggested as early as 1951 by Wrenn and colleagues [32]. At that time positron-emitting isotopes, such as carbon-11, nitrogen-13 and fluorine-18, were becoming available and were used for initial tracer development [33]. In 1953, Brownell and Sweet described the first planar positron scanner [34]. In 1962, Rankowitz and colleagues described the first planar positron scanner [35]. Much of the initial work and development of PET occurred simultaneously at the University of Pennsylvania and Washington University. David Kuhl and colleagues at the University of Pennsylvania described their initial studies using cross-sectional imaging with a single photon device [36]. In 1973 they described orthogonal reconstruction techniques, which became the basis for further development of PET as an imaging tool [37]. Ter-Pogossian and colleagues at Washington University began development of a positron emission tomograph with cross-sectional imaging capabilities in the early 1970s [38]. Their first scanner was PETT III, which used coincidence detection and modern image reconstruction techniques [39–41]. Since that time there has been continual and impressive development of PET hardware [42–45]. Today's tomographs (Fig. 1) typically include numerous rings of detectors [46,47] with the capability of producing 47 image planes in a field of view up to 16 cm. Hardware and software advancements have allowed for marked improvements in reconstruction time and display capabilities.

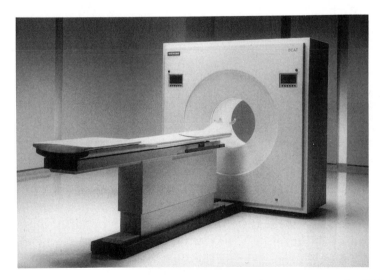

Fig. 1 The Siemens ECAT EXACT positron tomograph. This particular tomograph is of high resolution with a large field of view (16.0 cm) and has whole-body imaging capabilities. This particular scanner also has retractable septa, allowing for three-dimensional image acquisitions. (Courtesy of Siemens, Inc.)

I. PHYSICS

Positron decay, first described in the early 1900s, involves a nuclear decay with emission of a positron, a positively charged electron. The positron travels a short distance (the positron distance), typically a few millimeters in tissue, where it collides with an electron. The resulting annihilation produces two photons, which travel at the speed of light in opposite directions with an energy of 511 keV (Fig. 2). This process is known as positron annihilation and is the basis for imaging with PET (39). The detector design of the positron tomograph is able to simultaneously detect these events (coincidence detection). Thus, the positron annihilation can be located and registered as a coin-

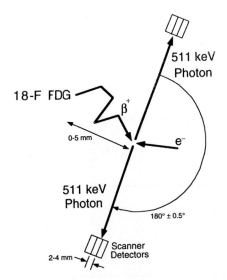

Fig. 2 Diagram showing positron decay and production of annihilation photons. In this case, the 18-F nuclide ejects a positron (β^+) from the nucleus. This particular particle travels a short distance before it collides with an electron (e^-) and annihilates it. The product of the annihilation reaction is two 511 Kev photons that travel in opposite directions. Coincidence detection, which allows for the simultaneous detection of each photon in the scanner detector pairs, is the basis for PET imaging. In this particular example, detection of the photons from the annihilation reaction took place somewhere along a line connecting the detector pairs. If a photon event is registered in a single detector and not registered as a coincidence event, then it is excluded from the information that is used to reconstruct the image. (Courtesy of John R. Votaw, Ph.D.)

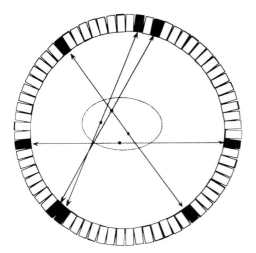

Fig. 3 Schematic diagram of an object to be imaged such as a brain or body in the tomographic field of view. Note that multiple coincidence annihilation events are registered in opposing detector pairs. A line drawn between the detector pairs is the line of response of where the annihilation occurred. This particular information is used to reconstruct the images from the coincidence events. Multiple rings of detectors are used in the design of the tomograph to obtain an adequate field of view for imaging. New state-of-the-art tomographs include thousands of detector pairs, the appropriate coincidence circuitry, and image reconstruction algorithms.

cidence event by a pair of opposing detectors (Fig. 3). New whole-body PET systems incorporate thousands of individual detectors into the design [46,47]. Detector blocks are arranged in a circular array around a central gantry opening. With complex electronics and coincidence circuitry, current generation tomographs are designed for high-resolution imaging in the X, Y, and Z directions. Earlier tomographs typically did not have symmetrical three-dimensional resolution; however, newer designs provide similar resolution and sampling in all directions.

PET tomographs use special detector material made with bismuth germinate. This detector material is well suited for PET imaging because of its high efficiency in trapping the high-energy annihilation photon and its high spatial resolution. Typically, several detector rings are incorporated into the design, making possible a large axial field of view imaging. Modern tomograph detector rings are primarily stationary; however, some designs incorporate wobble, which involves small motions of the detectors that enhance spatial resolution. The new tomographs provide high resolution, which is expressed as the full width at half-maximum (FWHM) of a radioactive line source in the field of view. Previous tomographs typically had resolution in the 10- to 20-mm range, whereas new tomographs have resolution approaching 4.0 mm. PET tomographs are complicated instruments, and the reader should refer to reviews for details concerning the instrument [33,42–45].

II. IMAGE RECONSTRUCTION

A requirement for any cross-sectional imaging technique is the capability of performing image reconstruction. In PET, the use of coincidence detection circuitry allows for detection of photons in opposite detectors, which are registered as coincident events. The information from the coincident events is used to reconstruct an image using the filtered backprojection technique [39,48]. This technique involves the mathematical process of deconvolution [49,50] and backprojecting the line data to form an image and is used in MRI, CT, SPECT, and PET. After the image is reconstructed, it can be filtered and smoothed for noise and the image displayed via computer or x-ray film.

Table 1 Characteristics of Positron-Emitting Radionuclides

Positron-emitting radionuclide	Half-life	Radiotracer	Application
^{18}F	109.7 min	Fluoro-2-deoxyglucose	Glucose metabolism
		Fluorodopa (FDOPA)	Dopamine metabolism
		Fluoroethylspiperone (FESP)	Dopamine receptor quantitation and binding
^{13}N	9.96 min	Ammonia (NH_3)	Cerebral perfusion
^{15}O	2.07 min	H_2O	Blood flow
		CO	Blood volume
		O_2	Oxygen metabolism
		CO_2	Blood flow
^{11}C	20.4 min	Deoxyglucose	Glucose metabolism
		Methionine	Amino acid uptake
		Leucine	Protein synthesis rate
		Aminoisobutyric acid	Blood-brain barrier permeability
		Spiperone compounds	Dopamine receptor activity
		CO	Blood volume
^{68}Ga	67.8 min	Ga-EDTA	Blood-brain barrier permeability

III. CHEMISTRY

The majority of currently used positron-emitting radionuclides are of biological importance and include oxygen-15, carbon-11, nitrogen-13, and fluorine-18 (Table 1). These radionuclides all require cyclotron production. The stable forms of these molecules are the backbone of all organic compounds. These particular positron-emitting radionuclides can then be appropriately incorporated into compounds such as glucose, water, amino acids, and other compounds with physiological properties for imaging with PET [1,45,51]. These positron-emitting radionuclides have very short half-lives (Table 1). Thus, if a wide array of available radiotracers is to be used, PET must be performed near a dedicated cyclotron for production of radionuclides. A major impediment to the widespread application of PET technology is the requirement for cyclotron-produced radionuclides. Advantages of the short half-life of the radiotracers are the low patient radiation dose received during a typical PET study and the possibility of performing numerous repeat studies on the same patient. The most widely used radiotracer in PET imaging is ^{18}F-2-fluoro-2-deoxyglucose (FDG) [52–54]. In this particular compound, a hydroxyl group is replaced with fluorine-18 (Fig. 4).

As with the development of the PET tomograph, tremendous advancements have been made in tracer production techniques for PET. Hospitals

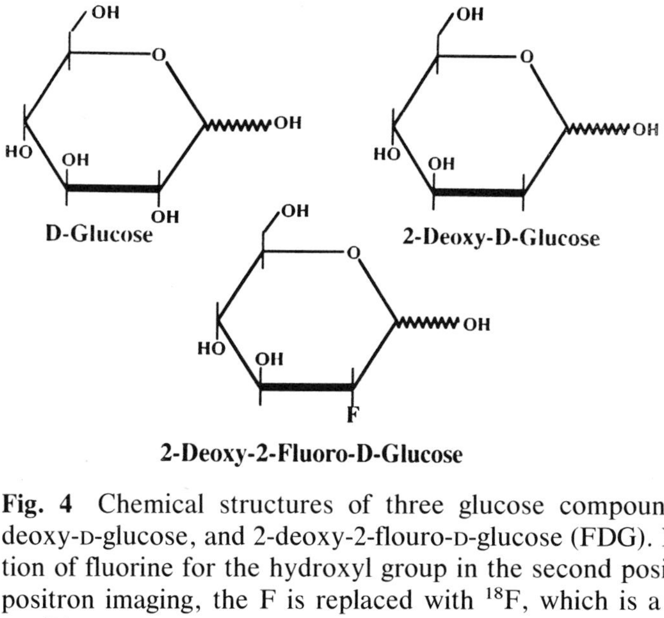

Fig. 4 Chemical structures of three glucose compounds: D-glucose, 2-deoxy-D-glucose, and 2-deoxy-2-flouro-D-glucose (FDG). Note the substitution of fluorine for the hydroxyl group in the second position in FDG. For positron imaging, the F is replaced with ^{18}F, which is a positron-emitting nuclide.

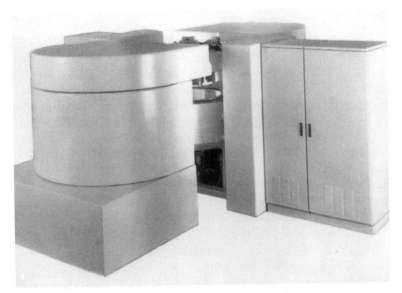

Fig. 5 A Siemens self-shielding cyclotron unit. This particular device is an 11 Mev cyclotron capable of producing all clinically relevant positron-emitting nuclides, including ^{18}F, ^{15}O, ^{13}N, and ^{11}C. Older versions of cyclotrons were extremely large and required a shielded vault and tremendous resources to maintain and operate. The newer, smaller cyclotrons are easily maintained in a hospital environment and allow for production of positron compounds on a routine, as-needed basis. (Courtesy of Siemens, Inc.)

can now purchase and maintain a small cyclotron. New cyclotrons are available that are self-shielded and do not require the large vault that was typically required for older medical cyclotrons (Fig. 5). The design improvements in hardware and computer control systems now make it possible for relevant positron-emitting radionuclides to be produced reliably and easily. In many clinically oriented PET centers, an array of important positron-emitting radiopharmaceuticals, such as FDG (Fig. 6), can be provided without a radiochemist on site. With continued improvements in radionuclide production and radiopharmaceutical synthesis techniques, PET certainly has the potential to be found at smaller institutions and be used for more clinical applications. In addition, with the 110-minute half-life of fluorine-18, FDG can be distributed from a central source on a regional basis.

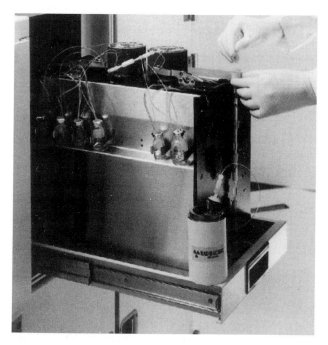

Fig. 6 FDG synthesis module from CTI, Inc. This particular device takes the 18-F produced by the cyclotron and using various chemical reactions, produces sterile, pyrogen-free, chemically pure FDG. Various chemical reactions occur, and the typical synthesis takes about one hour from the delivery of the 18-F. This particular device has been found to be extremely reliable and produces excellent yields of FDG. (Courtesy of CTI, Inc.)

IV. TRACER KINETIC MODELING

The PET tomograph measures the distribution of positron-labeled radiotracer. For quantitative PET studies, the time course of accumulation is used with information regarding the amount of activity in the blood in a tracer kinetic model, which is devised to describe a physiological process [55]. To date, the most widely used and studied tracer kinetic model is that of FDG. This particular model was originally described for ^{14}C-labeled–deoxyglucose by Sokoloff and colleagues in the early 1970s [52]. For PET, the initial carbon-14 deoxyglucose model was reformulated to be used with FDG [53,54]. FDG is transported into the cell and is not a substrate for further degradation after conversion to glucose-6-phosphate (Fig. 7). The fluorine-18 2-deoxy-D-glucose-6-PO$_4$ accumulates intracellularly and is not metabolized over the

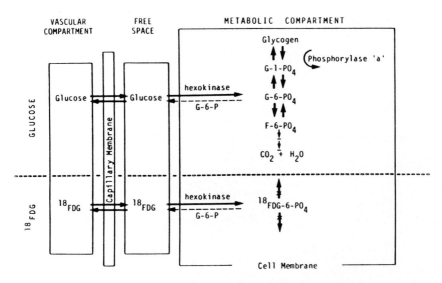

VASCULAR COMPARTMENT   FREE SPACE   METABOLIC COMPARTMENT

Fig. 7 Schematic diagram of the transport and metabolism of glucose and FDG in tissue. The FDG is transported across capillary and cell membranes and is competitively phosphorylated by hexokinase. FDG-6-PO$_4$ is not a significant substrate for further metabolism in the glycolytic pathway or for synthesis of glycogen. Because of the low membrane permeability of FDG-6-PO$_4$, it is trapped within cells in proportion to the net transport and phosphorylation of FDG. By the use of principles of competitive enzyme kinetics, the transport and phosphorylation rates of FDG can be converted to those of glucose. Glucose-6-PO$_4$ and FDG-6-PO$_4$ are eventually dephosphorylated by glucose-6-phosphatase. However, over the course of the typical FDG-PET study, this is not a significant problem. FDG's unique chemical composition thus allows the determination of the rate-limiting step of glucose metabolism, namely, the hexokinase reaction. (Used with permission, Courtesy of M. E. Phelps et al., UCLA School of Medicine.)

time course of a typical PET study. Positron-emitting fluorine-18 is measured by the PET tomograph. This particular information, when coupled with other information, can be used to determine the cerebral metabolic rate for glucose (LCMRGlc) using FDG. One of the variables required for determining the glucose metabolic rate involves determination of the input function, which is the plasma concentration of the FDG measured over time (Fig. 8). This input function is typically obtained by radial artery blood sampling or by heating the hand to arterialize venous blood [53]. The plasma radioactivity levels are used with the information obtained from the tomograph, the blood

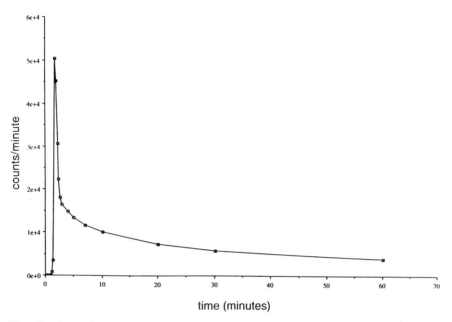

Fig. 8 A typical arterial input function for FDG. Rapid arterial sampling is performed at various intervals over the course of the study. Typically, approximately 12 2.0-mL samples are obtained over the first 2 minutes after injection of the tracer. This allows for determination of the distribution and absolute amount of radioactivity circulating in the blood. The whole blood samples are centrifuged, and plasma activity is measured. The arterial input function thus reflects the plasma activity of FDG measured over time. In this particular example, the y axis is in counts per minute, the measure of radioactive concentration. The x axis is in minutes. The characteristic shape of a very early and high peak with rapid reduction in plasma activity is typical for most physiologically relevant tracers.

glucose level, and the FDG tracer kinetic model to determine the glucose metabolic rate, which can be calculated on a regional basis or on a pixel-by-pixel basis. When the latter is performed, an image of absolute glucose metabolism is generated that is known as a parametric image. The mathematical description of the tracer kinetic model for FDG (Fig. 9) involves several rate constants for transport, conversion to glucose-6-phosphate, and efflux from the cell (Fig. 10) as well as the lumped constant, which is a ratio of net extraction of natural glucose to the extraction of FDG [56,57]. The tracer kinetic model for FDG is known as a compartmental model and is a very

$$LCMRGlc = \frac{Cp\left(C_i^*(T) - \frac{k_1^*}{\alpha_2 - \alpha_1}\left[\left(k_4^* - \alpha_1\right)e^{-\alpha_1 t} + \left(\alpha_2 - k_4^*\right)e^{-\alpha_2 t}\right] \otimes C_p^*(t)\right)}{LC\left(\frac{k_2^* + k_3^*}{\alpha_2 - \alpha_1}\right)\left(e^{-\alpha_1 t} - e^{-\alpha_2 t}\right) \otimes C_p^*(t)}$$

Fig. 9 The mathematical formula for the determination of local cerebral metabolic rate of glucose (LCMRGlc). This particular equation is rigorously derived and includes the unidirectional rate constants (k); the lumped constant (LC), which is the ratio of the arterial venous extraction fraction of FDG to that of glucose in steady-state condition; the cerebral concentration of FDG $C_{i(t)}$; and cerebral tissue concentration of FDG plus FDG-6-PO$_4$ $C_i^*(T)$ as a function of time. Cp refers to the capillary plasma glucose concentration. α_1, α_2 are the rate constants for response to an impulse change in FDG capillary plasma concentration. $\otimes$ refers to the operation of convolution.

standard approach to the modeling of physiological processes [55] (Fig. 10). Since the FDG model was described for normal brain, several assumptions are required in applying the model to cerebral pathology [58]. The lumped constant is assumed to be unchanged in pathological brain [56,57,59–61]. Furthermore, complicated issues such as delivery of tracer via blood flow, transport, and trapping are assumed to be unchanged with pathology.

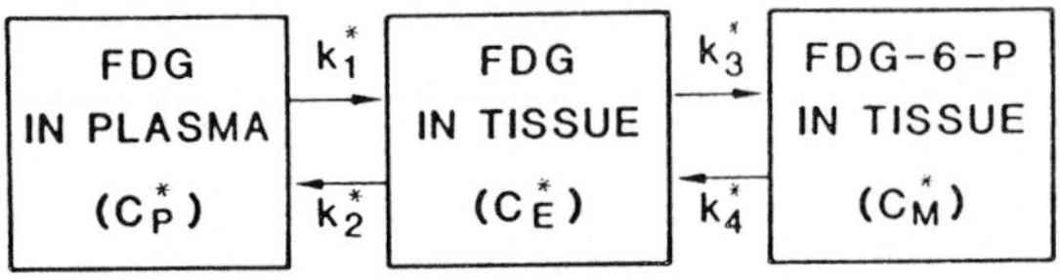

Fig. 10 A standard compartmental model for FDG kinetics in tissue. FDG in plasma is governed by the forward (k_1^*) rate constant for conversion to FDG in tissue (C_E^*). This particular reaction is reversible and is depicted by the rate constant k_2^*. In the case of FDG, there is phosphorylation to FDG-6-P (C_M^*), which is dependent upon the rate constant k_3^*. A small amount of dephosphorylation can occur and is measured by the rate constant k_4^*. This is a standard departmental model and is the basis for the mathematical formulation of the determination of cerebral metabolic rate, as noted in Figure 9.

V. PHYSIOLOGICAL IMAGING WITH PET

Several physiological variables can be determined with PET including cerebral glucose metabolism with FDG, cerebral blood flow with ^{15}O-labeled CO_2 or H_2O, protein synthesis rate with 18F-labeled amino acids [62], cerebral blood volume with ^{11}C- or ^{15}O-labeled CO, and quantitation of blood-brain barrier permeability [22] (Table 1). The unique property of PET is its ability to perform quantitative imaging. Extremely elegant and rigorous scientific evaluations of cerebral physiology can be performed in the normal [63] as well as the disease state [1,2]. For clinical studies, however, the relative distribution of the tracer is determined and the complicated quantitative techniques are avoided [64]. For qualitative clinical studies, the distribution of tracer is visually assessed and the images are typically interpreted much like CT or MRI images. Many of the early studies with PET involved absolute quantitation of physiological variables in small numbers of patients because of the complexity of the technique. More recent publications evaluating neurological and psychiatric disorders have relied on qualitative visual or semi-quantitative analysis of images. The distribution of the tracer such as FDG for metabolism (Fig. 11) and H_2O for CBF (Fig. 12) are examined in comparison to areas of known normal physiology.

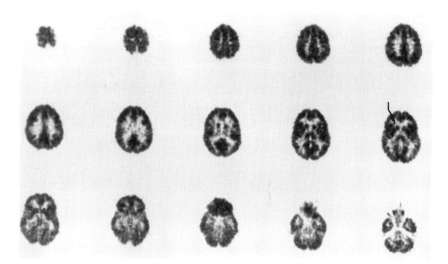

Fig. 11 Set of FDG-PET images of a 30-year-old, normal male volunteer. Note the high-resolution quality of the images. Sulcal and gyral patterns are apparent, and one can resolve the internal capsule (arrow).

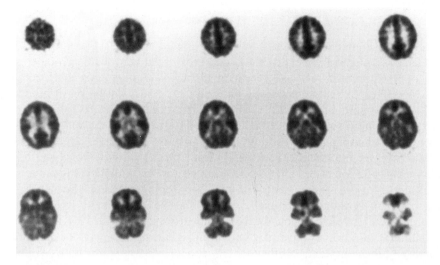

Fig. 12 Cross-sectional PET images of cerebral blood flow as determined with the tracer H_2 ^{15}O. Images appear very similar to FDG, and under typical situations, metabolism and blood flow are tightly coupled. Typically, blood flow images are slightly noisier than FDG images, and it is more difficult to resolve smaller brain structures.

VI. NORMAL STUDIES

The effects of variables such as age, handedness, and sex on brain function have long been of interest to neuroscientists [1,2]. Many of the initial research studies done with PET imaging were attempting to clearly define the normal magnitude and distribution of the LCMRGlc [63]. These early investigations provided a basis for the definition of the resting state [63,65], which was to serve as a reference for comparison to various neurological disorders. The initial studies examining the effects of age described gradual regional declines in LCMRGlc with age [23,66,67]. Glucose utilization in the hemispheres remained unchanged and symmetrical with advancing age. Other investigators have found no effects of age on glucose metabolism in healthy elderly subjects when compared to normal young subjects [68,69]. More recent investigations have examined larger numbers of subjects and have taken into account such variables as head size and brain atrophy [69,70]. The largest and most complete study of normal individuals using FDG-PET was performed on 76 normal volunteers and did note age-related changes particularly in the frontal, parietal, and temporal regions [69]. However, when these variables were corrected for brain volume and brain atrophy, no age-related effects were noted. The authors concluded that much of the variance in metabolic values in normal subjects is secondary to methodological differences between various studies.

The majority of studies have been performed on different types of tomographs with different resolutions, which have an effect on the absolute metabolic rates as well as the variance. With the development of newer, higher-resolution tomographs and methods for regional correction of atrophy, the effects of aging on glucose metabolism and cerebral blood flow can be answered. The discrepancies in age-related changes noted in previous studies may be entirely methodological.

Studies of cerebral glucose metabolism in children have revealed progressive changes from the neonatal period through young adulthood and regional changes that evolve over time [71]. These findings are in excellent agreement with behavioral, neuropsychological, and anatomic alterations, which are also occurring during infant development. Initially, the newborn demonstrates glucose metabolism that is symmetrically reduced in all brain regions. During infant development, regional variation in the metabolic rate of glucose occurs with an increase to the highest levels (approximately two to three times adult levels) noted around age 10. During adolescence there is a general reduction to adult levels. Regional changes follow developmental patterns, with the frontal lobes being the last to increase and eventually normalize to adult levels.

Since PET measures cerebral physiology (LCMRGlc or CBF), which is obviously dependent on conditions such as sensory input, motor activity, cognitive activity [65,72], level of consciousness, diet, and effects of drugs, these variables may have an effect on metabolism and blood flow. These particular variables, typically referred to as ambient test conditions, are important because they may affect both global and regional glucose metabolism and CBF.

VII. BRAIN-MAPPING AND ACTIVATION STUDIES

A tremendous amount of interest has been generated regarding the potential for PET to be used as a tool in brain-mapping studies [73–81]. Initial investigations with FDG by Mazziotta and colleagues examined the effects of sensory deprivation [82], auditory stimulation [83,84], visual stimulation [84,85], motor activity tasks [86], and cognitive processing [2,78,79] on glucose metabolism. The same ambient test conditions are necessary for performing patient studies as well as investigative studies. If the test conditions vary, then different regional and global determinations of glucose metabolism and CBF can occur, and the study is measuring the effects of various ambient conditions rather than the variable of interest.

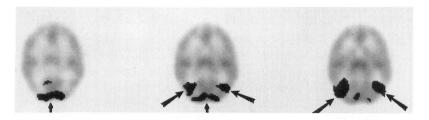

Fig. 13 Typical visual activation images obtained at three levels. A visual task of viewing various animals is performed. The control or baseline task involves the subject being blindfolded with no visual input. In these particular images, the black refers to significant (>8%) increase in CBF overlaid on the baseline PET image. Note activation of the primary (small arrow) and visual association cortex (large arrows). (Courtesy of John R. Votaw, Ph.D.)

Present brain-mapping techniques rely on CBF determination with $H_2{}^{15}O$. The basis for the PET methodology for brain mapping and activation studies is the fact that a stimulus causes an increase in neuronal activity with subsequent increase in cerebral blood flow [11,19,20,73,74]. The images are appropriately normalized for the amount of injected radioactive H_2O and

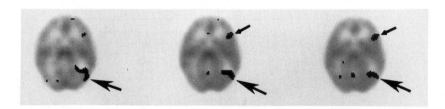

Fig. 14 Activation images of a language task obtained at three levels. The activation task involves viewing, then naming animals. The baseline task involves viewing various size figures. In the subtraction images, activation (>8% increase in CBF) is noted in specific left brain areas known to be responsible for naming (large arrow) and word generation (small arrow). The areas of activation are superimposed on the baseline blood flow image to better show localization. In this particular study, like that in Figure 13, visual input (animals and figures) are part of the task. However, when subtracted, the signal disappears since the visual aspect of the task is similar in the activation and baseline task. This shows the importance of careful selection of the activation and baseline task to examine and localize the specific function of interest. (Courtesy of John R. Votaw, Ph.D.)

task and control images subtracted to obtain task-specific areas of cerebral blood flow activation (Figs. 13, 14). Oxygen-15 H_2O, with its short half-life, is ideally suited to these types of studies, and repeat studies can be obtained about every 10–15 minutes. This allows for multiple acquisitions and paradigms with various cognitive, motor, and sensory activation tasks. The subtraction technique is elegant; however, careful design of the baseline or control condition and the specific activation task is imperative. The results of brain activation studies are complex and often difficult to interpret. Determining what is a significant change and its relationship to global brain function is somewhat controversial [87–103]. Newer techniques using three-dimensional PET acquisition techniques will improve statistical power [104,105]. Methods for registration of PET with MRI images [106–109] have allowed for the determination of structure-function relationships [88] and intersubject variability [91,101].

REFERENCES

1. J. M. Hoffman, M. W. Hanson, and R. E. Coleman, Clinical PET imaging, *Radiol. Clin. North Am. 31*(4):935 (1993).
2. J. C. Mazziotta and M. E. Phelps, Positron emission tomography studies of the brain, *Positron Emission Tomography and Autoradiography: Principles and Applications for the Brain and Heart* (M. E. Phelps, J. C. Mazziotta, and H. R. Schelbert, eds.), Raven Press, New York, 1986, pp. 493–579.
3. M. E. Raichle, Images of the mind: studies with modern imaging techniques, *Ann. Rev. Psychol. 45*:333 (1994).
4. ACNP/SNM Task Force on Clinical PET, Positron emission tomography: clinical status in the United States in 1987, *J. Nucl. Med. 29*:1136 (1988).
5. P. Horowicz and M. G. Larrabee, Glucose consumption and lactate production in a mammalian sympathetic ganglion at rest and in activity, *J. Neurochemistry 2*:102 (1958).
6. P. Horowicz and M. G. Larrabee, Oxidation of glucose in a mammalian sympathetic ganglion at rest and in activity, *J. Neurochemistry 9*:1 (1962).
7. C. S. Roy and C. S. Sherrington, On the regulation of the blood supply of the brain, *J. Physiol. (London) 11*:85 (1890).
8. L. Sokoloff, Relation between physiological function and energy metabolism in the central nervous system, *J. Neurochem. 19*:13 (1977).
9. S. S. Kety and C. E. Schmidt, The nitrous oxide method for the quantitative determination of cerebral blood flow in man: theory, procedure and normal values, *J. Clin. Invest. 27*:476 (1948).
10. S. S. Kety, Circulation and metabolism of the human brain in health and disease, *Am. J. Med. 8*:205 (1950).
11. L. Sokoloff, Mapping cerebral functional activity with radioactive deoxyglucose, *Trends Neurosci. 1*:75 (1978).
12. L. Sokoloff, Localization of functional activity in the central nervous system

by measurement of glucose utilization with radioactive deoxyglucose, *J. Cereb. Blood Flow Metab. 1*:7 (1981).

13. S. J. Frackowiak, G. L. Lenzi, T. Jones, and J. D. Heather, Quantitative measurement of regional cerebral blood flow and oxygen metabolism in man using $^{15}0$ and positron emission tomography: theory, procedure and normal values, *J. Comput. Tomogr. 4*:727 (1980).

14. M. E. Raichle, W. R. W. Martin, P. Herscovitch, et al., Brain blood flow measured with intravenous $H_2^{15}O$. II. Implementation and validation, *J. Nucl. Med. 24*:790 (1983).

15. P. Herscovitch, J. Markham, and M. E. Raichle, Brain blood flow measured with intravenous $H_2^{15}O$. I. Theory and error analysis, *J. Nucl. Med. 24*:782 (1983).

16. J. C. Baron, P. Lebrun-Grandie, P. Collard, C. Crouzel, G. Mestelan, and M. G. Bousser, Noninvasive measurement of blood flow, oxygen consumption, and glucose utilization in the same brain regions in man by positron emission tomography: concise communication, *J. Nucl. Med. 23*:391 (1982).

17. T. Jones, D. A. Chesler, and M. M. Ter-Pogossian, The continuous inhalation of oxygen-15 for assessing regional oxygen extraction in the brain of man, *B. J. Radiol. 49*:339 (1976).

18. S. C. Huang, M. E. Phelps, Carson, R. E., et al., Tomographic measurement of local cerebral blood flow in man with O-15 water, *J. Cereb. Blood Flow Metab. 1 (Suppl. 1)*:S31 (1981).

19. J. Greenberg, M. Reivich, A. Alavi, et al., Metabolic mapping of functional activity in human subjects with the [^{18}F]fluorodeoxyglucose technique, *Science 212*:678 (1981).

20. M. E. Raichle, R. L. Grubb, Jr., M. L. Gado, J. O. Eichling, and M. M. Ter-Pogossian, Correlation between regional cerebral blood flow and oxidative metabolism, *Arch. Neurol. 33*:523 (1976).

21. P. T. Fox and M. E. Raichle, Focal physiological uncoupling of cerebral blood flow and oxidative metabolism during somatosensory stimulation in normal subjects, *Proc. Natl. Acad. Sci. USA 83*:1140 (1986).

22. R. M. Kessler, J. C. Globe, J. H. Bird, et al., Measurement of blood-brain barrier permeability with positron emission tomography and [^{68}Ga]EDTA, *J. Cereb. Blood Flow Metab. 4*:323 (1984).

23. J. M. Hoffman, B. H. Guze, L. R. Baxter, et al., [^{18}F]-fluorodeoxyglucose (FDG) and positron emission tomography (PET) in aging and dementia: a decade of studies, *Eur. Neurol. 29 (Suppl. 3)*: (1989).

24. R. E. Coleman, J. M. Hoffman, M. W. Hanson, et al., Clinical application of PET for the evaluation of brain tumors, *J. Nucl. Med. 32*:616 (1991).

25. K. F. Hubner, J. T. Purvis, S. M. Mahaley, Jr, et al., Brain tumor imaging by positron emission computed tomography using 11C-labeled amino acids, *J. Comput. Assist. Tomogr. 6*:544 (1982).

26. J. Engel, Jr. The use of positron emission tomographic scanning in epilepsy, *Ann. Neurol. 15 (Suppl.)*:S180 (1984).

27. J. C. Mazziotta and J. Engel, Jr., The use and impact of positron computed tomography scanning in epilepsy, *Epilepsia 25(Suppl. 2)*:S86 (1984).

28. R. A. Radtke, M. W. Hanson, J. M. Hoffman, Crain B. J., T. S. Walszak, D. V. Lewis, C. Beam, R. E. Coleman, and A. H. Friedman, Temporal lobe hypometabolism on positron emission tomography: predictor of seizure control after temporal lobectomy, *Neurology 43*:1088 (1993).

29. G. L. Lenzi, R. S. J. Frackowiak, T. Jones, et al., $CMRO_2$ and CBF by the oxygen-15 inhalation technique: results in normal volunteers and cerebrovascular patients, *Eur. Neurol. 20*:285 (1981).

30. J. D. Brodie, A. P. Wolf, N. Volkow, et al., Evaluation of regional glucose metabolism with positron emission tomography in normal and psychiatric populations, *Positron Emission Tomography of the Brain* (W. D. Heiss and M. E. Phelps, eds.), Springer-Verlag, New York, 1983, pp. 201–206.

31. M. S. Buchsbaum, J. Cappelletti, R. Ball, E. Hazlett, A. C. King, J. Johnson, J. Wu, and L. E. DeLisi, Positron emission tomographic image measurement in schizophrenia and affective disorders, *Ann. Neurol. 15 (Suppl.)*:S157 (1984).

32. E. R. Wrenn, Jr., M. L. Good, and P. Handler, The use of positron-emission radioisotopes for the localization of brain tumors, *Science 113*:525 (1951).

33. M. M. Ter-Pogossian, The origins of positron emission tomography, *Semin. Nucl. Med. 22*(3):140 (1992).

34. G. L. Brownell and W. H. Sweet, Localization of brain tumors with positron emitters, *Nucleonics 1*:40 (1953).

35. S. Rankowitz, J. S. Robertson, W. A. Higinbotham, et al., Positron scanner for localization brain tumors, *IRE Int. Conven. Rec. 9*:49 (1962).

36. D. E. Kuhl and R. Q. Edwards, Image separation radioisotope scanning, *Radiology 80*:653 (1963).

37. D. E. Kuhl, R. Q. Edwards, A. R. Ricci, et al., Quantitative section scanning using orthogonal tangent correction, *J. Nucl. Med. 14*:196 (1973).

38. M. M. Ter-Pogossian, M. E. Phelps, E. J. Hoffman, et al., A positron-emission transaxial tomograph for nuclear imaging (PETT), *Radiology 114*:89 (1975).

39. M. E. Phelps, E. J. Hoffman, N. A. Mullani, et al., Application of annihilation coincidence detection to transaxial reconstruction tomography, *J. Nucl. Med. 16*:210 (1975).

40. M. E. Phelps, E. J. Hoffman, S. C. Huang, et al., Design and performance characteristics of the ECAT positron tomograph, *J. Comput. Assist. Tomogr. 2*:648 (1978).

41. M. E. Phelps, E. J. Hoffman, S. C. Huang, and D. E. Kuhl, ECAT: a new computerized tomographic imaging system for positron-emitting radiopharmaceuticals, *J. Nucl. Med. 19*:635 (1978).

42. E. J. Hoffman and M. E. Phelps, Positron emission tomography: principles and quantitation, *Positron Emission Tomography and Autoradiography: Principles and Applications for the Brain and Heart* (M. Phelps, J. Mazziotta, and H. Schelbert, eds.), Raven Press, New York, 1986, pp. 238–284.

43. R. A. Koeppe and G. D. Hutchines, Instrumentation for positron emission tomography: tomographs and data processing and display systems, *Semin. Nucl. Med. 22*:162 (1992).

44. F. Daghighian, R. Sumida, and M. E. Phelps, PET imaging: an overview and instrumentation, *J. Nucl. Med. 18*:5 (1990).

45. M. E. Phelps, J. C. Mazziotta, and H. R. Schelbert, *Positron Emission Tomography and Autoradiography: Principles and Applications for the Brain and Heart*, Raven Press, New York, 1986.
46. K. Wienhard, L. Eriksson, S. Grootoonk, M. Casey, U. Pietrzyk, and W.-D. Heiss, Performance evaluation of the positron scanner ECAT EXACT, *J. Comp. Assist. Tomogr. 16*(5):804 (1992).
47. T. R. DeGrado, T. G. Turkington, J. J. Williams, C. W. Stearnes, J. M. Hoffman, and R. E. Coleman, Performance characteristics of a whole-body PET scanner, *J. Nucl. Med. 35*:1398 (1994).
48. R. A. Brooks and G. DiChiro, Theory of image reconstruction in computed tomography, *Radiology 117*:561 (1975).
49. R. N. Bracewell and A. C. Riddle, Inversion of fan-beam scans in radioastronomy, *Astrophys. J. 150*:427 (1967).
50. L. A. Shepp and B. F. Logan, The Fourier reconstruction of a head section, *IEEE Trans. Nucl. Sci. NS-21*:21 (1974).
51. G. B. Saha, W. J. MacIntyre, and R. T. Go. Cyclotrons and positron emission tomography radiopharmaceuticals for clinical imaging, *Semin. Nucl. Med. 22*: 150 (1992).
52. L. Sokoloff, M. Reivich, C. Kennedy, et al., The [^{14}C]deoxyglucose method for the measurement of local cerebral glucose utilization: theory, procedure, and normal values in the conscious and anesthetized albino rat, *J. Neurochem. 28*:897 (1977).
53. M. E. Phelps, S. C. Huang, E. J. Hoffman, et al., Tomographic measurement of local cerebral metabolic rate in humans with (F-18) 2-fluoro-2-deoxy-D-glucose: validation of method, *Ann. Neuro. 6*:371 (1979).
54. S. C. Huang, M. E. Phelps, E. J. Hoffman, et al., Noninvasive determination of local cerebral metabolic rate of glucose in man, *Am. J. Physiol. 238*:E69 (1980).
55. S. C. Huang and M. E. Phelps, Principles of tracer kinetic modeling, in *Positron Emission Tomography and Autoradiography* (M. Phelps, J. Mazziotta, and H. Schelbert, eds.), Raven Press, New York, 1986, pp. 287–343.
56. M. Reivich, J. H. Greenberg, A. Wolf, J. Fowler, C. Arnett, R. Ferrieri, H. Atkins, R. Dann, and A. Alavi, The evaluation of the lumped constant for deoxyglucose and fluorodeoxyglucose in man, *J. Nucl. Med. 25*:P32 (1984).
57. M. E. Phelps, J. C. Mazziotta, R. A. Hawkins, et al., An alternate approach to the investigation of the lumped constant, *J. Cereb. Blood Flow Metab. 3(Suppl 1)*:S13 (1983).
58. A. M. Spence, M. M. Graham, M. Muzi, G. L. Abbott, K. A. Krohn, R. Kapoor, and S. D. Woods, Deoxyglucose lumped constant estimated in a transplanted rat astrocytic glioma by the hexose utilization index, *J. Cereb. Blood Flow Metab. 10*(2):190 (1990).
59. R. A. Hawkins, M. E. Phelps, S. C. Huang, et al., Effect of ischemia on quantification of local cerebral glucose metabolic rate in man, *J. Cereb. Blood Flow Metab. 1*:37 (1981).
60. R. A. Hawkins, J. C. Mazziotta, M. E. Phelps, et al., Cerebral glucose metabo-

lism as a function of age in man: Influence of the rate constants in the fluoro-deoxyglucose method, *J. Cereb. Blood Flow Metab. 3*:250 (1983).

61. S. C. Huang, M. E. Phelps, E. J. Hoffman, and D. E. Kuhl, Error sensitivity analysis for fluorodeoxyglucose method for measurement of cerebral metabolic rate of glucose, *J. Cereb. Blood Flow Metab. 1*:391 (1981).

62. M. E. Phelps, J. R. Barrio, S. C. Huang, R. Keen, H. Chugani, and J. C. Mazziotta, Criteria for the tracer kinetic measurement of protein synthesis in man with positron CT, *Ann. Neurol. 15(Suppl. 1)*:S192 (1984).

63. J. C. Mazziotta, M. E. Phelps, J. Miller, et al., Tomographic mapping of human cerebral metabolism: normal unstimulated state, *Neurology 31*:503 (1981).

64. G. Di Chiro and R. A. Brooks, PET quantitation: blessing and curse, *J. Nucl. Med. 29*:1603 (1988).

65. P. E. Roland, L. Eriksson, S. Stone-Elander, and L. Widen, Does mental activity change the oxidative metabolism of the brain?, *J. Neurosci. 7(8)*:2373 (1987).

66. D. E. Kuhl, E. J. Metter, W. H. Riege, and M. E. Phelps, Effects of human aging on patterns of local cerebral glucose utilization determined by the [(^{18}F)]fluorodeoxyglucose method, *J. Cereb. Blood Flow Metab. 2*:163 (1982).

67. J. M. Hoffman, B. H. Guze, T. C. Hawk, J. P. Pahl, R. Sumida, L. R. Baxter, J. C. Mazziotta, and M. E. Phelps, Cerebral glucose metabolism in normal individuals: effects of aging, sex, and handedness, *Neurology 38 (Suppl. 1)*: 371 (1988).

68. R. Duara, R. A. Margolin, E. A. Robertson-Tchabo, et al., Cerebral glucose utilization as measured with positron emission tomography in 21 resting healthy men between the ages of 21 and 83 years, *Brain 106*:761 (1983).

69. F. Yoshii, W. W. Barker, J. Y. Chang, et al., Sensitivity of cerebral glucose metabolism to age, gender, brain volume, brain atrophy, and cerebrovascular risk factors, *J. Cereb. Blood Flow Metab. 8*:654 (1988).

70. J. B. Chawluk, A. Alavi, R. Dann, H. I. Hurtig, S. Bais, M. J. Kushner, R. A. Zimmerman, and M. Reivich, Positron emission tomography in aging and dementia: effect of cerebral atrophy, *J. Nucl. Med. 28*:431 (1987).

71. H. T. Chugani and M. E. Phelps, Maturational changes in cerebral function in infants determined by [18]FDG positron emission tomography, *Science 231*: 840 (1986).

72. G.-J. Wang, N. D. Volkow, A. P. Wolf, J. D. Brodie, and R. J. Hitzemann, Intersubject variability of brain glucose metabolic measurements in young normal males, *J. Nucl. Med. 35*:1457 (1994).

73. P. T. Fox, M. A. Mintun, M. E. Raichle, and P. Herscovitch, A noninvasive approach to quantitative functional brain mapping with $H_2^{15}O$ and positron emission tomography, *J. Cereb. Blood Flow Metab. 4*:329 (1984).

74. J. C. Mazziotta, S-C. Huang, M. E. Phelps, R. E. Carson, N. S. MacDonald, and K. Mahoney, A noninvasive positron computed tomography technique using oxygen-15-labeled water for the evaluation of neurobehavioral task batteries, *J. Cereb. Blood Flow Metab. 5*:70 (1985).

75. U. Knorr, B. Weder, A. Kleinschmidt, A. Wirrwar, Y. Huang, H. Herzog, and

R. J. Seitz, Identification of task-specific rCBF changes in individual subjects: validation and application for PET, *J. Comput. Assist. Tomogr. 17*(4):517 (1993).

76. J. C. Mazziotta, M. E. Phelps, E. Halgren, R. E. Carson, S. C. Huang, and J. Bayer, Hemispheric lateralization and local cerebral metabolic and blood flow responses to physiologic stimuli, *J. Cereb. Blood Flow Metab. 3(Suppl. 1)*:S246 (1983).

77. J. R. Votaw and H. L. Hengli, Analysis of PET neurofunctional mapping studies, *J. Cereb. Blood Flow Metab. 15*:492 (1995).

78. M. Reivich, A. Alavi, and R. C. Gur, Positron emission tomographic studies of perceptual tasks, *Ann Neurol. 15(Suppl.)*:S61 (1984).

79. M. Reivich, R. Gur, and A. Alavi, Positron emission tomographic studies of sensory stimuli, cognitive processes and anxiety, *Human Neurobiol. 2*:25 (1983).

80. P. Roland, E. Meyer, Y. Yamamoto, et al., Dynamic positron emission tomography as a tool in neuroscience: functional brain-mapping in normal human volunteers, *J. Cereb. Blood Flow Metab. 1(Suppl. 1)*:S463 (1981).

81. J. A. Sanders and W. W. Orrison, Jr., Functional magnetic resonance imaging in: *Functional Magnetic Resonance Imaging* (W. W. Orrison, Jr., J. D. Lewine, J. A. Sanders, and M. F. Hartshorne, eds.), Mosby, St. Louis, MO, pp. 239–326 (1995).

82. J. C. Mazziotta and M. E. Phelps, Human sensory stimulation and deprivation. PET results and strategies, *Ann. Neurol. 15(Suppl. 1)*:S50 (1984).

83. J. C. Mazziotta, M. E. Phelps, R. E. Carson, et al., Tomographic mapping of human cerebral metabolism: auditory stimulation, *Neurology 32*:921 (1982).

84. J. C. Mazziotta, M. E. Phelps, and R. E. Carson, Tomographic mapping of human cerebral metabolism: subcortical responses to auditory and visual stimulation, *Neurology 34*:825 (1984).

85. J. C. Mazziotta, M. E. Phelps, and E. Halgren, Local cerebral glucose metabolic responses to audio-visual stimulation and deprivation: studies in human subjects with positron CT, *Human Neurobiol. 2*:11 (1983).

86. J. C. Mazziotta and M. E. Phelps, Positron computed tomography studies of cerebral metabolic responses to complex motor tasks, *Neurology 34(Suppl. 1)*:116 (1984).

87. J. C. Mazziotta and S. H. Koslow, Assessment of goals and obstacles in data acquisition and analysis from emission tomography: Report of a series of international workshops, *J. Cereb. Blood Flow Metab. 7(Suppl. 1)*:S1 (1987).

88. J. C. Mazziotta, C. C. Pelizzari, G. T. Chen, F. L. Bookstein, and F. L. Valentino, Region of interest issues: the relationship between structure and function in the brain, *J. Cereb. Blood Flow Metab. 11*:A51 (1991).

89. I. Ford, Confounded correlations: statistical limitations in the analysis of interregional relationships of cerebral metabolic activity, *J. Cereb. Blood Flow Metab. 6*:385 (1986).

90. I. Ford, J. H. McColl, A. G. McCormack, and S. J. McCrory, Statistical issues in the analysis of neuroimages, *J. Cereb. Blood Flow Metab. 11*:A89 (1991).

91. P. T. Fox, M. A. Mintun, E. M. Reiman, and M. E. Raichle, Enhanced detec-

tion of focal brain responses using intersubject averaging and change-distribution analysis of subtracted PET images, *J. Cereb. Blood Flow Metab. 8*:642 (1988).

92. K. J. Friston, C. D. Frith, P. F. Liddle, R. J. Dolan, A. A. Lammertsma, and R. S. J. Frackowiak, The relationship between global and local changes in PET scans, *J. Cereb. Blood Flow Metab. 10*:458 (1990).

93. K. J. Friston, A. P. Holmes, K. J. Worsley, J.-P. Poline, C. D. Frith, and R. S. J. Frackowiak, Statistical parametric maps in functional imaging: a general linear approach, *Human Brain Mapping 2*:189 (1995).

94. K. J. Friston, C. D. Frith, P. F. Liddle, and R. S. J. Frackowiak, Comparing functional (PET) images: the assessment of significant change, *J. Cereb. Blood Flow Metab. 11*:690 (1991).

95. K. J. Friston, C. D. Frith, P. F. Liddle, and R. S. J. Frackowiak, Functional connectivity: the principal-component analysis of large (PET) data sets, *J. Cereb. Blood Flow Metab. 13*:5 (1993).

96. K. J. Friston, Statistical parametric mapping: ontology and current issues, *J. Cereb. Blood Flow Metab. 15*:361 (1995).

97. B. Horwitz, Functional interactions in the brain: use of correlations between regional metabolic rates, *J. Cereb. Blood Flow and Metab. 11*:A114 (1991).

98. G. Pawlik, Statistical analysis of functional neuroimaging data: exploratory versus inferential methods, *J. Cereb. Blood Flow Metab. 11*:A136 (1991).

99. J.-B. Poline and B. M. Mazoyer, Analysis of individual positron emission tomography activation maps by detection of high signal-to-noise-ratio pixel clusters, *J. Cereb. Blood Flow and Metab. 13*:425 (1993).

100. J.-B. Poline and B. M. Mazoyer, Enhanced detection in brain activation maps using a multifiltering approach, *J. Cereb. Blood Flow Metab. 14*:639 (1994).

101. M. E. Raichle, M. A. Mintun, L. D. Shertz, M. J. Fusselman, and F. Miezen, The influence of anatomical variability on functional brain mapping with PET: a study of intrasubject versus intersubject averaging, *J. Cereb. Blood Flow and Metab. 11(Suppl. 2)*:S364 (1991).

102. D. A. Silbersweig, E. Stern, C. D. Frith, C. Cahill, L. Schnorr, S. Grootoonk, T. Spinks, J. Clark, R. S. J., Frackowiak, and T. Jones, Detection of thirty-second cognitive activations in single subjects with positron emission tomography: a new low-dose $H_2^{15}O$ regional cerebral blood flow three-dimensional imaging technique, *J. Cereb. Blood Flow Metab. 13*:617 (1993).

103. S. C. Strother, I. Kanno, and D. A. Rottenberg, Principal component analysis, variance partitioning, and "functional connectivity," *J. Cereb. Blood Flow Metab. 15*:353 (1995).

104. D. W. Townsend, A. Geissbuhler, M. Defrise, E. J. Hoffman, T. J. Spinks, D. L. Bailey, M-C Gilardi, and T. Jones, Fully three-dimensional reconstruction for a PET camera with retractable septa, *IEEE Trans. Med. Imaging 10*(4): 505 (1991).

105. S. R. Cherry, R. P. Woods, E. J. Hoffman, and J. C. Mazziotta, Improved detection of focal cerebral blood flow changes using three-dimensional positron emission tomography, *J. Cereb. Blood Flow Metab. 13*:630 (1993).

106. C. A. Pelizzari, G. T. Y. Chen, D. R. Spelbring, R. R. Weichselbaum, and C-T. Chen, Accurate three-dimensional registration of CT, PET, and/or MR images of the brain, *J. Comput. Assist. Tomogr. 13*(1):20 (1989).

107. R. P. Woods, S. R. Cherry, and J. C. Mazziotti, Rapid automated algorithm for aligning and reslicing PET images, *J. Comput. Assist. Tomogr. 16*(4):620 (1992).

108. R. P. Woods, J. C. Mazziotta, and S. R. Cherry, MRI-PET registration with automated algorithm, *J. Comput. Assist. Tomogr. 17*(4):536 (1993).

109. S. Minoshima, R. A. Koeppe, K. A. Frey, and D. E. Kuhl, Anatomic standardization: linear scaling and nonlinear warping of functional brain images, *J. Nucl. Med. 35*:1528 (1994).

3

Functional Brain Imaging: SPECT
Basic and Technical Considerations

Madhukar H. Trivedi, Mustafa M. Husain, and Michael Devous, Sr.
University of Texas Southwestern Medical Center, Dallas, Texas

Interest in studying metabolism in the living human brain has been renewed with the introduction of newer investigative tools that can be described as "functional imaging techniques." Functional brain imaging refers to a set of techniques that derive images reflecting biochemical, physiological, or electrical properties of the central nervous system (CNS). The most developed of these techniques are topographic electroencephalography (TEEG), positron emission tomography (PET), and single-photon emission computed tomography (SPECT). Of these three techniques; SPECT matured last but may eventually offer the most widely available and applicable measures of neuronal behavior. Functional magnetic resonance imaging (fMRI), which is still in its infancy, is rapidly becoming an important functional brain imaging tool as well.

SPECT's late maturation can be attributed to three primary factors. First, instrumentation for brain SPECT was initially inferior to that of PET. Although PET is still considered to provide the highest resolution tomographic images of brain function, SPECT images are currently comparable in resolution. Second, the development of radiopharmaceuticals for brain SPECT lagged behind those for PET, especially for metabolism and receptor imaging agents. Although this remains true, available perfusion and receptor tracers for SPECT imaging are expanding rapidly. Currently, the lack of a direct SPECT measure of metabolism is the only significant difference between SPECT and PET tracers; indeed, this may not be a critical factor since under most normal and pathological circumstances, especially in psychiatric disorders, perfusion and metabolism are tightly coupled in the CNS. In addition, there are emerging reports of iodine-123 (^{123}I)-labeled glucose analogs and SPECT ligands that bind to hypoxic tissue.

Increasing collaboration between nuclear medicine and clinical researchers is beginning to hasten the incorporation of this technology into clinical research and practice. With lower cost, increased availability, improved high-resolution systems, and the development of novel approaches to diagnosis, increased collaboration within the medical community will allow brain SPECT to achieve its greatest level of clinical utility.

I. TECHNICAL CONSIDERATIONS

In examining the technical aspects of SPECT functional brain imaging, several factors independent of pathology must be considered [1]:

1. The quality of the tomographic device.
2. Environmental conditions.
3. Characteristics of the subject (e.g., age, gender, handedness, etc.).
4. Radiopharmaceuticals utilized.
5. Format used for image presentation.
6. Image processing techniques.

A. Tomographic Devices

Historically, the conceptual origins of tomography can be traced to the work of the Austrian mathematician Radon. In 1917, Radon developed the mathematics of image reconstruction from projections for mapping gravitational fields [2]. Shortly thereafter, several pioneering radiologists deduced that if an x-ray tube and film are translated in opposite directions about a fulcrum or focal point within a patient, the longitudinal projection of only the focal plane remains in focus. The result, noncomputed tomography, remained the predominant means of tomographic imaging in medicine for 40 years until the development and explosive growth of computed tomography (CT).

Olendorf [3] was among the first to recognize the potential of image reconstruction from projections for medical imaging, constructing a prototype tomographic scanner in 1961. At about the same time, Kuhl and Edwards [4], the acknowledged originators of emission CT, adapted this image reconstruction technology to the field of nuclear medicine, particularly brain imaging, and constructed and evaluated a series of increasingly sophisticated devices, known as the "MARK" series [5].

Rapid development of new and more advanced systems throughout the 1970s and 1980s has culminated in the current variety of imaging systems capable of high-resolution brain SPECT that are now commercially available. These systems fall into two categories: non–camera-based and gamma–camera-based systems.

Non–camera-based systems include rotating detector arrays, multidetector scanners, and fixed rings. The rotating detector array group includes the Tomomatic two-, three-, and five-slice machines (Medimatic, A/S) and the Hitachi four-head system. The Tomomatic's outstanding characteristic is its capacity for xenon-133 (^{133}Xe) SPECT, which requires high sensitivity and the capacity for rapid, dynamic imaging (i.e., complete tomographic studies every 10 seconds) [6]. The Tomomatic, by changing collimators, can also produce images of relatively high resolution (9–10 mm). The Hitachi rotating detector array system is also capable of both ^{133}Xe and high-resolution (8–10 mm) static imaging [7].

The first multidetector scanner was the unit developed by Stoddart and colleagues [8], known as the Harvard multidetector scanner. This scanner is a slice-based tomograph, as are the Hitachi, Shimadzu, and Tomomatic, but is constructed with very thick crystals that operate much like pinhole cameras as they traverse through space obtaining tomographic data. Hill and colleagues [9] have demonstrated that this device can image technetium-99 (^{99m}Tc) and ^{123}I, as well as fluorodeoxyglucose-18 (^{18}F), in a single-photon (not PET) mode.

Fixed-ring systems are also commercially available. The original models were designed with fixed detectors or a circular annulus of sodium iodide with an internally rotating collimator. Currently, there are two available versions: the Shimadzu (Headtome) system and the CERASPECT. The Shimadzu (Headtome), available only in Japan, is capable of high-sensitivity ^{133}Xe studies and moderate resolution (10–12 mm) imaging using ^{123}I or ^{99m}Tc. The most widely available system is the CERASPECT [10], the first of the fixed sodium-iodide annulus/rotating collimator machines to come to commercial production. It does yield high-resolution images (8–10 mm) but cannot currently perform ^{133}Xe dynamic SPECT.

Gamma-camera–based systems are more common today than dedicated tomographs because they are capable of performing both head and body SPECT. In addition, modern tomographs have overcome many of the limitations of the original systems, including poor head alignment, magnetic field aberrations, and inadequate uniformity and linearity for tomography. There are currently two forms: single-head and multihead systems. A few of the modern single-head systems have been designed to circumvent shoulders, so that minimal radius scanning is possible. Most of these systems provide fairly high-resolution images with static tracers; unfortunately, they suffer from poor sensitivity and prolonged imaging times.

The first three-head gamma-camera–based SPECT systems were developed in the late 1980s. Today, three-head SPECT systems are considered the most sophisticated instruments for brain SPECT—approximately 500 units have been installed, indicating increasing acceptance of this technology [1].

1. Data Acquisition

The raw data acquired through SPECT studies emerge as a series of discrete planar or projection images at uniform angular increments about the longitudinal axis of the patient. On the basis of its location (as determined by conventional Anger logic), each detected event, or count, is assigned to the corresponding computer-defined bin address: the number of counts in each bin, or channel, represents the "ray sum" or line integral of the sampling line perpendicular to and extending from the detector surface through the patient. Collectively, the bin contents represent the raw data, which are then mathematically reconstructed to produce the transverse section images.

2. Collimation

The selection of collimation for SPECT studies is complicated by the issues of "high-resolution collimation" versus "high-sensitivity collimation." According to Keyes et al. [11], a 2-mm improvement in spatial resolution, typically associated with a 30–50% decrease in count sensitivity, may actually yield a three- to fourfold improvement in effective sensitivity (defined as the data acquisition time or the number of counts required to yield an image of a given visual quality [12,13]. In practice, therefore, higher-resolution, as opposed to higher-sensitivity, collimation appears preferable; this is particularly true when localization of small, high-contrast structures, rather than simple detection of lesions, is significant, as in brain SPECT. Dynamic ^{133}Xe SPECT is a striking exception to this principle.

The choice of high-resolution collimation over high-sensitivity collimation is easier to make when more efficient multidetector cameras are used. Other mechanical approaches to improving sensitivity and/or resolution, specifically for brain SPECT, include the use of a cut-off, or contoured, detector assembly or a specially designed head-holder to minimize the patient-to-collimator distance, allowing rotation unobstructed by the patient's shoulders [14].

3. Statistical Considerations

An important practical limitation of radionuclide imaging in general, and SPECT in particular, is the generally small numbers of counts, resulting in statistical uncertainties or noise [15]. In tomographic images, the reconstructed count value in a given pixel (i.e., picture element) is affected by the reconstructed count values in all the pixels intersected by all the rays or sampling lines that include that pixel. Specifically, in tomographic image reconstruction by filtered back-projection, the counts in a given bin in the projection image data are distributed among the pixels along the sampling line and then removed from the inappropriate pixels by mathematical filtering. However, the arithmetic operations composing back-projection propogate the random error in the projection image data among all of the pixels along the sampling line. Therefore, in order to obtain reconstructed tomographic images that are not excessively "noisy," the projection image data in SPECT must have larger numbers of counts than would be required for planar (two-dimensional) imaging. This increase is accomplished by acquiring a large number of projection views (typically 120 for brain SPECT).

4. Sampling Considerations

As previously discussed, projection image data in SPECT are not continuous, but discrete bin-by-bin samples, defined by the digital image matrix and the dimensions of the pixels, defining the "linear sampling interval." In addition, the projection images may not be acquired continuously, but at uniform angular increments about the longitudinal axis of the patient with the angular increment between successive projection images defining the "angular sampling interval." The linear and angular sampling intervals, together with the maximum spatial frequency of the filter function and the system spatial resolution, determine the resolution in the reconstructed tomographic images.

Finally, continuity or discontinuity of the detector rotation assembly must be considered in defining the angular sampling parameters. Many commercial SPECT systems offer the option of acquiring the projection image data continuously (continuous rotation) or only while stationary at predefined angular positions ("step-and-shoot"). Continuous rotation offers the advantage of greater "effective" sensitivity in that there is no time during the actual SPECT study when projection image data are not being acquired. In contrast, off-time (i.e., time when the detector assembly is rotating between successive angular positions) often exceeds 25% of the total duration of the study in "step-and-shoot" systems. In general, continuous rotation is preferred for many current gamma-camera–based SPECT systems.

In summary, modern SPECT instruments offer high resolution, reliable performance, and low cost. They function as full-body imaging devices yielding multiple angle, cross-sectional displays as well as three-dimensional representations. Their computer systems offer powerful image processing and valuable flexibility, including imaging opportunities (e.g., dual-isotope imaging) not available with PET systems. No longer a lesser substitute for more expensive PET systems, SPECT imaging offers a mature technology of independent merit.

B. Environmental Conditions

The environmental conditions experienced by a subject during radiotracer administration play a significant role in regional cerebral blood flow (rCBF) distribution. A variety of studies have reviewed the coupling of rCBF to regional metabolism under resting and cognitive or motoric activation. These studies have consistently shown that visual, auditory, and soma to sensory stimuli impact the regional level of neuronal activity and thus rCBF [16–22]. Unfortunately, there are not clearly established standards for environmental conditions during SPECT imaging. The majority of investigators use an "eyes-and-ears-open" imaging environment. In this scenario, subjects are seated, room lights are generally dimmed to provide a minimum and relatively standard visual stimulus, and personnel in the area are requested to control auditory and visual stimuli. Research data support these conditions as opposed to an "eyes-and-ears-closed" setting, which actually appears to produce greater variability in quantitative flow and metabolism values [23].

The duration of steady-state conditions necessary to ensure minimal variability induced by environmental conditions is also not well established, but appears to be dependent on the choice of radiotracer. For example, ^{99m}Tc-hexamethylpropyleneamineoxime (HMPAO) has very rapid first-pass extraction, while a component of ^{123}I-isopropyliodoamphetamine (IMP) is retained by the lung and may affect brain tracer distribution for 5–10 minutes after injection; ^{133}Xe is a dynamic tracer that must be imaged during administration. In each case, the specific requirements for environmental stability before and after tracer administration vary. In general, steady-state environmental conditions are required for 10 minutes prior and after tracer administration for injectables; there is no steady-state requirement after administration for ^{133}Xe.

C. Subject Characteristics

A variety of subject characteristics appear to affect rCBF, including age, gender, handedness, anxiety, time of day (diurnal variations), blood pressure, carbon dioxide levels, cognitive involvement (attention), and others. Several studies have confirmed both age [24–30] and gender [25,31–34] effects on whole brain blood flow; regional effects remain less well established. Furthermore, recent studies suggest that age may affect rCBF in complex ways, e.g., the decline in rCBF in elderly subjects is not as marked in the active elderly as in age-matched inactive individuals [35].

Patient motion can also significantly degrade high-resolution SPECT scans. Certain groups (e.g., patients with dementia and pediatric patients, particularly those with attention deficit disorders) can be so uncooperative that successful scanning is impossible. In these situations, mild sedatives can be administered prior to scanning (no sooner than 10 minutes after radiopharmaceutical administration), in which case these sedatives do not appear to alter radiopharmaceutical uptake. Mechanical restraints may also be used, but they do not inhibit small head movements, which will significantly degrade high-resolution SPECT images.

The impact of other pharmacological substances is only now being clarified. For example, caffeine, which may be present in subjects in various quantities, can lead to reductions in both global and regional cerebral blood flow. In general, it is advisable to eliminate all such complicating factors for as long as possible preceding a study. For caffeine, 24 hours of abstention may be sufficient, while some antidepressants may require up to 14 days for complete drug clearance—longer for fluoxetine and the monoamine oxidase inhibitors [36].

In general, consistency of environmental conditions is the greatest asset; attempts should be made to study all subjects under as identical a set of conditions as possible.

D. Radiopharmaceuticals

Since the late nineteenth century, it has been known that a close relationship exists among regional brain perfusion, metabolism, and neuronal activity [37]. Because neuronal activity is closely coupled to glucose utilization and blood flow, perfusion imaging studies should help explain which neuronal pathways are activated during sensory processing or disrupted during various diseases. Visualization and localization of activated brain regions are possible because neuronal stimulation increases brain uptake of the blood flow tracer in gray matter regions to a much greater extent than in white matter regions. The radiotracers used for SPECT studies must cross the blood-brain barrier, distribute proportionally to rCBF, and remain fixed in the brain for a time period sufficient for SPECT imaging. Alternatively, blood flow can be measured quantitatively from the clearance of the inert gas (^{133}Xe) with highly sensitive instrumentation that can image its distribution repeatedly during its rapid clearance from the brain.

For radiotracers that have a very slow clearance from the brain, quantitative estimates of rCBF are based on the microsphere model, which assumes that the radiotracer is freely diffusible from the blood pool, that it is completely extracted from the blood into the brain, and that it remains fixed within the brain without redistribution. Since most clinical applications of brain perfusion SPECT do not require quantification of rCBF, but rely on the generation of images that reflect *relative* rCBF only, available radiotracers follow rCBF closely enough to be clinically useful and correspond well with independent measures of rCBF over a wide range of flows.

Iodine-123-IMP (Spectamine) was the first brain perfusion tracer to be synthesized and remains the most ideal with respect to its kinetics [38,39]. The distribution of IMP reflects rCBF over a wide range of flows, but it may underestimate flow when plasma pH is low, as in cerebral ischemia or acidosis. Brain imaging must be completed fairly quickly after injection (peak activity is reached within 15–20 minutes) since redistribution is fairly rapid and significant changes can be observed after 60 minutes. With the standard injected dose of 3–6 mCi, the photon flux is low and image quality is not as good as that achieved with the ^{99m}Tc-labeled ligands, posing particular problems for high-resolution imaging systems. Finally, the fact that ^{123}I is a cyclotron product and must be transported daily from the production site to the imaging facility has caused difficulties in commercial development. At present, no ^{123}I brain-imaging agents are available in the United States.

Technetium-99m brain perfusion agents offer a number of advantages. They are easily produced (from ^{99}Mo) with a small on-site generator and ideally suited to the gamma cameras currently in use because of their 140 keV monoenergetic photon and 6-hour half-life. It is a highly soluble macrocyclic amine with rapid brain uptake, but only moderate first-pass extraction, resulting in underestimation of rCBF [40,41]. The tracer remains fixed in the brain following conversion to a hydrophilic compound in the presence of intercellular glutathione [42]. Because blood clearance is slow, perfusion defects are not as clear as with other blood flow tracers.

Technetium-99m-ECD (ethyl cysteinate dimer, Neurolite) [43,44], like ^{99m}Tc-HMPAO, has moderate cerebral extraction and underestimates rCBF. Brain uptake is rapid and clearance from the brain is very slow; blood clearance is also rapid, resulting in a higher brain-to-background activity ratio than with HMPAO.

The inert gas clearance technique estimates rCBF from the clearance of ^{133}Xe from the brain; it can be combined with SPECT using specially designed equipment [45,46]. Because of the rapid clearance of the tracer, multiple studies can be performed on the same day and quantitative measures can be obtained without arterial sampling. Limitations of this technique include the low photon energy of this tracer and its rapid clearance from the brain, producing poor spatial resolution. Overall, the inhalation technique is more complex and technically difficult than the intravenous method using brain perfusion radiotracers. Recently we have adapted this technique for use on triple-head SPECT systems and enhanced its spatial resolution [46].

E. Format for Image Presentation

The advances in tomographs and image processing permit the presentation of image data in a wide variety of formats. Transverse, sagittal, and coronal reconstructions are readily produced by most computer systems. However, certain brain structures are better understood when they are presented in nonconventional display orientations and/or in a variety of orientations. For example, evaluation of the orbital frontal cortex is better performed from sagittal cross sections than from transverse; evaluation of mesial temporal lobe hypoperfusion in epilepsy is easier in coronal than in sagittal or transverse views. SPECT studies should always be reviewed in at least three orthogonal orientations.

A second area for consideration is the modality employed for image review. The traditional film-and-lightbox format requires the viewer to consider the image data over a similar contrast range, often with a fixed degree of background subtraction. Direct viewing from a video display offers opportunities for gray scale adjustments and dynamic background subtraction. Yet another available option is the choice between gray scale and color image displays. Most reviewers of high-resolution images prefer gray scales, since the human visual system appears better suited to gray scale discrimination across structural boundaries than to color-based schemes. On the other hand, reviewers using poorer-resolution systems or foreshortened image data sets (minimum pixel density) find that color scales provide enhanced interpretation of abnormalities.

Three-dimensional surface-rendered displays are now commonplace. Surface-rendered images are helpful in assessing the distribution of cortical defects but do not allow visualization of either defect magnitude (count density) or subcortical abnormalities. Established standards for count-density threshold settings have not yet been established, and the "dial-a-lesion" format of most surface-rendered images currently limits their applicability. The development of more sophisticated three-dimensional displays of "see-through" or "smoked glass" images offers additional perspectives, but they are not yet widely available. Cinemagraphic displays of projection data provide a certain three-dimensional quality, but at this time they are primarily used to monitor patient motion as a source of image degradation.

F. Image-Processing Techniques

In SPECT, as in other forms of CT, the tomograph image is a thin, tissue-section image representing a two-dimensional mathematical reconstruction from multiple projections (line integrals) of a three-dimensional object [47]. A critical component, therefore, is the reconstruction of the tomographic image from the projection image data.

I. Reconstruction Filters

Filter function can dramatically affect the appearance of the reconstructed tomographic images. The filter function determines not only which spatial frequencies in the projection images are retained, but also their relative weighting when back-projected. In clinical SPECT studies, which are always count-limited, a cut-off spatial frequency (v_c) somewhat less than the Nyquist frequency (v_N) and a relatively gradual roll-off should generally be used, sacrificing some spatial resolution in principle, but further reducing noise in the reconstructed tomographic images. For a properly functioning SPECT system and a properly acquired SPECT study, a balance between "sharpening," or edge enhancement, and "smoothing," or noise reduction filters, will yield tomographic images that retain the most visualizable spatial detail while minimizing statistical artifact and distracting mottle. For high–spatial definition studies (such as brain blood flow imaging using ^{99m}Tc-HMPAO), a higher Butterworth-type filter may be preferable.

2. Attenuation Correction

Attenuation of radiation as it passes through overlying tissue to the patient surface is an unavoidable limitation of radionuclide imaging. It is a particular problem in SPECT imaging because the depth-related loss of counts may appear as a "hot rim" surrounding large distributed sources [14,48]. In addition, attenuation compromises the potential of SPECT imaging for radionuclide quantitation [49] because the apparent reconstructed number of counts in a structure of interest depends not only on the activity in the structure, but on its depth and composition as well, thereby affecting the attenuation coefficients of surrounding tissues.

Diverse techniques have been used for attentuation correction in SPECT. These attenuation correction algorithms can be classified as analytical, based on mathematical modeling of attenuation, or empirical, based on direct measurement of attenuation. Analytical methods introduce assumptions regarding the attenuation process (e.g., uniform activity distribution and/or a uniformly attenuating medium). To the extent that these assumptions differ from the actual situation, the resulting attenuation correction suffers. Nonetheless, analytical methods, particularly the Sorenson method [50] and Chang's first-order correction [51], remain the most widely available correction algorithms on commercial SPECT systems. On the other hand, empirical methods, based on direct measurement of regional attenuation factors in the patient, do not introduce any gross assumptions and are potentially more accurate and more generally applicable [52].

II. QUALITY CONTROL

The SPECT process compounds or magnifies gamma camera imperfections: since a tomographic image represents a complex product of multiple projection images, with any imperfections propagated and, in fact, amplified in the reconstructed image, an imperceptible defect in the projection images may very well appear as a prominent artifact in the tomographic image. In addition, the rotational motion of the SPECT system introduces another potential source of image artifact not encountered in non-SPECT studies. Accordingly, quality control procedures unique to SPECT are essential to its diagnostic utility and acceptance within the nuclear medicine community.

A. Center of Rotation

In order to reconstruct tomographic images accurately, it is necessary to know the location of the projection of the axis of rotation, referred to as the center of rotation (COR), on the projection image matrix so that each image may be properly oriented for filtered back-projection. If the mechanical and electrical CORs are aligned, the pixel location of the projection of the axis of rotation on the projection image matrix will be the same for all projection images. If, however, the mechanical and electrical CORs are misaligned, the pixel location of the projection image angle and the contents of each projection image bin will then be back-projected in incorrect locations across the tomographic image matrix. This will result in blurred tomographic images, with the degree of blurring related to the magnitude of the misalignment of the mechanical and electronic CORs [53,54]. Fortunately, modern SPECT systems monitor COR alignments robotically and automatically during routine quality control and service procedures, such that COR misalignment is now uncommon.

B. Field Uniformity

Uniformity of response over the entire useful field of view of the gamma camera is probably the single most important factor in obtaining high-quality tomographic images. Even small, nearly imperceptible nonuniformities of response may appear as severe "ring" or "bulls-eye" artifacts in reconstructed tomographic images. Factors adversely affecting uniformity of gamma camera responses may be intrinsic or extrinsic. Intrinsic factors include nonuniformities of sensitivity, linearity, and energy discrimination; extrinsic factors include nonuniformities caused by collimator defects, and inadequate differential linearity in the analog-to-digital converters of the camera-computer interface [55]. Nonuniformity defects at or near the center of rotation will produce more pronounced artifacts in the reconstructed image than those at the periphery of the field of view, with larger objects exhibiting more pronounced artifacts as well. In general, gamma-camera nonuniformity is measured and subsequently corrected using an extrinsic radionuclide- and collimator-specific flood image.

C. Overall System Performance

In general, all radionuclide-collimator combinations used in clinical practice should be evaluated every six months, using a water-fillable cylinder with non-radioactive inserts of varying sizes to evaluate visual scatter, image contrast, and transverse and longitudinal spatial resolution; it should also have a uniform-activity section to visually evaluate the accuracy of nonuniformity corrections.

D. Projection Images: Visual Inspection of Static and Cine Displays and of Sinograms

In addition to the periodic quality control procedures described above, each individual clinical SPECT study should be carefully evaluated for its overall technical quality. Perhaps the simplest method of evaluation is visual inspection of the static and cine displays.

Viewing all of the projection images in a single static display will immediately reveal variations in overall intensity and if any images are missing. Visual inspection of the cine display of the projected images, on the other hand, is particularly useful in detecting excessive patient motion, especially in the longitudinal direction. In addition, inspection of the cine display may reveal different overlying structures, passing between the organ of interest and the detector as it rotates about the patient, suddenly obscuring all or part of the target organ in various projection images. Another interesting way of inspecting the projection image data is the "sinogram" display: deviations from its characteristic sinusoidal appearance are easily detected and reflect a problem in the projection image data, such as gamma camera nonuniformity, the object falling outside the detector's field of view at certain projection angles, missing projection images, and patient motion [56].

III. CONCLUSIONS

After reviewing the technical advancements in SPECT functional brain imaging, the following conclusions and recommendations for future study can be offered:

1. Standard conditions for all SPECT scans should be established as a laboratory standard and maintained for all clinical and research studies. Currently, the most common standard is "ears and eyes open" in a dimly lit environment with a minimal level of "white noise."
2. The normal distribution of rCBF in such a setting shows symmetrical flow distribution between homologous regions.
3. Age and gender effects should be noted; currently, they are only well established for whole-brain blood flow.
4. Image presentation for SPECT rCBF studies should include transverse, coronal, and sagittal cross sections.

ACKNOWLEDGMENTS

This review was supported in part by a grant from NARSAD, The National Alliance for Research in Schizophrenia and Depression (Dr. Trivedi) and NIMH grants MH-41115 (Dr. Rush) and MH-52870 (Dr. Trivedi). Acknowledgments go to Dr. A. John Rush, Betty Jo Hay Distinguished Chair in Mental Health, and Dr. Kenneth Z. Altshuler, Stanton Sharp Distinguished Chair, Professor and Chairman, Department of Psychiatry, for administrative support.

REFERENCES

1. M. D. Devous, SPECT functional brain imaging, *Clinical SPECT Imaging* (E. L. Kramer and J. J. Sanger, eds.), Raven Press, Ltd., New York, 1995, p. 97.
2. J. Radon, Über die Bestimmung von Funktionen durch ihre Integralwerte langs gewisser Mannigfaltigkeiten, *Ber. Verh. 69*:262 (1917).
3. W. H. Olendorf, Isolated flying-spot detection of radiodensity discontinuities:

displaying the internal structural pattern of a complex object, *IRE Trans. Bio-Med. Electron 8*:68 (1961).

4. D. E. Kuhl and R. Edwards R, Image separation isotope scanning, *Radiology 80*:53 (1963).

5. D. E. Kuhl, R. Q. Edwards, A. R. Ricci, et al., The MARK IV system for radionuclide computed tomography of the brain, *Radiology 121*:405 (1976).

6. M. D. Devous Sr, E. M. Stokely, and F. J. Bonte, Quantitative imaging of regional cerebral blood flow in man by dynamic single-photon tomography. *Radionuclide Imaging of the Brain* (B. L. Holman, ed.), Churchill Livingstone, New York, 1985, p. 135.

7. K. Kimura, K. Hashikawa, H. Etani, et al., A new apparatus for brain imaging: four-head rotating gamma camera single-photon emission computed tomograph, *J. Nucl. Med. 31*:603 (1990).

8. H. F. Stoddart and H. A. Stoddart, A new development in single-gamma transaxial tomography. Union Carbide focused collimator scanner, *IEEE Trans. Nucl. Sci. 26*:2710 (1979).

9. T. C. Hill, H. F. Stoddart, M. D. Doherty MD, et al., Simultaneous SPECT acquisition of CBF and metabolism, *J. Nucl. Med. 29*:876 (1988).

10. A. P. Smith and S. Genna, Imaging characteristics of ASPECT, a single-crystal ring camera for dedicated brain SPECT, *J. Nucl. Med. 30*:796 (1989).

11. J. W. Keyes Jr., F. H. Fahey, and B. H. Harkness, Tips for high-quality SPECT. *Comput. Instrum. Council Newslett. 7*:1 (1990).

12. M. E. Phelps, S. C. Huang, and E. J. Hoffman, An analysis of signal amplification using small detectors in positron emission tomography, *J. Comput. Assist. Tomogr. 6*:551 (1982).

13. G. Muehllehner, Effect of resolution improvement on required count density in ECT imaging: a computer simulation, *Phys. Med. Biol. 30*:163 (1985).

14. R. J. English and S. G. Brown, *SPECT, Single Photon Emission Computed Tomography: A* Primer, 2nd ed., Society of Nuclear Medicine, New York, 1990; pp. 30, 50, 62–63, 69–91, 176–177, 181–183, 190–205, 208.

15. J. A. Sorenson and M. E. Phelps, *Physics in Nuclear Medicine*, 2nd ed., Grune & Stratton, Orlando, FL, 1987, p. 391.

16. G. C. Baron, P. Lebrun-Grandie, P. Collard, et al., Non-invasive measurement of blood-flow, oxygen consumption and glucose utilization in the same brain regions in man by positron emission tomography, *J. Nucl. Med. 23*:391 (1982).

17. D. H. Ingvar and J. Risberg, Increase of regional cerebral blood flow during mental effort in normals and in patients with focal brain disorders, *Exp. Brain Res. 3*:195 (1967).

18. S. S. Ketty and C. F. Schmidt, The nitrous oxide method for quantitative determination of cerebral blood flow in man: theory, procedure and normal values, *J. Clin. Invest. 27*:476 (1948).

19. J. C. Mazziotta, M. E. Phelps, R. E. Carson, et al., Tomographic mapping of human cerebral metabolism: auditory stimulation, *Neurology 32*:921 (1982).

20. M. E. Phelps, D. E. Kuhl, and J. C. Mazziotta, Metabolic mapping of the brain's response to visual stimulation: studies in humans, *Science 211*:1445 (1981).

21. M. E. Raichle, R. L. Grubb, M. H. Gado, et al., Correlation between regional cerebral blood flow and oxidative metabolism, *Arch. Neurol. 33*:523 (1976).
22. P. E. Roland, L. Eriksson, S. Stone-Elander, et al., Does mental activity change the oxidative metabolism of the brain?, *J. Neurosci. 7*:2373 (1987).
23. J. C. Mazziotta, M. E. Phelps, R. E. Carson, et al., Tomographic mapping of human cerebral metabolism: sensory deprivation, *Ann. Neurol. 12*:435 (1982).
24. S. S. Ketty and C. F. Schmidt, The nitrous oxide method for quantitative determination of cerebral blood flow in man: theory, procedure and normal values, *J. Clin. Invest. 27*:476 (1948).
25. M. D. Devous Sr., E. M. Stokely, H. H. Chehabi, et al., Normal distribution of regional cerebral blood flow measured by dynamic single-photon emission tomography, *J. Cereb. Blood Flow Metab. 6*:95 (1986).
26. R. C. Gur, R. E. Gur, W. D. Obrist, et al., Age and regional cerebral blood flow at rest and during cognitive activity, *Arch. Gen. Psychiatry 44*:617 (1987).
27. S. Hagstadius and F. Risburg, Regional cerebral blood flow characteristics and variations with age in resting normal subjects, *Brain Cogn. 10*:28 (1989).
28. D. E. Kuhl, E. J. Metter, W. H. Riege, et al., Effects of human aging on patterns of local cerebral glucose utilization determined by the ^{18}F fluorodeoxyglucose method, *J. Cereb. Blood Flow Metab. 2*:153 (1982).
29. R. J. Matthew, W. Wilson, and S. R. Tant, Determinants of resting regional cerebral blood flow in normal subjects, *Biol. Psychiatry 21*:907 (1986).
30. R. L. Rogers, J. S. Meyer, and K. F. Mortel, After reaching retireme»t age physical activity sustains cerebral perfusion and cognition, *J. Am. Geriatr. Soc. 38*:123 (1990).
31. L. R. Baxter, J. C. Mazziotta, M. E. Phelps ME, et al., Cerebral glucose metabolic rates in normal human females vs. normal males, *Psychiatry Res. 21*:237 (1987).
32. D. G. Daniel, R. J. Mattew, and W. H. Wilson, Sex roles and regional cerebral blood flow, *Psychiatry Res. 27*:55 (1988).
33. R. C. Gur, R. E. Gur, W. D. Obrist, et al., Sex and handedness differences in cerebral blood flow during rest and cognitive activity, *Science 217*:659 (1982).
34. G. Rodriguez, S. Warkentin, J. Risberg, et al., Sex differences in regional cerebral blood flow, *J. Cereb. Blood Flow Metab. 8*:783 (1988).
35. R. L. Rogers, J. S. Meyer, and K. F. Mortel, After reaching retirement age physical activity sustains cerebral perfusion and cognition, *J. Am. Geriatr. Soc. 38*:123 (1990).
36. A. J. Rush, J. W. Cain, J. Raese, et al., The neurobiological bases for psychiatric disorders, *Comprehensive Neurology* (R. N. Rosenberg, ed.), Raven Press, New York, 1991, p. 555.
37. C. S. Roy and C. S. Sherrington, On the regulation of blood supply, *J. Physiol. (Lond) 11*:85 (1980).
38. H. S. Winchell, R. M. Baldwin, and T. H. Lin, Development of I-123-labeled amines for brain studies: localization of I-123 iodophenyalkyl amines in rat brain, *J. Nucl. Med. 21*:947 (1980).
39. T. C. Hill, B. L. Holman, R. Lovett, et al., Initial experience with SPECT (single

photon emission computerized tomography) of the brain using N-isopropyl I-123 p-iodamphetamine, *J. Nucl. Med. 23*:191 (1982).

40. P. J. Ell, J. M. L. Hocknell, P. H. Jarritt, et al., A Tc-99m-labeled radiotracer for the investigation of cerebral vascular disease, *Nucl. Med. Commun. 6*:437 (1985).

41. A. R. Anderson, H. Friberg, D. M. B. Knudsen, et al., Extraction of Tc-99m-d,l, HM-PAO across the blood-brain barrier, *J. Cereb. Blood Flow Metab. 8*: S44 (1988).

42. R. D. Neirinckx, J. F. Burke, R. C. Harrison, et al., The retention mechanism of Tc-99m HMPAO: intracellular reaction with glutathione, *J. Cereb. Blood Flow Metab. 8*:S4 (1988).

43. B. L. Holman, R. S. Hellman, S. J. Goldsmith, et al., Biodistribution, dosimetry, and clinical evaluation of technetium-99m ethyl cysteinate dimer in normal subjects and in patients with chronic cerebral infarction, *J. Nucl. Med. 30*:1018 (1989).

44. R. C. Walovitch, T. C. Hill, S. T. Garrity, et al., Characterization of technetium-99m-l,l-ECD for brain perfusion imaging. Part I. Pharmacology of technetium-99m ECD in non-human primates, *J. Nucl. Med. 30*:1892 (1989).

45. W. D. Obrist, H. K. Thompson, H. S. Wang, et al., Regional cerebral blood flow estimated by xenon-133 inhalation, *Stroke 6*:245 (1975).

46. M. D. Devous Sr., W. Gong, J. K. Payne, and T. S. Harris, Dynamic quantitative Xe-133 rCBF SPECT on the PRISM 3-headed tomography, *Human Stud. J Nuc Med 34*:68P (1993).

47. G. T. Herman, *Image Reconstruction from Projections: The Fundamentals of Computerized Tomography*, Academic Press, New York, 1980, p. 4.

48. R. J. Jaszcak, R. E. Coleman, and F. R. Whitehead, Physical factors affecting quantitative measurements using camera-based single-photon emission computed tomography (SPECT), *IEEE Trans. Nucl. Sci. NS-28*:69 (1981).

49. T. E. Budinger, Physical attributes of single-photon tomography, *J. Nucl. Med. 21*:579 (1980).

50. J. A. Sorenson, Quantitative measurement of radioactivity in vivo by whole-body counting, *Instrum. Nucl. Med. 2*:311 (1974).

51. L. T. Chang, A method for attenuation correction in radionuclide computed tomography, *IEEE Trans. Nucl. Sci. NS25*:638 (1978).

52. B. M. W. Tsui, G. T. Gullberg, E. R. Edgerton, et al., Correction of nonuniform attenuation in cardiac SPECT imaging, *J. Nucl. Med. 30*:497 (1989).

53. K. Greer R. Jaszcak, C. Harris, et al., Quality control in SPECT, *J. Nucl. Med. Technol. 13*:76 (1985).

54. S. B. Saw, Effects of centre-of-rotation shift on contrast and spatial resolution of the SPECT system, *Nucl. Med. Commun. 7*:373 (1986).

55. B. A. Harkness, W. L. Rogers, N. H. Clinthorne, et al., SPECT: quality control and artifact identification, *J. Nucl. Med. Technol. 11*:55 (1983).

56. E. M. Woronowicz, R. L. Eisner, G. T. Gullberg, et al., Factors affecting single photon emission computed tomography image quality and recommended QC procedures, Publication 5407, General Electric Medical Systems, Milwaukee, WI, 1982.

4

Functional Neuroanatomy of the Limbic System and the Planum Temporale

Cynthia G. Wible, Martha E. Shenton, and Robert W. McCarley

Harvard Medical School, Boston; Brockton Veterans Affairs Medical Center, Brockton; Massachusetts Mental Health Center, Boston; and McLean Hospital, Belmont, Massachusetts

I. INTRODUCTION

A. The Limbic System: A Brain Circuit for Processing Emotion?

In 1937, James Papez [1] proposed a brain circuit for the expression and experience of emotion. He theorized that the hippocampus, mammillary bodies, hypothalamus, and cingulate gyri formed a neural system for processing emotion. MacLean [2] added other regions to the circuit, such as the amygdala, orbital frontal region, septal nuclei, and nucleus accumbens. The formulation of the limbic system has remained influential to this day. The term is still used by many researchers, although the specific brain areas presumed to form the system often vary. Much has been discovered about the function and anatomical connectivity of these areas since Papez's time. The brain areas originally designated as limbic have, at the very least, complex roles in brain functions such as memory, attention, and emotion. Furthermore, it is now known that there are dissociations of function between some of the regions, so that grouping them together as a single functional unit may be misleading. This chapter will review current views of the function and connectivity of several of the major components of this system, including the hippocampus, amygdala, cingulate, orbital frontal region, and anatomically and functionally related areas. In the anatomy sections, many of the regions referred to by number were assigned by Brodmann [3] (Fig. 1). Many of the brain regions discussed are shown in three-dimensional and slice representations in Figure 2.

B. The Planum Temporale and Language Function

The planum temporale is a triangular region posterior to the first transverse gyrus (Heschl's gyrus, the primary auditory cortex) on the superior plane of the superior temporal gyrus (STG). Geschwind and Levitsky [4] found that this area was asymmetrical, with the left surface being larger than the right. It has long been assumed that the region is involved in language function. Evidence concerning the function of the planum temporale and related regions in the superior temporal lobe will be surveyed in this chapter.

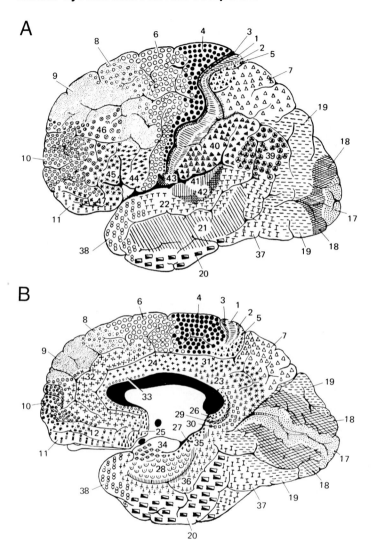

Fig. 1 Cytoarchitectural map of the human cortex. (A) Left lateral view. (B) Medial view of the right hemisphere. (From Ref. 3.)

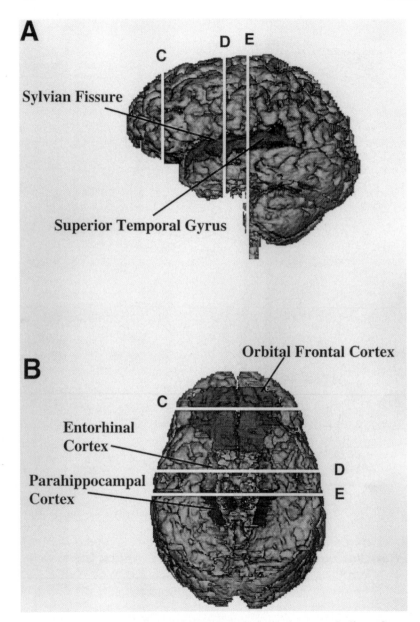

Fig. 2 Three-dimensional reconstructions and coronal slices from an MRI scan of a human brain. Coronal slices shown in panels C, D, and E were taken from the designated points in the brain. (A) Left hemisphere, lateral view of the superior temporal gyrus. (B) Ventral view of the orbital frontal

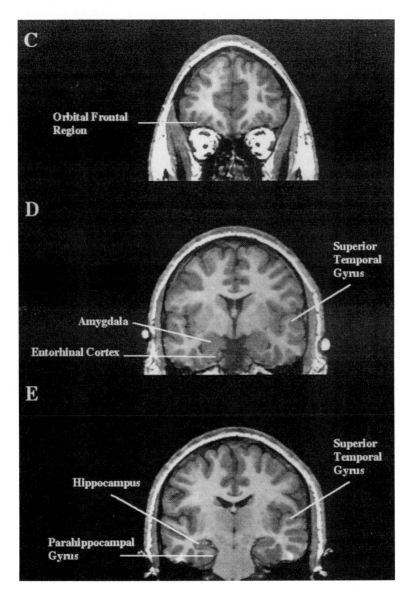

cortex, the entorhinal cortex, and the parahippocampal region. (C) Coronal section through the frontal lobe showing the orbital frontal region. (D) Coronal section through the brain at the level of the amygdala. (E) Coronal section through the brain at the level of the hippocampus.

C. Functional/Anatomical Circuits Involving Limbic Regions and Their Involvement in Psychiatric Disorders

The final section of this chapter will briefly review evidence showing that subsets of limbic regions play important roles in various psychiatric disorders such as schizophrenia and depression. The specific brain regions involved and the type of dysfunction may differ according to the disease. However, some of the regions that are designated as limbic structures (e.g., the cingulate, amygdala, and hippocampus) have physiological properties in common that may result in an increased vulnerability to certain types of dysfunction relative to other brain regions.

II. STRUCTURES OF THE LIMBIC SYSTEM

A. The Hippocampal System

I. Anatomy

The hippocampus and parahippocampal gyrus occupy the medial and ventral portion of the temporal lobe. The hippocampus is a tubelike structure that occupies most of the longitudinal extent of the temporal lobe (Fig. 3). Within

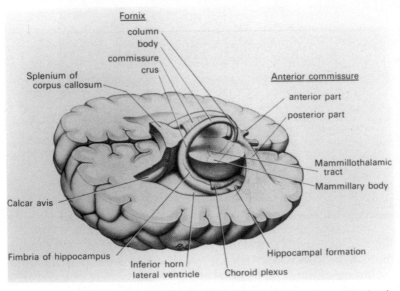

Fig. 3 Drawing of the hippocampus dissected out from the brain. (From Ref. 76.)

the coronal plane, the cornu ammonis (CA) fields and subiculum form a C-shaped structure and, together with the dentate gyrus, resemble two interdigitated C-shaped cellular fields (Fig. 4). The CA fields consist of pyramidal cells and are usually subdivided into four regions (CA1–CA4) (see Fig. 4). In the posterior end of the hippocampus, emerging axons form a white matter tract called the fimbria/fornix (Fig. 3).

The gyrus that is immediately ventral to the hippocampus is usually described as the parahippocampal gyrus in humans, but it actually consists of several subregions. The dorsal part of the gyrus (inferior to the hippocampal fissure), throughout its extent, is called the subiculum (Fig. 4). The subiculum is often subdivided into four subfields: parasubiculum, presubiculum, subiculum, and prosubiculum.

The posterior parahippocampal region can be subdivided into the cytoarchitechtonic areas TH (medially) and TF (laterally), which extend approximately from the posterior border of the entorhinal cortex to the posterior end of the hippocampus. These regions have a very complex configuration in humans and are simply designated as the parahippocampal gyrus on Figure 2.

The spatial configuration of the cortical regions in the anterior medial temporal lobe are shown in detail in Figures 5 and 6. The entorhinal and perirhinal cortices have approximately the same anterior-posterior extent and comprise the more anterior portion of the parahippocampal gyrus. The exact borders of these regions can only be determined histologically in humans, but approximate borders using surface landmarks have been determined [5]. The anterior entorhinal border begins adjacent to the most anterior portion of the amygdala and extends to approximately 10 mm posterior to the beginning of the hippocampal fissure (Figs. 5,6). The periamygdaloid cortex has approximately the same anterior-posterior boundaries as the

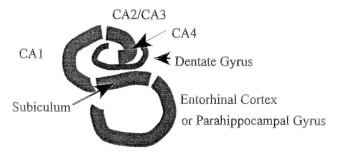

Fig. 4 Drawing of the intrinsic structure of the hippocampus.

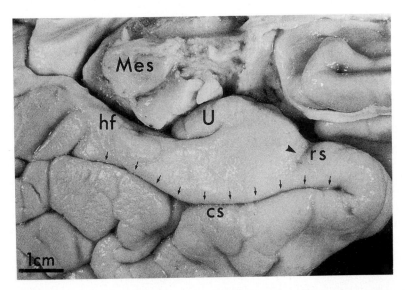

Fig. 5 Photograph of the human medial temporal lobe showing the location of the entorhinal cortex (arrows), the hippocampal fissure (hf), the collateral sulcus (cs), the uncus (U), the rhinal sulcus (rs) and the mesencephalon (Mes). (From Ref. 5.)

amygdala. The pyriform and perirhinal regions are situated in the most anterior portion of the medial temporal lobe (Fig. 6).

Early anatomical theories placed a great deal of emphasis on the fimbria/fornix output pathway of the hippocampus. This pathway contains direct outputs from the hippocampus proper to the septal region (see Ref. 6 for a historical review of hippocampal anatomy). In recent years, the importance of another set of connections has been emphasized. The hippocampus communicates with several regions of cortex through a group of highly interconnected brain regions in the medial temporal lobe that, together with the hippocampus, will be referred to as the hippocampal system. In this chapter we define the hippocampus as the dentate gyrus, the CA (coronu ammonis) layers, and the subiculum. The reader should note that the definition of the hippocampus varies, and that some authors include the CA fields and the dentate gyrus [6], and others also include the subicular fields.

The entorhinal, perirhinal, and parahippocampal cortices form the major pathways by which the hippocampus communicates with widespread cortical areas throughout the brain (Fig. 7). The entorhinal cortex provides the major input to the hippocampus and also receives output from the CA1 layer via

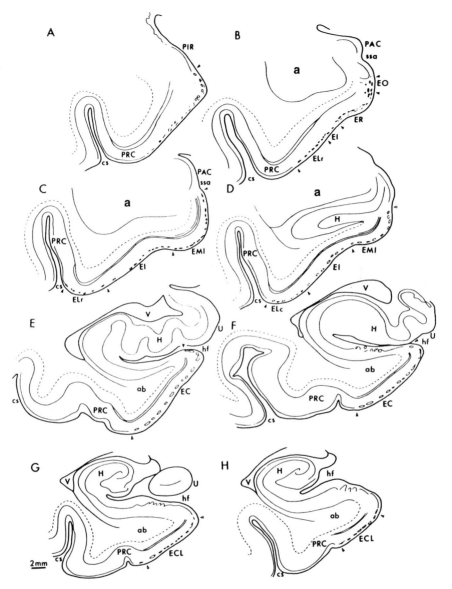

Fig. 6 Drawing of coronal sections through the human medial temporal region starting from a region anterior to the amygdala (a) to a more posterior region at the level of the hippocampus (H). Abbreviations: Piriform cortex (PIR), perirhinal cortex (PRC), collateral sulcus (cs), sulcus semiannularis (ssa), periamygdaloid cortex (PAC), amygdala (a), ventricle (v), hippocampus (H), hippocampal fissure (hf), uncus (U), angular bundle (ab). The entorhinal region is composed of the following subfields: caudal (EC), caudal limiting (ECL), intermediate (EI), lateral caudal (Elc), lateral rostral (Elr), medial intermediate (EMI), olfactory (EO), and rostral (ER). (From Ref. 5.)

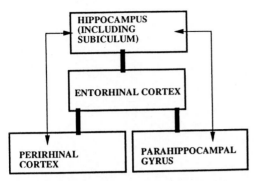

Fig. 7 Diagram showing the connectivity of the hippocampal system. The hippocampus and subiculum project primarily to the entorhinal cortex, which then projects primarily to the perirhinal and parahippocampal regions (thick lines). There are sparse projections directly from the hippocampus and subiculum to the perirhinal and parahippocampal regions (thin arrows). (Adapted from Ref. 10.)

the subiculum [7] (Fig. 8). Input to the hippocampus from the entorhinal cortex comes from two major pathways: one projecting from entorhinal layer II to the dentate gyrus and CA3 fields, and the other from entorhinal layer III to CA1; this projection also terminates in the subiculum. The subiculum then sends a major input back to the entorhinal cortex layers V and VI. Recent anatomical studies have found that the connections between the entorhinal cortex and the hippocampal formation are topographically organized and that cell layers within the hippocampus preserve this organization (see Ref. 8 for a current review of intrinsic hippocampal connectivity).

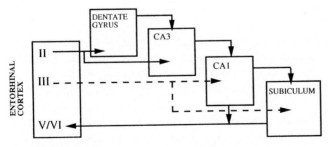

Fig. 8 Diagram showing the intrinsic connectivity of the hippocampus. (Modified from Ref. 8.)

The entorhinal cortex has its main reciprocal connections with the perirhinal and parahippocampal cortices. However, other prominent projections include the superior temporal gyrus, the orbital region of frontal cortex, and portions of the cingulate gyrus [9]. The perirhinal and parahippocampal regions in turn project to many areas of the cerebral cortex, including higher-order multimodal areas such as the cingulate gyrus and superior temporal sulcus (STS), higher-order visual areas in the temporal lobe and auditory areas in the superior temporal gyrus, visuospatial parietal areas, and dorsolateral prefrontal cortex (Fig. 1, area 46) [10].

2. Function

At the time that the theory of the limbic system was developed, the hippocampus was thought to mediate olfaction. The major pathways of the limbic system were thought to consist of efferent connections from the hypothalamus to the cingulate cortex, through the mammillary bodies and anterior thalamus, and a pathway from the fornix of the hippocampus to the mammillary bodies, anterior thalamus, and cingulate. In this conceptualization, the hippocampus was a relay station for perceptual representations from the cortex to reach the cingulate, which was thought to be the center for the conscious experience of emotion [1]. Subsequent research on the neuroanatomical connectivity and psychological function of the hippocampal system has dramatically altered this view. In fact, recent research shows that it is more likely that other areas, such as the amygdala, are involved in the processing of emotion.

Damage or surgical resection of the medial temporal lobe, that includes the hippocampus, results in a dense, circumscribed anterograde amnesia (inability to retain new information) concurrent with normal intellectual, perceptual, and motor functioning and normal short-term memory [11,12]. Recent studies of patients with damage limited to the hippocampal formation show that the damage is sufficient to result in amnesia [13]. The memory deficit affects stimuli from all modalities and can be described as a deficit in the consolidation of declarative, explicitly recalled memory. (Reminiscences about past experiences, the recollection that Martin Luther King was a civil rights leader, and the memory of what you had for breakfast are all examples of declarative memory.) Declarative memory ("knowing that") is available to conscious access, is flexible, and is retrievable in multiple contexts [14,15]. This memory system allows for the storage of concepts or percepts that are encoded in relationship to each other. This is in contrast to memory that is spared in amnesia, procedural memory ("knowing how"). Procedural memory is the type of memory thought to underlie the learning of skills, like riding a bike. This will be described in detail later. Unilateral temporal lobectomy also results in differential impairments on verbal and nonverbal memory tasks depending on the side of resection [16–19].

Patient H. M. was the first epileptic patient to undergo the experimental treatment of bilateral medial-temporal lobe removal for the treatment of intractable epilepsy [12]. Unfortunately, although the epilepsy was ameliorated, H. M. could no longer store any new declarative memories. However, his long-term memory for experiences before the surgery were intact, with the exception of memories from a period of 5–10 years before the surgery [20,21]. Now over four decades after the surgery, H. M. lives in a nursing home and still does not remember who his caretakers are or where he lives [21]. In a 1968 paper, Milner et al. wrote that H. M. would often describe his awareness from moment to moment as "like waking from a dream." For patients with bilateral medial temporal damage like H. M., each instance of experience is isolated, because they are not able to remember what came before [20].

Animal models of amnesia have been used extensively to help in the identification of the brain areas involved and to further specify the type of impairment. Monkeys and rats with hippocampal system damage show patterns of impairment similar to those found in amnesic patients, concurrent with a sparing of short-term memory and perceptual and motor abilities. Many of the tasks used with rats have been spatial memory tasks, and those used with monkeys have generally been nonspatial object memory tasks, sometimes resulting in disagreements about the nature of the memory impairment. However, several experiments have demonstrated that both rats and monkeys with hippocampal system damage are impaired on spatial and non-spatial tasks that require memory similar to that used in declarative memory tasks with human amnesics (e.g., Refs. 15,22,23). The delayed nonmatch to sample task has been used extensively to test declarative memory function in animals. In the basic version of this task, the animal is presented with an object for a few seconds during the "sample phase," a delay period then ensues, during which the animal is unable to see the object. During the "choice phase" the animal is presented with the previously shown object and a novel object and is rewarded for choosing the novel object. Performance of tasks such as the delayed nonmatch to sample and other object discriminations that require the memory of several objects, or several pairs of objects, over a delay is impaired with hippocampal system damage in both rats and monkeys [24–28] (see Ref. 29 for review).

A series of investigations with monkeys designed to pinpoint the specific regions involved in producing amnesia clarified several key issues. First, ischemic damage to the hippocampus alone in monkeys produced memory impairment [30]. Lesions of the amygdala, fornix, or mammillary nuclei did not produce a lasting memory impairment [26,31]. However, lesions limited to the perirhinal and parahippocampal cortex, the regions surrounding the amygdala, did produce severe memory deficits [32]. Together, these findings indicate that the hippocampus proper and surrounding entorhinal, perirhinal, and parahippocampal regions are the critical cites of damage in medial-temporal amnesia.

Not all forms of memory are impaired in medial temporal amnesia; patients show normal memory abilities on tasks that involve the learning of perceptual skills, perceptual-motor skills, priming, and many classical conditioning tasks [20,33] (see Ref. 14 for review). The type of memory that is spared in amnesia is procedural memory. This type of memory is involved in skills such as riding a bike or typing, but it can also include some of the components of psychological processes that are not normally thought of in the same way as motor skills, such as conceptual problem solving, categorization, and reading (e.g. Ref. 34). The term "nondeclarative memory" has been used more recently to reflect the idea that these disparate types of skill may not be of one category. Nondeclarative memory is unimpaired in amnesia, is not available to conscious access, and is expressible only via the activation of the processing structures used in the original learning experience, and stimuli are encoded individually instead of associatively [15]. Mirror tracing is an example of a perceptual-motor task used to assess nondeclarative memory. The subject is required to trace the outline of a geometric figure (often a star) while being able to see their hand movements only in a mirror. This skill develops after several trials of practice, after which subjects learn to trace the figure fairly quickly. Amnesic subjects show normal learning on mirror tracing, although a few minutes after completion they are completely unaware of ever having performed the task [11]. Monkeys with hippocampal system damage also show normal learning of perceptual-motor skills [23].

Performance of most types of priming tasks is also normal in amnesic subjects (see Ref. 35 for review). Priming tasks are based on the finding that if a stimulus is perceived and identified once, it will be identified faster the second time it is presented. The lexical decision paradigm is a common priming task. Words and nonwords are presented, one at a time, and the subject must decide if the stimulus is a word or not. The time to make this decision for a particular word is decreased by either showing the word repeatedly or by showing words that are semantically related to the target word (i.e., presenting the word bread first decreases the reaction time to identify the word butter). Another way of demonstrating priming is in a word-stem completion task, where a few letters of a word are presented and subjects are instructed to complete the word with the first word that comes to mind. Amnesiacs perform normally on most priming tasks, but they cannot recall the words that were presented during the task. Word-stem completion priming and priming with a semantically related word is also normal in amnesic subjects, with the exception that the word or the semantic relationship must have already existed in long-term memory before the amnestic incident [36,37].

Medial temporal amnesia is usually accompanied by a temporally limited retrograde amnesia, with more distant long-term memory intact [21,38]. Memories that were acquired long before the amnestic incident are intact, but memory for the years just prior to the incident are lost. These data suggest that the hippocampal system is not the (ultimate) site of storage of long-term memory, but participates in the consolidation and retrieval of memory for a time after learning. Monkeys with hippocampal system damage also show this pattern of a limited retrograde amnesia with an impairment of recent memories and sparing of more long-term memories [39].

Hippocampal unit activity reflects the fact that the hippocampus receives input from higher-order sensory and multimodal cortex. Single units show correlates in a variety of tasks that reflect the representation of percepts such as words and pictures in humans [40] and visual stimuli, odors, sounds, and spatial locations in animals [15,28,41,42]. Unit recording studies also show that although hippocampal system function may not be necessary for the maintenance of short-term memory or working memory, it is often active during the processing of these types of memory (e.g., Ref. 43).

The mechanisms used by the hippocampal system to participate in the consolidation of memory are not well understood. Psychological research has shown that the repetition and/or rehearsal of items will consolidate them in memory. The embedding of an item within an associative structure, either by elaboration or by presenting the item within a meaningful context, also improves memory for the item. The processing characteristics of the hippocampal system may underlie these psychological mechanisms of consolidation.

The hippocampus is plastic relative to most other brain areas and has been shown to undergo what is called long-term potentiation (LTP), which results in an increased efficacy of neural elements for a time after their initial activation [44]. LTP has been extensively investigated, not only at the molecular and cellular levels, but also in relationship to behavior and, in particular, to memory formation. It is likely that LTP plays an important role in enabling the hippocampus to participate in the consolidation of memory, and it has been shown to be related to memory function in animals [45]. However, memory is not ultimately stored only in the hippocampus. Given this paradox, what role might LTP play in memory consolidation? LTP may be used to store representations for a short time, allowing the hippocampus to act as a medium-term memory buffer. In this role as a memory buffer, the hippocampus would change quickly to retain a strong memory trace that decays rapidly, while the cortex would change in small increments to store the representation over repeated instances of activation [46]. It is assumed that each repetition or rehearsal of the stimulus results in a change in all of the neural elements throughout the brain that were used to process the representation, but that the change in the hippocampus would be incrementally larger than in other regions.

The facilitation of the distributed neural elements that represent an item could also allow for the association or linking of stimuli that are processed within a short time frame (Fig. 9). LTP may be part of a mechanism for creating associations between stimulus representations that are processed by the hippocampus within a short time frame [46]. Several possible mechanisms could underlie this computation. For example, the memory buffer could allow for the near-simultaneous activation of representations in cortex that were originally processed with a longer time gap between them. The timing of the activation of representations in cortical regions has been shown to be a major determinant of associative cortical storage [47].

Previously established associations could also be reorganized by these processing mechanisms. It is known from semantic priming studies that the perception of a stimulus automatically causes the partial activation of previously stored semantic associates. If semantic primes were strongly activated,

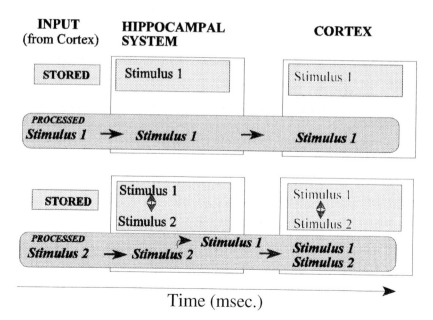

Fig. 9 Diagram showing the processing stages of the formation of associative networks and consolidation.

the representation would be processed by the hippocampus, just as stimuli from the environment are processed. This would allow for the creation of associations either between two or more internally activated stimuli or between an internally activated stimulus and incoming stimuli from the environment, resulting in the reorganization of existing associative networks. These processes probably occur in degrees, varying with the strength of the representations in question, and would not necessarily need to be conscious processes. The formation of associates, or the embedding of a representation within a network of associates, would consolidate an item by increasing the number of available retrieval routes, hence increasing the probability of recall.

In summary, the hippocampal system is essential for the consolidation of associative or declarative memory. The hippocampal system is thought to interact with other cortical areas to consolidate and organize information over time. In other words, the hippocampus is responsible for creating the associative networks that store experiences and that give percepts and concepts meaning.

B. The Amygdala

1. Anatomy

Amygdala is the word for almond in Latin; this structure is anterior to the hippocampus in the temporal lobe, and early anatomists named it for its shape (Fig. 10; see also Fig. 2d). A portion of the posterior amygdala is situated superior to the head of the hippocampus. Thirteen distinct nuclei make up the amygdaloid complex [48].

As a whole, the amygdaloid complex has strong reciprocal connections with the hypothalamus and autonomic nuclei of the brainstem, receives a strong input from the basal forebrain, and projects to the dorsal medial nucleus of the thalamus [49]. The strength of amygdalar input and output pathways to cortical regions is asymmetrical. The amygdala receives input primarily from higher-order sensory and multimodal areas, but has strong efferent connections to both higher-order and primary cortices [48].

Three nuclei—lateral, basal or basolateral, and central—form an important intrinsic pathway for sensory information coming in to the amygdala to be sent back out to the cortex, to the hypothalamus, and to autonomic nuclei [49,50] (Fig. 11). Sensory input from the cortex and thalamus come into the amygdala through the lateral nucleus. The lateral nucleus receives strong inputs from the orbital frontal (areas 13 and 14, and some of area 12), perirhinal, and insular regions [49]. It also receives input from the inferior frontal region (area 45), the anterior cingulate (area 24), the anterior inferotemporal cortex (TE), and the parahippocampal gyrus (TH, TF), as well as a light

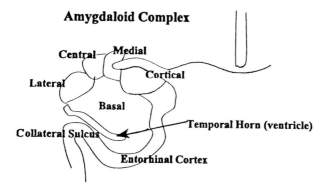

Fig. 10 A drawing of several amygdalar nuclei in a coronal section (Adapted from Ref. 104.)

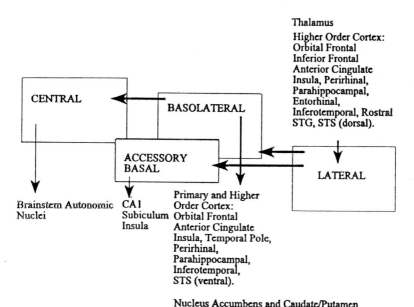

Fig. 11 Diagram of the connectivity of four key amygdalar nuclei. (Adapted from figure supplied by Dr. D. G. Rainnie.)

projection from dorsolateral prefrontal cortex (area 46) and other portions of the frontal lobe [49]. The lateral nucleus projects to both the basal and accessory basal nuclei. The basal nucleus in turn projects to many higher-order areas including the orbital frontal cortex (areas 12,14), the anterior cingulate (area 25), the insula, the anterior STG, the inferotemporal cortex (TE), the temporal pole (TG), and the perirhinal and parahippocampal regions [51]. The basal nucleus also has light projections to inferior and dorsolateral frontal regions (areas 45,46) and to the parietal lobe (area 7) [51]. In addition to projecting to higher-order regions, the basal nucleus also projects directly to primary sensory cortical areas, including somatosensory, auditory, and visual areas [48,49]. The nucleus accumbens and parts of the basal ganglia also receive projections from the basal nucleus. The accessory basal nucleus projects to the CA1, CA3, subiculum, and entorhinal portions of the hippocampal system [52]. The basal nucleus in turn projects to the central nucleus. The central nucleus then projects to the hypothalamus and to brainstem nuclei related to the autonomic system.

The amygdala is preferentially connected with the areas that process object (or nonspatial) information (ventral areas such as those in temporal cortex) rather than spatial information (dorsal areas such as parietal cortex) [48]. The temporal pole and perirhinal cortex constitute the strongest connections to the amygdala within the temporal lobe. The strongest connections to frontal cortex are with the orbitofrontal and anterior cingulate regions. It is also important to note that the right and left amygdala are somewhat segregated by a lack of commissural fibers and are thus interconnected with cortical areas within the same hemisphere [48].

2. Function

The extensive autonomic connections of the amygdala make it no surprise that lesions to this area in animals interfere with the ability to learn in conditioned fear and fear potentiated startle paradigms, because the autonomic nervous system mediates many aspects of the fear response (see Refs. 53–55 for reviews). Connections from the lateral nucleus to the basal ganglia and nucleus accumbens may also participate in the processing of the motor responses to fear and in representing the reward value of stimuli [56]. The circuit for conditioned fear has been carefully characterized and may provide information about the role of the amygdala in other types of emotional processing.

During fear conditioning using a tone, the tone representation is processed through the usual auditory pathways, from peripheral sensory receptors and brainstem nuclei to the thalamus, and then to primary auditory cortex. Simultaneously, the tone representation is also sent from the thalamus to the amygdala. During conditioning, this pathway to the amygdala is strengthened and facilitated. Conditioning increases the number of neurons responding to the tone, the magnitude of the responses, and synchronous firing in neurons of the lateral nucleus [57]. The lateral nucleus also receives information from the regions that process the unconditional stimulus (usually footshock) [58]. The amygdala may not only facilitate the relationship between a threatening stimulus coming into the lateral nucleus and the fear response (output from the central nucleus), but it may also store the association between the conditional and unconditional stimulus [58]. In addition, it is known that fear conditioning can result in memory that is easily reinstated after behavioral extinction. The synchronous firing of lateral nucleus neurons also persisted after extinction, perhaps as part of this persistent memory trace [57].

The projections from the basal nucleus of the amygdala to cortical regions put it in a position to modulate the response of cortical neurons to the tone [57]. In addition, it is known that the auditory pathways from the thalamus to the cortex and then amygdala are needed for conditioning paradigms where more than one stimulus is used or where the stimuli are more perceptually complex.

The amygdala is also involved in functional systems having to do with the processing of species-specific calls and facial expressions [59,60]. Single unit activity in the amygdala shows correlates with individual faces and also with various aspects of memory tasks during performance [42]. Stimulation of the amygdala in animals can produce "sham rage," a response similar to the characteristic aggressive response for that animal. Stimulation of the amygdala in human subjects can also produce aggressive behavior, affective states, or "memories" of interpersonal interactions [61,62].

For several years the amygdala was thought to participate in memory formation along with other medial temporal areas [63]. However, the development of more precise lesion techniques has shown that it was damage to surrounding cortical areas that produced the memory deficit (see Sec. B). A recent experiment using a conditioned emotional response paradigm with human subjects demonstrated the difference between the function of the amygdala and hippocampus. The subjects were patients with bilateral circumscribed amygdala damage, circumscribed hippocampal damage, or combined bilateral amygdala and hippocampal damage. Subjects were conditioned for several trials using a loud startling sound that was paired with a blue-colored slide but none of the other colored slides shown. Successful conditioning was measured as an increase in galvanic skin response after the blue slide, but no other slides, when the blue slide was no longer followed by the tone. A declarative memory test was also given and subjects were asked to explicitly recall information about the slides, including which one was followed by a sound. Subjects with amygdala damage failed to develop a conditioned response to the blue slide but performed normally on the declarative memory test. Subjects with hippocampal damage learned the conditioned response normally but failed to explicitly remember the testing situation and did not perform correctly on the declarative memory task. Subjects with damage to both areas failed on both the conditioning and declarative memory portions of the task [64].

Another study using subjects with circumscribed amygdala damage showed that although the amygdala may not be essential for the storage of declarative memory, it can affect the strength of this type of memory under emotional circumstances. Subjects with circumscribed amygdala damage and control subjects were tested for memory of a story containing an emotionally charged passage. Subjects with amygdala damage did not show, as did control subjects, better memory of the emotionally charged portion of the story [65].

These findings indicate that, although the amygdala is not necessary for the storage of declarative memory, it can modulate the strength of declarative memory, at least under some circumstances. During times of intense emotion, the sympathetic nervous system is activated and causes physiological changes in the body such as an increase in respiration rate and increased blood flow to muscles in order for the organism to respond quickly in the face of danger. One way of conceptualizing amygdala function would be to say that it does for the brain what the sympathetic system does for the muscles; it heightens, in a specific way, processing of representations that the organism perceives during strong emotional states. It facilitates the relationship between the stimulus coming into the amygdala and fear responses and may also store the association between the conditional stimulus and the aversive stimulus. In addition, it may heighten processing in primary cortex (aiding in identification) and in secondary and multimodal areas (further aiding in both identification and in semantic processing of the stimulus). This heightened processing may allow for the stimulus to be identified and acted upon faster and for memories associated with the stimulus to be retrieved more quickly, thus helping decision making. The longer-term result of this processing might be a strengthening of the normal processes underlying priming and memory consolidation for the particular stimuli processed during the emotional state.

C. The Cingulate Gyrus

1. Anatomy

The cingulate gyrus is the first major gyrus superior to the corpus callosum on the medial wall of each hemisphere (Fig. 12). The cingulate connections will be discussed in terms of anterior (areas 32, 25, and rostral 24) and poste-

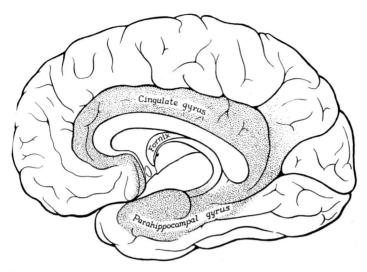

Fig. 12 Drawing showing the cingulate gyrus, fornix, and parahippocampal gyrus on the medial surface of the right hemisphere of a human brain. (From Ref. 76.)

rior (caudal areas 24,31,23,26, and 29) connections, as they differ in some cases. Both portions are interconnected with the parahippocampal gyrus, and both portions also project to multimodal temporal areas in the superior temporal sulcus. However, there are several differences in connectivity. For example, the anterior, but not posterior, portion of the cingulate projects to both motor and premotor cortex. There are also differences in connectivity with temporal and frontal regions. The anterior cingulate is also interconnected with the subiculum, the CA1 layer of the hippocampus, the amygdala, and the rostral superior temporal gyrus [66]. In terms of frontal lobe connections, the anterior cingulate is more heavily connected to the orbital region (areas 11,12, and 13) than is the posterior cingulate. The posterior cingulate is more heavily connected with the dorsolateral frontal cortex (areas 9 and 46) and posterior inferior parietal areas (PG and OPT) [66].

Cortical projections to the anterior cingulate include orbital (areas 11,12,13,14) and dorsolateral (areas 9,46) frontal cortex. The insula, amygdala, CA1 region of the hippocampus, subiculum, temporal pole (PG), parahippocampal gyrus, STS (the dorsal portion of the sulcus, or region TPO), and inferior dorsal temporal cortical regions (TS2,TS3) also project to the anterior cingulate [66]. The anterior cingulate sends projections back to most of these areas (although not to area 46, or to the parahippocampal gyrus) and in addition also projects to premotor areas (6,8), the anterior STG, and the perirhinal cortex [67].

Cortical projections to the posterior cingulate include the orbital frontal (areas 11,14), dorsolateral frontal (area 46), and frontal pole regions (area 10). The parahippocampal gyrus and STS (TPO), parietal (OPT) and occipital (area 19) regions also project to the posterior cingulate region [68]. The posterior cingulate projects back to the dorsolateral frontal region (areas 9,10,46), to the orbital frontal region (area 11), and to the parahippocampal gyrus region (TH, TF, retrosplenial, presubiculum) and parietal lobe (area 7) [67].

2. Function

The cingulate was thought by Papez to be the neural substrate for the experience of conscious emotion. Although this may not be a complete explanation of its role, some of the data on cingulate function does suggest a role in emotional processing. The cingulate is highly interconnected with areas that process emotion, social/emotional behavior, and drive states (i.e., amygdala, orbital frontal cortex, hypothalamus), with areas that participate in the consolidation and retrieval of memory (i.e., the hippocampal system), and with motor areas. This puts the cingulate in the position of processing integrated information about stimuli and their emotional/motivational context, in addition to providing output to motor areas. The right cingulate is also part of a circuit that is thought to subserve attention; this circuit involves parietal and dorsolateral frontal regions (see Ref. 69 for a review of cingulate function).

The cingulate, along with the dorsolateral prefrontal cortex and posterior parietal cortex in the right hemisphere, are the areas most often involved in producing neglect disorders [70]. Attention in relationship to cingulate function has also been studied using the Stroop task [71]. In this task, subjects are required to read the names of colors when the word is printed in a color different from the name to be read. In a PET study, the anterior cingulate region showed the highest level of activity related to the Stroop task [71]. Another PET study found that cingulate activity increased along with the number of targets to be detected [72].

The anterior cingulate may also participate in verbal processing or behavior. Neuroimaging studies showed that the anterior cingulate was active during verbal tasks [73]. Bilateral lesions of the cingulate can produce akinetic mutism, in which patients lack the motivation to speak or act [74]. Lesions of the anterior cingulate can also produce a syndrome in which patients believe that their thoughts or actions are controlled by someone else [75].

The cingulate is a region for the convergence of information from many of the higher-order processing systems of the brain. It is possible that the cingulate region can be further subdivided into functional modules. However, data from current research suggest a complex role for the cingulate in several processes, including attention, volition, and the processing of the emotional or motivational significance of stimuli in relationship to behavior.

D. The Orbital Frontal Cortex

1. Anatomy

McLean included the orbitofrontal cortex in his expansion of the concept of the limbic system [2]. The orbital area (corresponding approximately to Walker's areas 11,12,13, and 14) consists of a number of small gyri on the ventral surface of the frontal lobe (see Fig. 2b,c). The amygdala projects directly to the orbitofrontal cortex [51,76] and indirectly through the magnocellular portion of the dorsomedial nucleus of the thalamus [77]. The entorhinal cortex and perirhinal cortex project more heavily to the orbital region than any other areas of the prefrontal cortex [9,10]. The polar or anterior portion of the superior temporal gyrus also projects primarily to the orbital frontal area (in addition to the anterior cingulate region) [78,79].

2. Function

One general theory of prefrontal function is that it is a central executive system for the allocation of attention and the coordination of working memory. It is thought to interact with "slave systems" in the temporal, parietal, and occipital lobes. The phonological loop (verbal working memory) and the visuospatial sketch pad are separate working memory systems that have been postulated to be associated with temporal and parietal-occipital slave systems, respectively. These slave systems may be controlled by different portions of prefrontal cortex [80]. The prefrontal cortex may function in working memory by reactivating, or keeping active, those primary and association cortices in other cortical areas that are responsible for information storage.

Damage to the orbital cortex in humans is often reported to result in profound personality changes, without concomitant changes in intellectual function [81,82]. Orbitofrontal lesions often result in a syndrome where the patient exhibits poor judgment and inappropriate behavior in social situations. The famous patient Phineas Gage, who was injured in an explosion by an iron rod that penetrated his skull, is now thought to have had damage concentrated mainly in the orbital region [83]. Before the accident he was described as a responsible and socially well-adapted person. These characteristics changed radically, and for the rest of his life he was irreverent and irresponsible. Damasio et al. [83] reported that "his respect for the social conventions by which he once abided had vanished."

One theory of orbital function that accounts for this syndrome is that the aberrant behavior stems from a "defect in the activation of somatic markers that must accompany the internal and automatic processing of response options'' [81]. It is claimed that during decision making, response alternatives and their probable outcomes are evaluated. A somatic marker (an emotional state) is thought to automatically accompany these representations of response alternatives and the consequences being evaluated. The orbitofrontal cortex, through its connections with amygdala, hippocampus, and associated medial temporal cortices, is postulated to make possible the reactivation of emotional states previously associated with a behavioral context [81]. Patients with orbital frontal damage are therefore unable to evaluate or are unaware of the negative consequences of actions or decisions.

E. Superior Temporal Gyrus and Planum Temporale

1. Anatomy

The superior temporal gyrus is just ventral to the sylvian fissure. The planum temporale is a region on the superior surface of the superior temporal gyrus that is posterior to the first transverse gyrus (Heschl's gyrus) (Figs. 2a,13). The transverse gyri or Heschl's gyri comprise the primary auditory cortex within the superior temporal gyrus. In monkeys, the posterior superior temporal gyrus projects primarily to frontal regions 46, 8, and 6 (dorsolateral), the middle portion projects to areas 12 (orbital), 46, 9, (dorsolateral) and 10 (pole), and the anterior portion projects to 14 (orbital), 9 (dorsolateral) and 10 (pole)[78].

2. Function

The planum temporale has been assumed to be at least part of the neural substrate for language comprehension [84,85]. In general, lesions of the posterior superior temporal area are often associated with aphasia [86]. Wernicke's aphasia is characterized by deficits in language comprehension in the face of fluent and grammatical speech. These aphasic patients fail to comprehend the meaning of spoken or written words and also produce speech that is lacking in content or meaning. It has been shown that the representations of words themselves (lexical) are separate from the semantic representation (or meaning) of the words [87]. Some components of Wernicke's aphasia include the production of empty speech or speech that fails to convey meaning, paraphrasias, neologisms, and logorrhea, or excessive speech. These patients are also often unaware of their semantic deficits. This syndrome is in contrast to aphasia resulting from frontal damage (Broca's area), in which verbal output is markedly impaired, but the patient understands meaning. Broca's aphasics are usually aware of their deficits and experience frustration with their speech difficulties.

Data from brain stimulation and neuropsychological studies indicate not only that the temporal lobe (especially the superior temporal region) contains

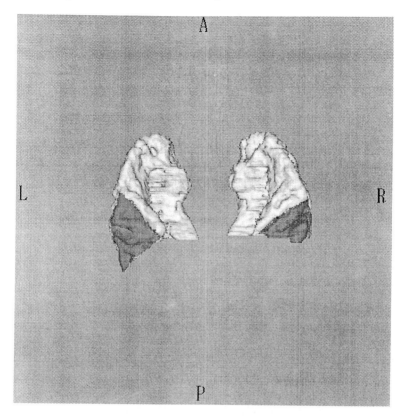

Fig. 13 Three-dimensional reconstruction of the superior plane of the superior temporal gyrus showing the planum temporale region (in dark gray) in the posterior extent.

areas involved in the processing of associative verbal and auditory memory, but that the semantic associations that underlie meaning are actually stored in this cortical region [88].

III. FUNCTIONAL/ANATOMICAL CIRCUITS INVOLVING LIMBIC REGIONS AND THEIR ROLE IN PSYCHIATRIC DISORDERS

A. Physiological Properties that Increase Susceptibility to Dysfunction

The cingulate, amygdala, and hippocampal system contain relatively high concentrations of the types of receptors [N-methyl-D-aspartate (NMDA)] that underlie the formation of LTP, making these regions more vulnerable to dysfunction relative to other areas of the brain. The anterior cingulate, perirhinal cortex, entorhinal cortex, amygdala, and hippocampus contain some of the highest concentrations of NMDA receptors in the brain [89]. The basal ganglia (including the nucleus accumbens), the dorsal lateral septum, and frontal cortex also contain relatively high concentrations of these receptors.

NMDA receptors are one type of glutamate receptor, and as stated previously, NMDA receptor activity underlies the formation of LTP. A synapse that has undergone LTP will be more likely to produce an action potential. Thus, regions that contain high concentrations of these receptors are relatively plastic relative to other brain regions. However, this plasticity comes with a price. LTP is also thought to underlie the excitotoxic mechanisms that make these regions relatively more vulnerable to neuronal damage than other regions. Under some circumstances, such as anoxia or ischemia, the cellular mechanisms that underlie plasticity can lead to activity-dependent excitotoxic damage or oxidative stress.

The vulnerability of the amygdala and hippocampal system makes these regions the most frequent cites of epileptic foci and of damage after anoxia or ischemia [90]. It is also important to note that glutamate is critically involved in brain development and that during critical periods of development glutamatergic abnormalities could result in developmental abnormalities in these and other regions of the brain.

Other physiological properties of these regions (especially the hippocampus) also make them likely candidates for dysfunction associated with psychiatric diseases. For example, the hippocampus contains the highest concentration of glucocorticoid receptors in the brain. Glucocorticoids are released by the adrenal glands during psychological stress. These compounds can regulate LTP in the hippocampus and may also increase the likelihood of excitotoxic cell death with prolonged exposure [91–93].

B. Schizophrenia

1. Introduction

In this section, we will use schizophrenia as an example of how advances in the understanding of the anatomy, physiology, and function of some of the "limbic" brain regions have been used to develop hypotheses about the brain abnormalities that underlie the disease. We will discuss hypotheses of brain dysfunction that are based on the anatomical connectivity and physiological properties of regions that have been implicated in schizophrenia. Information about the psychological function of these regions is used to make inferences about brain-symptom relationships. In addition, a specific physiological hypothesis is presented and tested using a neural network model.

2. Evidence

There is converging evidence that the hippocampal system, amygdala, superior temporal region, and some portions of the prefrontal cortex such as the anterior cingulate, and orbital frontal regions, especially in the left hemisphere, form at least part of a functional circuit that is disturbed in schizophrenia (Fig. 14). There are several reports of abnormalities of the hippocampal system and amygdala; in fact, these abnormalities are the most consistent findings in the schizophrenia literature (see Chapter 12). Histological studies of the cingulate have found abnormalities [94,95]. In addition, anterior cingulate and hippocampal hypometabolism were found in actively psychotic, drug-free schizophrenic patients in a PET study [96]. Recent MRI studies from our group show that in schizophrenic subjects, the volume of left temporal lobe regions that were reduced were correlated with the volumes of some portions of the prefrontal cortex [97]. Volumes of the orbital region in the prefrontal cortex were particularly strongly correlated with volumes of the anterior portions of temporal lobe structures, including the amygdala/hippocampal complex (amygdala and some anterior hippocampus), the parahippocampal gyrus (mostly entorhinal cortex), and the superior temporal

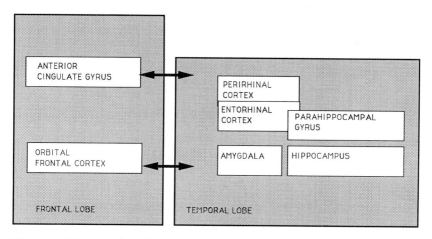

Fig. 14 Diagram showing several limbic brain regions. Every region shown in the diagram is highly interconnected with most of the other regions. These brain regions may also form part of a functional/anatomical circuit in schizophrenia.

gyrus. These temporal-prefrontal volume correlations were not present in the control group.

The volume correlations between structures in left temporal and left prefrontal cortex are consistent with a theory of developmental abnormality and/or excitotoxic or oxidative stress damage in these areas in schizophrenic patients. These types of abnormalities could result in correlated volume loss in brain regions that are closely anatomically and functionally connected. There is a striking correspondence between the frontal lobe regions showing high correlations with the anterior amygdala/hippocampal complex volume and those areas whose projections both to and from the amygdala use glutamate as a neurotransmitter [51]. As discussed above, NMDA receptors (a subset of glutamate receptors) exist throughout the brain, but the concentration of receptors varies. If NMDA abnormalities exist in proportion to the number of receptors in a region, then regions with the highest receptor concentrations may be relatively more abnormal. In addition, relatively higher levels of abnormalities might be expected in regions that have primary efferent/afferent glutamatergic connections with these regions of high NMDA concentration. It is also important to note that it is not known specifically what types of physiological effects NMDA or glutamate abnormalities could produce. Many types of abnormalities may occur, including cell loss, changes in cell processes (dendrites or axons), and/or many types of neurodevelopmental changes.

The prefrontal regions that are proposed to be a part of an abnormal circuit in schizophrenic subjects also had volumes that were correlated with clinical symptoms. Orbital volume was highly correlated with apathy and asociality, and anterior cingulate and right middle frontal gyrus volumes were highly correlated with attentional deficits.

3. A Proposed Model

Based on findings of abnormalities in MRI, histological, and functional studies, we have proposed a neural model for possible neurodevelopmental and/or neurodegenerative processes of schizophrenia due to abnormalities in NMDA, the neurotransmitter underlying the formation of LTP. This neural model is part of a first step in attempting to bridging findings from basic physiology at the molecular and neural levels and brain function at the systems level to clinical symptoms.

Several key properties of cortical circuit neurons have been included in the model and are important for understanding neuronal interactions. Neurons often have axons that branch off from the main axons, called collateral axons. Recurrent collateral axons provide a way for the neuron to influence its own firing and the firing of surrounding neurons. In the hippocampus, some primary neuronal projections (and specifically, for our purposes, the

Schaeffer collateral projections) have recurrent branches that synapse on inhibitory interneurons. These inhibitory interneurons then project back to the original neuron and also to surrounding neurons. Both the primary neuron and the recurrent branch of the axon have NMDA receptors, and both exhibit LTP (Fig. 15).

Our laboratory's in vitro work in the hippocampus indicates that cortical recurrent inhibition is much more susceptible to blockage by NMDA receptor blockers, such as APV, than primary neuron excitation [98]. This finding provides a sound physiological basis for the acute excitatory effects of phencyclidine (PCP), another NMDA receptor blocker. Although PCP blocks NMDA receptors, it paradoxically acts to excite neurons. The Grunze et al. [98] findings suggest that PCP blocks recurrent inhibitory pathways more strongly than the main excitatory pathways, leading to the disinhibition of principle neurons, and resulting in predominately excitatory effects. The symptoms of PCP intoxication are similar to those of schizophrenia, including bizarre speech and psychosis [99]. In addition, increased levels of the endogenous NMDA blocker N-acetyl-aspartyl-glutamate (NAAG) in schizophrenic brains, as reported by Tsai et al. [100], might be responsible for use-dependent excitotoxic damage or oxidative stress damage and the behavioral symptoms of schizophrenia.

Blocking NMDA receptors also blocks the formation of LTP. If recurrent inhibition was more sensitive to blockage by NMDA blockers than the principal projection, then LTP at the recurrent inhibitory circuit might also be more sensitive to blockage. The consequences of a selective antagonism of LTP of recurrent inhibitory circuits on the processing characteristics of hippocampal CA1 neuronal networks has been examined, and it was found,

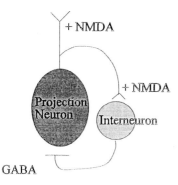

Fig. 15 Drawing of a hypothetical neuron showing a recurrent collateral inhibitory circuits.

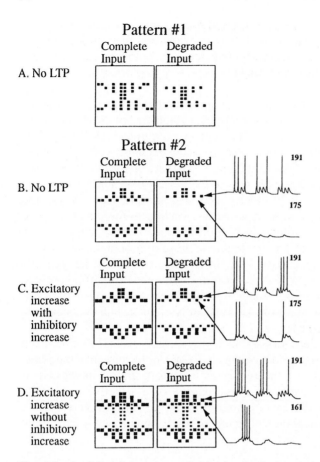

Fig. 16 Activity in a network biophysical simulation showing the significance of LTP of recurrent inhibition for recall of stored input patterns. This figure illustrates activity during recall. Activity during learning is not shown. (A) Spiking activity induced in a network of 240 pyramidal cells without any strengthening of excitatory intrinsic synapses. Each enclosed panel contains 240 neurons plotted in a 15 × 16 matrix. The size of the black squares represents the number of action potentials generated by each pyramidal cell during a 500-ms period of recall. For each pattern, the left panel shows the response to the complete input version of the pattern (with 40 neurons active) and the right square shows the response to a degraded input version of the pattern (with 24 neurons activated by afferent input). (B) Activity induced by pattern #2 (to the right of pattern #2, traces illustrate the membrane potential of neurons 191 and 175). For panels C and D, the network has been trained on both pattern #1 and pattern #2, but recall is only shown for

as predicted, that the recurrent inhibitory LTP was more sensitive to NMDA blockade [98]. In order to determine the computational consequences of these findings, computer simulations were done using networks whose neural elements have biophysical properties that are similar to the hippocampal CA1 pyramidal cells [98]. Although computational models are a valuable tool, caution must be used in interpreting the data from these models. It is important to note that even physiologically constrained neural networks are likely to be, at best, a simplistic model of neural processing. For example, a 1-mm-square region of cortex contains more than 20,000 neurons, each receiving input from hundreds, often thousands of other neurons.

The ability of this network to store and recall two different patterns of input (each activating 40 out of 240 total units) under two different conditions was evaluated: with LTP only at the excitatory synapses and with LTP at both the excitatory and recurrent inhibitory synapses. LTP in the network was modeled by strengthening of synaptic interactions between modeled neurons (Fig. 16). The full and degraded versions of patterns 1 and 2 are shown in Figure 16A and B.

During a learning phase, LTP of excitatory synapses was applied at synapses experiencing both pre and postsynaptic activity. During a separate recall phase, the network was capable of recalling specific patterns of action potential generation in modeled neurons. For example, the network was presented with degraded versions of the input patterns, which directly induced spiking in only 24 out of the original 40 neurons activated by the full input. After the learning phase, the spread of activity across strengthened synapses caused action potential generation in neurons not receiving afferent input from the degraded pattern but which were previously activated by the complete pattern, thus completing the pattern (Fig. 16).

The reproduction of the full pattern from a degraded input was carefully modulated using recurrent inhibition, and without it presentation of a partial input could cause the abnormal activation of neural elements that were previously associated with other learned patterns, causing confusion between pat-

---

pattern #2. (C) With both excitatory LTP and inhibitory LTP, the network responds to the complete pattern with no excess spread of activity and responds to the degraded input with activity spreading only into neurons that were a component of the original learned pattern. (D) With excitatory LTP in the absence of inhibitory LTP, the network responds to both the complete and degraded versions of pattern #2 with activity that spreads to components of the other stored pattern, pattern #1. This is due to the spread of activity from neurons which were components of both patterns. (Adapted from Ref. 98.)

terns. Strengthening of excitatory synapses from principal cells to inhibitory interneurons prevented this problem. During recall, the network was tested both with and without the strengthening of excitatory input onto inhibitory interneurons. With strengthening of this recurrent inhibition, the network effectively recalled missing components without the spread of activity into other neurons of the second pattern (Fig. 16C). Without strengthening of recurrent inhibition, during recall activity spread into neurons representing both patterns, thereby preventing the ability to distinguish between overlapping stored patterns (Fig. 16D).

The results of the simulation show that, as predicted, the blockage of recurrent inhibition caused the increased spread of lateral excitation, so that formerly distinct patterns of neural activity became merged. In terms of information processing, this abnormal excitatory activity resulted in the erroneous activation of neural units that had participated in previously stored input patterns (Fig. 16).

4. Relationship of Abnormalities to Symptomotology

If this type of glutamatergic abnormality were present in the hippocampus, then it also would be likely to present in neocortical regions, but to a lesser extent. It is proposed that a dysfunctional or overactive hippocampus, acting in concert with dysfunctional neocortical regions, could produce at least some of the symptoms of the schizophrenic syndrome [101].

For example, it was suggested in an earlier section that the hippocampus acts as a memory buffer, allowing for the near-simultaneous activation of representations in cortex that were originally processed with a longer time gap between them. It is also known that any stimulus that is processed will cause a slight activation of previously stored associated concepts (semantic priming). An overactivation of the hippocampal system would also result in an overactivation of cortical regions, resulting in above normal activation of semantically associated representations. Overactivation of the left hippocampal system and/or the superior temporal gyrus could cause the normally present partial activation of semantically related representations to become supernormal, creating the erroneous addition of semantically related words to the stream of thought, resulting in thought disorder. In addition, a dysfunction of the medial temporal lobe–dependant mechanisms used to create associations in memory could result in the formation or retrieval of abnormal associations between concepts or to the spurious activation and recall of distantly related words, resulting in disordered thought and speech. Overactivation might also cause a stronger than normal activation of inner thought, causing verbal stimuli to be perceived when there is no external activation or stimulus (verbal hallucinations).

The amygdala is also known to contain pathways that use glutamate as a neurotransmitter and that can undergo LTP. Overexcitation of amygdalar pathways would be expected to contribute a negative affective tone to processing or perhaps to result in higher than normal anxiety levels, or even paranoid thoughts.

C. Other Psychiatric Disorders

Limbic regions may be involved in other psychiatric diseases. Depression, obsessive compulsive disorder, and posttraumatic stress syndrome all may involve abnormalities of subsets of "limbic" structures. For example, patients with familial pure depressive disease were shown in PET experiments to have abnormalities in the amygdala and anterior cingulate, as well as other regions such as parts of the frontal cortex [102]. Cingulotomy is sometimes performed on patients to alleviate stress due to chronic pain or as a treatment for severe obsessive-compulsive disorder [103]. PET imaging of individuals with obsessive compulsive disorder showed abnormalities in orbital and cingulate regions [102]. In addition, posttraumatic stress syndrome is likely to involve abnormalities in the hippocampus, which has relatively high concentrations of stress hormone receptors [91,92].

IV. CONCLUSIONS

In conclusion, the hippocampal system, amygdala, orbital frontal cortex, anterior cingulate, and superior temporal regions form a set of highly interconnected brain regions that may participate in functional systems subserving memory, emotion, social behavior, attention, communication, and verbal processing. Several of these regions also have special physiological properties that make them especially vulnerable to dysfunction. The dysfunction may not necessarily reflect the symptoms found when the region is lesioned when the function of the region is "missing." The symptoms will likely be better characterized by understanding the mechanisms involved in the on-line processing of representations and then trying to understand how these mechanisms would act if they were dysfunctional or abnormal, but not absent. In other words, the characterization of the consequences or symptoms of dysfunction will require detailed processing theories of the functional interactions between brain systems in normal individuals. Progress in understanding the anatomy, physiology, and function of these regions has allowed for the development of hypotheses about the relationship of brain abnormalities to symptoms in psychiatric populations. The integration of neuroscience, cognitive neuroscience, and the clinical sciences will allow these fields or levels of analysis to inform each other.

ACKNOWLEDGMENTS

The investigators were supported by the National Institute of Mental Health (40,799)[RWM], K02-MH-01110 [MES], and 1R29MH50740 [MES] and by the Department of Veterans Affairs Schizophrenia Center [RWM], the Stanley Foundation [MES], the Commonwealth of Massachusetts Research Center, [RWM], and a Health and Education Fund Award from the Massachusetts Mental Health Center [CGW].

REFERENCES

1. J. W. Papez, A proposed mechanism of emotion, *Arch. Neurol. Psychiatry* *38*:725 (1937).
2. P. MacLean, The limbic system ("visceral brain") and emotional behavioral, *Arch. Neurol. Psychiatry 73*:130 (1955).
3. K. Brodmann, *Vergleichende Lokalisationslehre der Grosshirnrinde in ihren Prinzipien dargestellt auf Grund des Zellenbaues*, Barth, Leipzig, 1909.
4. N. Geschwind and W. Levitsky, Human brain: left-right asymmetries in temporal speech region, *Science 161* (837):186 (1968).
5. R. Insausti, T. Tunon, T. Sobreviela, A. M. Insausti, and L. M. Gonzalo, The human entorhinal cortex: a cytoarchitectonic analysis, *J. Comp. Neurol. 355*: 171 (1995).
6. J. O'Keefe and L. Nadel, *The Hippocampus as a Cognitive Map*, Clarendon Press, Oxford University Press, Oxford, 1978.
7. M. P. Witter and D. G. Amaral, Entorhinal cortex of the monkey: V. Projections to the dentate gyrus, hippocampus, and subicular complex, *J. Comp. Neurol. 307*:437 (1991).
8. D. Amaral, Emerging principles of intrinsic hippocampal organization, *Curr. Opin. Neurobiol. 3*:225 (1993).
9. R. Insausti, D. G. Amaral, and W. M. Cowan, The entorhinal cortex of the monkey: II. Cortical afferents, *J. Comp. Neurol. 264*:356 (1987).
10. W. A. Suzuki and D. G. Amaral, Perirhinal and parahippocampal cortices of the macaque monkey: cortical afferents, *J. Comp. Neurol. 350*:497 (1994).
11. B. Milner, Disorders of learning and memory after temporal lobe lesions in man, *Clin. Neurosurg. 19*:421 (1972).
12. W. B. Scoville and B. Milner, Loss of recent memory after bilateral hippocampal lesions, *J. Neurol. Neurosurg. Psychiatry 20*:11 (1957).
13. S. Zola-Morgan, L. R. Squire, and D. G. Amaral, Human amnesia and the medial temporal region: memory impairment following a bilateral lesion limited to field CA1 of the hippocampus, *J. Neurosci. 6*:2950 (1986).
14. N. J. Cohen, Preserved learning capacity in amnesia: evidence for multiple memory systems, *Neuropsychology of Memory* (L. R. Squire and N. Butters, eds.), Guilford Press, New York, 1984, p. 83.
15. H. Eichenbaum, N. J. Cohen, T. Otto, and C. G. Wible, Memory representation in the hippocampus: functional domain and functional organization, *Memory: Organization and Locus of Change* (L. R. Squire, G. Lynch, N. M. Wein-

berger, and J. L. McGaugh, eds.), Oxford University Press, New York, 1992, p. 163–204.

16. V. Frisk and B. Milner, The role of the left hippocampal region in the acquisition and retention of story content, *Neuropsychologia 28*:349 (1990).

17. M. Jones-Gotman, Memory for designs: the hippocampal contribution, *Neuropsychologia 24*(2):193 (1986).

18. M. L. Smith, Recall of spatial location by the amnesic patient H. M., *Brain Cogn. 7*:178 (1988).

19. M. L. Smith and B. Milner, The role of the right hippocampus in the recall of spatial location, *Neuropsychologia 19*:781 (1981).

20. B. Milner, S. Corkin, and H. Teuber, Further analysis of the hippocampal amnesic syndrome: 14 year follow-up study of H. M., *Neuropsychologia 6*: 215 (1968).

21. S. Corkin, Lasting consequences of bilateral medial temporal lobectomy: clinical course and experimental findings in H. M., *Semin. Neurol. 4*:249 (1984).

22. L. Squire, S. Zola-Morgan, and K. Chen, Human amnesia and animal models of amnesia: performance of amnesic patients on tests designed for the monkey, *Behav. Neurosci. 102*:201 (1988).

23. S. Zola-Morgan and L. R. Squire, Preserved learning in monkeys with medial temporal lesions: Sparing of motor and cognitive skills, *J. Neurosci. 4*:1072 (1984).

24. J. Rawlins, G. Lyford, R. Seferiades, M. Deacon, and H. Cassaday, Critical determinants of nonspatial working memory deficits in rats with conventional lesions of the hippocampus or fornix, *Behav. Neurosci. 107*:420 (1993).

25. M. Moss, H. Mahut, and S. Zola-Morgan, Concurrent discrimination learning in monkeys after hippocampal, entorhinal or fornix lesions, *J. Neurosci. 1*:227 (1981).

26. S. Zola-Morgan, L. R. Squire, and D. G. Amaral, Lesions of the hippocampal formation but not lesions of the fornix or the mammillary nuclei produce long-lasting memory impairment in monkeys, *J. Neurosci. 9*(3):898 (1989).

27. K. C. Raffaele and D. S. Olton, Hippocampal and amygdaloid interaction in working memory for nonspatial stimuli, *Behav. Neurosci. 102*:349 (1988).

28. C. G. Wible, J. R. Shiber, and D. S. Olton, Hippocampus, fimbria-fornix, amygdala and memory: object discriminations in rats, *Behav. Neurosci. 106*(5): 751 (1992).

29. L. R. Squire, Memory and the hippocampus: a synthesis from findings with rats, monkeys, and humans, *Psychol. Rev. 99*(2):195 (1992).

30. S. Zola-Morgan, L. R. Squire, N. L. Rempel, R. P. Clower, and D. G. Amaral, Enduring memory impairment in monkeys after ischemic damage to the hippocampus, *J. Neurosci. 12*(7):2582 (1992).

31. S. Zola-Morgan, L. R. Squire, and D. G. Amaral, Lesions of the amygdala that spare adjacent cortical regions do not impair memory or exacerbate the impairment following lesions of the hippocampal formation, *J. Neurosci. 9*(6): 1922 (1989).

32. S. Zola-Morgan, L. R. Squire, D. G. Amaral, and W. A. Suzuki, Lesions of perirhinal and parahippocampal cortex that spare the amygdala and hippocam-

pal formation produce severe memory impairment, *J. Neurosci.* *9*(12):4355 (1989).

33.   N. Cohen and L. R. Squire, Preserved learning and retention of pattern analyzing skill in amnesia: dissociation of knowing how and knowing that, *Science* *210*:207 (1980).

34.   B. Knowlton and L. Squire, The learning of categories: parallel brain systems for item memory and category knowledge, *Science 262*:1747 (1993).

35.   E. Tulving and D. L. Schacter, Priming and human memory systems, *Science* *247*:301 (1990).

36.   B. Postle and C. Suzanne, H. M. shows impaired word-stem completion priming with novel words (in press).

37.   A. Shimamura and L. Squire, Impaired priming of new associations in amnesia, *J. Exp. Psychol. 15*:721 (1989).

38.   L. R. Squire, F. Haist, and A. P. Shimamura, The neurology of memory: quantitative assessment of retrograde amnesia in two groups of amnesic patients, *J. Neurosci. 9*(3):828 (1989).

39.   S. M. Zola-Morgan and L. R. Squire, The primate hippocampal formation: evidence for a time-limited role in memory storage, *Science 250*:228 (1990).

40.   G. Heit, M. E. Smith, and E. Halgren, Neural encoding of individual words and faces by the human hippocampus and amygdala, *Science 261*:1054 (1993).

41.   M. A. Wilson and B. L. McNaughton, Dynamics of the hippocampal ensemble code for space, *Science 261*:1055 (1993).

42.   E. T. Rolls, A theory of emotion and consciousness, and its application to understanding the neural basis of emotion, *The Cognitive Neurosciences* (M. S. Gazzaniga, ed.), MIT Press, Cambridge, MA, 1995, p. 1091.

43.   T. Watanabe and H. Niki, Hippocampal unit activity and delayed response in the monkey, *Brain Res. 325*:241 (1985).

44.   T. V. P. Bliss and T. Lømo, Long lasting potentiation of synaptic transmission in the dentate area of the anaesthetized rabbit following stimulation of the perforant path input patterns, *J. Physiol. 232*:331 (1973).

45.   C. A. Barnes, Involvement of LTP in memory: Are we "searching under the street light"? *Neuron 15*:751 (1995).

46.   C. G. Wible, R. Sarrafezadeh, and D. S. Olton. Memory function and the hippocampus: towards an integrated theory. *Soc. Neurosci. Abstracts, 12*(2): 554 (1986).

47.   M. M. Merzenich and K. Sameshima, Cortical plasticity and memory, *Curr. Opin. Neurobiol. 3*:187 (1993).

48.   D. G. Amaral, J. L. Price, A. Pitkanen, and S. T. Charmichael, Anatomical organization of the primate amygdaloid cortex, *The Amygdala* (J. P. Aggleton, ed.), Wiley-Liss, New York, 1992, p. 1.

49.   D. G. Amaral and J. L. Price, Amygdalo-cortical projections in the monkey, *J. Comp. Neurol. 230*:465 (1984).

50.   A. Pitkanen, L. Stefanacci, C. L. Farb, G. G. Go, J. E. LeDoux, and D. G. Amaral, Intrinsic connections of the rat amygdaloid complex: projections originating in the lateral nucleus, *J. Comp. Neurol. 356*:288 (1995).

51. D. G. Amaral and R. Insausti, Retrograde transport of D-[³H]-aspartate injected into the monkey amygdaloid complex, *Exp. Brain Res. 88*:375 (1992).
52. R. C. Saunders, D. L. Rosene, and G. W. Van Hoesen, Comparison of the efferents of the amygdala and the hippocampal formation in the rhesus monkey: II. Reciprocal and non-reciprocal connections, *J. Comp. Neurol. 271*:185 (1988).
53. M. Davis, The role of the amygdala in conditioned fear, *The Amygdala* (J. P. Aggleton, ed.), Wiley-Liss, New York, 1992, p. 255.
54. J. LeDoux, Emotion: clues from the brain, *Annu. Rev. Psychol. 46*:209 (1995).
55. S. Maren and M. S. Fanselow, The amygdala and fear conditioning: Has the nut been cracked?, *Neuron 16*:237 (1996).
56. M. Davis, D. Rainne, and C. Martin, Neurotransmission in the rat amygdala related to fear and anxiety, *Trends Neurosci. 17*(5):208 (1994).
57. G. J. Quirk, J. C. Repa, and J. E. LeDoux, Fear conditioning enhances short-latency auditory responses of lateral amygdala neurons: parallel recordings in the freely behaving rat, *Neuron 15*:1029 (1995).
58. L. M. Romanski, M. C. Clugnet, F. Bordi, and J. E. LeDoux, Somatosensory and auditory convergence in the lateral nucleus of the amygdala, *Behav. Neurosci. 107*:444 (1993).
59. J. Allman and L. Brothers, Faces, fear and the amygdala, *Nature 372*:613 (1994).
60. R. Adolphs, D. Tranel, H. Damasio, and A. Damasio, Impaired recognition of emotion in facial expressions following bilateral damage to the human amygdala, *Nature 372*:669 (1994).
61. P. Gloor, Role of the amygdala in temporal lobe epilepsy, *The Amygdala* (J. P. Aggleton, ed.), Wiley-Liss, New York, 1992, p. 505.
62. V. H. Mark, F. R. Ervin, and W. H. Sweet. Deep temporal lobe stimulation in man, *The Neurobiology of the Amygdala* (B. E. Eleftheriou, ed.), Plenum Press, New York, 1972, pp. 485–507.
63. M. Mishkin, Memory in monkeys severely impaired by combined but not by separate removal of amygdala and hippocampus, *Nature 273*:297 (1978).
64. A. Bechara, D. Tranel, H. Damasio, R. Adolphs, C. Rockland, and A. R. Damasio, Double dissociation of conditioning and declarative knowledge relative to the amygdala and hippocampus in humans, *Science*:1115 (1995).
65. L. Cahill, R. Babinsky, H. Markowitsch, and J. McGaugh, The amygdala and emotional memory (letter), *Nature 377*:295 (1995).
66. B. A. Vogt and M. Gabriel, *Neurobiology of Cingulate Cortex and Limbic Thalamus: A Comprehensive Handbook*, Birkhauser, Boston, 1993.
67. D. M. Pandya, G. W. Van Hoesen, and M. M. Mesulam, Efferent connections of the cingulate gyrus in the rhesus monkey, *Exp. Brain Res. 42*:319 (1981).
68. B. Vogt and D. Pandya, Cingulate cortex of the rhesus monkey: II. Cortical afferents, *J. Comp. Neurol. 262*:271 (1987).
69. O. Devinsky and D. Luciano, The contributions of the cingulate cortex to human behavior, *Neurobiology of the Cingulate Cortex and Limbic Thalamus: A Comprehensive Handbook* (B. A. Vogt and M. Gabriel, eds.), Birkhauser: Boston, 1993, p. 527.

70. M. M. Mesulam, Large-scale neurocognitive networks and distributed processing for attention, language, and memory, *Ann. Neurol.* 28(5):597 (1990).
71. J. V. Pardo, P. J. Pardo, K. W. Janer, and M. E. Raichle, The anterior cingulate cortex mediates processing selection in the Stroop attentional conflict paradigm, *Proc. Natl. Acad. Sci.* 87:256 (1990).
72. M. I. Posner, S. E. Petersen, P. T. Fox, and M. E. Raichle, Localization of cognitive operations in the human brain, *Science 240*:1627 (1988).
73. S. E. Peterson, P. T. Fox, M. I. Posner, M. Mintun, and M. E. Raichle, Positron emmission tomographic studies of the cortical anatomy of single-word processing, *Nature 331*:585 (1988).
74. A. R. Damasio and G. W. Van Hoesen, Emotional disturbances associated with focal lesions of the limbic frontal lobe, *Neuropsychology of Human Emotion* (K. Heilman and P. Satz, eds.), Guilford, New York, 1983, p. 85.
75. G. Goldberg, Medial frontal cortex infraction and the alien hand sign, *Neurology 38*:683 (1981).
76. M. B. Carpenter, *Core Text of Neuroanatomy*, Williams & Wilkins, Baltimore, 1991.
77. J. E. Krettek and J. L. Price, A direct input from the amygdala to the thalamus and the cerebral cortex, *Brain Res.* 67:169 (1974).
78. A. M. Galaburda and D. N. Pandya, The intrinsic architechtonic and connectional organization of the superior temporal region of the rhesus monkey, *J. Comp. Neurol.* 221:169 (1983).
79. M. Petrides and D. N. Pandya, Association fiber pathways to the frontal cortex from the superior temporal region in the rhesus monkey, *J. Comp. Neurol.* 228:105 (1988).
80. A. Baddely, *Working Memory*, Oxford University Press, Oxford, 1986.
81. A. R. Damasio, D. Tranel, and H. Damasio, Somatic markers and the guidance of behavior: theory and preliminary testing, *Frontal Lobe Function and Dysfunction* (H. S. Levin, H. M. Eisenberg, and A. L. Benton, eds.), Oxford University Press, New York, 1991, p. 217.
82. P. J. Elinger and A. R. Damasio, Severe disturbance of higher cognition after bilateral frontal lobe ablations: patient EVR, *Neurology 35*:1731 (1985).
83. H. Damasio, T. Grabowski, R. Frank, A. M. Galaburda, and A. R. Damasio, The return of Phineas Gage: clues about the brain from the skull of a famous patient. *Science 264*:1102 (1994).
84. A. Galburda and F. Sanides, Cytoarchitechtonic organization of the human auditory cortex, *J. Comp. Neurol. 190*:597 (1980).
85. B. Kolb and I. Q. Whishaw, *Fundamentals of Human Neuropsychology*, Freeman, New York, 1990.
86. H. Goodglass and E. Kaplan, *The Assessment of Aphasia and Related Disorders*, Lea and Febiger, Philadelphia, 1983.
87. B. C. Rapp and A. Caramazza, Disorders of lexical processing and the lexicon, *The Cognitive Neurosciences* (M. S. Gazzaniga, ed.), MIT Press, Cambridge, MA, 1995, p 901.
88. G. A. Ojemann, Cortical organization of language, *J. Neurosci. 11*(8):2281 (1991).

89. C. W. Cotman, Excitatory amino acids in the brain—focus on NMDA receptors, *Trends Neurosci. 10*(7):263 (1987).

90. D. P. Cain, Kindling and the amygdala, *The Amygdala* (J. P. Aggleton, ed.), Wiley-Liss, New York, 1992, p. 539.

91. R. M. Sapolsky, H. Uno, C. S. Rebert, and C. E. Finch, Hippocampal damage associated with prolonged glucocorticoid exposure in primates, *J. Neurosci. 10*(9):2897 (1990).

92. R. Sapolsky, Glucocorticoids, stress and exacerbation of excitotoxic neuron death, *Sem. Neurosci. 6*:323 (1994).

93. B. McEwen, Introduction: stress and the nervous system, *Sem. Neurosci. 6*: 195 (1994).

94. F. M. Benes, J. Davidson, and E. D. Bird, Quantitative cytoarchitectural studies of the cerebral cortex of schizophrenics, *Arch. Gen. Psychiatry 43*:31 (1986).

95. F. M. Benes, J. McSparren, E. D. Bird, J. P. SanGiovanni, and S. L. Vincent, Deficits in small interneurons in prefrontal and cingulate cortex of schizophrenic and schizoaffective patients, *Arch. Gen. Psychiatry 48*(11):996 (1991).

96. C. A. Tamminga, G. K. Thaker, R. Buchanan, B. Kirkpatrick, L. D. Alphs, T. N. Chase, and W. T. Carpenter, Limbic system abnormalities identified in schizophrenia using positron emission tomography with fluorodeoxyglucose and neocortical alterations with deficit syndrome, *Arch. Gen. Psychiatry 49*(7): 522 (1992).

97. C. G. Wible, M. E. Shenton, R. Kikinis, F. A. Jolesz, D. Metcalf, D. V. Iosifescu, and R. W. McCarley, Parcellation of the human prefrontal cortex in schizophrenia: a quantitative MRI study, submitted.

98. H. C. R. Grunze, D. G. Rainnie, M. E. Hasselmo, E. Barkai, E. F. Hearn, R. W. McCarley, and R. W. Greene, NMDA-dependent modulation of CA1 local circuit inhibition, *J. Neurosci. 16*(6):2034 (1996).

99. J. Krystal, L. Karper, J. Seibyl, G. Freeman, et al., Subanesthetic effects of the noncompetitive NMDA antagonist, ketamine, in humans, *Arch. Gen. Psychiatry 51*:199 (1994).

100. G. Tsai, L. A. Passani, B. S. Slusher, R. Carter, L Baer, J. E. Kleinman, and J. T. Coyle, Abnormal excitatory neurotransmitter metabolism in schizophrenic brains, *Arch. Gen. Psychiatry 52*:829 (1995).

101. C. G. Wible, M. E. Shenton, R. W. McCarley. Do positive symptoms in schizophrenia result from abnormalities of functionally linked temporal lobe structures? A new theory. Society of Biological Psychiatry Annual Meeting, Washington, DC, 1992.

102. W. C. Drevets and M. E. Raichle, Positron emission tomographic imaging studies of human emotional disorders, *The Cognitive Neurosciences* (M. S. Gazzaniga, ed.), MIT Press, Cambridge, MA, 1995, p. 1153.

103. H. T. Ballantine Jr., A. J. Bouckoms, E. K. Thomas, and I. E. Giriunas, Treatment of psychiatric illness by stereotactic cingulotomy, *Biol. Psychiatry 22*:807 (1987).

104. H. M. Duvernoy, *The Human Brain: Surface, Three-Dimensional Sectional Anatomy and MRI*, Springer-Verlag, New York, 1991.

5

Normal Brain Development: Ages 4–18

Jay N. Giedd
National Institute of Mental Health, Bethesda, Maryland

I. INTRODUCTION

An understanding of normal brain development is necessary to interpret the often subtle neuroanatomical deviations observed in childhood-onset neuropsychiatric disorders. Prior to the advent of magnetic resonance imaging (MRI), which allows in vivo studies without the use of ionizing radiation,

103

data regarding brain anatomy of healthy subjects between the ages of 4 and 18 years were sparse. Mortality is low for this age group, with accidents being the leading cause of death, and autopsies are seldom performed. Much of the postmortem literature is derived from the Yakovlev Brain Collection in Washington, DC, where only 13 of 483 normal brains are from subjects aged 3–18 years. The dangers of ionizing radiation in conventional radiography, computerized tomography, or positron emission tomography precludes their use in healthy children.

Even with the advent of MRI, studies of healthy children in this age range have been infrequent. Most studies use as controls children who were referred clinically and whose scans were subsequently read as normal. This is less than ideal because children in diagnostic groups under study, such as attention-deficit/hyperactivity disorder (ADHD), are overrepresented in clinical referrals. Also, excluding healthy children who have scans read as abnormal confounds comparisons to diagnostic groups.

For these reasons direct recruitment of healthy children from the community is preferable. Even with community recruitment care must be taken during screening to account for several factors that have been shown to influence brain morphometry in children, including psychiatric history [1–21], intelligence [22,23], handedness [24,25], and infection with Group A β-hemolytic streptococci or other infections, which may affect brain structure size through an autoimmune phenomenon [19,26].

Brain development is most active in utero where the dramatic overproduction and then selective elimination of neurons and synaptic connections prepare the brain for its lifelong task of adaptation to the environment. Although the basic foundation of the brain is fairly well established in the preschool years, processes of competitive elimination, myelination, and dendritic and axonal arborization continue throughout adolescence and beyond [27,28], as indicated in Figure 1.

Brain structure size is determined by the number, size, and packing density of its constituent neuronal and glial cells. The maximum number of neurons is obtained during gestation [29]. The size and physical characteristics of the neurons undergo cyclic changes throughout development [30] as axonal thickness and the number of synaptic connections and dendrites vary with age [31] and in response to environmental factors. An example of environmental factors affecting neuronal development and connectivity is the irreversible cortical blindness that can occur in children with cataracts who do not receive treatment prior to age 1 year [32].

Unlike neurons, glial cells, which outnumber neurons by ratios ranging from 1.7 to 10 [33], continue to actively proliferate and die postnatally. Myelination by oligodendrocytes, a subclass of glial cells, is a major determinant of increases in structure size during childhood and adolescence. Structure

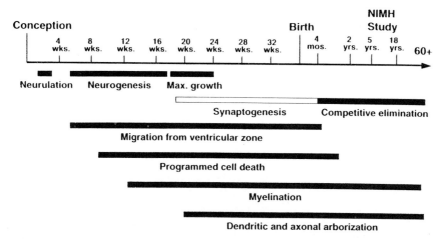

Fig. 1 Time course of critical events in the determination of human brain morphometry.

size is ultimately determined by a dynamic balance between size and number of glial cells, size of neurons, and changes in vasculature. One of the major processes in brain development, synaptic pruning, may have little impact on overall structure size. Postmortem research on the primary visual cortex of the macaque monkey indicates that a total loss of all boutons would result in only a 1–2% decrease in volume [34]. However, the effect synaptic pruning may have on the thickness of the parent axon or dendritic branches is not accounted for in this calculation. Packing density also influences structure size and is affected by the degree of hydration, vascularity, and extracellular fluid volumes.

Structure size is influenced by genetics, hormones, growth factors, nutrients in the developing nervous system, diet, infections, toxins, trauma, stress, or degree of enriched environment [27,35]. Interpretation of the clinical significance of gross structural volume changes should be evaluated in light of the complex interactions among all of these parameters.

As previously indicated, literature regarding neuroimaging of normal development from ages 4 to 18 is not abundant, but a few studies have identified important developmental themes. In a study of 39 subjects aged 8 to 35, cerebrospinal fluid (CSF) volumes increased with age and both cortical and subcortical gray matter decreased with age [36]. Another study [37] of 88 subjects aged 3 months to 30 years found no changes in CSF but confirmed age-related decreases in gray matter and increases in cortical white matter as well. PET studies of clinical pediatric populations demonstrate dynamic

Table 1 Characteristics of Healthy MRI Subjects, Ages 4–18, Participating in the NIMH Normal Brain Development Study

	Male	Female
Sample Size	78	51
Age (y)	10.6 (3.9)	10.9 (3.9)
Height (cm)	144.8 (23.9)	144.3 (21.3)
Weight (kg)	40.0 (17.7)	40.1 (15.9)
Tanner Stage	2.2 (1.6)	2.4 (1.6)
Handedness	86% right-handed	90% right-handed
Vocabulary[a]	13.6 (3.1)	12.7 (2.5)
Block Design[a]	13.3 (3.1)	12.7 (3.5)
Digit Span[a]	11.2 (2.9)	11.4 (2.5)
Woodcock-Johnson	516 (34)	498 (70)

[a] Subtests of the Wechsler Intelligence Scale for Children–Revised.
No significant differences between sexes on any of these variables.

developmental changes with cerebral metabolic rates increasing sharply during the first years of life, peaking during childhood, and then declining to adult levels during adolescence [38].

The majority of normative data presented for this chapter is from an ongoing pediatric MRI brain imaging project at the Child Psychiatry Branch of the National Institute of Mental Health. For this project subjects are recruited from the community and undergo an extensive battery of testing, including physical and neurological exams, clinical interviews and family history assessment, and neuropsychological testing in which only about one in six initial contacts is accepted for study. Longitudinal scans are being acquired at 2-year intervals. Subject characteristics are presented in Table 1.

The resulting sample had higher-than-average vocabulary and block design subtests of the Wechsler Intelligence Scale for Children—Revised [39]. This finding is not unexpected given the strictness of inclusion criteria, but it does limit the generalizability of findings. The following data will be in reference to NIMH data set unless otherwise indicated.

II. AGE-RELATED CHANGES IN BRAIN SIZE

A. Total Cerebral Volume

In the NIMH sample of 119 children and adolescents, total cerebral volume changed surprisingly little from ages 4 to 18 (Fig. 2). Babies have dispropor-

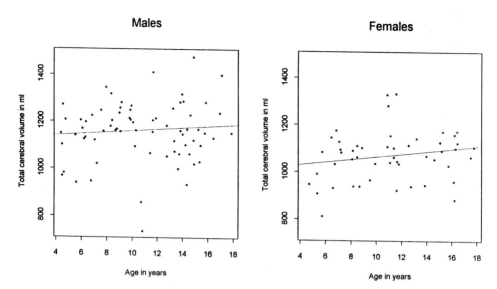

Fig. 2 Scatterplots with least-squares fit lines of total cerebral volume vs. age for healthy male (N = 73) and female (N = 50) children and adolescents: ages 4–18 years.

tionately larger heads than adults. At birth head size accounts for approximately 25% of height, whereas in adults it is only 11% [40]. Postmortem and in vivo imaging studies indicate that the brain is about 95% of its adult size by age 5 [41,42]. This seems improbable to anyone who has seen an adult's hat falling over the eyes of a child. It is true that head circumference increases across this age span (approximately, 2.0 inches in boys and 1.9 inches in girls), however, the increase is not due to an enlarging brain volume but to an increase in skull thickness [43] and less so to an increase in ventricular volume [44].

The lack of increase in total brain volume should not be interpreted as a sign of completed maturation. Indeed, as indicated in the following sections, the stability of total brain volume represents a dynamic equilibrium between active forces of growth and degeneration in the complexly interacting components of the brain.

Gender differences in brain morphology are striking, with male brains being approximately 9% larger than those of females across all ages. This difference remains statistically significant when controlling for height and weight. The size difference appears to be relatively uniform across brain structures. Of course, sexually dimorphic differences in neuronal connectivity or receipt density may not be reflected in gross size of structures. Increased size alone should not be interpreted as imparting any sort of functional advantage or disadvantage.

B. Gray Matter/White Matter

From an MRI perspective healthy brain tissue can be categorized as gray matter (consisting mostly of cell bodies and dendrites), white matter (composed mostly of myelinated axons), vasculature, or CSF. The relative amount of white matter increases during childhood and adolescence [37,45]. This is driven by the ongoing process of myelination, which, although most pronounced in the first 2 years of life, continues throughout adolescence and even into adulthood [46]. Gray matter tends to decrease throughout the life span [36,37], possibly related to pruning or cell death.

C. Ventricles

Lateral ventricular volume increased robustly with age in the NIMH sample. The increase was 0.62 mL/y for males and 0.39 mL/y for females. In males, the rate of enlargement increased significantly after age 11 (Fig. 3).

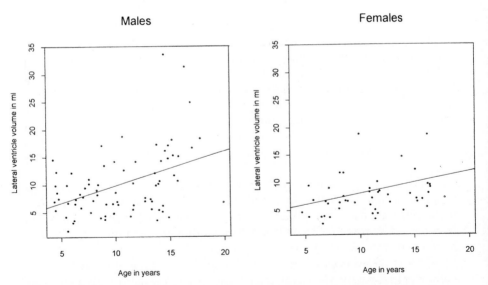

Fig. 3 Scatterplots with least-squares fit lines of lateral ventricle volume vs. age for healthy male (N = 77) and female (N = 50) children and adolescents: ages 4–18 years.

This phenomenon is widely observed in adult aging studies but is not widely appreciated for children and adolescents. That this occurs in healthy adolescents adds to the complexity of interpreting findings of ventricular enlargement in a variety of neuropsychiatric conditions.

D. Corpus Callosum

The corpus callosum (CC) consists of approximately 200 million myelinated fibers, which connect homologous areas of the cortex. It is well visualized on midsagittal MRI images and maintains a roughly topographic pattern with fibers from the anterior cortical regions traversing through the anterior CC segments, fibers from the middle cortical regions traversing through the middle CC segments, and fibers from the posterior cortical regions traversing through the posterior CC.

The corpus callosum's primary role is integrating the activities of the left and right cerebral hemispheres. This includes unifying sensory fields [47,48], aiding memory storage and retrieval [49], facilitating language and auditory functions [50], and allocating attention and arousal [51]. These capacities all improve during childhood and adolescence, making morphological exploration of this structure intriguing.

CC maturation continues to progress throughout childhood and adolescence [52–55], and several neuropsychiatric disorders of childhood onset have reported anomalies of the CC [6,10,56–60]. Gender effects have been inconsistently identified in CC morphology, with some authors finding gender-related differences [53,61–63] and others not [64–70]. In the NIMH sample midsagittal corpus callosum area increased robustly from ages 4 to 18, but neither areas nor age-related increases in area demonstrated sexual dimorphism. The increase in CC area was most robust for mid and posterior regions. The rostrum and genu (anterior regions) were at adult sizes by age 8 [71] (Fig. 4).

E. Basal Ganglia

The basal ganglia are a collection of subcortical gray matter nuclei involved in circuits mediating higher cognitive functions, affective states, and attention as well as playing a central role in the control of movement and muscle tone. The basal ganglia are comprised of the caudate, putamen, globus pallidus, subthalamic nucleus, and substantia nigra [72]. Only the first three of these are readily quantifiable by MRI.

Basal ganglia anomalies in size or symmetry have been implicated in a variety of childhood-onset neuropsychiatric disorders, including ADHD [8,11,12], early-onset schizophrenia [13,73–76], Sydenham's chorea [19], and Tourette's syndrome [21,77,78]. All of these disorders have marked sex dif-

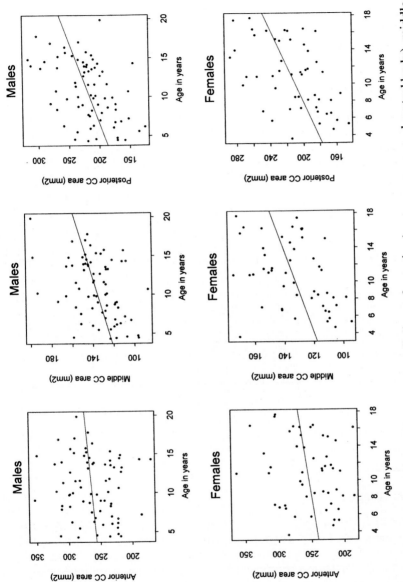

Fig. 4 Scatterplots with least-squares fit lines of anterior (rostrum, genu, and rostral body), middle (anterior midbody and posterior midbody), and posterior (isthmus and splenium) midsagittal corpus callosum area vs. age for healthy male (N = 74) and female (N = 50) children and adolescents: ages 4–18 years.

ferences in prevalence, and so it is of note that the basal ganglia are among the most sexually dimorphic structures of the brain. After adjusting for total brain size, the caudate is relatively larger in females whereas the putamen and globus pallidus are larger in males. A robust right-greater-than-left asymmetry of the caudate and left-greater-than-right asymmetry of the putamen, which did not change with age, was noted for both males and females.

The relationship between basal ganglia size and neuropsychiatric disorders is also interesting from an evolutionary perspective. One way to assess evolutionary changes across species is to adjust brains from several different species to a standard size. This so-called progression index reveals that the basal ganglia of humans are 16.4 times larger than those of a comparably sized primitive insectivore would be [79]. This is the largest of any species and second only to the neocortex (progression index = 156) in terms of evolutionary brain changes. Perhaps more recently acquired anatomical substrates or attributes are more genetically vulnerable, as is supported by the high rates of disorders for the evolutionary recent capacity of language.

F. Temporal Lobe

The temporal lobes and related medial structures, such as the amygdala and hippocampus, are integral players in the realms of emotion, language, and memory [80]. Because our capacities for these functions change markedly from age 4 to 18, examination of developmental changes in their neuroanatomical substrates is of interest.

In the NIMH study total temporal lobe volume remained constant, while amygdala volume increased, most robustly in males, and hippocampal volume increased, most robustly in females [81] (Fig. 5). This gender-specific pattern is consistent with the distribution of sex hormone receptors for these structures, with the amygdala having mostly androgen receptors [82, 83] and the hippocampus having mostly estrogen receptors [84]. That estrogen may influence hippocampal size is supported by studies indicating that women with gonadal hypoplasia have smaller hippocampi [85] and gonadectomized female rats have lower density of dendritic spines and decreased fiber outgrowth in the hippocampus, which can be alleviated with hormone replacement [84,86].

Also consistent with these findings is an MRI study of 20 young adults showing proportionately larger hippocampal volumes in females [87] and a postmortem study revealing ongoing myelination in the subicular and presubicular regions of the hippocampus throughout adolescence and into adulthood [88]. In the postmortem study females showed a greater degree of myelin staining from 6 to 29 years, but no significant gender differences thereafter.

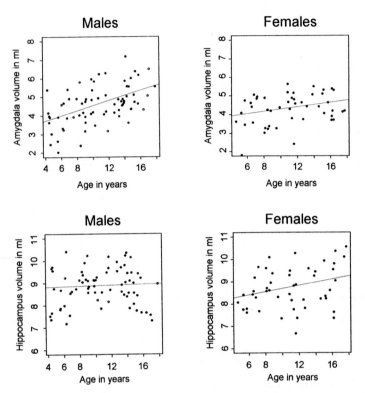

Fig. 5 Scatterplots with least-squares fit lines of amygdala and hippocampus volume vs. age for healthy male (N = 73) and female (N = 48) children and adolescents: ages 4–18 years.

The hippocampus is noteworthy as the only structure for which straightforward relationships between size and performance on specific cognitive tasks have been consistently found. Such relationships are complicated by the myriad of afferent and efferent connections to the many distinct nuclei of most structures as well as the intricacy of their various neurochemical systems. Despite this complexity, relationships between hippocampal size and memory function have been noted in birds, voles, and humans. In birds, species that store food, which requires excellent spatial memory for retrieval, have larger hippocampi than related species that do not store food [89,90]. In voles, males of the polygamous species, who travel considerable distances in search of mates, perform better than their female counterparts on laboratory measures of spatial ability and have significantly larger hippocampi [91].

Table 2 NIMH Pediatric Brain MRI Study (N = 129):
Volume Measures Showing Significant Maturational Changes

Measure	Direction	Sex
Amygdala	↑	M
Hippocampus	↑	F
Corpus callosum	↑	M and F
Ventricles	↑	M (F trend)

No differences in hippocampal size are observed in the monogamous vole species, which do not show male-female differences in spatial ability [92]. In humans, correlations between memory for stories and left hippocampal volume have been noted [93,94].

These characteristics of medial temporal structures encourage further study of healthy and neuropsychologically impaired subjects.

III. SUMMARY

A summary of developmental brain morphometry is presented in Tables 2, 3, and 4.

Total cerebral volume approaches adult size around the time children begin the first grade. However, this relative stability of total cerebral volume overlies a storm of maturational activity in which gender-specific changes occur in the basal ganglia, corpus callosum, ventricles, amygdala, hippocampus, and regional distribution of gray and white matter.

It is noteworthy that the regions undergoing the greatest change in normal development are by and large the same regions most often anomalous in developmental disorders. The relationship between these sexually dimorphic

Table 3 NIMH Pediatric Brain MRI Study (N = 129):
Volume Measures Showing Significant Gender Effects

Measure	Direction	p-value
Total cerebrum	M > F	0.001
Caudate[a]	F > M	0.01
Globus pallidus[a]	M > F	0.05
Ventricles[a]	M > F	0.03

[a] After ANCOVA adjusting for total cerebral volume.

Table 4   NIMH Pediatric Brain MRI Study (N = 129):
Volume Measures Showing Significant Laterality Effects

Measure	Direction	% Difference	p-value
Amygdala	R > L	6.84	0.0004
Caudate	R > L	3.08	0.0001
Cerebrum	R > L	1.82	0.0001
Hippocampus	R > L	5.32	0.0001
Putamen	L > R	3.89	0.0001
Temporal lobe	R > L	4.30	0.0001
Ventricle	L > R	9.70	0.0001

patterns of normal brain development and the observed gender differences in prevalence, age of onset, and symptom profiles of nearly all pediatric neuropsychiatric disorders deserves further study.

Variability of size was high for all brain structures examined in the NIMH study, as is evident in the scatterplots of total cerebral and ventricular volume (Figs. 2 and 3). This enormous variability calls for large sample longitudinal studies to characterize the heterochronous developmental changes of the pediatric population. Stability of morphological measures from scans acquired at 2- to 4-week intervals, indicating that changes seen would not be due to variability related to the scan acquisition itself, supports the feasibility of longitudinal MRI studies [95]. Large sample studies may require multisite collaborations and some standardization of image acquisition and analysis.

The rapid advances in imaging technology offering greater spatial resolution, shorter acquisition times, and the capacity for functional imaging hold great promise for increasing our understanding of the relationship between brain and behavior in healthy and ill children and adolescents.

REFERENCES

1. E. Courchesne, R. Yeung-Courchesne, G. A. Press, J. R. Hesselink, and T. L. Jernigan, Hypoplasia of cerebellar vermal lobules VI and VII in autism, *N. Engl. J. Med. 318*:1349 (1988).
2. J. Piven, E. Nehme, J. Simon, P. Barta, G. Pearlson, and S. E. Folstein, Magnetic resonance imaging in autism: measurement of the cerebellum, pons, and fourth ventricle, *Biol. Psychiatry 31*:491 (1992).
3. E. Courchesne, G. A. Press, and R. Yeung-Courchesne, Parietal lobe abnormalities detected with MR in patients with infantile autism, *AJR 160*:387 (1993).
4. E. Courchesne, J. Townsend, and O. Saitoh, The brain in infantile autism:

posterior fossa structures are abnormal (see comments), *Neurology 44*:214 (1994).

5. J. M. Rumsey, G. R. Lyon, and J. M. Rumsey. Neuroimaging studies of autism, *Neuroimaging: A Window to the Neurological Foundations of Learning and Behavior in Children* (G. R. Lyon and J. M. Rumsey, ed.),

6. G. W. Hynd, M. Semrud-Clikeman, A. R. Lorys, E. S. Novey, and D. Eliopulos, Brain morphology in developmental dyslexia and attention deficit disorder/hyperactivity, *Arch. Neurol. 47*:919 (1990).

7. G. W. Hynd, M. Semrud-Clikeman, A. R. Lorys, E. S. Novey, D. Eliopulos, and H. Lyytinen, Corpus callosum morphology in attention deficit-hyperactivity disorder: morphometric analysis of MRI, *J. Learn. Disabilities 24*:141 (1991).

8. G. W. Hynd, K. L. Hern, E. S. Novey, D. Eliopulos, R. Marshall, and J. J. Gonzalez, Attention deficit hyperactivity disorder (ADHD) and asymmetry of the caudate nucleus, *J. Child Neurol. 8*:339 (1993).

9. M. Semrud-Clikeman, P. A. Filipek, J. Biederman, R. Steingard, D. Kennedy, P. Renshaw, and K. Bekken, Attention-deficit hyperactivity disorder: magnetic resonance imaging morphometric analysis of the corpus callosum, *J. Am. Acad. Child. Adolesc. Psychiatry 33*:875 (1994).

10. J. N. Giedd, F. K. Castellanos, B. J. Casey, P. L. Kozuch, A. C. King, S. D. Hamburger, and J. L. Rapoport, Quantitative morphology of the corpus callosum in attention deficit hyperactivity disorder, *Am. J. Psychiatry 151*:665 (1994).

11. F. X. Castellanos, J. N. Giedd, P. Eckburg, W. L. Marsh, A. C. King, S. D. Hamburger, and J. L. Rapoport, Quantitative morphology of the caudate nucleus in attention-deficit hyperactivity disorder, *Am. J. Psychiatry 151*(12):1791 (1994).

12. F. X. Castellanos, J. N. Giedd, W. L. Marsh, S. D. Hamburger, A. C. Vaituzis, J. W. Snell, N. Lange, D. P. Dickstein, Y. C. Vauss, D. Kaysen, G. F. Ritchie, J. C. Rajapakse, and J. L. Rapoport, Quantitative brain magnetic resonance imaging in attention-deficit/hyperactivity disorder, *Arch. Gen. Psychiatry 53*: 607 (1996).

13. J. A. Frazier, J. N. Giedd, S. D. Hamburger, K. E. Albus, D. Kaysen, A. C. Vaituzis, J. C. Rajapakse, M. C. Lenane, K. McKenna, L. K. Jacobsen, C. T. Gordon, A. Breier, and J. L. Rapoport, Brain anatomic magnetic resonance imaging in childhood onset schizophrenia, *Arch. Gen. Psychiatry 53*:617 (1996).

14. R. Duara, A. Kushch, K. Gross-Glenn, W. Barker, B. Jallad, S. Pascal, D. A. Loewenstein, J. Sheldon, M. Rabin, B. Levin, and H. Lubs, Neuroanatomic differences between dyslexic and normal readers on magnetic resonance imaging scans, *Arch. Neurol. 48*:410 (1991).

15. J. M. Rumsey, R. Dorwart, M. Vermess, M. B. Denckla, M. J. P. Kruesi, and J. L. Rapoport, Magnetic resonance imaging of brain anatomy in severe developmental dyslexia, *Arch. Neurol. 43*:1045 (1986).

16. G. W. Hynd and M. Semrud-Clikeman, Dyslexia and brain morphology, *Psychol. Bull. 106*:447 (1989).

17. J. P. Larsen, T. Hoien, I. Lundberg, and H. Odegaard, MRI evaluation of the size and symmetry of the planum temporale in adolescents with developmental dyslexia, *Brain Lang. 39*:289 (1990).

18. R. G. Laessle, J. C. Krieg, and M. M. Fichter, Cerebral atrophy and vigilance performance in patients with anorexia nervosa and bulemia nervosa, *Neuropsychobiology 21*:187 (1989).
19. J. N. Giedd, J. L. Rapoport, M. J. P. Kruesi, C. Parker, M. B. Schapiro, A. J. Allen, H. L. Leonard, D. Kaysen, D. P. Dickstein, W. L. Marsh, P. L. Kozuch, A. C. Vaituzis, S. Hamburger, and S. E. Swedo, Sydenham's chorea: magnetic resonance imaging of the basal ganglia, *Neurology 25*:11 (1995).
20. B. Peterson, M. A. Riddle, D. J. Cohen, L. D. Katz, J. C. Smith, M. T. Hardin, and J. F. Leckman, Reduced basal ganglia volumes in Tourette's syndrome using three-dimensional reconstruction techniques from magnetic resonance images, *Neurology 43*:941 (1993).
21. H. S. Singer, A. L. Reiss, J. E. Brown, E. H. Aylward, B. Shih, E. Chee, E. L. Harris, M. J. Reader, G. A. Chase, R. N. Bryan, and M. B. Denckla, Volumetric MRI changes in basal ganglia of children with Tourette's syndrome, *Neurology 43*:950 (1993).
22. N. C. Andreasen, M. Flaum, V. Swayze, 2d, D. S. O'Leary, R. Alliger, G. Cohen, J. Ehrhardt, and W. T. Yuh, Intelligence and brain structure in normal individuals (see comments), *Am. J. Psychiatry 150*:130 (1993).
23. L. Willerman, R. Schultz, J. N. Rutledge, and E. D. Bigler, In vivo brain size and intelligence, *Intelligence 15*:223 (1991).
24. A. Kertesz, M. Polk, S. E. Black, and J. Howell, Anatomical asymmetries and functional laterality, *Brain 115*:589 (1992).
25. S. F. Witelson, Hand and sex differences in the isthmus and genu of the human corpus callosum, *Brain 112*:799 (1989).
26. J. N. Giedd, J. L. Rapoport, H. L. Leonard, D. Richter, and S. E. Swedo, Acute basal ganglia enlargement and obsessive compulsive symptoms in an adolescent boy, *J. Am. Acad. Child. Adol. Psychiatry 35*:913 (1996).
27. M. Jacobson, *Developmental Neurobiology*, Plenum Press, New York, 1991.
28. P. R. Huttenlocher, Morphometric study of human cerebral cortex development, *Neuropsychologia 28*:517 (1990).
29. T. Rabinowicz, F. Falkner, and J. M. Tanner. The differentiated maturation of the cerebral cortex, *Human Growth, Vol. 2* (F. Falkner and J. M. Tanner, eds.), Plenum Press, New York, p. 385.
30. R. W. Thatcher, Cyclic cortical reorganization during early childhood, *Brain Cogn. 20*:24 (1992).
31. S. M. Blinkov and I. I. Glezer, *The Human Brain in Figures and Tables. A Quantitative Handbook*, Plenum Press, New York, 1968.
32. T. L. Lewis, D. Maurer, and H. P. Brent, Effects on pereceptual development of visual deprivation during infancy, *Br. J. Opthalmol. 70*:214 (1986).
33. K. R. Brizzee, J. Vogt, and X. Kharetehko, Postnatal changes in glia neuron index with a comparison of methods of cell enumeration in the white rat, *Proc. Brain Res. 4*:136 (1964).
34. J. P. Bourgeois and P. Rakic, Changes of synaptic density in the primary visual cortex of the macaque monkey from fetal to adult stage, *J. Neurosci. 13*:2801 (1993).
35. M. C. Diamond, D. Krech, and M. R. Rosenzweig, The effects of an enriched

environment on the histology of the rat cerebral cortex, *J. Comp. Neur. 123*: 111 (1964).

36. T. L. Jernigan, D. A. Trauner, J. R. Hesselink, and P. A. Tallal, Maturation of human cerebrum observed in vivo during adolescence, *Brain 114*:2037 (1991).

37. A. Pfefferbaum, D. H. Mathalon, E. V. Sullivan, J. M. Rawles, R. B. Zipursky, and K. O. Lim, A quantitative magnetic resonance imaging study of changes in brain morphology from infancy to late adulthood, *Arch. Neurol. 51*:874 (1994).

38. H. T. Chugani, M. E. Phelps, and J. C. Mazziotta, Positron emission tomography study of human brain functional development, *Ann. Neurol. 22*:487 (1987).

39. D. Wechsler, *Wechsler Intelligence Scale for Children—Revised*, The Psychological Corporation, New York, 1974.

40. V. C. Vaughan, I. S. Litt, R. E. Behrman, and W. E. Nelson. Developmental pediatrics, *Nelson's Textbook of Pediatrics* (R. E. Behrman, V. C. Vaughan, and W. E. Nelson, eds.), W. B. Saunders, Philadelphia, 1987, p. 6.

41. A. S. Dekaban, Tables of cranial and orbital measurements, cranial volume, and derived indexes in males and females from 7 days to 20 years of age, *Ann. Neurol. 2*:485 (1977).

42. A. S. Dekaban and D. Sadowsky, Changes in brain weight during the span of human life: relation of brain weights to body heights and body weights, *Ann. Neurol. 4*:345 (1978).

43. R. Shapiro and A. H. Janzen, *The Normal Skull*, Paul B. Hoeber, Inc., New York, 1960.

44. J. N. Giedd, J. W. Snell, N. Lange, J. C. Rajapakse, D. Kaysen, A. C. Vaituzis, Y. C. Vauss, S. D. Hamburger, P. L. Kozuch, and J. L. Rapoport, Quantitative magnetic resonance imaging of human brain development: ages 4–18, *Cerebral Cortex 6*:551 (1996).

45. J. C. Rajapakse, C. DeCarli, A. McLaughlin, J. N. Giedd, A. L. Krain, S. D. Hamburger, and J. L. Rapoport, Cerebral magnetic resonance image segmentation using data fusion. *J. Comput. Assist. Tomogr. 20*:206 (1996).

46. P. I. Yakovlev and A. R. Lecours, The myelogenetic cycles of regional maturation of the brain, *Regional Development of the Brain in Early Life* (A. Minkowski, ed.), Blackwell Scientific, Oxford, 1967, p. 3.

47. G. Berlucchi, Interhemispheric asymmetries in visual discrimination: a neurophysiological hypothesis, *Doc. Opthal. Proc. Ser. 30*:87 (1981).

48. M. F. Shanks, A. J. Rockel, and T. P. S. Powel, The commissural fiber connections of the primary somatic sensory cortex, *Brain Res. 98*:166 (1975).

49. D. Zaidel and R. W. Sperry, Memory impairment after commissurotomy in man, *Brain 97*:263 (1974).

50. N. D. Cook, *The Brain Code. Mechanisms of Information Transfer and the Role of the Corpus Callosum*, Methuen, London, 1986.

51. J. Levy, Interhemispheric collaboration: single mindedness in the asymmetric brain, *Hemisphere Function and Collaboration in the Child* (C. T. Best, ed.), Academic Press, New York, 1985, p. 11.

52. L. S. Allen, M. F. Richey, Y. M. Chai, and R. A. Gorski, Sex differences in the corpus callosum of the living human being, *J. Neurosci. 11*:933 (1991).

53. P. E. Cowell, L. S. Allen, N. S. Zalatimo, and V. H. Denenberg, A developmental study of sex and age interactions in the human corpus callosum, *Dev. Brain Res. 66*:187 (1992).

54. J. Pujol, P. Vendrell, C. Junque, J. L. Marti-Vilalta, and A. Capdevila, When does human brain development end? Evidence of corpus callosum growth up to adulthood, *Ann. Neurol. 34*:71 (1993).

55. R. A. Rauch and J. R. Jinkins, Analysis of cross-sectional area measurements of the corpus callosum adjusted for brain size in male and female subjects from childhood to adulthood, *Behav. Brain Res. 64*:65 (1994).

56. C. Njiokiktjien, *Pediatric Behavioral Neurology, Vol. 3, The Child's Corpus Callosum* (G. Ramaekers and C. Njiokiktjien, eds.), Suyi Publications, Amsterdam, 1991.

57. G. W. Hynd, M. Semrud-Clikeman, A. R. Lorys, E. S. Novey, D. Eliopulos, and H. Lyytinen, Corpus callosum morphology in attention deficit-hyperactivity disorder: morphometric analysis of MRI, *J. Learn. Disabil. 24*:141 (1991).

58. L. H. Bigelow, H. A. Nasrallah, and F. P. Rauscher, Corpus callosum thickness in chronic schizophrenia, *Br. J. Psychiatry 142*:284 (1983).

59. R. Rosenthal and L. Bigelow, Quantitative brain measurements in chronic schizophrenia, *Br. J. Psychiatry 121*:259 (1972).

60. B. S. Peterson, J. F. Leckman, J. S. Duncan, R. Wetzles, and M. A. Riddle, Corpus callosum morphology from magnetic resonance images in Tourette's syndrome, *Psychiatry Res. Neuroimaging 55*:85 (1994).

61. M. C. de Lacoste, R. L. Holloway, and D. J. Woodward, Sex differences in the fetal human corpus callosum, *Human Neurobiol. 5*:93 (1986).

62. R. L. Holloway and M. C. de Lacoste, Sexual dimorphism in the human corpus callosum: an extension and replication study, *Human Neurobiol. 5*:87 (1986).

63. S. Clarke, R. Kraftsik, H. Van Der Loos, and G. M. Innocenti, Forms and measures of adult and developing human corpus callosum: is there sexual dimorphism? *J. Comp. Neurol. 280*:213 (1989).

64. A. D. Bell and S. Variend, Failure to demonstrate sexual dimorphism of the corpus callosum in childhood, *J. Anat. 143*:143 (1985).

65. S. F. Witelson, On hemisphere specialization and cerebral plasticity from birth, *Hemisphere Function and Collaboration in the Child* (C. T. Best, ed.), Academic Press, Orlando, FL, 1985, p. 33.

66. S. F. Witelson, The brain connection: the corpus callosum is larger in left-handers, *Science 229*:665 (1985).

67. J. S. Oppenheim, A. B. Benjamin, C. P. Lee, R. Nass, and M. S. Gazzianga, No sex-related differences in human corpus callosum based on magnetic resonance imagery, *Ann. Neurol. 21*:604 (1987).

68. S. Weis, G. Weber, E. Wenger, and M. Kimbacher, The human corpus callosum and the controversy about sexual dimorphism, *Psychobiology 16*:411 (1988).

69. W. Byne, R. Bleier, and L. Houston, Variations in human corpus callosum do not predict gender: a study using magnetic resonance imaging, *Behav. Neurosci. 102*:222 (1988).

70. S. Weis, G. Weber, E. Wenger, and M. Kimbacher, The controversy about

sexual dimorphism of the human corpus callosum, *Int. J. Neurosci. 47*:169 (1989).

71. J. N. Giedd, J. M. Rumsey, F. X. Castellanos, J. C. Rajapakse, D. Kaysen, A. C. Vaituzis, Y. C. Vauss, S. D. Hamburger, and J. L. Rapoport, A quantitative MRI study of the corpus callosum in children and adolescents, *Brain Res. Dev. Brain Res. 91*:274 (1996).

72. J. Nolte, Basal ganglia, *The Human Brain: An Introduction to Its Functional Anatomy* (R. Farrell, ed.), Mosby Year Book, Inc., St. Louis, 1993, p. 319.

73. A. M. Elkashef, R. W. Buchanan, F. Gellad, R. C. Munson, and A. Breier, Basal ganglia pathology in schizophrenia and tardive dyskinesia: an mri quantitative study, *Am. J. Psychiatry 151*:752 (1994).

74. M. S. Keshavan, W. W. Bagwell, G. L. Haas, J. A. Sweeney, N. R. Schooler, and J. W. Pettegrew, Changes in caudate volume with neuroleptic treatment, *Lancet 344*:1434 (1994).

75. M. H. Chakos, J. A. Lieberman, R. M. Bilder, M. Borenstein, G. Lerner, B. Bogerts, H. Wu, B. Kinon, and M. Ashtari, Increase in caudate nuclei volumes of first-episode schizophrenic patients taking antipsychotic drugs, *Am. J. Psychiatry 151*:1430 (1994).

76. J. A. Frazier, J. N. Giedd, D. Kaysen, K. Albus, S. Hamburger, J. Alaghband-Rad, M. C. Lenane, A. Breier, and J. L. Rapoport, Childhood onset schizophrenia: brain magnetic resonance imaging rescan after two years of clozapine maintenance, *Am. J. Psychiatry 153*:564 (1996).

77. B. Peterson, M. A. Riddle, D. J. Cohen, L. D. Katz, J. C. Smith, M. T. Hardin, and J. F. Leckman, Reduced basal ganglia volumes in Tourette's syndrome using three-dimensional reconstruction techniques from magnetic resonance images, *Neurology 43*:941 (1993).

78. T. M. Hyde, M. E. Stacey, R. Coppola, S. F. Handel, K. C. Rickler, and D. R. Weinberger, Cerebral morphometric abnormalities in Tourette's syndrome: a quantitative MRI study of monozygotic twins, *Neurology 45*:1176 (1995).

79. S. I. Rapoport, Integrated phylogeny of the primate brain, with special reference to humans and their diseases, *Brain Res. Rev. 15*:267 (1990).

80. J. Nolte, Olfactory and limbic systems, *The Human Brain. An Introduction to Its Functional Anatomy* (R. Farrell, ed.), Mosby Year Book, Inc., St. Louis, 1993, p. 397.

81. J. N. Giedd, A. C. Vaituzis, J. C. Rajapakse, D. Kaysen, Y. C. Vauss, S. D. Hamburger, N. Lange, and J. L. Rapoport, Quantitative MRI of the temporal lobe, amygdala, and hippocampus in normal human development: ages 4–18, *J. Comp. Neurol. 366*:223 (1995).

82. A. S. Clark, N. J. MacLusky, and P. S. Goldman-Rakic, Androgen binding and metabolism in the cerebral cortex of the developing rhesus monkey, *Endocrinology 123*:932 (1988).

83. S. A. Sholl and K. L. Kim, Estrogen receptors in the rhesus monkey brain during fetal development, *Dev. Brain Res. 50*:189 (1989).

84. J. K. Morse, S. W. Scheff, and S. T. DeKosky, Gonadal steroids influence axonal sprouting in the hippocampal dentate gyrus: a sexually dimorphic response, *Exp. Neurol. 94*:649 (1986).

85. D. G. M. Murphy, C. D. DeCarli, E. Daly, J. V. Haxby, G. Allen, B. J. White, C. M. Powell, B. Horowitz, S. I. Rapoport, and M. B. Schapiro, X chromosome effects on female brain: a magnetic resonance imaging study of Turner's Syndrome, *Lancet 342*:1197 (1993).

86. E. Gould, C. S. Woolley, M. Frankfurt, and B. S. McEwen, Gonadal steroids regulate dendritic spine density in hippocampal pyramidal cells in adulthood, *J. Neurosci. 10*:1286 (1990).

87. P. A. Filipek, C. Richelme, D. N. Kennedy, and V. S. Caviness, Jr. The young adult human brain: an MRI-based morphometric analysis, *Cereb. Cortex 4*:344 (1994).

88. F. M. Benes, M. Turtle, Y. Khan, and P. Farol, Myelination of a key relay zone in the hippocampal formation occurs in the human brain during childhood, adolescence, and adulthood, *Arch. Gen. Psychiatry 51*:477 (1994).

89. J. R. Krebs, D. F. Sherry, S. D. Healy, V. H. Perry, and A. L. Vaccarino, Hippocampal specialization of food-storing birds, *Proc. Natl. Acad. Sci. USA 86*:1388 (1989).

90. D. F. Sherry, A. L. Vaccarino, K. Buckenham, and R. S. Herz, The hippocampal complex of food-storing birds, *Brain Behav. Evol. 34*:308 (1989).

91. D. F. Sherry, L. F. Jacobs, and S. J. Gaulin, Spatial memory and adaptive specialization of the hippocampus (see comments), *Trends Neurosci. 15*:298 (1992).

92. L. F. Jacobs, S. J. Gaulin, D. F. Sherry, and G. E. Hoffman, Evolution of spatial cognition: sex-specific patterns of spatial behavior predict hippocampal size, *Proc. Natl. Acad. Sci. USA 87*:6349 (1990).

93. T. E. Goldberg, E. F. Torrey, K. F. Berman, and D. R. Weinberger, Relations between neuropsychological performance and brain morphological and physiological measures in monozygotic twins discordant for schizophrenia, *Psychiatry Res. 55*:51 (1994).

94. T. Lencz, G. McCarthy, R. A. Bronen, T. M. Scott, J. A. Inserni, K. J. Sass, R. A. Novelly, J. H. Kim, and D. D. Spencer, Quantitative magnetic resonance imaging in temporal lobe epilepsy: relationship to neuropathology and neuropsychological function, *Ann. Neurol. 31*:629 (1992).

95. J. N. Giedd, P. Kozuch, D. Kaysen, A. C. Vaituzis, S. D. Hamburger, J. J. Bartko, and J. L. Rapoport, Reliability of cerebral measures in repeated examinations with magnetic resonance imaging, *Psychiatr. Res. Neuroimaging 61*: 113 (1995).

6

Developmental Disorders

Jay N. Giedd and F. Xavier Castellanos
National Institute of Mental Health, Bethesda, Maryland

I. INTRODUCTION

Many neuropsychiatric disorders of childhood onset may reflect deviations along the complex path of normal brain development. A neurodevelopmental perspective is increasingly being applied to adult psychiatric illnesses as well [1,2]. However, there is no identified "lesion" common to all, or even most,

Table 1 Psychiatric Indications for Pediatric Cerebral MRI Scans

1. Movement disorder of uncertain etiology
2. Anorexia nervosa
3. Severe psychotic or mood disorder not responding, or responding atypically, to conventional treatment
4. First episode of a psychotic disorder

children with the most frequently studied disorders of autism, attention deficit/hyperactivity disorder (ADHD), dyslexia, fragile X syndrome, early-onset schizophrenia, Sydenham's chorea, or Tourette's syndrome. At the time of this writing, neuroimaging investigations of these childhood-onset neuropsychiatric disorders are not of diagnostic utility except to rule out possible central nervous system (CNS) insults such as tumors, intracranial bleeds, or congenital anomalies as etiologies for the symptoms. Accepted neuropsychiatric indications for obtaining MRI or CT scans in children are indicated in Table 1. Despite this limited diagnostic utility, neuroimaging of childhood-onset neuropsychiatric disorders is useful for shedding light on the neurobiological bases and pathogenesis of these illnesses. This information may lead to greater understanding of the underlying pathophysiology and genetic influences of the diseases, which may ultimately lead to more efficacious treatment, prevention, or cure.

II. DEVELOPMENTAL DISORDERS

A. Attention Deficit/Hyperactivity Disorder

Attention deficit/hyperactivity disorder is a disorder affecting domains of attention, impulsivity, and motor activity. Found in approximately 5% of school age children [3], ADHD accounts for over 40% of clinic referrals [4–6].

Functional imaging studies of ADHD began with Xenon blood flow studies finding decreased perfusion in the striatal region, particularly on the right [7]. Interestingly, this hypoperfusion was reversed by the administration of methylphenidate. An early ^{18}fluorodeoxyglucose positron emission tomography (PET) study [8] indicated decreased glucose consumption in ADHD adults, particularly in frontal regions. However, this was not replicated for adolescents with ADHD [9,10]. PET studies of acute and chronic stimulant drug treatment in ADHD adults have not revealed consistent changes [11,12].

Early qualitative CT studies of ADHD reported nonspecific abnormalities [13,14]. However, these were not confirmed by a subsequent CT study using a more valid contrast group and quantitative techniques [15]. Hynd et al. in MRI studies with 7–11 ADHD children reported a decreased width of the right frontal cortex [16], smaller total midsagittal corpus callosum (CC) area [17], and, based on a single 5-mm axial slice, a right-greater-than-left caudate asymmetry (normal in this study reported to left-greater-than-right) [18]. Smaller CC areas in ADHD were also reported by two other groups: one finding decreased areas of the rostrum and rostral body (anterior regions) in 18 subjects [19] and the other decreased area only in the splenium (posterior region) of 15 subjects [20]. A larger study of the basal ganglia in 50 ADHD boys and 48 matched controls found, in contrast to Hynd, a normal right-greater-than-left caudate asymmetry which was absent in ADHD subjects [21]. An expansion of that study quantifying the basal ganglia, corpus callosum, ventricles, amygdala, hippocampus, temporal lobes, cerebellum, and cortical regions in a sample of 57 boys with ADHD and 55 matched controls found that total cerebral volume was 4.7% smaller in the ADHD group [22]. After adjusting for total cerebral volume by analysis of covariance, right globus pallidus, right anterior frontal region, and cerebellum were all significantly smaller in the ADHD group. In addition to the previously reported loss of right-greater-than-left caudate asymmetry a reversal of the normal left-greater-than-right ventricular asymmetry was noted as well. The normal age-related decreases in caudate volume and increases in lateral ventricular volume were not seen in the ADHD group.

These results are consistent with hypothesized right-sided prefrontal-striatal dysfunction in ADHD. Longitudinal studies, functional MRI studies, and studies of females with ADHD, drug-naive subjects, and twins discordant for ADHD are underway.

B. Autism

Autism is a behavioral syndrome characterized by impairments in communication and social interaction and a markedly restricted repertoire of activities and interests. The onset of autism occurs by definition prior to age 3 and prevalence is estimated at 2–5 per 10,000 [23].

Postmortem studies in autism have most consistently revealed anomalies of the limbic system (increased cell packing density and decreased nerve cell size bilaterally in the hippocampus, subiculum, entorhinal cortex, amygdala, mammillary body, and medial septal nucleus) or cerebellum (loss of Purkinje and granule cells in the neocerebellar cortex) [24,25]. PET studies in autism have not identified a consistent pattern of abnormal blood flow or brain metabolism. In a patient sample of 10 unusually high functioning autistic adults, nonlocalized elevation of glucose metabolism was noted [26]. A subsequent correlational study after increasing the sample size to 14 subjects found reduced intercorrelations within and between frontal and parietal lobes and frontoparietal neocortex and subcortical regions [27]. However, a series of studies by Buchsbaum et al. [28–30], also in high functioning autistic, and a study of 18 autistic children [31] did not find hypermetabolism in autistic subjects. SPECT studies indicated either normal cerebral blood flow in a sample of 21 subjects [32[or decreased blood flow in smaller sample studies [33,34].

Magnetic resonance spectroscopy (MRS) studies of autism revealed low levels of phosphocreatine (Pcr) in the prefrontal cortex, suggesting a hypermetabolic state in which Pcr is used to maintain adenosine triphosphate (ATP) levels [35]. Decreased levels of esterified ends on alpha-ATP were also consistent with lower synthesis and higher degradation of cell membranes, the significance of which is not well understood. In the autistic group scores on neuropsychological tests designed to involve the prefrontal cortex correlated in the expected directions with the MRS metabolite levels. Early in vivo imaging studies using CT looked at cerebral asymmetries and sizes of the lateral ventricles, basal ganglia, and thalamus, but except for nonspecific findings of enlarged ventricles they yielded inconsistent findings [36].

In a qualitative MRI study of 13 high functioning adult men with autism, 5 were noted to have polymicrogyria, one had macrogyria, and one had both macrogyria and schizencephaly [37]. Similar cortical findings of poly- and microgyria were reported for two patients with Asperger's syndrome [38]. These anomalies most likely reflect problems in neural migration during the first 6 months of pregnancy, which may indicate a particularly vulnerable time for external factors such as infections to contribute to the pathogenesis of autism. Other reports of cortical abnormalities include decreased parietal lobe volumes, manifest by sulcal widening, which was found in 9 of 21 autistic subjects versus none in 12 controls [39].

Because of the previously mentioned postmortem data and a series of MRI studies by Courchesne and colleagues, the cerebellum has become an active area of investigation in autism research. An initial case study demonstrated incomplete development of vermal lobules VI and VII in a young autistic man [40]. This was followed by a study of 18 autistic subjects indicating a 19% reduction in these lobules compared to 12 controls [41]. A report on a subsample of these subjects indicated more widespread involvement of the cerebellum with a 12% reduction in cerebellar volume [42]. In a more recent report of the sample enlarged to 50 patients and 53 controls, mean sizes of vermal lobules VI and VII were not different. However, in contrast to the Gaussian distribution of values in the control group, the values in the autistic group were bimodally distributed. Based on this distribution, two distinct subgroups were proposed; one including 86% of the patients having a mean midsagittal area of vermal lobules VI and VII 16% smaller than the control group, and the other including 12% of the patients having a 34% larger mean area.

In contrast to these studies, a number of investigators found no differences in the midsagittal area of vermal lobules VI and VII in autism [43–48]. The importance of controlling for IQ on this measure was exemplified by a study of 15 high functioning autistic males who had smaller vermal lobules VI and VII when compared to a group matched for age and parental socioeconomic status, but did not when compared to a group matched for nonverbal IQ [49].

Although cerebellar MRI findings in autism remain controversial, accumulating evidence of the cerebellum's role in learning and cognition and its extensive connections to the rest of the brain [50] make for an intriguing hypotheses in the pathogenesis of autism. Other structural brain anomalies reported for autism include smaller brainstems [51], gray matter heterotopia [52], altered asymmetries of frontal lobe volumes [53], and a smaller right lenticular nucleus [54].

In summary, a variety of functional and structural brain anomalies have been reported in autistic subjects, although rarely are the same anomalies reported from one study to the next. These heterogeneous findings may reflect a heterogeneous nature of the syndrome itself in addition to confounds related to different inclusion criteria for patients in different studies, different imaging hardware, software, and measuring protocols, and differences in control groups.

C. Dyslexia

Reading disorder, or developmental dyslexia, is characterized by substantial deficits in reading accuracy, speed, or comprehension based on an individual's age, intelligence, and education [23]. In order to meet DSM-IV diagnostic criteria, the deficit must also significantly interfere with academic achievement or with activities of daily living and if sensory deficits are present the reading difficulties must be more severe than usually associated with those sensory deficits. The disorder is fairly common, affecting about 4% of U.S. school age children. It is diagnosed more often (60–80%) in males, although controversy exists as to whether this reflects a truly greater prevalence or is the result of referral biases.

Imaging studies have been informed by earlier postmortem work of four dyslexic men and three dyslexic women indicating a loss of the usual left-greater-than-right asymmetry of the planum temporale [55,56]. Interestingly, the loss of normal asymmetry in dyslexic subjects was due to an increased size of the right planum temporale, not a decrease on the left. The planum temporale lies along the superior surface of the superior temporal gyrus and is thought to be involved in language functions, particularly phonetic processing [57]. Also noted in this postmortem sample were neural ectopias and distortions of cytoarchitecture in the cortex [55], medial geniculate nucleus and lateral posterior nucleus of the thalamus [58], and magnocellular layers of the lateral geniculate nucleus [59].

Loss of normal brain asymmetries has also been the predominant theme of CT studies (primarily assessing parieto-occipital regions) [60–63] and MRI studies. MRI studies of reversed or diminished normal asymmetry include loss of the usual left-greater-than-right asymmetry of the lateral ventricles and right-greater-than-left asymmetry temporal lobes [64], loss of the normal left-greater-than-right asymmetry of the planum temporale in adolescents which correlated with degree of phonological decoding deficits [65], reversal of the normal left-greater-than-right asymmetry of the angular gyrus in familial dyslexics, driven by an increase on the right, which correlated with severity of dyslexia [66], and loss of normal right-greater-than-left asymmetry of the frontal cortices and bilaterally smaller size of the frontal cortices in children with dyslexia [67]. Another study, extending the measurement of the planum along its ascending parietal extension, found a larger proportion of the planum on the right parietal bank in dyslexia, raising questions as to the most appropriate method to assess this region [68]. This study also noted bilateral anomalies, such as multiple Heschl's gyri (a key component of auditory processing), in the dyslexic group.

However, a more recent study controlling for IQ, handedness, and gender did not find asymmetry differences [69]. Overall, despite methodological differences in image acquisition, slice orientation and thickness, definition of boundaries, and control and patient group criteria, the preponderance of evidence points to altered hemispheric symmetry in dyslexia, although the precise nature of these difference awaits clarification with more precise imaging protocols.

Consistent with the hypothesis of altered hemispheric symmetries, the CC, the largest interhemispheric commissure, has also been the target of dyslexia neuroimaging studies. A larger splenium (posterior) of the CC was reported in a study of adult familial dyslexics [66] but not replicated in a sample of dyslexic adolescents using similar measures [70]. Another study also found no difference in the splenium but did find a reduction in the genu (anterior) [71]. A study of 21 dyslexic adult men dividing the CC into thirds found the posterior third larger in the dyslexic than in the control group [72].

Functional imaging studies in dyslexia have used Xenon inhalation, [18]fluorodeoxyglucose PET, and O^{15} PET. These studies have only been conducted in adults. A Xenon inhalation study including a semantic classification task designed to activate the left hemisphere and a line orientation task designed to activate the right hemisphere showed exaggerated asymmetries of blood flow in the dyslexic group [73]. This was interpreted to imply difficulties in integration of the two hemispheres or in allocation of cognitive resources in the dyslexic group. A Xenon inhalation study of 83 subjects using the task of identifying which concrete nouns contained four letters found performance positively correlated with blood flow in Wernicke's area [74]. This correlation held both for the control group and those with childhood histories of poor reading ability. Blood flow in a more posterior temporoparietal region showed a negative correlation with childhood reading level, leading to the hypothesis that neurons targeted for Wernicke's area may improperly synapse in more posterior regions in the dyslexic group.

[18]Fluorodeoxyglucose PET studies have indicated increased glucose utilization in the inferior occipital cortex in dyslexic men reading single words aloud [75] and in the medial temporal lobes bilaterally during a task requiring the detection of a target syllable [76]. Increased glucose utilization was hypothesized to reflect activation of compensatory pathways or inefficient metabolic processing.

A series of studies using O[15] PET (which has greater temporal resolution than [18]fluorodeoxyglucose PET) to assess regional cerebral blood flow were conducted by Rumsey and colleagues. During a task in which subjects indicate when paired words rhyme, the left temporoparietal and posterior temporal regions (near Wernicke's area) were activated in the control, but not the dyslexic group [77]. A sentence comprehension task in which subjects decide whether two sentences have the same meaning activated left temporal (anterior and middle) and the inferior frontal cortex in both dyslexics and controls, despite a mild performance deficit in the dyslexic group [78]. Dyslexics showed significant performance deficits when choosing which of a series of paired tones were identical. During this task frontotemporal activation was greater in controls than in dyslexics [79].

Taken together, the functional imaging studies of dyslexia generally indicate dysfunction of left posterior regions, although it is of note that right hemisphere deficits, particularly of the medial and lateral temporal cortex, have been reported as well.

D. Fragile X Syndrome

Fragile X syndrome is the most common heritable cause of a developmental neuropsychiatric disorder [80], and is second only to trisomy 21 as a genetic cause of mental retardation. It is of enormous interest to developmental neurobiologists because the well-characterized mutation [81], specific behavioral and cognitive profile [82], and identified neuroanatomical findings offer a rare opportunity to explore the relationship between genes, behavior, and brain anatomy.

Males, having only one X chromosome, tend to suffer more severe impairments than females who are heterozygous for the disorder. This varying degree of genetic vulnerability allows an exploration of "dose" effects of the fragile X mutation on brain anatomy and clinical manifestation. For instance, size of cerebellar vermal lobules VI and VII was found to be smallest in fragile X males, intermediate in fragile X females, and largest in controls [83,84].

Bilaterally enlarged hippocampal volume in the fragile X group, possibly related to abnormal neuronal pruning, was noted in a study of six male and nine female subjects [85]. These findings are consistent with a study of the mouse homologue of the fragile X gene (fragile X mental retardation 1 gene), which demonstrates greatest expression in the granular layers of the cerebellum and hippocampus [86].

Etiological heterogeneity is inherent in the other disorders discussed in this chapter. The advantages offered from the study of a more homogeneous sample with a known genetic defect may unveil important links between brain and behavior. This, in turn, may have widespread application to the understanding and treatment of other disorders.

E. Childhood-Onset Schizophrenia

Childhood-onset schizophrenia (COS), defined as onset of psychotic symptoms prior to age 12, occurs less than one-fiftieth as frequently as the adult-onset type [87–91]. Despite its rarity, COS is an important clinical group to study because it may be caused by a more severe genetic and/or environmental insult or an earlier process of the brain maturational changes, which trigger the onset of psychosis, the understanding of which may shed light on the neurodevelopmental etiology of its more common adult counterpart. COS appears to be clinically continuous with adult-onset schizophrenia [90,92–94], although premorbid impairments tend to be more severe [95].

Structural neuroimaging studies of adult schizophrenia have most consistently found enlarged ventricles and basal ganglia structures and smaller total cerebral volume and mesial temporal lobe structures [96–107]. Thalamic anomalies have also been reported [108,109]. A review of functional imaging studies in adult schizophrenia is presented in Chapter 12.

As might be expected for such a rare disorder, few large sample imaging studies have been conducted for COS. An MRI case study of a 10-year-boy with COS reported ventriculomegaly and a small left cerebellum [110]. A study that included six children with schizophrenia, schizophreniform disorder, or other psychosis found larger ventricular volume in three of the subjects [111]. A third study likewise found enlarged ventricles in a group of 15 schizophrenic or schizophreniform disorder adolescents (mean age 16.5 years) [112].

The largest sample of COS subjects is from an ongoing study at the Child Psychiatry Branch of the National Institute of Mental Health. Subjects are recruited nationally for participation in a 3- to 6-month inpatient pharmacology study. To date 30, subjects have been recruited, screened from over 500 chart reviews and patient/family interviews.

An MRI study involving the first 21 of these subjects found a lack of normal right-greater-than-left asymmetry of the hippocampus, but no mean difference in the volume of the temporal lobe, amygdala, hippocampus, or superior temporal gyrus [113]. A study of 24 of these subjects reported a smaller total cerebral volume and midsagittal thalamic area, larger basal ganglia structures (caudate, putamen, and globus pallidus), and a trend towards larger ventricular volume in the COS group [114].

Because of controversy related to the effect of neuroleptics on reported basal ganglia enlargement in schizophrenia [104,105,115] a 2-year follow-up study was done with eight patients taking typical neuroleptics at the time of the first scan and maintained on clozapine for 2 years prior to the second scan [116]. On follow-up the clozapine-maintained COS group, but not eight age- and gender-matched controls also receiving a 2-year follow-up scan, demonstrated decreased caudate and putamen volumes over time. These findings are consistent with the hypothesis that basal ganglia enlargement in COS is secondary to medication effects. Study of the CC in these subjects revealed a relatively larger midsagittal area in the COS group consistent with other studies indicating a relative sparring of white matter with decreased cortical volume in schizophrenia [117–119].

Overall, results of neuroimaging investigations add to the data from clinical and neuropsychological reports indicating a continuity between COS and adult-onset schizophrenia [90–93,120,121]. An examination of effect sizes for adult-onset and COS neuroanatomical studies indicates that the degree of anomalies is generally similar. This does not support the notion of a more severe fetal "lesion" in COS, at least as reflected in gross neuroanatomical measures. Perhaps the early onset is related to the processes by which brain maturation triggers the onset of psychosis in susceptible individuals.

F. Sydenham's Chorea

Sydenham's chorea is a semi-acute disorder usually presenting in childhood or early adolescence characterized by sudden, involuntary, arrhythmic, aimless movements, often accompanied by muscular weakness and psychological symptoms including emotional lability, obsessive-compulsive disorder, anxiety, impulsivity, and inattentiveness [122–124]. It is sometimes referred to as St. Vitus dance in reference to the masses of afflicted people who made pilgrimages to the shrine of St. Vitus in medieval Europe seeking cure. The purported powers of St. Vitus were reinforced by the self-limiting nature of the illness, as many of the sufferers' symptoms abated coincident with their arrival to the shrine. Although uncommon, the severe and often dramatic presentation of symptoms has maintained the interest of physicians.

Sydenham's chorea follows infection with Group A β-hemolytic strepto-cocci (GABHS) and is a "major" criterion of rheumatic fever [125]. The proposed mechanism is that antibodies directed against antigens on GABHS cross-react with certain host tissues in the cardiac, skeletal, or central ner-vous system (CNS) [126–128]. It is involvement with the CNS, particularly of the basal ganglia, that is thought to be related to the movement and behavioral manifestations of Sydenham's chorea.

Basal ganglia involvement is supported by postmortem, functional, and structural imaging studies. Postmortem studies of Sydenham's chorea have identified swollen and eccentric nuclei in corpus striatum cells [129,130] and diffuse basal ganglia changes [131]. Specific cross-reactivity of IgG antibod-ies to neuronal cytoplasmic antigens of the caudate and subthalamic nuclei have been noted using immunofluorescent staining [132]. An ^{18}fluorodeoxyg-lucose PET study of a 15-year-old girl scanned shortly after onset and a 74-year-old woman with residual hyperkinesis following Sydenham's chorea in adolescence found increased glucose consumption in the caudate and lenti-form nuclei [133]. On a scan done after symptom resolution, the 15-year-old's striatal glucose consumption returned to normal. Swelling of the cau-date, which returned to normal 2 weeks later after symptoms had abated, was observed in a computed tomography of an 18-year-old male with Sydenham's chorea [134]. Three separate MRI case reports (four subjects total) found basal ganglia hyperintensities on T_2-weighted images of Sydenham's chorea subjects [135–137]. T_2 hyperintensities may be indicative of inflammatory or exudative processes, which is consistent with an immunologically mediated pathophysiology. Finally, in a study comparing 24 subjects with Sydenham's chorea to 48 matched controls volumes of the caudate, putamen, and globus pallidus, but not of the thalamus, total brain, prefrontal, or midfrontal re-gions, were significantly increased in the Sydenham's chorea group [138].

Basal ganglia dysfunction may underlie a common thread between Syde-nham's chorea and obsessive-compulsive disorder (OCD). Obsessive-com-pulsive symptomatology is common in Sydenham's chorea [139] and some children with OCD (and Tourette's syndrome) experience symptom onset or exacerbation following GABHS infections [140]. A case report of serial MRI brain scans to monitor basal ganglia volumes during plasmapheresis in a 12-year-old boy with a postinfectious exacerbation of his OCD found dramatic changes in caudate and globus pallidus volumes in relation to plasmapheresis and severity of obsessive-compulsive symptoms [141]. Caudate volume decreased 24% and globus pallidus volume 28% during effective treatment with plasmapheresis. The magnitude of these changes well exceeds the error expected from the processes of rescanning and remeasuring these structures (4% for the caudate and 6% for the globus pallidus) [142]. These data provide support for immunological treatments in certain subgroups of patients with neuropsychiatric presentations.

G. Tourette's Syndrome

Tourette's syndrome (TS) is characterized by chronic motor and vocal tics and is often associated with ADHD, OCD, or learning disorders [23]. Prevalence is 4–5 per 10,000, and vulnerability seems to be transmitted via an autosomal dominant pattern.

Three independent groups have reported basal ganglia anomalies in MRI studies of TS [143–145], consistent with the role of motor control attributed to these structures. Peterson et al., in a study of 14 adult TS subjects and 14 controls, found no statistically significant mean differences in left or right caudate, putamen, or globus pallidus measures, but the sum of the putamen and globus pallidus, comprising the lenticular nucleus, was significantly smaller on the left in the TS group [143]. Singer et al., in a study of 37 children and 18 controls, also found no statistically significant mean differences in left or right caudate, putamen, or globus pallidus measures and found a loss of lenticular asymmetry driven by decreases on the left side. However, further analysis assessing comorbidity of ADHD in the sample revealed that TS subjects without ADHD did not differ from controls on any measure [144]. Hyde et al., in a study of 10 monozygotic twins discordant for tic severity, found a reduction in right anterior caudate volume in the more severely affected twin [145]. This study may also have been confounded by the high proportion of subjects with ADHD. A study assessing the effect of comorbid TS on right-sided reductions of corticostriatal-pallidal structures in 26 subjects with ADHD alone, 14 subjects with ADHD and TS, and 29 controls found no significant effect related to the TS comorbidity [146]. These results highlight the importance of controlling for comorbid ADHD in studies of TS. Other TS structural imaging studies have noted a decreased size of the CC [147], possibly related to anomalies in lateralization noted earlier and nonspecific findings such as mild ventricular enlargement [148].

Functional imaging studies of TS have implicated involvement of the basal ganglia and related frontal structures. A PET study indicated hypometabolism in the ventromedial caudate, left anterior putamen, and nucleus accumbens [149], supporting an earlier PET study finding hypometabolism in the basal ganglia as well as frontal, cingulate, and insular cortices [150]. SPECT studies also indicate involvement of basal ganglia structures, as well as frontal and temporal cortices [151–153].

IV. SUMMARY

As stated in the introduction, the clinical utility of neuroimaging in pediatric neuropsychiatric disorders is quite limited. None of the common psychiatric disorders of childhood-onset disease can be diagnosed by imaging studies, although neurological conditions included in the differential diagnoses may be assessed. The most likely clinically relevant next advance is for imaging studies to help identify biologically homogeneous subgroups of disorders, which may respond preferentially to different treatment interventions. The noted gender differences in age of onset, prevalence, and symptom profiles in all of the disorders covered in this chapter and their relationship to the sexually dimorphic differences in normal brain maturation deserve further study.

The abundance of reported neuroanatomical findings has been more notable than the consistency of the findings. Differences in image acquisition, image analysis, patient and control characteristics, and statistical interpretation contribute to the discordance of the findings, although continued improvements in imaging technology and study design may pave the way for greater agreement in future studies. Theoretical limitations in spatial resolution of MRI scans have not been reached, and functional MRI, which is still in its infancy, shows tremendous promise for brain studies of children and adolescents.

REFERENCES

1. F. E. Bloom, Advancing a neurodevelopmental origin for schizophrenia, *Arch. Gen. Psychiatry 50*:224 (1993).
2. D. R. Weinberger, From neuropathology to neurodevelopment, *Lancet 346*: 552 (1995).
3. P. Szatmari, The epidemiology of attention-deficit hyperactivity disorder, *Child Adolesc. Psychiatr. Clin. North Am. 1*:361 (1992).
4. J. C. Anderson, S. Williams, R. McGee, and P. A. Silva, DSM-III disorders in preadolescent children. Prevalence in a large sample from the general population, *Arch. Gen. Psychiatry 44*:69 (1987).
5. H. R. Bird, G. Canino, M. Rubio-Stipec, M. S. Gould, J. Ribera, M. Sesman, M. Woodbury, S. Huertas-Goldman, A. Pagan, and A. Sanchez-Lacay, Estimates of the prevalence of childhood maladjustment in a community survey

in Puerto Rico. The use of combined measures, *Arch. Gen. Psychiatry 45*:1120 (1988).

6. D. R. Offord, M. H. Boyle, P. Szatmari, N. I. Rae-Grant, P. S. Links, D. T. Cadman, J. A. Byles, J. W. Crawford, H. M. Blum, and C. Byrne, Ontario Child Health Study. II. Six-month prevalence of disorder and rates of service utilization, *Arch. Gen. Psychiatry 44*:832 (1987).

7. H. C. Lou, L. Henriksen, P. Bruhn, H. Borner, and J. B. Nielsen, Striatal dysfunction in attention deficit and hyperkinetic disorder, *Arch. Neurol. 46*: 48 (1989).

8. A. J. Zametkin, T. E. Nordahl, M. Gross, A. C. King, W. E. Semple, J. Rumsey, S. Hamburger, and R. M. Cohen, Cerebral glucose metabolism in adults with hyperactivity of childhood onset, *N. Engl. J. Med. 323*(20):1361 (1990).

9. A. J. Zametkin, L. L. Liebenauer, G. A. Fitzgerald, A. C. King, D. V. Minkunas, P. Herscovitch, E. M. Yamada, and R. M. Cohen, Brain metabolism in teenagers with attention deficit hyperactivity disorder, *Arch. Gen. Psychiatry 50*:333 (1993).

10. M. Ernst, L. L. Liebenauer, A. C. King, G. A. Fitzgerald, R. M. Cohen, and A. J. Zametkin, Reduced brain metabolism in hyperactive girls, *J. Am. Acad. Child Adoles. Psychiatry 33*:858 (1994).

11. J. A. Matochik, T. E. Nordahl, M. Gross, W. E. Semple, A. C. King, R. M. Cohen, and A. J. Zametkin, Effects of acute stimulant medication on cerebral metabolism in adults with hyperactivity, *Neuropsychopharmacology 8*:377 (1993).

12. J. A. Matochik, L. L. Liebenauer, A. C. King, H. V. Szymanski, R. M. Cohen, and A. J. Zametkin, Cerebral glucose metabolism in adults with attention deficit hyperactivity disorder after chronic stimulant treatment, *Am. J. Psychiatry 151*:658 (1994).

13. K. Bergstrom and B. Bille, Computed tomography of the brain in children with minimal brain damage: a preliminary study of 46 children, *Neuropaediatrie 9*: 378 (1978).

14. B. K. Caparulo, D. J. Cohen, S. L. Rothman, J. G. Young, J. D. Katz, S. E. Shaywitz, and B. A. Shaywitz, Computed tomographic brain scanning in children with developmental neuropsychiatric disorders, *J. Abnorm. Child Psychol. 20*:338 (1981).

15. B. A. Shaywitz, S. E. Shaywitz, T. Byrne, D. J. Cohen, and S. Rothman, Attention deficit disorder: quantitative analysis of CT, *Neurology 33*:1500 (1983).

16. G. W. Hynd, M. Semrud-Clikeman, A. R. Lorys, E. S. Novey, and D. Eliopulos, Brain morphology in developmental dyslexia and attention deficit disorder/hyperactivity, *Arch. Neurol. 47*:919 (1990).

17. G. W. Hynd, M. Semrud-Clikeman, A. R. Lorys, E. S. Novey, D. Eliopulos, and H. Lyytinen, Corpus callosum morphology in attention deficit-hyperactivity disorder: morphometric analysis of MRI, *J. Learn. Disabilities 24*:141 (1991).

18. G. W. Hynd, K. L. Hern, E. S. Novey, D. Eliopulos, R. Marshall, and J. J. Gonzalez, Attention deficit hyperactivity disorder (ADHD) and asymmetry of the caudate nucleus, *J. Child Neurol. 8*(4):339 (1993).

19. J. N. Giedd, F. X. Castellanos, B. J. Casey, P. L. Kozuch, A. C. King, S. D. Hamburger, and J. L. Rapoport, Quantitative morphology of the corpus callosum in attention deficit hyperactivity disorder, *Am. J. Psychiatry 151*:665 (1994).

20. M. Semrud-Clikeman, P. A. Filipek, J. Biederman, R. Steingard, D. Kennedy, P. Renshaw, and K. Bekken, Attention-deficit hyperactivity disorder: magnetic resonance imaging morphometric analysis of the corpus callosum, *J. Am. Acad. Child Adolesc. Psychiatry 33*:875 (1994).

21. F. X. Castellanos, J. N. Giedd, P. Eckburg, W. L. Marsh, A. C. King, S. D. Hamburger, and J. L. Rapoport, Quantitative morphology of the caudate nucleus in attention-deficit hyperactivity disorder, *Am. J. Psychiatry 151*:1791 (1994).

22. F. X. Castellanos, J. N. Giedd, W. L. Marsh, S. D. Hamburger, A. C. Vaituzis, J. W. Snell, N. Lange, D. P. Dickstein, Y. C. Vauss, D. Kaysen, G. F. Ritchie, J. C. Rajapakse, and J. L. Rapoport, Quantitative brain magnetic resonance imaging in attention-deficit/hyperactivity disorder, *Arch. Gen. Psychiatry 53*:607 (1996).

23. American Psychiatric Association, *Diagnostic and Statistical Manual of Mental Disorders*, Washington, DC, (1994).

24. M. L. Bauman and T. L. Kemper, Histoanatomic observations of the brain in early infantile autism, *Neurology 35*:866 (1985).

25. E. R. Ritvo, B. J. Freeman, A. B. Scheibel, P. T. Duong, R. Robinson, D. Guthrie, and A. Ritvo, Lower Purkinje cell counts in the cerebella of four autistic subjects: initial findings of the UCLA-NSAC autopsy research project, *Am. J. Psychiatry 13*:862 (1986).

26. J. M. Rumsey, R. Duara, C. Grady, J. L. Rapoport, R. A. Margolin, S. I. Rapoport, and N. R. Cutler, Brain metabolism in autism: resting cerebral glucose utilization rates as measured with positron emission tomography, *Arch. Gen. Psychiatry 42*:448 (1985).

27. B. Horwitz, J. Rumsey, C. Grady, and S. I. Rapoport, The cerebral metabolic landscape in autism: intercorrelations of regional glucose utilization, *Arch. Neurol. 45*:749 (1988).

28. M. S. Buchsbaum, B. V. Siegel, J. C. Wu, Jr., E. Hazlett, N. Sicotte, and R. Haier, Attention performance in autism and regional metabolic rate assessed by positron emission tomography, *J. Autism Dev. Disord. 22*:115 (1992).

29. C. Heh, R. Smith, J. Wu, E. Hazlett, A. Russell, R. Asarnow, P. Tanguay, and M. Buchsbaum, Positron emission tomography of the cerebellum in autism, *Am. J. Psychiatry 146*:242 (1989).

30. B. V. Siegel, Jr., R. Asarnow, P. Tanguay, J. D. Call, L. Abel, A. Ho, I. Lott, and M. S. Buchsbaum, Regional cerebral glucose metabolism and attention in adults with a history of childhood autism, *J. Neuropsychiatry Clin. Neurosci. 4*:406 (1992).

31. A. DeVolder, A. Bol, C. Michel, M. Congneau, and A. M. Goffinet, Brain glucose metabolism in children with the autistic syndrome: positron tomography analysis, *Brain Dev. 9*:581 (1987).

32. M. Zilbovicius, B. Garreau, N. Tzourio, B. Mazoyer, B. Bruck, J. Martinot, C. Raynaud, Y. Samson, A. Syrota, and G. Lelord, Regional cerebral blood flow in childhood autism: a SPECT study, *Am J Psychiatry 149*:924 (1992).

33. M. S. George, D. C. Costa, K. Kouris, H. A. Ring, and P. J. Ell, Cerebral blood flow abnormalities in adults with infantile autism, *J Nerv. Ment. Dis. 180*:413 (1992).

34. K. Ozbayrak, O. Kapucu, E. Erdem, and T. Aras, Left occipital hypoperfusion in a case with the Asperger syndrome, *Brain Dev. 13*:454 (1991).

35. N. J. Minshew, G. Goldstein, S. M. Dombrowski, K. Panchalingam, and J. W. Pettegrew, A preliminary 31P MRS study of autism: evidence for undersynthesis and increased degradation of brain membranes, *Biological Psychiatry 33*:762 (1993).

36. N. J. Minshew and B. S. Dombrowski, In vivo neuroanatomy of autism: neuroimaging studies, *The Neurobiology of Autism* (M. Bauman et al., eds.), The Johns Hopkins University Press, Baltimore, 1994, p. 66.

37. J. Piven, M. L. Berthier, S. E. Starkstein, E. Nehme, G. Pearlson, and S. Folstein, Magnetic resonance imaging evidence for a defect of cerebral cortical development in autism, *Am. J. Psychiatry 147*:734 (1990).

38. M. L. Berthier, S. E. Starkstein, and R. Leiguarda, Developmental cortical anomalies in Asperger's syndrome: neuroradiological findings in two patients, *J. Neuropsychiatry 2*:197 (1990).

39. E. Courchesne, G. A. Press, and R. Yeung-Courchesne, Parietal lobe abnormalities detected with MR in patients with infantile autism [see comments], *Am. J. Roentgenol. 160*:387 (1993).

40. E. Courchesne, J. R. Hesselink, T. L. Jernigan, and R. Yeung-Courchesne, Abnormal neuroanatomy in a nonretarded person with autism. Unusual findings with magnetic resonance imaging, *Arch. Neurol. 44*:335 (1987).

41. E. Courchesne, R. Yeung-Courchesne, G. A. Press, J. R. Hesselink, and T. L. Jernigan, Hypoplasia of cerebellar vermal lobules VI and VII in autism, *N. Engl. J. Med. 318*:1349 (1988).

42. J. W. Murakami, E. Courchesne, G. A. Press, R. Yeung-Courchesne, and J. R. Hesselink, Reduced cerebellar hemisphere size and its relationship to vermal hypoplasia in autism, *Arch. Neurol. 46*:689 (1989).

43. T. Hashimoto, K. Murakawa, M. Miyazaki, M. Tayama, and Y. Kuroda, Magnetic resonance imaging of the brain structures in the posterior fossa in retarded autistic children, *Acta Paediatr. 81*:1030 (1992).

44. T. Hashimoto, M. Tayama, M. Miyazaki, K. Murakawa, and Y. Kuroda, Brainstem and cerebellar vermis involvement in autistic children, *J. Child Neurol. 7*:149 (1992).

45. T. Hashimoto, M. Tayama, M. Miyazaki, K. Murakawa, S. Shimakawa, Y. Yoneda, and Y. Kuroda, Brainstem involvement in high functioning autistic children, *Acta Neurol. Scand. 88*:123 (1993).

46. J. R. Holtum, N. J. Minshew, R. S. Sanders, and N. E. Phillips, Magnetic resonance imaging of the posterior fossa in autism, *Biol. Psychiatry 32*:1091 (1992).
47. M. D. Kleinman, S. Neff, and N. P. Rosman, The brain in infantile autism: are posterior fossa structures abnormal? *Neurology 42*:753 (1992).
48. M. A. Nowell, D. B. Hackney, A. S. Muraki, and M. Coleman, Varied MR appearance of autism: fifty-three pediatric patients having the full autistic syndrome, *Magn. Resonance Imaging 8*:811 (1990).
49. J. Piven, E. Nehme, J. Simon, P. Barta, G. Pearlson, and S. E. Folstein, Magnetic resonance imaging in autism: measurement of the cerebellum, pons, and fourth ventricle, *Biol. Psychiatry 31*:491 (1992).
50. H. C. Leiner, A. L. Leiner, and R. S. Dow, Does the cerebellum contribute to mental skills? *Behav. Neurosci. 100*:443 (1986).
51. T. Hashimoto, M. Tayama, M. Miyazaki, N. Sakurama, T. Yoshimoto, K. Murakawa, and Y. Kuroda, Reduced brainstem size in children with autism, *Brain Dev. 14*:94 (1992).
52. G. R. Gaffney and L. Y. Tsai, Magnetic resonance imaging of high level autism, *J. Autism Dev. Disord. 17*:433 (1987).
53. T. Hashimoto, M. Tayama, K. Mori, K. Fujino, M. Miyazaki, and Y. Kuroda, Magnetic resonance imaging in autism: preliminary report, *Neuropediatrics 20*:142 (1989).
54. G. R. Gaffney, S. Kuperman, L. Y. Tsai, and S. Minchin, Forebrain structure in infantile autism, *J. Am. Acad. Child Adol. Psychiatry 28*:534 (1989).
55. A. M. Galaburda, G. F. Sherman, G. D. Rosen, F. Aboitiz, and N. Geschwind, Developmental dyslexia: four consecutive patients with cortical anomalies, *Ann. Neurol. 18*:222 (1985).
56. P. Humphreys, W. E. Kaufman, and A. M. Galaburda, Developmental dyslexia in women: neuropathological findings in three patients, *Ann. Neurol. 28*:727 (1990).
57. A. M. Galaburda, J. Corsiglia, G. D. Rosen, and G. F. Sherman, Planum temporale asymmetry, reappraisal since Geschwind and Levitsky, *Neuropsychologia 25*:853 (1982).
58. A. M. Galaburda and D. Eidelberg, Symmetry and asymmetry in the human posterior thalamus. II. Thalamic lesions in a case of developmental dyslexia, *Arch Neurol. 39*:333 (1982).
59. M. S. Livingstone, C. D. Rosen, F. W. Drislane, and A. M. Galaburda, Physiological and anatomical evidence for a magnocellular defect in developmental dyslexia, *Proc. Natl. Acad. Sci. 88*:7943 (1991).
60. R. H. A. Haslam, J. T. Dalby, R. D. Johns, and A. W. Rademaker, Cerebral asymmetry in developmental dyslexia, *Arch. Neurol. 38*:679 (1981).
61. D. B. Hier, M. LeMay, P. B. Rosenberger, and V. P. Perlo, Developmental dyslexia. Evidence for a subgroup with a reversal of cerebral asymmetry, *Arch. Neurol. 35*:90 (1978).
62. G. Leisman and M. Ashkenazi, Aetiological factors in dyslexia: IV. Cerebral hemispheres are functionally equivalent, *Int. J. Neurol. 11*:157 (1980).

63. P. B. Rosenberger and D. B. Hier, Cerebral asymmetry and verbal intellectual deficits, *Ann. Neurol. 8*:300 (1980).

64. J. M. Rumsey, R. Dorwart, M. Vermess, M. B. Denckla, M. J. P. Kruesi, and J. L. Rapoport, Magnetic resonance imaging of brain anatomy in severe developmental dyslexia, *Arch. Neurol. 43*:1045 (1986).

65. J. P. Larsen, T. Hoien, I. Lundberg, and H. Odegaard, MRI evaluation of the size and symmetry of the planum temporale in adolescents with developmental dyslexia, *Brain Lang. 39*:289 (1990).

66. R. Duara, A. Kushch, K. Gross-Glenn, W. Barker, B. Jallad, S. Pascal, D. A. Loewenstein, J. Sheldon, M. Rabin, B. Levin, and H. Lubs, Neuroanatomic differences between dyslexic and normal readers on magnetic resonance imaging scans, *Arch. Neurol. 48*:410 (1991).

67. G. W. Hynd, M. Semrud-Clikeman, A. R. Lorys, E. S. Novey, and D. Eliopulos, Brain morphology in developmental dyslexia and attention deficit disorder/hyperactivity, *Arch. Neurol. 47*:919 (1990).

68. C. M. Leonard, K. K. S. Voeller, L. J. Lombardino, M. K. Morris, G. W. Hynd, A. W. Alexander, H. G. Andersen, M. Garofalakis, J. C. Honeyman, J. Mao, O. F. Agee, and E. V. Staab, Anomalous cerebral structure in dyslexia revealed with magnetic resonance imaging, *Arch. Neurol. 50*:461 (1993).

69. R. T. Schultz, N. T. Cho, L. H. Staib, L. E. Kier, J. M. Fletcher, S. E. Shaywitz, D. P. Shankweiler, L. Katz, J. C. Gore, J. S. Duncan, and B. A. Shaywitz, Brain morphology in normal and dyslexic children: the influence of sex and age, *Ann. Neurol. 35*:732 (1994).

70. J. P. Larsen, T. Hoien, and H. Odegaard, Magnetic resonance imaging of the corpus callosum in developmental dyslexia, *Cogn. Neuropsychol. 9*:123 (1992).

71. G. W. Hynd, J. Hall, E. S. Novey, D. Eliopulos, K. Black, J. J. Gonzalez, J. E. Edmonds, C. Riccio, and M. Cohen, Dyslexia and corpus callosum morphology, *Arch. Neurol. 52*:32 (1995).

72. J. M. Rumsey, M. Casanova, G. B. Mannheim, N. Patronas, N. DeVaughn, S. D. Hamburger, and T. Aquino, Corpus callosum morphology, as measured with MRI, in dyslexic men, *Biol. Psychiatry 39*:769 (1996).

73. J. M. Rumsey, K. F. Berman, M. B. Denckla, S. D. Hamburger, M. J. Kruesi, and D. R. Weinberger, Regional cerebral blood flow in severe developmental dyslexia, *Arch. Neurol. 44*:1144 (1987).

74. D. L. Flowers, F. B. Wood, and C. E. Naylor, Regional cerebral blood flow correlates of language processes in reading disability, *Arch. Neurol. 48*:637 (1991).

75. K. Gross-Glenn, R. Duara, W. W. Barker, D. Loewenstein, J. Y. Chang, F. Yoshi, A. M. Apicella, S. Pascal, T. Boothe, S. Sevush, B. J. Jallad, L. Novoa, and H. A. Lubs, Positron emission tomograpic studies during serial word reading by normal and dyslexic adults, *J. Clin. Exp. Neuropsychol. 13*:531 (1991).

76. J. O. Hagman, F. Wood, M. S. Buchsbaum, P. Tallal, L. Flowers, and W. Katz, Cerebral brain metabolism in adult dyslexic subjects assessed with PET during performance of an auditory task, *Arch. Neurol. 49*:734 (1992).

77. J. M. Rumsey, P. Andreason, A. J. Zametkin, T. Aquino, A. C. King, S. D.

Hamburger, A. Pikus, J. L. Rapoport, and R. M. Cohen, Failure to activate the left temporoparietal cortex in dyslexia, *Arch. Neurol. 49*:527 (1992).

78. J. M. Rumsey, A. J. Zametkin, P. Andreason, A. P. Hanahan, S. D. Hamburger, T. Aquino, A. C. King, A. Pikus, and R. M. Cohen, Normal activation of frontotemporal language cortex in dyslexia, as measured with oxygen 15 positron emission tomography, *Arch. Neurol. 51*:27 (1994).

79. J. M. Rumsey, P. Andreason, A. J. Zametkin, A. C. King, S. D. Hamburger, T. Aquino, A. P. Hanahan, A. Pikus, and R. M. Cohen, Right frontotemporal activation by tonal memory in dyslexia, an 015 PET study, *Biol. Psychiatry 36*:171 (1994).

80. S. Sherman, Epidemiology, *The Fragile X Syndrome* (R. J. Hagerman et al., eds,) Johns Hopkins University Press, Baltimore, MD, 1991, pp. 69–86.

81. A. J. Verkerk, M. Pieretti, J. S. Sutcliffe, and Y. H. Fu, Identification of a gene (FMR-1) containing CGG repeat coincident with a breakpoint cluster region exhibiting length variation in fragile X syndrome, *Cell 65*:905 (1991).

82. A. L. Reiss and L. Freund, Fragile x syndrome, *Soc. Biol. Psychiatry 27*:223 (1990).

83. L. A. Reiss, E. Aylward, L. S. Freund, P. K. Joshi, and R. N. Bryan, Neuroanatomy of fragile X syndrome: the poterior fossa, *Am. Neurol. Assoc. 29*:26 (1991).

84. L. A. Reiss, L. Freund, J. E. Tseng, and P. K. Joshi, Neuroanatomy in fragile x females: the posterior fossa, *Hum. Genet. 49*:179 (1991).

85. A. L. Reiss, J. Lee, and L. Freund, Neuroanatomy of fragile X syndrome: the temporal lobe, *Neurology 44*:1317 (1994).

86. H. L. Hinds, C. T. Ashley, J. S. Sutcliffe, and D. L. Nelson, Tissue specific expression of FMR-1 provides evidence for a functional role in fragile X syndrome, *Nature Genetics 3*:36 (1993).

87. J. H. Beitchman, Childhood schizophrenia: a review and comparison with adult-onset schizophrenia, *Psychiatr. Clin. North Am. 8*:793 (1985).

88. M. Kramer, Population changes and schizophrenia, *The Nature of Schizophrenia: New Approaches to Research and Treatment* (L. C. Wynne et al., eds.), John Wiley and Sons, New York, 1978, pp. 1970–1985.

89. M. Karno and G. S. Norquist, Schizophrenia: epidemiology, *Comprehensive Textbook of Psychiatry V* (H. I. Kaplan et al., eds.), Williams and Wilkins, Baltimore, MD, 1989, p. 699.

90. W. H. Green, M. Padron-Gayol, A. S. Hardesty, and M. Bassiri, Schizophrenia with childhood-onset: a phenomenological study of 38 cases, *J. Am. Acad. Child Adol. Psychiatry 31*:976 (1992).

91. F. Volkmar, D. Cohen, V. Hoshino, R. Rende, and R. Paul, Phenomenology and classification of the childhood psychoses, *Psychol. Med. 18*:191 (1988).

92. A. T. Russell, L. Bott, and C. Sammons, The phenomenology of schizophrenia occuring in childhood, *J. Amr. Acad. Child Adol. Psychiatry 28*:399 (1989).

93. C. T. Gordon, J. A. Frazier, K. McKenna, J. Giedd, A. Zametkin, T. Zahn, D. Hommer, W. Hong, D. Kaysen, and K. E. Albus, Childhood-onset schizophrenia: an NIMH study in progress, *Schizophr. Bull. 20*:697 (1994).

94. E. K. Spencer and M. Campbell, Children with schizophrenia: diagnosis, phenomenology, and pharmacotherapy, *Schizophr. Bull. 20*:713 (1994).

95. J. Alaghband-Rad, K. McKenna, C. T. Gordon, K. Albus, S. D. Hamburger, J. M. Rumsey, J. A. Frazier, M. C. Lenane, and J. L. Rapoport, Childhood-onset schizophrenia: the severity of premorbid course, unpublished.

96. L. Marsh, R. L. Suddath, N. Higgins, and D. R. Weinberger, Medial temporal lobe structures in schizophrenia: relationship of size to duration of illness, *Schizophr. Res. 11*:225 (1994).

97. M. E. Shenton, R. Kikinis, F. A. Jolesz, S. D. Pollak, M. LeMay, C. G. Wible, H. Hokama, J. Martin, D. Metcalf, and M. Coleman, Abnormalities of the left temporal lobe and thought disorder in schizophrenia. A quantitative magnetic resonance imaging study, *N. Engl. J. Med. 327*:604 (1992).

98. N. C. Andreasen, H. A. Nasrallah, V. Dunn, S. C. Olson, W. M. Grove, J. C. Ehrhardt, J. A. Coffman, and J. H. W. Crossett, Structural abnormalities in the frontal system in schizophrenia: a magnetic resonance imaging study, *Arch. Gen. Psychiatry 43*:136 (1986).

99. N. C. Andreasen, J. C. Ehrhardt, V. W. Swayze, 2d, R. J. Alliger, W. T. Yuh, G. Cohen, and S. Ziebell, Magnetic resonance imaging of the brain in schizophrenia. The pathophysiologic significance of structural abnormalities, *Arch. Gen. Psychiatry 47*:35 (1990).

100. A. Breier, R. W. Buchanan, A. Elkashef, R. C. Munson, B. Kirkpatrick, and F. Gellad, Brain morphology and schizophrenia. A magnetic resonance imaging study of limbic, prefrontal cortex, and caudate structures, *Arch. Gen. Psychiatry 49*:921 (1992).

101. D. R. Weinberger and R. J. Wyatt, Cerebral ventricular size: a biological marker for subtyping schizophrenia, *Biological Markers in Psychiatry and Neurology* (E. Usdin et al., eds.), Pergamon Press Inc, Elmsford, NY, 1982, pp. 505–512.

102. L. E. DeLisi, A. L. Hoff, J. E. Schwartz, G. W. Shields, S. N. Halthore, S. M. Gupta, F. A. Henn, and A. K. Anand, Brain morphology in first-episode schizophrenic-like psychotic patients: a quantitative magnetic resonance imaging study [published erratum appears in Biol Psychiatry 1991 Mar 1;29(5): 519], *Biol. Psychiatry 29*:159 (1991).

103. R. M. Bilder, H. Wu, B. Bogerts, G. Degreef, M. Ashtari, J. M. Alvir, P. J. Snyder, and J. A. Lieberman, Absence of regional hemispheric volume asymmetries in first-episode schizophrenia, *Am. J. Psychiatry 151*:1437 (1994).

104. M. H. Chakos, J. A. Lieberman, R. M. Bilder, M. Borenstein, G. Lerner, B. Bogerts, H. Wu, B. Kinon, and M. Ashtari, Increase in caudate nuclei volumes of first-episode schizophrenic patients taking antipsychotic drugs, *Am. J. Psychiatry 151*:1430 (1994).

105. A. M. Elkashef, R. W. Buchanan, F. Gellad, R. C. Munson, and A. Breier, Basal ganglia pathology in schizophrenia and tardive dyskinesia: an mri quantitative study, *Am. J. Psychiatry 151*:752 (1994).

106. V. W. Swayze, 2d, N. C. Andreasen, R. J. Alliger, W. T. Yuh, and J. C. Ehrhardt, Subcortical and temporal structures in affective disorder and schizo-

phrenia: a magnetic resonance imaging study (see comments), *Biol. Psychiatry 31*:221 (1992).

107. T. L. Jernigan, S. Zisook, R. K. Heaton, J. T. Moranville, J. R. Hesselink, and D. L. Braff, Magnetic resonance imaging abnormalities in lenticular nuclei and cerebral cortex in schizophrenia, *Arch. Gen. Psychiatry 48*:881 (1991).

108. N. C. Andreasen, S. Arndt, V. Swayze, T. Cizadlo, M. Flaum, D. O'Leary, J. C. Ehrhardt, and W. T. C. Yuh, Thalamic abnormalities in schizophrenia visualized through magnetic resonance image averaging, *Science 266*:294 (1994).

109. M. Flaum, V. W. Swayze, 2nd, D. S. O'Leary, W. T. Yuh, J. C. Ehrhardt, S. V. Arndt, and N. C. Andreasen, Effects of diagnosis, laterality, and gender on brain morphology in schizophrenia, *Am. J. Psychiatry 152*:704 (1995).

110. R. C. Woody, K. Bolyard, G. Eisenhauer, and L. Altschuler, CT scan and MRI findings in a child with schizophrenia, *J. Child. Neurol. 2*:105 (1987).

111. R. L. Hendron, J. E. Hodde-Vargas, L. A. Vargas, W. W. Orrison, and L. Dell, Magnetic resonance imaging of severely disturbed children: a preliminary study, *J. Am. Acad. Child Adol. Psychiatry 30*:466 (1991).

112. S. C. Schultz, M. M. Koller, R. R. Kishore, R. M. Hamer, J. J. Gehl, and R. O. Friedel, Ventricular enlargement in teenage patients with schizophrenia spectrum disorder, *Am. J. Psychiatry 140*:1592 (1983).

113. L. K. Jacobsen, J. N. Giedd, A. C. Vaituzis, S. D. Hamburger, J. C. Rajapakse, J. A. Frazier, D. Kaysen, M. C. Lenane, K. McKenna, C. T. Gordon, and J. L. Rapoport, Temporal lobe morphology in childhood onset schizophrenia, *Am. J. Psychiatry 153*:355 (1996).

114. J. A. Frazier, J. N. Giedd, S. O. Hamburger, K. E. Albus, D. Kaysen, A. C. Vaituzis, J. C. Rajapakse, M. C. Lenane, K. McKenna, L. K. Jacobsen, C. T. Gordon, A. Breier, and J. L. Rapoport, Brain anatomic magnetic resonance imaging in childhood onset schizophrenia, *Arch. Gen. Psychiatry 53*:617 (1996).

115. M. S. Keshavan, W. W. Bagwell, G. L. Haas, J. A. Sweeney, N. R. Schooler, and J. W. Pettegrew, Changes in caudate volume with neuroleptic treatment, *Lancet 344*:1434 (1994).

116. J. A. Frazier, J. N. Giedd, D. Kaysen, K. Albus, S. Hamburger, J. Alaghband-Rad, M. C. Lenane, A. Breier, and J. L. Rapoport, Childhood onset schizophrenia: brain magnetic resonance imaging rescan after two years of clozapine maintenance, *Am. J. Psychiatry 153*:564 (1996).

117. R. B. Zipursky, K. O. Lim, E. V. Sullivan, B. W. Brown, and A. Pfefferbaum, Widespread cerebral gray matter volume deficits in schizophrenia, *Arch. Gen. Psychiatry 49*:195 (1992).

118. H. A. Nasrallah, N. C. Andreasen, J. A. Coffman, S. C. Olson, V. O. Dunn, J. C. Ehrhardt, and S. M. Chapman, A controlled magnetic resonance imaging study of corpus callosum thickness in schizophrenia, *Biol. Psychiatry 21*:274 (1986).

119. K. O. Lim, D. Harris, M. Beal, A. L. Hoff, K. Minn, J. G. Csernansky, W. O. Faustman, L. Marsh, E. V. Sullivan, and A. Pfefferbaum, Gray matter deficits in young onset schizophrenia are independent of age of onset, *Biol. Psychiatry 40*:4 (1996).

120. J. M. Watkins, R. F. Asarnow, and P. E. Tanguay, Symptom development in childhood onset schizophrenia, *J. Am. Acad. Child Adol. Psychiatry 6*:865 (1988).

121. R. M. Murray, E. O'Callaghan, D. J. Castle, and S. H. Lewis, Neurodevelopmental approach to the classification of schizophrenia, *Schizophr. Bull. 18*:319 (1992).

122. F. G. Ebaugh, Neuropsychiatric aspects of chorea in children, *JAMA 87*:1083 (1926).

123. S. E. Swedo, H. L. Leonard, M. B. Schapiro, B. J. Casey, G. B. Mannheim, M. C. Lenane, and D. C. Rettew, Sydenham's chorea: physical and psychological symptoms of St. Vitus dance, *Pediatrics 91*:706 (1993).

124. G. H. Stollerman, Rheumatic fever, *Harrison's Principles of Internal Medicine* (J. O. Wilson et al., eds), McGraw-Hill, New York, 1991, p. 935.

125. Guidelines for the diagnosis of rheumatic fever. Jones Criteria, 1992 update. Special Writing Group of the Committee of Rheumatic Fever, Endocarditis, and Kawasaki Disease of the Council on Cardiovascular Disease of the Young of the American Heart Association, *JAMA 268*:2069 (1992).

126. A. Taranta and G. H. Stollerman, The relationship of Sydenham's chorea to infection with group A streptococci, *Am. J. Med. 20*:170 (1956).

127. J. Goldenberg, M. B. Ferraz, A. S. M. Fonseca, M. O. Hilario, W. Bastos, and S. Sachetti, Sydenham chorea: clinical and laboratory findings. Analysis of 187 cases, *Rev. Paul. Med. 110*(4):152 (1992).

128. E. M. Ayoub and L. W. Wannamaker, Streptococcal antibody titers in Sydenham's chorea, *Pediatrics 38*(6):946 (1966).

129. L. H. Ziegler, The neuropathological findings in a case of acute Sydenham's chorea, *J. Nerv. Mental Dis. 65*:273 (1927).

130. J. G. Greenfield and J. M. Wolfsohn, The pathology of Sydenham's chorea, *Lancet 32*:603 (1922).

131. R. Kolb and I. Whishaw, *Fundamentals of Human Neuropsychology*, Freeman, New York, 1990.

132. G. Husby, I. Van De Rijn, J. B. Zabriskie, Z. H. Abdin, and R. C. Williams, Antibodies reacting with cytoplasm of subthalamic and caudate nuclei neurons in chorea and acute rheumatic fever, *J. Exp. Med. 144*:1094 (1976).

133. S. Goldman, D. Amrom, H. B. Szliwowski, D. Detemmerman, L. M. Bidaut, E. Stanus, and A. Luxen, Reversible striatal hypermetabolism in a case of Sydenham's chorea, *Movement Disord. 8*(3):355 (1993).

134. M. Jergas, N. Heye, D. Pohlau, and J. Schaffstein, Computertomographische Befunde bei Chorea minor (Sydenham) [Computed tomographic findings in chorea minor (Sydenham's chorea)], *Fortsch. Rontgenst. 157*:288 (1992).

135. G. D. Kienzle, R. K. Breger, R. W. M. Chun, M. L. Zupanc, and J. F. Sackett, Sydenham chorea: MR manifestations in two cases, *Am. J. Neuroradiol. 12*: 73 (1991).

136. M. Konagaya and Y. Knoagaya, MRI in hemiballism due to Sydenham's chorea, *J. Neurol. Neurosurg. Psychiatry 55*(3):238 (1992).

137. N. Heye, M. Jergas, H. Hotzinger, J. Farahati, D. Pohlau, and H. Przuntek,

Sydenham chorea: clinical, EEG, MRI and SPECT findings in the early stage of the disease, *J. Neurol. 240*:121 (1993).

138. J. N. Giedd, J. L. Rapoport, M. J. P. Kruesi, C. Parker, M. B. Schapiro, A. J. Allen, H. L. Leonard, D. Kaysen, D. P. Dickstein, W. L. Marsh, P. L. Kozuch, A. C. Vaituzis, S. Hamburger, and S. E. Swedo, Sydenham's chorea: magnetic resonance imaging of the basal ganglia, *Neurology 25*:11 (1995).

139. S. E. Swedo, J. L. Rapoport, D. L. Cheslow, H. L. Leonard, E. M. Ayoub, D. M. Hosier, and E. R. Wald, High prevalence of obsessive-compulsive symptoms in patients with Sydenham's chorea, *Am. J. Psychiatry 146*(2):246 (1989).

141. J. N. Giedd, J. L. Rapoport, H. L. Leonard, D. Richter, and S. E. Swedo, Acute basal ganglia enlargement and obsessive compulsive symptoms in an adolescent boy, *J. Am. Acad. Child Adol. Psychiatry 35*(7):913 (1995).

142. J. N. Giedd, P. Kozuch, D. Kaysen, A. C. Vaituzis, S. D. Hamburger, J. J. Bartko, and J. L. Rapoport, Reliability of cerebral measures in repeated examinations with magnetic resonance imaging, *Psychiatry Res. Neuroimaging 61*:113 (1995).

143. B. Peterson, M. A. Riddle, D. J. Cohen, L. O. Katz, J. C. Smith, M. T. Hardin, and J. F. Leckman, Reduced basal ganglia volumes in Tourette's syndrome using three-dimensional reconstruction techniques from magnetic resonance images, *Neurology 43*:941 (1993).

144. H. S. Singer, A. L. Reiss, J. E. Brown, E. H. Aylward, B. Shih, E. Chee, E. L. Harris, M. J. Reader, G. A. Chase, R. N. Bryan, and M. B. Denckla, Volumetric MRI changes in basal ganglia of children with Tourette's syndrome, *Neurology 43*:950 (1993).

145. T. M. Hyde, M. E. Stacey, R. Coppola, S. F. Handel, K. C. Rickler, and D. R. Weinberger, Cerebral morphometric abnormalities in Tourette's syndrome: a quantitative MRI study of monozygotic twins, *Neurology 45*:1176 (1995).

146. F. X. Castellanos, J. N. Giedd, S. D. Hamburger, W. L. Marsh, and J. L. Rapoport, Brain morphometry in Tourette's syndrome: the influence of comorbid attention-deficit/hyperactivity disorder, *Neurology* (in press).

147. B. S. Peterson, J. F. Leckman, J. S. Duncan, R. Wetzles, and M. A. Riddle, Corpus callosum morphology from magnetic resonance images in Tourette's syndrome, *Psychiatry Res. Neuroimaging 55*:85 (1994).

148. D. F. Harcherik, D. J. Cohen, S. Ort, et al. Computed tomographic brain scanning in four neuropsychiatric disorders of childhood, *Am. J. Psychiatry 142*:731 (1985).

149. A. R. Braun, B. Stoetter, C. Randolph, et al. The functional neuroanatomy of Tourette's syndrome: an FDG-PET study. I. Regional changes in cerebral glucose metabolism differentiating patients and controls, *Neuropsychopharmacology 9*:277 (1993).

150. T. N. Chase, V. Geoffrey, M. Gillespie, and G. H. Burrows, Structural and functional studies of Gilles de la Tourette syndrome, *Rev. Neurol. 142*:851 (1986).

151. M. Hall, D. C. Costa, J. Shields, J. Heavens, M. Robertson, and P. J. Ell, Brain perfusion patterns with Tc-99mHMPAO/SPECT in patients with Gilles de la Tourette syndrome, *Eur. J. Nuclear Med. 16*:56 (1990).

152. M. S. George, M. R. Trimble, D. C. Costa, M. M. Robertson, H. A. Ring, and P. J. Ell, Elevated frontal cerebral blood flow in Gilles de la Tourette syndrome: a 99Tcm-HMPAO SPECT study, *Psychiatry Res. Neuroimaging* *45*:143 (1992).

153. K. G. Sieg, D. Buckingham, G. R. Gaffney, D. F. Preston, and K. G. Sieg, Tc-99m HMPAO SPECT brain imaging of Gilles de la Tourette's syndrome, *Clin. Nuclear Med. 18*:255 (1993).

7

The Neuromorphometry of Affective Disorders

Kelly N. Botteron

Washington University School of Medicine, St. Louis, Missouri

Gary S. Figiel
Emory University, Atlanta, Georgia

I. INTRODUCTION

In the past, neurobiological research in affective disorders has focused on neuroendocrinology, neurochemistry, metabolism, cognitive function, and treatment response. Recently there has been renewed interest in the anatomical neuropathology associated with affective disorders, and structural neuroimaging techniques using computerized tomography (CT) and magnetic resonance imaging (MRI) have enabled the quantitative examination of neuromorphometry in vivo. These quantitative neuromorphometric techniques are being widely applied to investigate psychiatric disorders—largely schizophrenia and, to a lesser degree, affective disorders. Understanding the cerebral structural correlates of affective disorder will add significantly to our understanding of the pathophysiology of affective disorders for several reasons. First, it has been established in several other neuropsychiatric disorders that the size of a brain region reflects its function [1,2], indicating that neuromorphometric investigations are an important complement to functional investigating such as PET or SPECT studies. Second, morphometric analysis can help to characterize underlying neurodevelopmental versus neurodegenerative processes through both longitudinal and cross-sectional investigations. Third, structural studies can serve as a framework to direct or interpret other types of investigation such as receptor imaging, neuropathological, and histopathological studies.

Many neuroimaging investigations have reported structural differences in subjects with affective disorders, however, conflicting results are common in the limited number of available investigations, thus the structural correlates of affective disorders remain poorly understood. Early investigations using CT examined gross structural differences such as cerebral atrophy, ventricular enlargement, or cerebellar atrophy. Many of these investigations reported significant differences in these features from comparison controls, however, results from other studies were negative. More recent MRI investigations have employed increasingly sophisticated imaging and research methodology, allowing for the quantitative examination of specific defined brain regions. Because neuropsychological and functional studies suggest abnormalities in frontal, temporal, and subcortical regions, many investigators have focused MRI neuromorphometric studies on these temporal limbic structures. However, the number of investigations examining each of these regions remains small and conflicting results continue to be reported. It does appear clear that for many brain regions the structural changes from normal may be subtle, and that differences in research methodologies between studies and across centers may lead to differences in reported results.

This chapter will review neuromorphometric imaging studies of affective disorders published to date. As noted earlier, methodological issues are critical in interpreting the results of imaging studies. Several issues are specifically pertinent to this review, because they are present in many of the affective disorder studies reported to date. First, until very recently estimates of structural volumes have largely consisted of linear and area measures, structured rating scales, and a few volumetric estimates. The first three estimates all have significant problems as volume estimators. The few available volumetric studies reported to date were completed with scanning sequences with image slice thickness of 5 mm or more, compared with current protocols, which easily obtain 1.0- to 1.5-mm-thick slices. The thicker 5-mm slices have substantially greater partial volume effects, which decreases the measurement precision and reliability, potentially obscuring small volumetric differences between groups. (All volumetric studies discussed in this chapter were based on ≥5-mm-thick slices unless otherwise indicated.) Second, many studies have not used screened normal comparison controls, but rather samples of convenience such as scans read as normal on individuals being scanned for evaluation of headaches, seizure, and trauma. Additionally many studies have examined heterogeneous populations of affective disorder subjects, and this heterogeneity may have the effect of masking potentially true differences.

II. GLOBAL CHANGES: VENTRICLES, CEREBRAL VOLUME, AND ATROPHY

A. Lateral Ventricles

1. Controlled CT and MRI Investigations

Ventricular size in affective disorders has now been examined in over 30 studies and remains poorly defined. Early investigations beginning in the 1980s examined lateral ventricular size using CT scans to determine ventricular brain ratios (VBR) [3]. Many studies using CT have demonstrated that, compared to controls, lateral ventricular size is increased in patients with affective disorders [4–17]. Consistent with these findings, several studies have also examined the lateral ventricular size in affective disordered subjects compared to schizophrenic subjects and have not shown statistically significant differences in VBRs between the two groups [4,5,11,18–25]. Lateral ventricular enlargement is established as a highly consistent finding in schizophrenia [26]. In contrast, there have also been reports of no observed increases in VBR in patients with affective disorders compared with controls [18,20,24,25,27–30]. However, many of the studies that found no overall increase in the VBR of patients with affective disorders reported that subgroups of patients had enlarged VBRs or demonstrated significant correlations between increased VBR and specific clinical characteristics.

The CT scan–based literature on ventricular enlargement has numerous methodological problems. For example, in the majority of these studies the ventricular size estimates were based on VBRs that sample only one portion of the ventricular system with the assumption that this measurement reflects total ventricular volume [31]. Area measures based on a single slice are subject to errors related to differences in head positioning. As a result of these methodological problems, few conclusions or comparisons between studies can be drawn. Many studies also used comparison groups using not strictly normal controls, but at times patients being evaluated for headaches or other neurological complaints who were not screened for possible psychiatric or other illnesses. Finally, in many studies patient groups were often mixed including all as ages as well as bipolar, unipolar, and psychotic patients without diagnostic groups examined separately. Despite these significant methodological issues, a review of the literature prior to 1988 by Jeste et al. [27] calculated from all the available studies that the mean ratio of VBRs in affective disorder patients was 1:1 to schizophrenic patients and 1.5:1 to control subjects and noted that there was ventricular enlargement in 11–29% of unipolar and bipolar patients.

Recent controlled MRI studies have also reported conflicting findings for overall ventricular size (Table 1). Unfortunately these studies have used varying methods of assessing ventricular size including traditional axial VBR area measures, coronal VBR measures, semistructured rating scales, and ventricular volume measures. Besson et al. [32] compared 10 bipolar patients to 10 screened controls and found no significant difference in VBRs based on a single axial image. Johnstone et al. [33] compared the right and left ventricular area as determined from a single coronal MRI image in bipolar, schizophrenic, and normal controls and found no significant group differences. Figiel et al. [34] examined ventricular size on MRIs in bipolar subjects compared to a group of normal controls using a visual rating scale and reported that 40% of their bipolar group had mildly to severely enlarged lateral ventricles compared to 0% in the control population. Lesser et al. [35] calculated VBRs using MRI scans to compare late-age-onset psychotic depressives to normal controls and found no significant differences in ventricular size. Rabins et al. [36] compared lateral ventricular size based on visual rating scales in elderly depressed patients compared to age-matched controls and found that the depressed subjects had significantly larger ventricles. More recent investigations have included measurement of ventricular volume. Swayze et al. [37] calculated lateral ventricular volumes based on seven coronal slices (1-cm thickness with no interslice gap) in bipolar, schizophrenic, and normal controls. They found no significant group differences, but reported a trend for male bipolar patients to have enlarged ventricles. This was the first study done measuring total ventricular volume. A subsequent report by Coffey et al. [38] estimated ventricular volumes from coronal images (5-mm-thick contiguous slices) in 48 depressed subjects and 76 normal controls. After partialing out effects of age, sex, cranial size, and years of education, no significant difference was detected, although they reported that examination of their confidence intervals reveals that the volume may be as much as 50% larger in the depressed population and that their sample size may have been inadequate to detect differences. Strakowski et al. [39] studied a group of 17 patients with their first episode of mania to explore whether prolonged illness, treatment effects, or comorbid conditions such as substance abuse were significantly contributing to ventricular enlargement and other structural changes in bipolar disorder. They compared their first-episode manics to screened normal controls using coronal MRI images (6-mm-thick contiguous slices). Ventricular volumes were determined using a combination of semi-automated threshholding and manually outlining the structures of interest. They reported a trend for increased lateral ventricular volume in the manic patients.

Elkis et al. [40] recently reported a review with meta-analysis of the available studies examining ventricular size in affective disorder. Meta-analyses are particularly appropriate for examining for potential Type II errors in a series of adequately designed studies, which may have missed a positive finding secondary to examining a variable with a small effect size with a small number of subjects. This could accurately characterize many of the investigations of ventricular size in affective disorder. Their recent meta-analytic review included all available studies with appropriately controlled design for which an effect size could be calculated, and their summary of 29 published MRI and CT studies reported a moderate to small effect size of $+0.437$. This composite effect size was highly statistically significant ($p < 0.001$), suggesting that studies to date support that ventricular size is significantly different in an affectively disordered population as compared to controls.

2. Clinical Correlates of Lateral Ventricular Enlargement

Many studies have reported significant clinical correlates to increased VBRs in affective disorders. Some studies have demonstrated a correlation with

Table 1 MRI Studies of Lateral Ventricular Size in Patients with Affective Disorders

Source	Affective disorder subjects		Ventricular measure used	Controls		Ventricular size	Significant group differences	Clinic correlates
	N	Age		N	Age			
Besson et al., 1987	10 BP (8F, 2M)	48.5 ± 9.5	Axial VBR area (4.49 ± 82)	10C (8F, 2M)	42.3 ± 8.9	4.26 ± 0.3	None	Limited exam, none reported
Johnstone et al., 1989	20 BP (8F, 12M)	38.9 ± 8.1	Coronal ventricular area	21 C	34.3	Coronal ventricular area	None	Age (<0.01)
Figiel et al., 1991	18 BP (13F, 5M)	37.5	Structured rating scale 44% mild to severe ventricular enlargement	18C (15F, 3M)	34.7	No ventricular enlargement	BP > controls	Not related to T2 weighted MRI, DWMH
Swayze et al., 1990	48 BP (19F, 29M)	34.0	Volume: coronal tracings summed (48 cm^3)	47C (19F, 28M)	34.4	47 cm^3	Schizophrenics vs. controls ($p < 0.05$)	Trend for male BP increased volume; trend for T2-weighted DWMH
				54S (18F, 36M)	33.3	52 cm^3		

Study	Subjects	Age	Method	Controls	Control age	Control volume/VBR	Findings
Lesser et al., 1991	14 MDD, LAOP (10F, 4M)	56.9 ± 6.0 (all > 45)	Axial VBR (10.0 ± 4.9)	72C (44F, 28M)	61.5 ± 9.9	8.5 ± 4.0 (VBR)	None related to increased ventricles None
Rabins et al., 1991	21 MDD elderly		Structured rating scale	14C 16A			Elderly depressed and A.D. vs. controls ($p < 0.05$)
Risch et al., 1992	8 BP 19 MDD	39.6 ± 8.7 43.0 ± 10.9	Axial VBR	94C	32.8 ± 8.9		None
Coffey et al., 1993	48 MDD (31F, 17M)	62.4 ± 16.4	21.2 mL (adjusted volume)	76C (51F, 25M)	61.6 ± 15.9	18.01 mL (Adjusted volume)	None
Strakowski et al., 1993	17 BP first episode (10F, 7M)	28.4 ± 6.8	Volume: semiautomated coronal segmentation	15C (8F, 7M)	30.9 ± 7.3		None

BP, bipolar disorder; MDD, major depressive disorder; LAOP, late-age-onset psychosis; C, indicates community control, clinically screened; S, schizophrenic control; M, medical control; A, Alzheimer control; DWMH, deep white matter hyperintensities.

increasing age [4,13,14,16,28,33,36] for patients over the age of 50, but there is no reported significant relationship to age for younger subjects. There has been very little examination of ventricular (or other structural) changes over time. No prospective investigations have yet been reported. Vita et al. [41] reported a significant increase in ventricular size over a mean of 35 months in middle-aged affective disordered patients. This increase was not found in schizophrenic patients. In contrast, Woods et al. [42] with a retrospective design found no significant increase in VBR in bipolar patients. A significant relationship between increased VBR and psychoses has been reported by five groups [6,10,11,16,41,43,44]. Several groups were unable to find a relationship with psychoses [45,46]. No specific relationship has been found to treatment response although most analyses are retrospective [7,12,14,15,44,46–50]. Two exceptions, Nasrallah et al. [46] and Roy-Byrne et al. [45], reported a negative correlation between VBRs and number of hospitalizations in females and length and number of episodes in males. Follow-up studies have also demonstrated no differences in number of hospitalizations or in treatment response, however, treatments were variable and not controlled [11,17,50,51]. Some authors have reported a significant effect of sex [14,16,25,36,37], while others have reported no significant effect of sex on ventricular size [12,22,24]. Several groups have demonstrated neuropsychological deficits in affective disordered patients, and there are reports of an association of Halsted Reitan deficits to increased VBRs in middle-aged [44,48,52] and elderly depressed patients [17,50]. Other reported clinical correlates of increased VBRs which require further study include unemployment [22], negative symptoms [22,43,44,48] psychomotor retardation, emotional blunting [43], and hypothyroidism [53].

The literature on increased ventricular size in the elderly depressed is more consistent. The majority of studies have reported increased lateral ventricular size as estimated by CT scan VBRs [17,28,54] and MRI ratings of ventricular size [36], although there have been some negative reports [35]. Increased ventricular size in elderly depressed patients has been associated with higher mortality rates [55], later onset of illness [36], decreased CT attenuation values [17,51,56], "pseudodementia" [17], and the presence of severe white matter hyperintensities on brain MRI images [57]. Similar to reports in younger affective disorder patients, several studies have replicated an association with increased ventricular size and statistically significant deficits on neuropsychological testing in elderly depressed patients: slowed speed in delayed matching and digit copying [54] and decreased immediate verbal recall [17]. Also, some neuropsychological deficits on Halsted Reitan that persist after resolution of depression, including slowing, errors made, and spatial recognition, are related to increased ventricular size [54].

The relationship between cortisol status and ventricular enlargement has been examined by several different authors. All but three studies [47,58,59] reported that dexamethasone suppression test (DST) suppression status is unrelated to VBR [10,16,60,61]. Two groups using different experimental approaches have demonstrated significant correlations between basal cortisol status and increased VBR. Kellner et al. [62] found a significant relationship between 24-hour urine free cortisol and ventricular size in depressed patients, and Schlegel et al. [58] reported a significant correlation between baseline plasma cortisol levels (collected every 20 minutes over a 3-hour period) and ventricular size. Dewan et al. [60] could not find a significant relationship to cortisol when using only two baseline cortisol levels. Rothschild et al. [47], however, did report a trend for VBR to correlate with baseline cortisol levels and dexamethasone nonsuppression. Other hypercortisolemic states, such as Cushing's disease, are associated with demonstrable ventricular dilation, which has been shown to resolve with resolution of the hypercortisolemic state [63]. These findings raise additional questions about the stability or state dependency of ventricular findings in affective disorders and their potential relationship to cortisol status. Coffey et al. [61] found no relationship between DST status and ventricular volume (or other brain regional volumes) after correction for the effects of age, sex, and cranial volume. Several of their subjects receiving serial MRI and DST exams had no significant change in volumes following resolution of their affective disorder and normalization of their DST status. This study did not support a relationship between cortisol status and ventricular volume, but only used the DST as a measure of cortisol status.

Several additional biochemical correlates of ventricular enlargement have been reported. Meltzer et al. [64] demonstrated a significant inverse relationship between serum levels of dopamine-β-hydroxylase and ventricular enlargement; this relationship was also reported in schizophrenics with ventricular enlargement. Standish-Barry et al. [49] found a significant correlation between ventricular CSF 5HIAA levels and ventricular enlargement and a negative correlation to plasma free tryptophan levels in a series of patients who were referred and underwent neurosurgical procedures for intractable mood disorders.

B. Third Ventricle

Enlarged third ventricles in patients with affective disorders were first observed in pneumoencephalographic studies by Nagy [65] and Otsuki et al. [66], who described a subgroup of affective disordered patients with enlarged third ventricles. All studies that have examined third ventricular size by CT have reported an increased third ventricular width in affective disorder subjects compared to controls (Table 2) [16,24,29,44,67]. Two MRI studies have also reported an increased third ventricular size in a sample of elderly depressives [36] and a sample of first-onset manic subjects [39]. One MRI

Table 2   Investigations of Third Ventricular Size in Affective Disorder

Source	Imaging method	Affective disorder subjects	Control subjects	Group differences
Tanaka et al., 1982	CT	9 BP 31 MDD	40 N	BP/MDD > control
Schlegal and Kretschmar, 1987/1989	CT	60 MDD/BP	60 C	MDD/BP > control
Dewan et al., 1988	CT	26 BP	22 C	BP > control
Iacono et al., 1988	CT	18 BP 16 MDD	44 C 51 S 30 M	BP/MDD > control
Rabins et al., 1991	MRI	21 MDD (elderly)	14 C 14 A	MDD > normal
Coffey et al., 1993	MRI	44 MDD 4 BP	76 C	No differences
Strakowski et al., 1993	MRI	17 BP	16 C	BP > control

BP, bipolar disorder; MDD, major depressive disorder; C, indicates community control, clinically screened; S, schizophrenic control; M, medical control; A, Alzheimer control; N, neurological control.

investigation examining individuals with major depression found no significant difference in third ventricular volume in comparison to controls [38]. Two investigators have reported third ventricular size to be significantly correlated to psychosis [38,44,68], and Schlegal et al. also found correlations with increased age, later age of onset, male gender, unipolarity, positive DST testing and motor and verbal retardation [44]. Most other investigators have not reported clinical correlates of third ventricular size, thus these correlations have not yet been replicated.

In summary, if all the studies on ventricular size in affective disorders are taken in perspective, it appears that enlarged lateral ventricles are seen in a subgroup of young affective disordered patients and are more consistently seen in older patients. In younger individuals, it is possible that the enlargement of the lateral ventricles may be related to hypercortisolemia, although recent investigations are providing less support for this theory [61]. The ventricular enlargement observed in some elderly depressed patients may reflect a progressive shrinkage of subcortical white and gray matter, which potentially could lead to a secondary "ex vacuo" expansion of the lateral ventricles. However, in the absence of postmortem data, these observations remain speculative. In addition, the presence of similar increases in ventricular size in patients with schizophrenia, dementia, and other neuropsychiatric disorders reveals the lack of specificity for these findings. Despite the lack of specificity, ventricular enlargement serves as an indicator of reduced tissue volume in other brain regions and is a marker of clear neuropathology in affective disorders. For example, increased third ventricular volume could represent decreased thalamic nuclei volume, and increased lateral ventricular volume could reflect changes in the volume of adjacent basal ganglia structures. Future work will need to examine larger numbers of homogeneous patient populations using brain MRI volumetric analyses to help further understand the potential structural and clinical correlates of ventricular enlargement in patients with affective disorders.

C. Cortical Atrophy

The majority of controlled studies examining cortical atrophy by CT scan report no significant differences between affective disorders and controls [16,18–21,24,28,58]. One MRI study also reported no significant atrophy [69]. These studies have used variable rating scales to evaluate overall cortical atrophy. Despite their individual negative reported results, a recent meta-analysis of the existing studies reported a composite effect size of 0.42, which was stated to be moderate to small and statistically significant [40]. Individual studies that have reported significant differences have noted regional atrophy in patients with major depression and bipolar disorder in the temporal lobes [16,67,70], the occipital lobes [47], inferior parietal areas [47,70], frontal lobes [16,70], and the interhemispheric fissures [16]. Two reports have found an increased incidence of atrophy in elderly depressed patients when compared to normal controls and younger depressed patients [21,36].

Many of these studies are limited by small sample size and diverse patient populations. In addition, the results of these studies are difficult to compare due to the use of different imaging protocols.

Quantitative volumetric reconstructions from MRI should provide a more definitive answer to the question of whether cortical atrophy exists in subgroups of patients with affective disorder. In fact, a few recent investigations have reported on overall cerebral volume and have not noted significant differences between normal controls, subjects with major depression and subjects with bipolar disorder [38,71–73].

III. THE CEREBELLUM

At least 10 studies have examined the cerebellum in affective disorders (Table 3). The majority of the studies examined cerebellar vermian atrophy

Table 3 Neuroimaging Investigations of the Cerebellum in Affective Disorder

Source	Imaging method	Affective disorder		Controls		Significant group differences	Clinical correlates
		N	Mean age	N	Mean age		
Heath et al., 1979	CT ratings of vermian atrophy	31 MDD + BP		65 S		29% MDD/BP patients and 34% schizophrenics with cerebellar abnormalities	None examined
Heath et al., 1982	CT ratings of atrophy	64 MDD/BP psychotic		50 S, 1541 M		BP/MDD > comparison schizophrenic > comparison	None
Lippman et al., 1982	CT blind ratings of vermian atrophy	18 BP		54 S, 79 C		BP vs. controls schizophrenics vs. controls	Alcohol abuse in BP patients ($p < 0.001$)
Nasrallah et al., 1982	CT blind ratings of 5 factors for overall cerebellar atrophy	24 BP (24M 0F)	30.8 ± 7.5	55 S / 27 T	29.9 ± 8.2 / 28.7 ± 5.8	Cerebellar atrophy in bipolars (24.8%) vs. schizophrenics (9.1%) vs. controls (3.7%) but no statistically significant difference	VBR ($p < 0.05$)
Weinberger et al., 1982	CT vermian atrophy	23 MDD (15F 8M)	30.3 ± 10.1	17 S (6F 11M)	28.3 ± 9.7	Atrophy in MDD (9%) and schizophrenia (12%) significantly greater than	None examined

Reference	Method	Patients	Age	Controls	Control age	Difference from controls	Comments
Yates et al., 1987	CT blind ratings of 5 factors for overall cerebellar atrophy	24 BP (12F 12M); 26 MDD (14F 12M)	35.5 ± 14.3; 37.3 ± 13.3	35 SA (16F 19M); 26 N; 108 S (43F 65M); 74 C	20.7 ± 6.2; 30.3 ± 6.9; 31.7 ± 10.4	other disorders and controls ($p < 0.03$); None	Trend for BP and age >50 to be associated with atrophy
Dewan et al., 1988	CT cerebellar density	26 BP (7F 19M)	32.7	22 N controls		None	
Reider et al., 1983	CT	19 BP (9F 10M)	43.6 ± 14.6	28 C (15F 13M)	25.9 ± 8.1	None	Small number in BP group showed atrophy; all BP with atrophy >50 years of age
Shah et al., 1992	MRI, anterior posterior, total vermian area	36 MDD	54.7 ± 19	30 C (20F 16M)	55.8 ± 19	MAD vs. controls, significantly smaller total, anterior ($p = 0.002$) and posterior ($p = 0.028$) vermis areas	Decline in size with age in affective disorder

BP, bipolar disorder; MDD, major depressive disorder; C, indicates community control, clinically screened; S, schizophrenic control; M, medical control; A, Alzheimer control; N, neurological control; T, trauma control.

in bipolar affective disorder compared to schizophrenics or controls and found significant atrophy in both groups compared to controls [20,74,75] and no difference between schizophrenics and bipolars [20,21,74–78]. Only two reports have observed no significant difference in cerebellar vermian atrophy between normal controls and bipolar patients [77,78]. All of these studies were done using visual rating scales of CT scans. There have been few tested or reported clinical correlates, but several groups found that elderly bipolars were more likely to exhibit cerebellar atrophy [21,78]. Nasrallah et al. [77] found a significant correlation to increased VBR, and one group found a significant correlation to alcohol consumption [75]. Dewan et al. [29] examined the CT density of the cerebellum and reported no significant difference from controls.

MRI has advantages over CT for posterior fossa structures because of high tissue contrast resolution, lack of bone artifact, and the ability to visualize structures in multiple planes. Shah et al. [79] were the first group to report on cerebellar structure in subjects with major affective disorder using MRI. They studied cerebellar vermian areas in 37 depressed subjects and 37 age- and sex-matched controls. They reported with MRI visual rating scales that the anterior, posterior, and total cerebellar vermian size is significantly smaller in depressed subjects as compared to controls, and that total and posterior vermis size declined with age significantly more in depressed subjects than in controls.

Recently, Shah et al. [79] reported that the brainstem and medulla areas were smaller in depressed patients compared with controls. In addition, they observed a striking age-related decline in the midbrain area of both groups. These findings are of interest, given the extensive neural interconnections between the brainstem and the cerebellum.

In conclusion, the majority of studies to date suggest that the cerebellum may be smaller in patients with affective disorders compared to controls but may not differ significantly from schizophrenic patients. These findings are of interest given that recent works have suggested a role for the cerebellum in vegetative functions, emotional behavior, and some higher cognitive tasks [79]. Clearly, additional MRI studies are needed that attempt to replicate Shah et al.'s findings and to further examine the potential clinical and structural correlates of reduced cerebellar size in patients with affective disorders.

IV. INTERHEMISPHERIC CONNECTIVITY: THE CORPUS CALLOSUM

The development of MRI has permitted visualization of the corpus callosum with high resolution. Three studies to date have examined corpus callosum dimensions in affective disorders. Hauser et al. [80] performed brain MRI scans on 24 schizophrenic patients, 22 bipolar patients, and 25 normal controls. Examining a midsagittal slice, specific collosal regions and the cerebral areas were measured. No significant differences in collosal widths, collosal area, and cerebral areas were found among diagnostic groups. Husain et al. [81] using midsagittal brain MRI slices, measured the cross-sectional area of the corpus callosum and the cerebral cortex in 20 depressed patients and 20 age-matched controls. They reported no significant group differences in any of these measurement. Coffman et al. [82] examined the potential neuropsychological correlates of corpus callosal area in 29 controls and 25 bipolar patients. They observed a smaller mean area for the corpus callosum in the bipolar patients. In addition, they reported that a reduction in callosal area was associated with global neuropsychological impairment. Wu et al. [83] studied 20 young adult patients with major depressive disorder (MDD) in comparison to 16 normal controls. A midsagittal slice was analyzed using a semi-automated edge finding algorithm, and the corpus callosum was subdivided into quarters. The corpus callosum was larger in the anterior and posterior quadrants in the depressed subjects.

To date, MRI studies are conflicting regarding the role of the corpus callosum in the pathophysiology of affective disorders. Additional studies are needed before any definitive conclusions can be reached.

V. SUBCORTICAL WHITE MATTER

A. Computed Tomography Attenuation

Before the advent of the more sophisticated technology of MRI, several investigators noted differences in subcortical white matter when studying differences in gray and white matter tissue properties by measuring CT attenuation values. Coffman et al. [84] compared subjects with bipolar affective disorder and schizophrenia and found the bipolar subjects to have increased white matter density. This finding was replicated by Dewan et al. [29], who compared bipolar patients to headache controls and found an increased white matter density in bipolar patients compared to controls in all areas and significant differences in several regions including the anterior white matter, right temporal lobe, bilateral caudate and thalamic nuclei. Neither of these investigators found any significant clinical correlations [85].

Pearlson et al. recently examined two groups of elderly depressed patients [17,56] and reported in both studies that elderly patients with dementia of depression had significantly decreased white matter attenuation values compared to controls. They also found that decreased attenuation values correlated with lower cognitive test scores on neuropsychological evaluation [51].

These brain density changes currently have unknown neuropathological correlates in affective disorders. However, in other disorders decreased CT density is related to increased tissue water content or decreased lipid tissue content. The reports of changes in white matter density on brain CT scans are of interest given the increasingly consistent finding of MRI white matter hyperintensities in patients with affective disorders.

B. Brain MRI Subcortical Hyperintensities

1. Elderly Depressed

   a. Rate and Severity of Hyperintensities With the advent of brain MRI, in vivo analysis of subcortical anatomy is now possible. Early research found a high incidence of subcortical hyperintensities in elderly depressed patients on T_2-weighted brain MRI scans. The potential significance of these early reports [86] was difficult to interpret due to the fact that subcortical hyperintensities were also reported to occur on 18–61% of brain MRI scans in healthy, nondemented elderly subjects. However, many of these studies with elderly populations were confounded by the inclusion of control subjects with cardiac, psychiatric, or neurological diseases.

   To more carefully examine the potential significance of subcortical hyperintensities on brain MRI in the elderly depressed, several groups compared the occurrence and severity of subcortical hyperintensities in elderly depressed patients with healthy elderly adults who had no history of significant psychiatric or neurological disorder.

   Coffey et al. [86] examined 51 elderly depressed subjects and 22 sex- and age-matched elderly volunteers recruited from the community. All brain MRI scans were performed on a General Electric 1.5 Tesla Signa System. Periventricular hyperintensities (PVH) were graded as follows: 0 = absent, 1 = caps or pencil-thin halo, 2 = smooth halo, 3 = irregular extension in the deep white matter. Deep white matter hyperintensities (DWMH) were graded as follows: 0 = absent, 1 = punctate foci, 2 = beginning confluence of foci, 3 = large confluent areas (Fig. 1). The rating scale was modified from Fazekas et al. [87]. Subcortical gray matter hyperintensities were noted by site (basal ganglia, thalamus, etc.) and side (Fig. 1). They found that grade 2 and grade 3 PVH were more common in depressed patients (62%) compared to controls (23%). Grade 2 and 3 deep white matter hyperintensities were also more common in the depressed group (55%) than in controls (14%). Hyperintensities of the basal ganglia were present in 51% of depressed patients and in 5% of controls. The occurrence of PVH, DWMH, and basal ganglia hyperintensities was associated with risk factors for cerebrovascular disease. Since vascular risk factors were more prevalent in depressed patients compared to control subjects, the potential differences could have

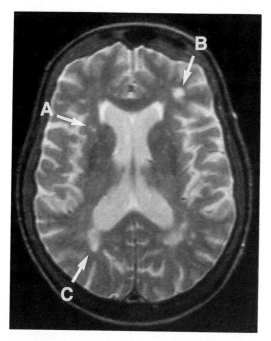

Fig. 1 T$_2$-weighted MR image from a 71-year-old female with late-onset major depression. This image demonstrates mild ventricular dilatation along with periventricular, deep white matter, and subcortical hyperintensities. (A) Multipunctate basal ganglia hyperintensities; (B) large confluent frontal DWMH; (C) periventricular capping and large confluent DWMH in the occipital lobe.

been related primarily to a difference in risk factors between the two groups. However, because lesions of the deep gray nuclei and large PVH or DWMH (grade 3) were not seen in any of the control subjects, they concluded that the site and size of the lesions may play a role in rendering some individuals vulnerable to developing depression.

Rabins et al. [36], using a rating scale for PVH, DWMH, and basal ganglia lesions similar to Coffey, compared 21 elderly depressed patients with 14 normal controls. Consistent with Coffey's findings [86], they observed a significant increase in basal ganglia lesions and DWMH in the elderly depressed compared with the healthy controls.

Figiel et al. [88] examined a group of 19 elderly depressed patients and 20 age- and sex-matched healthy elderly controls. All controls received a structured medical and neuropsychiatric evaluation prior to receiving a brain MRI, and any subject with a significant neurological or psychiatric history was excluded from the study. All brain MRI scans were performed on 1.5 Tesla General Electric systems. In this study the size and location of deep white matter and caudate nucleus hyperintensities were recorded. The two groups did not differ in atherosclerotic risk factors. Large (>1 cm) DWMH were observed in 2 of 20 (10%) control subjects and in 7 of 19 (37%) elderly depressed patients. In addition, caudate hyperintensities were observed in 2 of 20 (10%) control subjects and in 7 of 19 (37%) elderly depressed patients. Interestingly, the majority of large (>1 cm) DWMH and caudate hyperintensities were found in the group of elderly depressed patients who experienced their first episode of depression after the age of 60 ("late age onset"). The DWMH were commonly observed in the frontal lobes.

Lesser et al. [35] measured the volume of white matter hyperintensities in 14 patients with psychotic depression (mean age = 56.8 years) compared with 72 healthy controls (mean age of 61.5). All 14 patients had the onset of their psychotic symptoms after the age of 45. The two groups were significantly different. Seven of the 14 patients (50%) had a total volume of white matter hyperintensities (PVH and DWMH) of >3 cm compared to only 7 of 72 controls (9.7%).

Finally, Zubenko et al. [69] reported an increased prevalence of white matter hyperintensities in 67 elderly depressed patients compared with 44 healthy controls. The authors did not use a severity rating scale, nor did they comment on basal ganglia hyperintensities.

In summary, all studies to date have consistently found a more extensive area of deep white matter hyperintensities in elderly depressed patients compared with age-matched healthy elderly controls. Several investigators have noted the lesions to be more common in the frontal lobes. In addition, both Coffey and Figiel's studies observed a higher incidence of caudate hyperintensities in the elderly depressed. Given that frontal-basal ganglia pathways are believed to be important in mood regulation [89], it is speculated that frontal and caudate hyperintensities may play a role in the development of some late-age-onset depressions. The results of these studies emphasize the need for using standardized rating scales whenever examining differences in white matter hyperintensities between two groups. For example, no differences between the depressed elderly and control subjects would have been revealed if comparisons had been based solely on the neuroradiologists's clinical report for the presence or absence of hyperintensities. In addition, it is imperative that whenever comparing groups that atherosclerotic risk factors and age are recorded and considered in the analysis of data.

b.   Clinical Correlates of Subcortical Hyperintensities in the Depressed Elderly   Subcortical hyperintensities have been noted to have prognostic significance for the treatment of elderly depressives. Elderly depressed patients with caudate hyperintensities appear to be more sensitive toward developing delirium from ECT [90,91] and antidepressants [92]. Consistent with these reports it has been reported that patients with more severe subcortical hyperintensities tended to require longer reorientation time post-ECT [88]. However, the presence of subcortical hyperintensities in the depressed elderly does not appear to be associated with a past history of ECT [86]. In addition, patients with caudate hyperintensities may be at risk for developing neuroleptic-induced parkinsonism [93]. A recent study has demonstrated that shortened rapid eye movement sleep in elderly depressed patients is associated with pontine hyperintensities [94]. An inverse relationship may exist between the presence of white matter hyperintensities and the number of platelet [3H]-imipramine binding sites (a measure of the presynaptic 5HT transporter) in depressed patients [95].

Preliminary studies have suggested that subcortical hyperintensities may be related to cognitive impairment. However, the role that subcortical hyperintensities may play in the cognitive dysfunction found in the depressed elderly remains unknown. Additional work is needed in the depressed elderly that examines the potential effect of subcortical hyperintensities on response to treatment and on long-term prognosis.

2. Early-Onset Major Depression

Early works suggested that severe white matter hyperintensities are more commonly found in elderly depressed patients with late-age-onset depression. To further examine this, Figiel et al. [96] compared the incidence and severity of subcortical hyperintensities in 10 late-age-onset (LAO) elderly depressed patients with nine early-age-onset (EAO) elderly depressed patients. The two groups were similar in age and for the presence of atherosclerotic risk factors. Large (>10 mm diameter) deep white matter hyperintensities were observed in 6 of 10 (60%) LAO patients compared with only 1 of 9 (11%) EAO patients. In addition, caudate hyperintensities were found in 6 of 10 (60%) LAO patients compared with only 1 of 9 (11%) EAO patients. Nine of 10 LAO patients had either a caudate hyperintensity and/or a large (>1 cm) deep white matter hyperintensity, while only one EAO patient had either of these structural hanges. Subsequently, several investigators have reported an increased incidence of DWMH in nonelderly adults with recurrent major depression. Brown et al. [97] found that their patients with major depression (all ages included) had increased incidence of DWMH, and Coffey et al. [38] reported an increased incidence of white matter hyperintensities (specifically periventricular hyperintensities) in a sample of 48 MDD subjects not restricted by age in comparison to controls. The mean age of this sample was in the early sixties. Thus, although DWMH appear to be more pervasive

and severe in late-onset affective disorder subjects, they may also be significantly elevated in younger populations with major depression.

3. Bipolar Patients

   a. Frequency of Hyperintensities   More than five independent groups
have now reported a higher incidence of subcortical hyperintensities on brain
MRI in bipolar patients compared with age-matched controls (Fig. 2; Table
4). Dupont et al. [98] observed subcortical hyperintensities in 9 of 19 middle-
aged bipolar patients, while no hyperintensities were observed in 10 age-
matched controls. In addition, 7 of the bipolar patients with hyperintensities
received repeat brain MRI scans one year later, and in all 7 patients the
subcortical hyperintensities were found to be unchanged. Figiel et al. [34]
observed DWMH on brain MRI in 8 of 18 (44%) middle-aged bipolar patients
compared with only 1 of 18 (6%) age-matched controls. In the bipolar patients

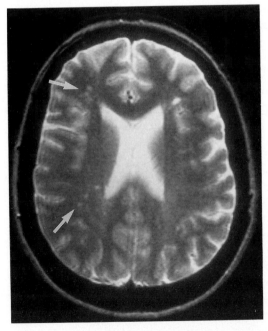

Fig. 2   T₂-weighted MR image from a 42-year-old female with bipolar affective disorder. Her first episode (depression) occurred in her mid-twenties.
Multifocal small confluent DWMH are evident in the frontal and parietal-
occipital regions.

Table 4 Investigations of Subcortical Hyperintensities (DWMH) as Visualized by MRI in Bipolar Affective Disorder

Source	Bipolar subjects (N)	% DWMH	Control subjects (N)	%DWMH	Significant group differences
Dupont et al., 1990	19	47	10 C	0	BP > normal
Swayze et al., 1990	48	15	47 C 54 S	4	BP > normal
Figiel et al., 1991	18	44	18 C	6	BP > normal
Brown et al., 1992	22	5	154 C 114 S	8	No differences
Strakowski et al., 1993	18	22	15 C	13	N.S.
Aylward et al., 1994	33	34	32 C	3	BP > normal
Botteron et al., 1995	8 (child and adolescent)	25	5 C	0	N.S.
Dupont et al., 1995	36	(volume) 3279 voxels	26 C	(volume) 2656 voxels	BP > normal (volume of hyperintensities)

C indicates community control, clinically screened; S, schizophrenic control.

the subcortical hyperintensities were observed predominantly in the frontal and parietal lobes. In 4 of the 8 bipolar patients with hyperintensities, the hyperintensities were large, ranging from 5 to 16 mm in diameter. Swayze et al. [37] found DWMH in 9 of 48 (15%) bipolar patients compared with only 2 of 47 (4%) control subjects and 5 of 54 (9%) schizophrenic patients. The authors found a weak trend toward an association between the presence of hyperintensities and ventricular enlargement in the bipolar patients. However, using a visual analog rating scale of ventricular size, Figiel et al. [34] did not find the hyperintensities to be related to the presence or severity of lateral ventricular enlargement in their patients. Aylward et al. [72] also reported an elevated rate of hyperintensities (34%) in their study of 33 bipolars and 32 normal controls. In contrast to all other studies, Brown et al. [97] reported no significant difference between bipolar patients and normal controls and reported only a 5% rate of DWMH in their bipolar sample.

Dupont et al. [73] used an automated image analysis method to estimate the volume of abnormal white matter hyperintensities in a sample of 36 bipolars, 30 MDDs, and 26 clinically screened, age- and sex-matched controls. The subjects were relatively young, with mean ages in the mid-thirties. The method for quantifying the volume of DWMH was based on computer-assisted pixel segmentation of the images into gray matter, white matter, CSF, and white matter hyperintensities based on pixel intensity classification using two image acquisitions. The reliability of the analytic method was established for CSF gray and white matter [99], but had not been established for white matter hyperintensities. Using this method they reported that bipolar subjects had a significantly increased volume of white matter hyperintensities, while young MDD subjects were not significantly different from controls. The volume of white matter hyperintensities roughly correlated with the frequency and severity of lesions noted by rating scale. There was an increased incidence of DWMH in frontal regions in bipolar subjects, and the volume of white matter hyperintensities was correlated with ventricular enlargement.

Taken together, these investigations clearly indicate that significant, confluent subcortical hyperintensities occur with increased frequency in relatively young individuals with bipolar disorder. In the positive studies the cumulative rate of hyperintensities was 30% in bipolars and 4% in the normal controls. However, it is unclear from these studies if the hyperintensities were present very early in the course of illness or if they were associated with factors related to repeated episodes, treatment effects, or the result of comorbid conditions. Two studies addressed these issues by examining first-episode patients and very young bipolars. Strakowski et al. [100] studied first-onset bipolar subjects and reported a 22% rate of hyperintensities, however, in their sample this was not significantly different from the 13% rate in the controls. Botteron et al. [101] studied a small sample of child and adolescent bipolars and found that 2 of 8 demonstrated confluent DWMHs in comparison to none of the 5 controls. These pilot investigations reported rates of hyperintensities very similar to the overall rate of 30%, but did not find statistically significant differences among their small number of subjects. Additional research will help to clarify if hyperintensities increase in frequency or severity over the course of bipolar illness.

b. Clinical Correlates of Subcortical Hyperintensities in Bipolar Patients   In both Dupont and Figiel's studies, the hyperintensities were found not to be associated with the patient's age or history of psychotic symptoms [34,98]. Figiel et al. found no relationship to family history of psychiatric disorder or age at onset of illness [34]. In bipolar patients, the hyperintensities do not appear to be associated with atherosclerotic risk factors or a prior exposure to lithium, neuroleptics, or electroconvulsive therapy [34,37,72,98,100]. Dupont found that bipolar patients with hyperintensities had significantly lower verbal fluency scores and digit symbol scores than did patients without hyperintensities [98]. In addition, the patients with hyperintensities scored more poorly on the recall measures of the California Verbal Learning Test and the Line Orientation Task. Subsequent studies by Dupont et al. [73] reported a relationship between increased volume of DWMH and higher rates of psychiatric disorder in family members and later onset of bipolar illness. They also reported a trend for relationship of DWMH to impairment on neuropsychological tests of fluency, psychomotor speed, and free recall.

4. Etiology of Subcortical Hyperintensities

In the elderly, subcortical hyperintensities are age-dependent, associated with atherosclerotic risk factors, and are felt to reflect several pathological changes (e.g., edema, dilated perivascular spaces, and sometimes lacunar infarction), resulting from ischemia to the subcortical brain regions [102,103]. The hyperintensities are most prevalent in regions that correspond to the distribution of penetrating arterioles of the lenticulostriate, thalamoperforate, and medullary arteries. These small arterioles are vulnerable to atherosclerotic compromise. However, the lesions observed in young bipolar subjects appear to be neither age-dependent nor associated with atherosclerotic risk factors in the majority of studies. (One exception is a positive relationship to age and atherosclerotic risk factors as reported by Alyward et al. [72].) These results suggest that the underlying pathophysiologies of the lesions may be different in bipolar and elderly depressed patients. Age appears to have a significant relationship to the severity of white matter lesions in normals and depressed subjects [73]. Cigarette smoking has been hypothesized as a potential correlate for white matter hyperintensities, and smoking has been reported to be significantly related to lesions in depression but has not been correlated with lesions in bipolar subjects in most [34,37,73,98] but not all studies [72]. Additionally, evidence of a similar percentage of white matter lesions in a small population of nonsmoking child and adolescent bipolar subjects argues against any significant relationship to smoking or other substance abuse [101].

In addition to ischemic disease, other diverse disease processes may produce signal characteristics similar to the lesions seen in psychiatric patients [104]. Examples of these include posttraumatic, anoxic, infectious, perinatal, demyelinating, or genetic factors. The role that any of these factors may play in the pathophysiology of the lesions observed in psychiatric patients requires further examination.

VI. NEUROENDOCRINE DYSFUNCTION AND PITUITARY SIZE IN DEPRESSION

Hypothalamic pituitary–adrenal axis hyperactivity is frequently observed in depressed patients, and hypothalamic function has been associated with the modulation of neurovegatative symptoms such as sleep, appetite, and sex drive. A number of studies have suggested that there is a central overdrive by CRF in patients with depression. In addition, animal studies have shown that chronic administration of CRF can lead to a marked increase in the number and volume of pituitary corticotroph cells (and therefore, pituitary volume) [105]. Given these findings, Krishnan et al. [106] compared pituitary gland areas and volumes using brain MRI in 19 depressed patients and 39 normal controls. They found that depressed patients had significantly larger pituitary gland area ($p = 0.0009$), volume ($p = 0.007$), and length ($p = 0.04$) compared to age- and sex-matched controls. These findings are the first to suggest that some depressed patients may have not only functional but also structural abnormalities in the neuroendocrine axis. Subsequently, Krishnan et al. [107] found a significant correlation between postdexamethasone cortisol levels and pituitary size in depressed patients. Whether the pituitary enlargement observed in depressed patients is reversible is unknown. Further work is underway to examine the clinical, neuroendocrine, and structural correlates of pituitary enlargement in depressed patients.

VII. FRONTAL LIMBIC CIRCUIT STRUCTURES

A. Temporal Lobe

In vivo examination of temporal lobe structures has only become available with the advent of MRI techniques. Earlier neuropathological work by Brown et al. [108], which focused on temporal lobe abnormalities in schizophrenics, reported a decreased parahippocampal cortical thickness in schizophrenics and bipolars that was not significantly different between groups. More recently, Bowen et al. [109] in a postmortem morphological study compared depressed subjects to patients with Alzheimer's disease and normal controls. They reported significant differences in temporal lobe structures between the normal controls and the affective disorder subjects. Depressed subjects had significantly decreased temporal pole and parahippocampal gyrus weights, which correlated with a loss of protein and decreased 5HT-2 binding in these areas. They concluded that the postmortem findings were consistent with a loss of cortical neurons and interneurons in these areas. In the only CT study to report on temporal lobe pathology, Dewan et al. [29] found that CT density as measured in Houndsfield units was significantly increased in the left and right temporal lobe of 26 bipolar patients in comparison to a group of 22 "headache controls."

Several MRI studies have been reported in the last 5 years examining different aspects of temporal lobe pathology (Table 5). Johnstone et al. [33], in an investigation primarily designed to study schizophrenia, compared 21 schizophrenic subjects, 20 bipolar subjects and 21 normal controls. Using coronal MRI scans they calculated the temporal lobe area and the temporal horn area from the one MRI image that demonstrated these structures at their largest. They reported that schizophrenic subjects but not bipolar subjects were statistically significantly different in temporal lobe size compared to normal controls. They reported a significant relationship between age and temporal lobe size. In addition, they found that bipolar subjects were similar

Table 5 MRI Investigations of Temporal Lobe Structures in Affective Disorders

Source	Structure/ method used	Affective disorder subjects	Control subjects	Significant group differences
Johnstone et al., 1989	Temporal lobe area	20 BP	21 C 21 S	Schiz < normal BP vs. schiz N.S.
Hauser et al., 1989	Temporal lobe area	17 MDD	21 C	MAD < normal
	Hippocampal complex	17 MDD	21 C	None
Altschuler et al., 1990	Temporal lobe volume	10 BP	10 C	BAD < normal
Swayze et al., 1992	Temporal lobe/ coronal tracings summed for volume	48 BP	55 S 47 C	Schiz < normal BAD (female)— no normal assymmetry
Coffey et al., 1993	Temporal lobe volume	44 MDD 4 BP	76 C	None
	Amygdala hippocampus			None BAD < control—R hippocampus

BP, bipolar disorder; MDD, major depressive disorder; C, indicates community control, clinically screened; S, schizophrenic control; M, medical control; A, Alzheimer control; N, neurological control.

to controls, with the right temporal lobe being smaller than the left temporal lobe. Hauser et al. [110] used multiple coronal MRI scans to measure the temporal lobe area and hippocampal area as expressed by ratios to total cerebral or total temporal lobe area. They reported significant differences between 17 depressed patients and 21 controls, with the depressed patients showing significantly smaller temporal lobe to cerebrum ratios in the right and left hemispheres. The effect persisted when controlled for age and education level. They found no significant differences in hippocampal ratios. They reported that the temporal lobe size did not correlate with the presence of psychosis, age of onset, or length of illness. Altschuler et al. [111] was the first to report temporal lobe volumes in 10 bipolar patients compared to 10 normal controls. Volumes were determined from manual planimetric tracing of coronal MRI scans (10 mm thickness) in subjects with bipolar affective disorder. They reported significantly decreased temporal lobe volumes bilaterally in the bipolar patients. Swayze et al. [71] subsequently examined temporal lobe volumes in a larger sample based on 10-mm coronal MRI slices and found no overall difference in volume, but did find a significant effect of cerebral laterality. Normal right-handed individuals have a larger right than left temporal lobe volume [112]. Bipolar men had significantly greater temporal lobe asymmetry (R > L) than normal controls, while bipolar women lacked the normal temporal lobe asymmetry. Coffey et al. [38] examined temporal lobe volumes in 48 MDD subjects in comparison to 76 matched normal controls based on manual computer-assisted tracings from 5-mm-thick coronal MR images. They completed a multivariate analysis of covariance, which included age, sex, years of education, and cranial area as covariates, and reported no significant difference in temporal lobe volume between the groups. They noted, however, that examination of the confidence intervals revealed that temporal lobe volumes could be as much as 7% smaller in the depressed subjects.

B. Amygdala and Hippocampus

Measurement of more specific temporal lobe structures is technically demanding, and it can be difficult to achieve highly reliable volumetric measures. There have been very few investigations of temporal lobe subregions reported in affective disorder. Krishnan et al. [113] measured MRI T_1 relaxation times in the hippocampus and in the temporal lobe white matter and found that depressed subjects had significantly shorter T_1 relaxation times in the hippocampus compared to normal controls. Age correlated with decreased T_1 values in normals but not depressed subjects. A decrease in T_1 values is reported to correspond to decreased water content, and the authors speculate that their findings are suggestive of atrophy in these structures.

Subsequently this group examined hippocampal volume based on 5-mm coronal MR images using a systematic stereological sampling method and reported no significant difference in hippocampal volume between depressed subjects and controls [114]. However there were significant relationships in the depressed subjects between hippocampal volume and some measures of cortisol status, age of depressive onset, and number of previous hospitalizations.

Two other groups have also reported on investigations of hippocampal volume. Swayze et al. [71] estimated hippocampal volume (based on area tracings in four select 10-mm coronal images) in 48 subjects with bipolar disorder and demonstrated decreased right hippocampal volume in comparison to normal controls. There was no reported difference in amygdala volume (estimated based on one slice). Coffey et al. [38] also estimated the volume of the amygdala/hippocampal complex based on 5-mm coronal slices in their sample of 48 depressed subjects and found no significant difference from the 76 controls, although again the confidence intervals indicated that the depressed subjects could have had up to a 10% reduction in volume in this region.

All of the MRI studies reported above have significant limitations. Often these exams were completed with clinical scanners and used 5- to 10-mm-thick slices, creating significant partial voluming effects, which can obscure subtle differences, make it difficult to determine boundaries of structures, and decrease the reliability of measurements. In spite of these limitations, which may obscure true differences, it is interesting that the majority of the imaging studies to date have reported temporal lobe abnormalities in patients with affective disorders. These findings are consistent with theories indicating that medial temporal lobe structures play a major role in the behavioral expression of emotion [89]. Substantial improvements in image acquisition and image analysis are now enabling the precise and reliable measurement of small complex structures [115]. Clearly, additional MRI studies that examine the extent and nature of structural abnormalities in the temporal lobes of depressed patients are needed.

C. Basal Ganglia Nuclei

Preliminary imaging studies have identified a high incidence of caudate nucleus structural changes in the elderly depressed. Based upon these observations, Krishnan et al. [116] examined caudate nuclei volumes using serial axial brain MRI images and an unbiased stereological technique in 50 depressed patients and 50 normal controls (Table 6). Both left ($p < 0.0006$) and right ($p < 0.007$) side caudate nuclei were smaller in depressed patients compared to controls. Cerebral hemisphere volumes were also measured,

Table 6   MRI Investigations of the Basal Ganglia in Affective Disorders

Source	Structure	Method used	Affective disorder subjects	Control subjects	Significant group difference
Husain et al., 1991	Putamen	5-mm axial images stereologic volumes	44 MDD	41 C	MDD < control
Krishnan et al., 1992	Caudate	5-mm axial images stereologic volumes	50 MDD	50 C	MDD < control
Swayze et al., 1992	Caudate putamen	1-cm coronal images manual outlining	48 BP	47 C	N.S.
Aylward et al., 1994	Caudate putamen globus pallidus	5-mm axial images manual outlining	33 BP	32 C	Caudate volume: BP > control
Dupont et al., 1995	Caudate lenticular nucleus thalamus	5-mm axial images, semi-automated segmentation based on pixel intensity classification	36 BP 30 MDD	26 C	Thalamic volume: BP > control > MDD

BP, bipolar disorder; MDD, major depressive disorder; C, indicates community control, clinically screened.

and the caudate nuclei/cerebral hemisphere volume ratio was calculated. This ratio was also significantly smaller ($p < 0.0006$) in depressed patients compared to controls. The caudate nuclei volumes of both young and older depressed subjects were smaller compared with controls. In addition, Husain et al. [117] have reported a reduction in size of the putamen nuclei bilaterally in depressed patients compared with controls. Aylward et al. [72] examined caudate, putamen, and globus pallidus volume in 33 bipolar subjects in comparison to 32 normal controls and reported that caudate volume was significantly increased in male bipolar subjects. They tested for deviations in the normal asymmetry of basal ganglia structures and found none in the individuals with bipolar disorder. Aylward et al. [72] also found an increased incidence of white matter hyperintensities, but these were uncorrelated with basal ganglia volumes. However, Dupont et al. [73] using an automated segmentation method reported no significant difference in caudate or lenticular nucleus volumes between bipolar, depressed, and normal controls. Each group had approximately 30 subjects. They reported an intriguing finding with the thalamus being larger than controls in bipolar patients and smaller than controls in depressed patients. Swayze et al. [71] also found no significant differences in caudate or putamen volume in 48 bipolars in comparison to 47 normal controls.

In summary, there appear to be conflicting results for basal ganglia structures in affective disorders. Some studies have demonstrated decreased volumes in individuals with recurrent major depression, whereas in bipolar disorder there are reports of increased volume or no significant differences. It is interesting that bipolar disorder has been reported to have increased caudate volume, similar to some reports in schizophrenics. More recent research with schizophrenics has also revealed that increased caudate volume may be secondary to neuroleptic medication. This was demonstrated when first-episode schizophrenics, prior to receiving any medication, were found to have no significant increase in caudate volume, however, after several months of treatment (including neuroleptics) their caudate volume was significantly larger than controls [118]. Most bipolar subjects who were studied were being clinically treated, and it is unclear how many were receiving neuroleptics prior to the study. Strakowski et al. [39] studied a group of first-onset manic subjects and reported no significant difference in their caudate or thalamus volumes in comparison to normal controls. However, a growing body of evidence (neuroanatomic, neurological, MRI, and PET) suggests that the basal ganglia may play an important role in the pathophysiology of affective disorders. Doraiswamy et al. [119] reexamined their depressed sample [116], separating the depressed patients into those who were receiving (or had received) antipsychotic therapy and those who were not, and reported that the MDD subjects who had received neuroleptic therapy had significantly larger caudates than the depressed subjects who had not received antipsychotic treatment. Both groups had smaller caudates than the comparison normal controls. The authors noted that this further supported the hypothesis that plastic hypertrophy of striatal synaptic or somal elements occurs in vivo and could be related to dopaminergic D_2 receptor blockade [118]. Given that results have been mixed thus far, further studies are needed to try to replicate the findings of differences in basal ganglia structure and further examine the potential clinical and functional correlates in affective disorders.

D. Frontal Lobe

Regions of the prefrontal lobe have been implicated in the pathophysiology of affective disorders based on functional PET investigations [89] and neuro-psychological studies. Coffey et al. [38] examined middle-aged subjects with recurrent MDD in comparison to age- and sex-matched screened normal controls and demonstrated a significant decrease (approximately 7%) in bilateral frontal lobe volume in the MDD subjects in comparison to controls. They defined the frontal lobe as gray and white matter anterior to the optic chiasm on 5-mm-thick coronal images. Strakowski et al. [39], in their sample of 17 first-episode manics, reported no significant difference in frontal lobe volume (defined as anterior to the genu of the corpus callosum) from normal controls. However, this investigation did not report any standardization for head positioning and did not reformat the imaging data into standardized position prior to image analysis. Given that frontal lobe volumes are defined by a plane (the slices anterior to the specified landmark), even slight differences in head positioning could bias the reported results. Botteron et al. [101], in a small sample of very young bipolars, also found support for frontal lobe abnormalities with a trend for bipolars not to demonstrate the usual frontal lobe asymmetry (right frontal lobe protrudes ahead of the left-right frontal petalia) in comparison to screened controls. Subsequently, Botteron et al. also demonstrated in a younger sample of prepubertal MDD subjects that they also lacked the usual asymmetry of prefrontal lobe volume (R > L) and instead exhibited nearly equivalent right and left prefrontal lobe volumes. This supports neurodevelopmental hypotheses and suggests that at least some structural changes are present quite early in the course of illness.

VIII. OTHER BRAIN REGIONS: THE PINEAL GLAND

Enlarged pineal calcifications (>1 cm) have been reported in 25% of institutionalized bipolar patients by Sandyk et al. [120,121]. Although no normal controls were included, this observation is reportedly 25 times the expected frequency in the general population. They reported that larger calcifications were significantly associated with axial tardive dyskinesia and a poorer response to ECT. This finding needs further replication.

IX. DISCUSSION

Imaging studies of affective disorders are beginning to report a diverse array of structural brain changes in multiple brain regions. However, due to small sample sizes and methodological limitations in many of these studies, the evidence is inconclusive as to which if any of these structural changes are specific to affective disorders. It also remains to be defined how these structural changes may relate to the pathophysiology of affective disorders. Although early studies tended to be somewhat atheoretical in the regions examined, more recent investigations are focusing on regions hypothesized to have some specific role in affective disorders. Increasing evidence from other lines of investigation suggests that affective disorders may be related to dysfunction within specific neural networks. Several authors have hypothesized that circuits involving the ventral and medial prefrontal cortex along with limbic structures such as the amygdala, and portions of the striatum and thalamus play a central role in affective disorders [89,122–124]. Based upon an impressive integration of experimental results from anatomy, neurochemistry, neurophysiology, animal behavioral, psychopharmacological and clinical psychiatry investigations, Swerdlow and Koob [124] have presented strong support for the potential importance of limbic-cortical-striatal-pallidal-thalamic circuits in the pathophysiology of affective disorders. Subsequent investigations, including structural and functional neuroimaging studies, have added support for their hypothesis.

The issue of diagnostic heterogeneity is an important concern for neurobiological investigation of affective disorders and is clearly pertinent to imaging investigations as well. The degree to which this has not been addressed in structural imaging studies to date could have a significant role in reports of conflicting results. Homogeneity of subject populations is necessary to detect potentially significant effects related to the pathophysiology specific to disorders. It is clear that affective disorders represent a heterogeneous group of disorders, which include recurrent depressive disorders, sporadic major depression, manic depressive disorders, affective disorders secondary to medical or other psychiatric conditions, etc. However, many studies, especially older ones, did not attempt to study uniform populations and included unipolar, bipolar, and other subtypes in their analyses. The lack of a homogeneous population could have a profound effect on reported results and needs to be kept in mind when reviewing the results of neurobiological research with affectively disordered populations. The importance of this has been illustrated by the observation that subtyping of depressive disorders in functional imaging studies has reduced the variability of image data [125]. Lesion studies and functional imaging studies have indicated that dysfunction or disruption of different regions within cortico-striatal-limbic circuits can lead to similar clinical pictures of affective disorders. Future structural MRI studies will require larger homogeneous patient groups using standardized imaging protocols to maximize the ability to detect specific but subtle structural differences in subgroups of affectively ill patients.

Little is known of the potential clinical or neurobiological correlates of the observed structural brain changes in the affectively ill. Some studies have revealed clear clinical utility, such as the demonstration that basal ganglia lesions in elderly depressed patients are associated with more severe post-ECT delirium [90,91]. Clinical studies will need to examine the potential impact of various structural brain changes on phenomenology, treatment response, and sensitivity to the development of side effects. Likewise, neurobiological studies should examine the potential metabolic, neuroendocrine, neurochemical, genetic, developmental, pharmacological, and neuropathological correlates of structural brain changes in the affectively ill.

The ability of MRI to safely produce high-resolution images that can be reliably quantified provides a methodology to address unresolved neuroanatomical issues related to etiology, course, and prognosis. Longitudinal investigations with MRI could help to resolve whether neuropathological changes are related to neurodevelopmental or neurodegenerative processes, or an interaction of the two. Investigations with children and younger populations will be necessary to confirm neurodevelopmental theories and will provide the opportunity to study populations longitudinally to examine for potential interactions with normal developmental processes. Such investigations are currently in progress. Additionally neuroanatomic variables may provide additional information to clarify diagnostic heterogeneity and provide prognostic information.

In conclusion, it appears that a number of affectively ill patients have a diverse array of structural brain changes. Although the significance of these observations in many cases remains undetermined, it is not unreasonable to believe that we are at the threshold of beginning to understand the neuroanatomic substrate of the affective disorders. Clearly, future imaging studies will address many important and exciting topics in the area of affective disorders.

REFERENCES

1. M. E. Shenton, R. Kikinis, F. A. Jolesz, S. D. Pollak, M. LeMay, C. G. Wible, H. Hokama, J. Martin, D. Metcalf, M. Coleman, and R. W. McCarley, Abnormalities of the left temporal lobe and thought disorder in schizophrenia, *N. Engl. J. Med. 327*:604 (1992).
2. F. Cendes, F. Andermann, P. Gloor, A. Evans, M. Jones-Gotman, C. Watson, D. Melanson, A. Olivier, T. Peters, I. Lopes-Cendes, and G. Leroux, MRI volumetric measurement of amygdala and hippocampus in temporal lobe epilepsy, *Neurology 43*:719 (1993).
3. V. Synek and J. R. Reuben, The ventricular-brain ratio using planimetric measurement of EMI scans, *Br. J. Radiol. 49*:233 (1976).
4. E. C. Johnstone, D. G. C. Owens, T. J. Crow, and R. Jagoe, A CT Study of 188 Patients with schizophrenia, affective psychosis and neurotic illness, *Biol. Psychiatry 16*:237 (1981).
5. G. D. Pearlson, A. E. Veroff, and P. R. McHugh, The use of computed tomog-

raphy in psychiatry: recent applications to schizophrenia, manic depressive illness and dementia syndromes, *Johns Hopkins Med. J. 149*:194 (1981).

6. G. D. Pearlson and A. E. Veroff, Computerized tomographic scan changes in manic depressive illness, *Lancet 71*:470 (1981).

7. H. A. Nasrallah, M. McCalley-Whitters, and C. G. Jacoby, Cerebral ventricular enlargement in young manic males: a controlled CT study, *J. Affect. Disord. 4*:15 (1982).

8. M. Luchins, Ventricular size and psychosis in affective disorder, *Biol. Psychiatry 18*:1197 (1983).

9. M. L. Scott, C. J. Golden, and S. L. Ruedrich, Ventricular enlargement in major depression, *Psychiatry Res. 8*:91 (1983).

10. S. D. Targum, L. N. Rosen, and L. E. DeLisi, Cerebral ventricular size in major depressive disorder: Association with delusional symptoms, *Biol. Psychiatry 18*:329 (1983).

11. D. J. Luchins, R. R. J. Lewine, and H. Y. Meltzer, Lateral ventricular size, psychopathology, and medication response in the psychoses, *Biol. Psychiatry 19*:29 (1984).

12. G. D. Pearlson, D. J. Garbacz, R. H. Tompkins, H. S. Ahn, D. F. Gutterman, A. E. Veroff, and J. R. DePaulo, Clinical correlates of lateral ventricular enlargement in bipolar affective disorder, *Am. J. Psychiatry 141*:253 (1984).

13. S. Shima, T. Shikano, and T. Kitamura, Depression and ventricular enlargement, *Acta Psychiatr. Scand. 70*:275 (1984).

14. R. J. Dolan, S. P. Calloway, and A. H. Mann, Cerebral ventricular size in depressed subjects, *Psychol. Med. 15*:873 (1985).

15. H. Kolbeinsson, O. S. Arnaldsson, H. Petursson, and S. Skulason, Computed tomographic scans in ECT-patients, *Acta Psychiatr. Scand. 73*:28 (1986).

16. S. Schlegel and K. Kretzschmar, Computed tomography in affective disorders. Part I: Ventricular and sulcal measurements., *Biol. Psychiatry 22*:4 (1987).

17. G. D. Pearlson, P. V. Rabins, and W. S. Kim, Structural brain CT changes and cognitive deficits in elderly depressives with and without reversible dementia, *Psychol. Med. 19*:573 (1989).

18. A. Rossi, P. Stratta, and V. Michele, A computerized tomographic study in patients with depressive disorder: a comparison with schizophrenic patients and controls, *Acta Psychiatr. Belg. 89*:56 (1989).

19. H. A. Nasrallah, M. McCalley-Whitters, and C. G. Jacoby, Cortical atrophy in schizophrenia and mania: a comparative CT study, *J. J. Clin. Psychiatry 43*:439 (1982).

20. D. R. Weinberger, L. E. DeLisi, and G. P. Perman, Computed tomography in schizophreniform disorder and other acute psychiatric disorders, *Arch. Gen. Psychiatry 39*:778 (1982).

21. R. O. Reider, L. S. Mann, and D. R. Weinberger, Computed tomographic scans in patients with schizophrenia, schizoaffective and bipolar affective disorder, *Arch. Gen. Psychiatry 40*:735 (1983).

22. G. D. Pearlson, D. J. Garbacz, W. R. Breakey, H. S. Ahn, and J. R. DePaulo, Lateral ventricular enlargement associated with persistent unemployment and

negative symptoms in both schizophrenia and bipolar disorder, *Psychiatry Res.* *12*:1 (1984).

23. D. G. Owens, E. C. Johnstone, and T. J. Crow, Lateral ventricular size in schizophrenia: relationship to the disease process and its clinical manifestations., *Psychol. Med.* *15*:27 (1985).

24. W. G. Iacono, G. N. Smith, M. Moreau, M. Beiser, J. A. E. Fleming, T. Lin, and B. Flak, Ventricular and sulcal size at the onset of psychosis, *Am. J. Psychiatry* *145*:820 (1988).

25. N. C. Andreasen, V. Swayze, M. Flaum, R. Alliger, and G. Cohen, Ventricular abnormalities in affective disorder: clinical and demographic correlates, *Am. J. Psychiatry* *147*:893 (1990).

26. J. Zigun and D. Weinberger, In vivo studies of brain morphology in schizophrenia, *New Biological Vistas on Schizophrenia* (J. P. Lindenmayer and S. R. Kay, eds.), Brunner/Mazel, New York, 1992, pp. 57–81.

27. D. V. Jeste, J. B. Lohr, and F. K. Goodwin, Neuroanatomical studies of major affective disorders, *Br. J. Psychiatry* *153*:444 (1988).

28. R. J. Jacoby and R. Levy, Computed tomography in elderly affective disorder, *Br. J. Psychiatry* *136*:270 (1980).

29. M. J. Dewan, C. V. Haldipur, E. E. Lane, A. Ispahani, M. F. Boucher, and L. F. Major, Bipolar affective disorder I. Comprehensive quantitative computed tomography, *Acta Psychiatr. Scand.* *77*:670 (1988).

30. A. Rossi, P. Stratta, and C. Petruzzi, A computerized tomographic study in DSM-III affective disorders, *J. Affect. Disord.* *12*:259 (1987).

31. L. M. Zatz and T. L. Jernigan, The ventricular-brain ratio on computed tomography scans: validity and proper use, *Psychiatry Res.* *8*:207 (1983).

32. J. A. Besson, J. G. Henderson, and E. I. Foreman, An NMR study of lithium responding manic depressive patients, *Magnet. Resonance Imag.* *5*:273 (1987).

33. E. C. Johnstone, D. G. Owens, and T. J. Crow, Temporal lobe structure as determined by nuclear magnetic resonance in schizophrenia and bipolar affective disorder, *J. Neurol. Neurosurg. Psychiatry* *52*:736 (1989).

34. G. S. Figiel, K. R. R. Krishnan, and V. P. Rao, Subcortical hyperintensities on brain magnetic resonance imaging: a comparison of normal and bipolar subjects, *J. Neuropsychiatry* *3*:18 (1991).

35. I. M. Lesser, B. L. Miller, and K. B. Boone, Brain injury and cognitive function in late-onset psychotic depression, *J. Neuropsychiatry* *3*:33 (1991).

36. P. V. Rabins, G. D. Pearlson, and E. Aylward, Cortical magnetic resonance imaging changes in elderly inpatients with major depression, *Am. J. Psychiatry* *148*:617 (1991).

37. V. W. Swayze, N. C. Andreasen, and R. J. Alliger, Structural brain abnormalities in bipolar affective disorder, *Arch. Gen. Psychiatry* *47*:1057 (1990).

38. C. E. Coffey, W. E. Wilkinson, R. D. Weiner, I. A. Parashos, W. T. Djang, M. C. Webb, G. S. Figiel, and C. E. Spritzer, Quantitative cerebral anatomy in depression, *Arch. Gen. Psychiatry* *50*:7 (1993).

39. S. M. Strakowski, D. R. Wilson, M. Tohen, B. T. Woods, A. W. Douglass, and A. L. Stoll, Structural brain abnormalities in first-episode mania, *Biol. Psychiatry* *33*:602 (1993).

40. H. Elkis, L. Friedman, A. Wise, and H. Y. Meltzer, Meta-analyses of studies of ventricular enlargement and cortical sulcal prominence in mood disorders, *Arch. Gen. Psychiatry 52*:735 (1995).

41. A. Vita, E. Saccleti, and C. Cazzullo, A CT scan follow-up study of cerebral ventricular size in schizophrenia and major affective disorder, *Schizophrenia Res. 1*:165 (1988).

42. B. T. Woods, D. Yurgelun-Todd, F. M. Benes, F. R. Frankenburg, H. G. Pope, and J. McSparren, Progressive ventricular enlargement in schizophrenia: comparison to bipolar affective disorder and correlation with clinical course, *Biol. Psychiatry 27*:341 (1990).

43. S. Schlegel, U. Frommberger, and R. Buller, Computerized tomography in affective disorders: relationship with psychopathology, *Psychiatry Res. 29*:271 (1989).

44. S. Schlegel, W. Maier, and M. Phillip, Computed tomography in depression: association between ventricular size and psychopathology, *Psychiatry Res. 29*:221 (1989).

45. P. P. Roy-Byrne, R. M. Post, and C. H. Kellner, Ventricular-brain ratio and life course of illness in patients with affective disorder., *Psychiatry Res. 23*: 277 (1988).

46. H. A. Nasrallah, M. McCalley-Whitters, and B. Pfohl, Clinical significance of large cerebral ventricles in manic males, *Psychiatry Res. 13*:151 (1984).

47. A. J. Rothschild, F. Benes, and N. Hebben, Relationships between brain CT scan findings and cortisol in psychotic and nonpsychotic depressed patients, *Biol. Psychiatry 26*:565 (1989).

48. G. D. Pearlson, D. J. Garbacz, P. J. Moberg, H. S. Ahn, and J. R. DePaulo, Symptomatic, familial, perinatal and social correlates of computerized axial tomography (CAT) changes in schizophrenics and bipolars, *J. Nerv. Ment. Dis. 173*:42 (1985).

49. H. M. Standish-Barry, N. Bouras, and A. S. Hale, Ventricular size and CSF transmitter metabolite concentrations in severe endogenous depression, *Br. J. Psychiatry 148*:386 (1986).

50. M. J. Dewan, C. V. Haldipur, M. F. Boucher, T. Ramachandran, and L. F. Major, Bipolar affective disorder II. EEG, neuropsychological and clinical correlates of CT abnormality, *Acta Psychiatr. Scand. 77*:677 (1988).

51. R. J. Jacoby, R. J. Dolan, R. Levy, and R. Baldy, Quantitative computed tomography in elderly depressed patients, *Br. J. Psychiatry 143*:124 (1983).

52. C. H. Kellner, D. R. Rubinow, and R. M. Post, Cerebral ventricular size and cognitive impairment in depression, *J. Affect. Disord. 10*:215 (1986).

53. E. C. Johnstone, D. G. C. Owens, T. J. Crow, N. Colter, C. A. Lawton, R. Jagoe, and L. Kreel, Hypothyroidism as a correlate of lateral ventricular enlargement in manic-depressive and neurotic illness, *Br. J. Psychiatry 148*: 317 (1986).

54. M. A. Abas, B. J. Sahakian, and R. Levy, Neuropsychological deficits and CT scan changes in elderly depressives, *Psychol. Med. 20*:507 (1990).

55. R. J. Jacoby, R. Levy, and J. M. Bird, Computed tomography and the outcome

of affective disorder: a follow-up study of elderly patients, *Br. J. Psychiatry* *139*:288 (1981).

56. G. D. Pearlson, P. V. Rabins, and A. Burns, Centrum semiovale white matter CT changes associated with normal aging, Alzheimer's disease and late life depression with and without reversible dementia, *Psychol. Med. 21*:321 (1991).

57. C. E. Coffey, G. S. Figiel, W. T. Djang, W. B. Saunders, and R. D. Weiner, White matter hyperintensity on magnetic resonance imaging: clinical and neuroanatomic correlates in the depressed elderly, *J. Neuropsychiatry Clin. Neurosci. 1*:135 (1989).

58. S. Schlegel, U. Bardeleben, and K. Wiedemann, Computerized brain tomography measures compared with spontaneous and suppressed plasma cortisol levels in major depression, *Psychoneuroendocrinology 14*:209 (1989).

59. V. P. Rao, K. R. R. Krishnan, V. Goli, W. B. Saunders, E. H. Ellinwood, D. G. Blazer, and C. B. Nemeroff, Neuroanatomical changes and hypothalamo-pituitary-adrenal axis abnormalities, *Biol. Psychiatry 26*:729 (1989).

60. M. J. Dewan, C. V. Haldipur, M. Boucher, and L. F. Major, Is CT ventriculomegaly related to hypercortisolemia?, *Acta Psychiatr. Scand. 77*:230 (1988).

61. C. E. Coffey, W. E. Wilkinson, R. D. Weiner, J. C. Ritchie, and M. Aque, The dexamethasone suppression test and quantitative cerebral anatomy in depression, *Biol. Psychiatry 33*:442 (1993).

62. C. H. Kellner, D. R. Rubinow, P. W. Gold, and R. M. Post, Relationship of cortisol hypersecretion to brain CT scan alterations in depressed patients, *Psychiatry Res. 8*:191 (1983).

63. T. Okuno, M. Ito, and Y. Konishi, Cerebral atrophy following ACTH therapy, *J. Comput. Assist. Tomogr. 4*:20 (1980).

64. H. Y. Meltzer, C. Tong, and D. J. Luchins, Serum dopamine-B-hydroxylase activity and lateral ventricular size in affective disorders and schizophrenia, *Biol. Psychiatry 19*:1395 (1984).

65. K. Nagy, Pneumencephalographische befunde bei endogenen psychosen, *Nervenarzt 34*:543 (1963).

66. S. Otuski, T. Hiramatsu, and K. Hosokawa, Pneumoencephalographic studies on the various psychiatric and neruological disorders—with special reference to the relationship between the enlargement of the third ventricle and the psychic symptoms, *Psychiat Neurol. Jap. 67*:711 (1965).

67. Y. Tanaka, H. Hazama, and T. Fukuhara, Computerized tomography of the brain in manic-depressive patients—a controlled study, *Folia Psychiatr. Neurol. 36*:137 (1982).

68. S. Schlegel and K. Kretzschmar, Computed tomography in affective disorders. Part II: Brain density, *Biol. Psychiatry 22*:15 (1987).

69. G. S. Zubenko, P. Sullivan, and J. P. Nelson, Brain imaging abnormalities in mental disorders of late life, *Arch. Neurol. 47*:1107 (1990).

70. F. M. Benes, M. E. Swigar, S. L. G. Rothman, C. Opsahl, and M. Dowds, CT scan studies of superficial cerebral regions: frequency and distribution of abnormalities in elderly psychiatric patients, *Neurobiol. Aging 4*:289 (1983).

71. V. W. Swayze, N. C. Andreasen, and R. J. Alliger, Subcortical and temporal

structures in affective disorder and schizophrenia: a magnetic resonance imaging study, *Biol. Psychiatry 31*:221 (1992).

72. E. H. Aylward, J. V. Roberts-Twillie, P. E. Barta, A. J. Kumar, G. J. Harris, M. Geer, C. E. Peyser, and G. D. Pearlson, Basal ganglia volumes and white matter hyperintensities in patients with bipolar disorder, *Am. J. Psychiatry 151*:687 (1994).

73. R. M. Dupont, T. L. Jernigan, W. Heindel, N. Butters, K. Shafer, T. Wilson, J. Hesselink, and J. C. Gillin, Magnetic resonance imaging and mood disorders, *Arch. Gen. Psychiatry 52*:747 (1995).

74. R. G. Heath, D. E. Franklin, C. F. Walker, and J. J. W. Keating, Cerebellar vermal atrophy in psychiatric patients, *Biol. Psychiatry 17*:569 (1982).

75. S. Lippman, M. Manshadi, H. Baldwin, G. Drasin, J. Rice, and S. Alrajeh, Cerebellar vermis dimensions on computerized tomographic scans of schizophrenic and bipolar patients, *Am. J. Psychiatry 139*:667 (1982).

76. R. G. Heath, D. E. Franklin, and D. Shraberg, Gross pathology of the cerebellum in patients diagnosed and treated as functional psychiatric disorders, *J. Nerv. Ment. Dis. 167*:585 (1979).

77. H. A. Nasrallah, C. G. Jacoby, and M. McCalley-Whitters, Cerebellar atrophy in schizophrenia and mania, *Lancet 1(8229)*:1102 (1981).

78. W. R. Yates, C. G. Jacoby, and N. C. Andreasen, Cerebellar atrophy in schizophrenia and affective disorder, *Am. J. Psychiatry 144*:465 (1987).

79. S. A. Shah, P. M. Doraiswamy, M. M. Husain, P. R. Escalona, C. Na, G. S. Figiel, L. J. Patterson, E. H. Ellinwood, W. M. McDonald, O. B. Boyko, and K. R. Krishnan, Posterior fossa abnormalities in major depression: A controlled magnetic resonance imaging study, *Acta Psychiatr. Scand. 85*:474 (1992).

80. P. H. Hauser, D. Dauphinais, and W. Berrettini, Corpus callosum dimensions measured by magnetic resonance imaging in bipolar affective disorder and schizophrenia, *Biol. Psychiatry 26*:659 (1989).

81. M. M. Husain, G. S. Figiel, and S. N. Lurie, MRI of corpus callosum and septum pellucidum in depression, *Biol. Psychiatry 29*:300 (1991).

82. J. A. Coffman, R. A. Bornstein, S. C. Olson, S. B. Schwarzkopf, and H. A. Nasrallah, Cognitive impairment and cerebral structure by MRI in bipolar disorder, *Biol. Psychiatry 27*:1188 (1990).

83. J. C. Wu, M. S. Buchsbaum, J. C. Johnson, T. G. Hershey, E. A. Wagner, C. Teng, and S. Lottenberg, Magnetic resonance and positron emission tomography imaging of the corpus callosum: size, shape and metabolic rate in unipolar depression, *J. Affect. Disord. 28*:15 (1993).

84. J. A. Coffman and H. A. Nasrallah, Brain density patterns in schizophrenia and mania, *J. Affect. Disord. 6*:307 (1984).

85. J. A. Coffman and H. A. Nasrallah, Relationships between brain density, cortical atrophy and ventriculomegaly in schizophrenia and mania, *Acta Psychiatr. Scand. 72*:126 (1985).

86. C. E. Coffey, G. S. Figiel, and W. I. Djang, Leukoencephalopathy in elderly depressed patients referred for ECT, *Biol. Psychiatry 24*:143 (1988).

87. F. Fazekas, K. Niederkorn, and R. Schmidt, White matter signal abnormalities in normal individuals: correlation with carotid ultrasonography, cerebral blood flow measurements and cerebrovascular risk factors, *Stroke 19*:1285 (1988).

88. G. S. Figiel, C. E. Coffey, and R. D. Weiner, Brain magnetic resonance imaging in elderly depressed patients receiving electroconvulsive therapy, *Convulsive Ther. 5*:26 (1989).

89. W. C. Drevets, T. O. Videen, J. L. Price, S. H. Preskorn, S. T. Carmichael, and M. E. Raichle, A functional anatomical study of unipolar depression, *J. Neurosci. 12*:3628 (1992).

90. G. S. Figiel, C. E. Coffey, and W. T. Djang, Brain magnetic resonance imaging findings in ECT-induced delirium, *J. Neuropsychiatry 2*:53 (1990).

91. G. S. Figiel, K. R. R. Krishnan, and P. M. Doraiswamy, Subcortical structural changes in ECT induced delirium, *J. Geriatr. Psychiatry Neurol. 3*:172 (1991).

92. G. S. Figiel, K. R. R. Krishnan, and J. C. Breitner, Radiologic correlates of antidepressant induced delirium: the possible significance of basal-ganglia lesions, *J. Neuropsychiatry 1*:188 (1989).

93. G. S. Figiel, K. R. R. Krishnan, and P. M. Doraiswamy, Caudate hyperintensities in elderly depressed patients with neuroleptic induced parkinsonism, *Geriatr. Psychiatry Neurol. 4*:86 (1991).

94. C. W. Erwin, C. E. Coffey, and G. R. Marsh, Polysomnographic findings in elderly depressed patients with unsuspected MRI abnormalities of the pons, *Sleep Res. 18*:174 (1989).

95. M. M. Husain, D. Knight, and P. M. Doraiswamy, Platelet imipramine binding and leukoencephalopathy in geriatric depression, *Biol. Psychiatry 29*:655 (1991).

96. G. S. Figiel, K. R. R. Krishnan, and P. M. Doraiswamy, Subcortical hyperintensities on brain magnetic resonance imaging: a comparison between late age onset and early onset elderly depressed subjects, *Neurobiol. Aging 26*:245 (1991).

97. F. W. Brown, R. J. Lewine, P. A. Hudgins, and S. C. Risch, White matter hyperintensity signals in psychiatric and non-psychiatric subjects, *Am. J. Psychiatry 149*:620 (1992).

98. R. M. Dupont, T. L. Jernigan, and N. Butters, Subcortical abnormalities detected in bipolar affective disorder using magnetic resonance imaging, *Arch. Gen. Psychiatry 47*:55 (1990).

99. T. L. Jernigan, G. A. Press, and J. R. Hesselink, Methods for measuring brain morphologic features on magnetic resonance images: Validation and normal aging, *Arch. Neurol. 47*:27 (1990).

100. S. M. Strakowski, B. T. Woods, M. Tohen, D. R. Wilson, A. W. Douglass, and A. L. Stoll, MRI subcortical signal hyperintensities in mania at first hospitalization, *Biol. Psychiatry 33*:204 (1993).

101. K. N. Botteron, M. W. Vannier, B. Geller, R. Todd, and B. C. Lee, Magnetic resonance imaging in childhood and adolescent bipolar affective disorder: a pilot investigation, *J. Am. Acad. Child Adol. Psychiatry 34*:742 (1995).

102. F. Fazekas, R. Kleinert, H. Offenbacher, F. Payer, R. Schmidt, G. Kleinert,

H. Radner, and H. Lechner, The morphologic correlate of incidental punctate white matter hyperintensities on MR images, *A.J.N.R. 12*:915 (1991).

103. I. A. Awad, P. C. Johnson, and R. J. Spetzler, Incidental subcortical lesions identified on magnetic resonance imaging in the elderly, II: Postmortem pathological correlations, *Stroke 17*:1090 (1986).

104. B. A. Holland, Diseases of white matter, *Magnetic Resonance Imaging of the Central Nervous System* (M. Brant-Zawadski and D. Norman, eds.), Raven Press, New York, 1987, pp. 259–277.

105. K. N. Westlund, A. Aguilera, and G. V. Childs, Quantification of morphological changes in pituitary corticotropes produced by in vivo corticotropin-releasing factor stimulation and adrenalectomy, *Endocrinology 116*:439 (1985).

106. K. R. R. Krishnan, P. M. Doraiswamy, and S. N. Lurie, Pituitary size in depression, *J. Clin. Endocrinol. Metab. 72*:256 (1991).

107. D. A. Axelson, P. M. Doraiswamy, O. B. Boyko, P. Rodrigo Escalona, W. M. McDonald, J. C. Ritchie, L. J. Patterson, E. H. Ellinwood, C. B. Nemeroff, K. R. R. Krishnan, In vivo assessment of pituitary volume with magnetic resonance imaging and systematic stereology: relationship to dexamethasone suppression test results in patients, *Psychiatry Res. 44*:63 (1992).

108. R. Brown, N. Colter, and J. Corsellis, Postmortem evidence of structural brain changes in schizophrenia: differences in brain weight, temporal horn area, and parahippocampal gyrus compared with affective disorder, *Arch. Gen. Psychiatry 43*:36 (1986).

109. D. M. Bowen, A. Najlerahim, A. W. Procter, P. T. Francis, and E. Murphy, Circumscribed changes of the cerebral cortex in neuropsychiatric disorders of later life, *Proc. Natl. Acad. Sci. 86*:9504 (1989).

110. P. H. Hauser, D. Dauphinais, and W. Berrettini, Temporal lobe measurement in primary affective disorder by magnetic resonance imaging, *J. Neuropsychiatry 1*:128 (1989).

111. L. L. Altschuler, A. Conrad, and P. Hauser, Reduction of temporal lobe volume in bipolar disorder: a preliminary report of magnetic resonance imaging, *Arch. Gen. Psychiatry 48*:482 (1992).

112. C. R. Jack, C. K. Twomey, A. R. Zinsmeister, F. W. Sharbrough, R. C. Petersen, and G. D. Cascino, Anterior temporal lobes and hippocampal formations: normative volumetric measurements from MR images in young adults, *Radiology 172*:549 (1989).

113. K. R. R. Krishnan, P. M. Doraiswamy, G. S. Figiel, M. M. Husain, S. A. Shah, C. Na, O. B. Boyko, W. M. McDonald, C. B. Nemeroff, and E. H. Ellinwood, Hippocampal abnormalities in depression, *J. Neuropsychiatry 3*: 387 (1991).

114. D. A. Axelson, P. M. Doraiswamy, W. M. McDonald, and O. B. Boyko, Hypercortisolemia and hippocampal changes in depression, *Psychiatry Res. 47*:163 (1993).

115. J. Haller, K. N. Botteron, B. Brunsden, Y. Sheline, R. Walkup, K. Black, M. Gado, and M. Vannier, Hippocampal MR volumetry, *Int. Soc. Optical Eng. Proc. 2359*:660 (1994).

116. K. R. R. Krishnan, W. M. McDonald, P. R. R. Escalona, P. M. Doraiswamy, C. Na, M. M. Husain, G. S. Figiel, O. B. Boyko, E. H. Ellinwood, and C. B. Nemeroff, Magnetic resonance imaging of the caudate nuclei in depression, *Arch. Gen. Psychiatry 49*:553 (1992).

117. M. M. Husain, W. M. McDonald, P. M. Doraiswamy, G. S. Figiel, C. Na, P. R. Escalona, O. B. Boyko, C. B. Nemeroff, and K. R. R. Krishnan, A magnetic resonance imaging study of putamen nuclei in major depression, *Psychiatry Res. 40*:95 (1991).

118. M. S. Keshavan, W. W. Bagwell, G. L. Haas, J. A. Sweeney, N. R. Schooler, and J. W. Pettegrew, Changes in caudate volume with neuroleptic treatment, *Lancet 344*:1434 (1994).

119. P. M. Doraiswamy, L. A. Tupler, and K. R. R. Krishnan, Neuroleptic treatment and caudate plasticity, *Lancet 345*:734 (1995).

120. R. Sandyk and R. Pardeshi, The relationship between ECT nonresponsiveness and calcification of the pineal gland in bipolar patients, *Int. J. Neurosci. 54*: 301 (1990).

121. R. Sandyk, The relationship of pineal calcification to subtypes of tardive dyskinesia in bipolar patients, *Int. J. Neurosci. 54*:307 (1990).

122. S. E. Folstein, Diseases of the caudate: a model for manic depressive disorder, *Function and Dysfunction in the Basal Ganglia* (A. J. Franks, ed.), Manchester University Press, Manchester, England, 1990.

123. P. R. McHugh, The neuropsychiatry of basal ganglia disorders, *Neuropsychiatry Neuropsychol. Behav. Neurol. 2*:239 (1989).

124. N. R. Swerdlow and G. F. Koob, Dopamine, schizophrenia, mania and depression: toward a unified hypothesis of cortico-striato-pallido-thalamic function, *Behav. Brain Sci. 10*:197 (1987).

125. W. C. Drevets and M. E. Raichle, Neuroanatomical circuits in depression: implications for treatment mechanisms, *Psychopharmacol. Bull. 28*:261 (1992).

8

Magnetic Resonance Spectroscopy Studies of Affective Disorders

Constance M. Moore and Perry F. Renshaw
Brain Imaging Center, McLean Hospital, Belmont, and Harvard Medical School, Boston, Massachusetts

I. INTRODUCTION

In this chapter the application of in vivo magnetic resonance spectroscopy (MRS) to the study of patients with affective disorders will be discussed. The first section will briefly describe the nuclei most commonly used in MRS studies of subjects with affective disorders: in particular, proton (^{1}H) and phosphorus (^{31}P) for determining alterations of brain biochemistry, and fluorine (^{19}F) and lithium (^{7}Li) for assessing brain drug levels. While the physical principles that underlie in vivo MRS techniques are presented in another chapter, a short description will be included here with a focus on how different methodologies may be better suited than others for the study of a particular nucleus.

The second section will describe the use of MRS for evaluation of cerebral metabolism using ^{1}H and ^{31}P MRS. The compounds that can be detected using ^{1}H and ^{31}P MRS will be described in relation to current theories on the biochemical abnormalities associated with affective disorders.

Finally, a third section will detail the role of MRS in measuring the levels and effects of ^{19}F- and ^{7}Li-containing drugs that have been used for the treatment of affective disorders. In particular, the utility of these studies in the evaluation and development of treatment strategies for affective disorders will be highlighted.

II. MAGNETIC RESONANCE SPECTROSCOPY

MRS is unique in clinical medicine as a noninvasive technique that provides information regarding tissue biochemistry in vivo. The main elements found in the human body are hydrogen (H), phosphorus (P), carbon (C), oxygen (O), sodium (Na), and potassium (K). The naturally occurring isotopes of hydrogen and phosphorus are the proton (^{1}H), with an abundance of 99.98%, and ^{31}P, with an abundance of 100%, respectively. Both of these isotopes are MR detectable and have relatively high sensitivities: ^{31}P has a sensitivity of 8.3%, compared to a proton sensitivity of 100%, at constant field [1]. The naturally occurring isotope of carbon is ^{12}C (natural abundance of 98.9%) and that of oxygen is ^{16}O (natural abundance of 99.8%). Neither of these isotopes produces an MR signal, and in order to carry out an MRS study of carbon or oxygen metabolism, it is necessary to introduce ^{13}C (natural abundance of 1.1%)– or ^{17}O (natural abundance of 0.038%)–labeled compounds into the human system [2,3]. However, labeling compounds with these isotopes is very expensive, especially when doses for the study of human subjects are involved. The naturally abundant isotope of sodium, ^{23}Na (100% abundance), is present in the body as an ion and, as such, produces a spectrum with a single resonance. Potassium, ^{39}K (natural abundance of

93.2%), is also present as an ion, and has a relatively low MR sensitivity of 0.1%. For these reasons the most commonly used endogenous isotopes for human MRS studies are ^{31}P and [1]H [1].

Additionally, two naturally occurring isotopes not found in the human body but which are MR visible are [7]Li and [19]F. Both of these are of interest in the study of affective illness. Lithium salts are commonly used in the treatment of patients with bipolar disorder, and fluorinated serotonin reuptake inhibitors, such as fluoxetine, are used in the treatment of depression [4,5]. [7]Li has both a high natural abundance (92.58%) and a sensitivity relative to ^{1}H of 29% [6,7]. [19]F is 100% naturally abundant, with a sensitivity of 83% relative to [1]H. [19]F also has a large chemical shift range (500 ppm), making it an ideal isotope for MRS studies [8].

A. ^{31}P MRS

Some of the earliest in vivo MRS assessments of tissue biochemistry involved the evaluation of ^{31}P metabolism using surface coils [9]. The geometry and size of the surface coil defines the sensitive volume from which the spectral signals arise. Depth resolved surface coil spectroscopy (DRESS) [10] allows for localized signal detection from slices at different distances from the surface coil.

It is now possible to use ^{31}P volume coils for MRS studies of human brain. Volume coils provide more homogeneous radiofrequency excitation and are commonly used in conjunction with a localizing pulse sequence. One of the earliest localization methods proposed was image selective in vivo spectroscopy (ISIS) [11]. With ISIS, signals arising from a cubic volume may be selected as a result of the addition and subtraction of eight separate acquisitions. The ISIS technique allows for the volume of interest (VOI) to be selected from a standard MR proton image. Both ISIS and DRESS are well suited for ^{31}P spectroscopy as the delay time between excitation of the nuclei and signal detection for these sequences is quite short, allowing for the detection of short T_2 metabolites. The T_2s of the α-, β-, and γ-nucleotide triphosphate (NTP) resonances, at 1.5 T, have been reported to be in the range of 15–28 ms [12] and 62–89 ms [13] in the brain. The T_2s of the PME and PDE signals are even less: 33 and 11 ms, respectively [12].

Spectra can also be acquired using chemical shift imaging (CSI). CSI provides a two- or three-dimensional map of metabolite distribution as a matrix of spectra acquired over the VOI [14]. CSI may be very time consuming, and the signal-to-noise ratio (SNR) of the individual spectra may be too low for quantitation.

Phosphorus spectra provide important information with respect to phospholipid metabolism, tissue energetics, and pH. In particular, ^{31}P spectra can identify (a) phosphomonoesters (PMEs) and phosphodiesters (PDEs), (b) the high-energy phosphates phosphocreatine (PCr), α-, β-, and γ-nucleotide triphosphate (NTP), and (c) inorganic phosphate (Pi) (Fig. 1).

Brain membranes are largely composed of phospholipid bilayers. The primary anabolites and catabolites of phospholipids are PME and PDE, respectively [15]. The ^{31}P PME resonance arises from phosphoethanolamine (PEt), phosphocholine (PC), and sugar phosphates. The total in vivo PME signal has been reported to be of the order of 3.0 ± 0.3 mM/L [16]. PEt is a precursor of the membrane phospholipid phosphatidylethanolamine (PtdEt) [17]. The principal components of the PDE resonance are more mobile phospholipids and the freely soluble molecules glycerophosphocholine and glycerophosphoethanolamine [18]. The total in vivo PDE signal has been estimated as 11.4 ± 0.6 mM/L [16]. In vivo ^{31}P MRS brain spectra are dominated by a broad baseline resonance arising from the bilayer phospholipids; this "hump" is generally removed by postprocessing prior to data analysis [18].

Information on alterations in high-energy metabolism may be gained by measuring the relative levels of PCr ($\approx 4.1 \pm 0.7$ mM/L), NTP ($\approx 2.8 \pm 0.5$ mM/L), and Pi ($\approx 1.4 \pm 0.6$ mM/L) [15]. The brain NTP resonance is primar-

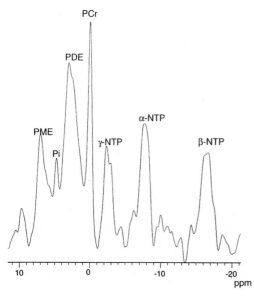

Fig. 1 ^{31}P MRS spectrum from the bilateral basal ganglia of a subject with major depression.

ily derived from adenosine triphosphate (ATP), which is found universally in living systems and performs the essential function of storing energy for various cellular activities [19]. When the phosphate group is hydrolyzed to adenosine diphosphate (ADP), the reaction liberates a great deal of energy ($\Delta G^{\circ\prime}$ = 7.3 kcal/mol; pH: 7.0).

$$ATP \Longleftrightarrow ADP + Pi \tag{1}$$

The energy supplied by the conversion of ATP to ADP is constantly being used by the cell. Since the supply of ATP at any given time is limited, a mechanism exists to replenish it: a phosphate group is added to ADP to produce ATP.

$$ADP + PCr \Longleftrightarrow ATP + Cr \tag{2}$$

The energy for this reaction ($\Delta G^{\circ\prime}$ = -3.0 kcal/mol; pH: 7.0) is supplied from oxidation-reduction reactions in the electron transfer chain and is catalyzed by creatine kinase [20]. These are aerobic reactions and cannot be carried out without oxygen. Since the creatine kinase reaction is near equilibrium in human brain [21], changes in ATP concentration are most likely associated with changes in the level of adenosine diphosphate (ADP), thus maintaining a constant ratio of ATP/ADP, as well as with changes in the total adenosine pool.

The Pi peak contains both H_2PO_4 and HPO_4^{2-} ions. Each of these ions has a slightly different chemical shift, but the in vivo resonance typically occurs as one peak, due to fast exchange. Depending on the equilibrium between these two ions, which has a pK$'$ of 7.2, the Pi resonance frequency will change as a function of tissue pH. Conversely, the pH of the tissue of interest may then be measured by comparing the chemical shift of Pi to that of a compound with a fixed chemical shift (usually PCr) [22]. However, under normal physiological conditions, the concentration of inorganic phosphate is low and the chemical shift of the Pi resonance may be difficult to interpret due to overlap with other peaks [23].

B. ^{1}H MRS

^{1}H spectroscopy is complicated by the fact that the signals from most metabolites of interest are 10^5 times smaller than the signals arising from tissue water and lipid. However, using specially developed sequences, it has become possible in recent years to effectively suppress the water signal. Using water-suppressed localized ^{1}H spectroscopy it is therefore possible to acquire ^{1}H spectra from a region where there are no large lipid signals present.

Techniques commonly used for localized, water-suppressed proton spectroscopy include stimulated echo acquisition mode spectroscopy (STEAM)

[24] and point resolved spectroscopy (PRESS) [25]. STEAM produces a stimulated echo from a cubic VOI within a single experiment. As with ISIS, the location of the VOI may be selected from an MR image. A major advantage of this sequence is that it permits variation of the echo time (TE), so the sequence may be optimized to investigate metabolites with short T_2 values. PRESS is a similar technique to STEAM; however, the PRESS sequence samples the entire signal while STEAM, as a stimulated echo technique, samples only half the signal originating from within the VOI. PRESS is also less sensitive to motion artifacts. However, STEAM allows for shorter echo times to be used [26]. CSI may also be used to acquire a map of metabolite distribution in conjunction with either STEAM or PRESS.

Using water-suppressed, in vivo proton spectroscopy it is possible to observe a number of cerebral metabolites. These include N-acetyl aspartate (NAA), creatine/phosphocreatine (Cr/PCr), cytosolic choline compounds (Cho), and *myo*-inositol (Ino) (Fig. 2). NAA contributes the largest signal to water-suppressed cerebral spectra and is primarily found in neurons [27,28]. The NAA resonance intensity has frequently been used as a neuronal marker. PCr is a high-energy phosphate, and the Cr/PCr resonance is often used as a reference standard as the total concentration of Cr and PCr remains

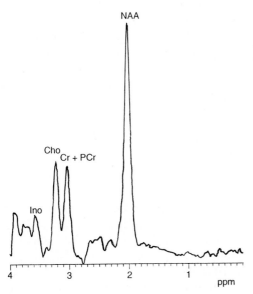

Fig. 2 272 ms ¹H MRS STEAM spectrum from the occipital lobe of an elderly subject.

approximately the same throughout the brain, although it is slightly higher in cerebral cortex than in white matter [29]. Most of the choline in the brain is in the form of the membrane phospholipid phosphatidylcholine [30]. However, as the motion of this molecule is restricted, it is largely invisible to in vivo ^{1}H MRS [31]. The major contributors to the Cho peak are phosphorylcholine and glycerophosphorylcholine [32], as well as small amounts of choline and acetylcholine [33,34]. Phosphorylcholine and glycerophosphorylcholine are involved in phospholipid metabolism. Choline is a precursor of acetylcholine, which serves as a neurotransmitter. Ino is also involved in phospholipid metabolism and plays an important role in intracellular message transduction through its role in the phosphatidylinositol cycle [4]. It is also important in the maintenance of osmotic equilibrium within the brain [35].

Other metabolites that are ^{1}H MR visible are present at lower concentrations and typically require short echo time acquisitions (TE: 20–65 ms) (Fig. 3). These include the amino acids alanine (Ala), acetate (Ace), glutamate (Glu), glutamine (Gln), aspartate (Asp), taurine (Tau), and γ-amino butyrate (GABA). Glu and Asp are also excitatory neurotransmitters, while GABA is an inhibitory neurotransmitter. However, it is very difficult to separate these resonances from the larger resonance lines that overlie them (i.e.,

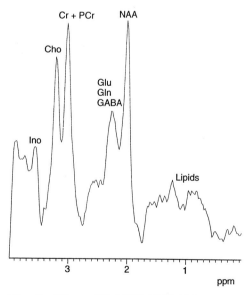

Fig. 3 30 ms ^{1}H MRS STEAM spectrum from the basal ganglia of a euthymic subject with bipolar depression.

NAA, Cr(PCr), and Cho) using conventional spectroscopy sequences, and special techniques need to be employed [36].

C. ^{19}F and ^{7}Li MRS

In vivo ^{19}F and ^{7}Li MRS have the potential to trace the distribution and concentration of fluorine and lithium containing psychopharmacological agents. In turn, this may provide insights into the mechanisms that underlie their clinical efficacy.

^{19}F is found in the trifluoromethyl group of the serotonin reuptake inhibitor fluoxetine. Fluoxetine has been used successfully to treat major depression, obsessive-compulsive disorder (OCD), and bulimia [5,37,38]. Lithium salts are commonly used for the treatment of bipolar disorder [4].

^{19}F and ^{7}Li MRS are limited by the same factors that occur in ^{31}P and ^{1}H MRS. The main technical problem associated with in vivo drug studies is that the drugs are present in relatively small concentrations ($\leq$1.0 mM) and a large VOI must be used. Initial studies of these isotopes relied on the localization provided by the limited excitation volume of surface coils. Surface coils placed over a "brain" region will excite and detect signal from skull, scalp, fat, and musculature. Quantitation of drug levels is complicated by the inhomogeneous excitation and detection profiles of these coils [39]. More recently, volume coils have been used in association with localizing sequences for spectral quantitation using in vivo ^{19}F and ^{7}Li MRS.

III. ^{1}H AND ^{31}P MAGNETIC RESONANCE SPECTROSCOPY STUDIES

A. ^{31}P MRS Studies

The earliest studies of cerebral metabolism in patients with affective disorders utilized ^{31}P MRS. One of the first studies in bipolar disorder was reported by Kato et al. in 1991 [40]. They examined 11 lithium-medicated bipolar patients, 7 of whom were studied during both the manic and euthymic states. Using a DRESS sequence, they acquired ^{31}P MR spectra from a 30-mm coronal slice centered in the frontal lobe. Spectra were also acquired from nine comparison subjects. The PME-to-total peak ratio was significantly higher in the patients during the manic state compared with bipolar patients in the euthymic state ($\uparrow$ 55%; $p < 0.01$) or the comparison subjects ($\uparrow$ 27%; $p < 0.01$) (Table 1). The PME-PDE ratio in patients in the manic state was also significantly higher than that observed for patients in the euthymic state ($\uparrow$ 55%; $p < 0.01$) or for normal controls ($\uparrow$ 33%; $p < 0.05$). As with all MRS results expressed as ratios, it should be noted that the PME-PDE increase may be due to a reduction in PDE. However, the authors did not report a statistically significant reduction in the PDE-to-total peak ratio.

Table 1 Comparison of Different Cerebral PME and PCr Levels in Subjects with Bipolar Disorder Measured with ^{31}P MRS

Subjects	PME	PCr	Ref.
Bipolar disorder ($n = 11$)	↑ 55% $p < 0.01$: manic vs. euythmic ↑ 27% $p < 0.01$: manic vs. control		40
Major depression ($n = 12$)	↑ 25% $p < 0.05$: bipolar depressed vs. bipolar euythmic	Severe depressed vs. mild depressed: ↓ 12% $p < 0.05$	44
Bipolar disorder ($n = 10$)	↓ 23% $p < 0.002$: bipolar euythmic vs. control ↓ 25% $p < 0.05$: bipolar euythmic vs. unipolar euythmic		
Bipolar disorder ($n = 17$)	↑ 20% $p < 0.01$: manic vs. euythmic ↓ 10% $p < 0.05$: manic vs. control		48
Bipolar I disorder ($n = 14$)	↑ 18% $p < 0.05$: bipolar I depressed vs. bipolar I euythmic	↓ 11%: $p < 0.01$: bipolar II depressed vs. control	49
Bipolar II disorder ($n = 15$)	↓ 21% $p < 0.05$: bipolar I euythmic vs. bipolar II euythmic ↓ 14% $p < 0.01$: bipolar I euythmic vs. control ↑ 11% $p < 0.05$: bipolar II hypomanic vs. control ↑ 10% $p < 0.05$: bipolar II depressed vs. control	↓ 10.5% $p < 0.05$: bipolar II euythmic vs. control ↓ 10%: $p < 0.05$: bipolar II hypomanic vs. control	
Bipolar disorder ($n = 40$)	↓ 5.4%: euythmic vs. control		50
Bipolar disorder ($n = 12$)	↓ 25% left frontal: bipolar euythmic vs. control ↓ 14% right frontal: bipolar euythmic vs. control ↓ 21% left temporal: bipolar euythmic vs. control ↓ 25% right temporal: bipolar euythmic vs. control	↑ 20% $p < 0.02$: right vs. left frontal bipolar euythmic	52,53

The increase in PME observed in this study was interpreted as evidence for an increase in brain myo-inositol-1-phosphate (I-1-P) as a consequence of lithium treatment in patients. After lithium administration, I-1-P is known to accumulate in rat brain [41], and lithium administration causes an increase in the ^{31}P MRS PME resonance in cat brain [42]. The accumulation of PME in the manic state may provide indirect evidence in support of the "monoamine hypothesis" [43]. Brain phosphoinositide (PI) turnover may be increased in the manic state, due to an instability of monoamine neuronal activity, leading to an increase in I-1-P, which is augmented in the presence of lithium.

In 1992, Kato et al. [44] extended this work to include subjects with major depression. Using the same coronal slice measurement protocol, they acquired ^{31}P spectra from the frontal cortex in 22 subjects—12 with major depression and 10 with bipolar disorder—and 22 controls. All subjects were examined in the depressed and euthymic states and were receiving medication (lithium, antidepressants, hypnotics, and/or antipsychotics). For the bipolar subjects, both PME and pH were higher in the depressed than the euthymic state ($\uparrow 25\%$; $p < 0.05$ and $\uparrow 0.86\%$; $p < 0.05$, respectively). The bipolar subjects also had lower PME and pH in the euthymic state compared with the normal controls ($n = 10$) ($\uparrow 23\%$; $p < 0.002$ and $\downarrow 1\%$; $p < 0.002$, respectively) and compared with the subjects with major depression in the euthymic state ($\downarrow 25\%$; $p < 0.05$ and $\downarrow 1.4\%$; $p < 0.01$, respectively).

In their initial study [40], the authors suggested that increases in PME in the manic state may be a result of lithium treatment. In this subsequent study, they report an increased PME level in bipolar patients in the depressed state. However, 7 of the 10 bipolar subjects who participated in this study were not on lithium. Thus, the PME increase in depressed subjects would appear to arise as function of mood state, rather than as an effect of lithium treatment.

Changes in brain energy metabolism were also reported. The depressed bipolar and unipolar subjects were evaluated as two groups, chosen according to the severity of depression [severe: HAM-D > 20 ($n = 11$); mild: HAM-D $\leq$ 20 ($n = 11$)]. PCr was significantly lower in the severe group ($\downarrow 12\%$; $p < 0.05$) than in the mild group. These results suggest that there may be alterations in brain high-energy phosphate metabolism related to severity of depression, an assumption that is supported by radionuclide imaging studies. Positron emission tomography (PET) [45] and single photon emission computed tomography (SPECT) [46,47] have shown decreases in fluorodeoxyglucose metabolic rates and blood flow, respectively, in the frontal lobes of patients with unipolar depression relative to comparison subjects.

In 1993 Kato et al. [48] performed a multinuclear study, acquiring both ^{31}P and [7]Li spectra from subjects with bipolar disorder. The [31]P ($n = 17$) spectra were acquired from the frontal cortex as in their previous studies.

The ^{7}Li (n = 9) spectra were acquired using a double-tuned surface coil. Each bipolar subject was examined a total of one to eight times in the manic and euthymic states. All were receiving lithium. Some were also receiving antipsychotics and/or hypnotics. Six subjects were examined in the manic state before commencing lithium treatment. ^{31}P spectra were also acquired from an age- and sex-matched group of controls (n = 17).

PME was significantly increased ($\uparrow$ 20%; $p < 0.01$) in the manic state compared with the euthymic state and PME in the euthymic state was lower ($\downarrow$ 10%; $p < 0.05$) than in the normal controls. These results are consistent with the authors' previous reports. In nine subjects whose brain lithium concentration was measured, PME did not correlate with brain lithium concentration, and in the six subjects with mania, who were examined before and after commencing lithium treatment, PME did not change with lithium treatment. The time between initiation of lithium treatment and the repeat MRS exam was not reported. Similarly, no data were provided with regard to treatment response.

Subsequently Kato and colleagues investigated the effects of medication in patients with bipolar depression [49]. They did not note any significant difference in frontal lobe PME levels between the medicated depressed (n = 12) and drug-free depressed (n = 13) patients. In this study, Kato and colleagues also investigated differences between the ^{31}P MR spectra of subjects with bipolar I disorder (n = 14) and bipolar II disorder (n = 15). Bipolar II disorder subjects were examined in the depressive (n = 12), euthymic (n = 9) and hypomanic (n = 10) states. Eleven bipolar I disorder subjects were examined in the depressive and the euthymic state. The ^{31}P spectra were acquired as before and compared to values from 59 control subjects.

PME was lower in the euthymic subjects with bipolar I disorder compared to normal controls ($\downarrow$ 14%; $p < 0.01$) and was higher in the depressive state compared to the euthymic state ($\uparrow$ 18%; $p < 0.05$). PME in the euthymic subjects with bipolar I disorder was significantly lower than that observed in the patients with bipolar II disorder in the euthymic state ($\downarrow$ 21%; $p < 0.05$). PME was higher in the subjects with bipolar II disorder, in the hypomanic state ($\uparrow$ 11%; $p < 0.05$) and the depressive state ($\uparrow$ 10%; $p < 0.05$), than the normal controls.

PCr was lower in the bipolar II disorder subjects in all three states (depressive— $\downarrow$ 11%: $p < 0.01$; euthymic— $\downarrow$ 10.5%; $p < 0.05$; hypomanic— $\downarrow$ 10.%: $p < 0.05$) compared with the normal controls. In the patients with bipolar I disorder, there was a trend for PCr to be lower in the depressed state compared with the euthymic state ($p < 0.1$).

Kato and colleagues have measured reduced PME signal intensity in the frontal lobes of euthymic subjects with bipolar I disorder. The reason for this change has been difficult to interpret. However, a reduction in PME may arise as a result of altered membrane phospholipid metabolism. The authors hypothesized that this may, in turn, be associated with cerebral atrophy and ventricular enlargement. Therefore, they used ^{31}P MRS to determine whether this reduction in PME was associated with ventricular enlargement in 40 patients with bipolar disorder (31 with bipolar I disorder and 9 with bipolar II disorder) and 60 controls [50]. All of the patients were examined in the euthymic state, and the PME signal intensity was reduced in the patient group compared with the normal controls ($p < 0.05$).

Overall, the ventricular size in the subjects with bipolar disorder was greater than in controls (Evans ratio: ↑ 4.6%; $p < 0.05$). This is in agreement with studies by Swayze et al. [51], who report increased ventricular volume in 48 bipolar males ($p < 0.05$) compared with a control group ($n = 47$), using MRI. However, no correlation was found between ventricular size and PME level. Those patients with psychotic features had significantly increased ventricular size compared to patients without psychotic features (Evans ratio: ↑ 10%; $p < 0.05$).

Other research groups have also used ^{31}P MRS to evaluate possible biochemical changes in patients with bipolar disorder. Deicken et al. reported the results of a ^{31}P CSI study in 12 unmedicated euthymic male subjects with bipolar disorder and 16 matched controls. For ^{31}P CSI, a volume head coil was used and the effective volume of each voxel was 25 cm^3. They examined abnormalities in the frontal [52] and temporal lobes [53]. The bipolar subjects were medication free for one week prior to the study. The euthymic bipolar subjects had significantly lower PME and significantly higher PDE values in both the left (PME: ↓ 25%; PDE: ↑ 12%) and right (PME: ↓ 14%; PDE: ↑ 10%) frontal lobes compared with the control subjects. Also, PCr was higher (↑ 20%; $p < 0.02$) in the right frontal lobe of the patient group compared with the left. In the temporal lobe, PME level was lower in both the left (↓ 21%) and right (↓ 25%) temporal lobes of the patient group compared with the control group ($p < 0.006$: group difference).

The finding of reduced PME in the frontal lobe of euthymic subjects with bipolar disorder is similar to the results of Kato and colleagues. This finding appears to be mood state dependent and not a result of lithium treatment or cerebral atrophy. However, reduced PME has also been noted in the frontal cortex of subjects with schizophrenia [16,54]. This raises the question of whether or not these two disorders may share some common pathophysiological features.

While there have been several studies of ^{31}P MRS in bipolar disorder, there have been few in patients with unipolar disorder. At this center we have measured reduced β-NTP (↓ 21%; $p < 0.02$) in a 45 cm^3 voxel encompassing the bilateral basal ganglia of unmedicated subjects with major depression ($n = 36$) compared with normal controls ($n = 17$), using ^{31}P ISIS MRS

[55]. The observed decrease in β-NTP in the depressed subjects, in the presence of a constant PCr-to-Pi ratio, is consistent with the presence of metabolic abnormalities within neurons and/or glial cells. This profile of metabolite changes is unusual, since NTP concentration is usually maintained at the expense of PCr. Decreases in ATP are most likely associated with decreases in adenosine diphosphate (ADP), thus maintaining a constant ratio of ATP to ADP, as well as with decreases in the total adenosine pool. The decrease in β-NTP reported here is also similar to the reduction in β-NTP reported by Deicken et al. [56] in the basal ganglia of subjects with schizophrenia. This is an interesting result as patients with schizophrenia [57] and major depression [45,46] both appear to show reductions in flourodeoxyglucose metabolic rates and blood flow in the basal ganglia.

B. ^{1}H MRS Studies

Relatively little ^{1}H MRS has been done in subjects with affective disorders. One of the earliest studies was by Sharma et al. [58], who used STEAM to acquire ^{1}H spectra from the basal ganglia and occipital cortex of four subjects with bipolar disorder, one with major depression, and nine comparison subjects. The ratios of NAA to Cr, Cho to Cr and Ino to Cr were increased by 46, 28, and 39%, respectively, in the basal ganglia of subjects with bipolar disorder taking lithium ($n = 4$) compared with controls. The small number of patients studied makes it difficult to draw any definite conclusions, although the reported effect sizes are quite large in comparison to those noted in other ^{1}H MRS studies. Additionally, it is difficult to assess whether the results are primarily due to the diagnosis of bipolar disorder, to changes in mood state, or to the effects of lithium treatment.

Proton MRS has also been used to study treatment response. Charles et al. [33] used ^{1}H spectroscopy (1D CSI with STEAM) to study elderly subjects with major depression both before ($n = 7$) and after treatment ($n = 4$) with the antidepressant nefazadone (500 mg/day). The scan was repeated once the symptoms of depression had ceased (2–3 months after starting treatment). Spectra were also acquired from 10 comparison subjects. The Cho:Cr ratio was increased in a 27 cc VOI, which contained white matter, thalamus, and putamen, in the depressed patients pre-therapy compared with post-therapy ($\uparrow$ 60%; $p < 0.03$) and control subjects ($\uparrow$ 17%; $p < 0.02$). The post-therapy Cho:Cr ratio was lower than that observed in control subjects ($\downarrow$ 27%; $p < 0.01$).

Changes in choline concentration have been related to alterations in cholinergic function [59]. In 1973, Janowsky et al. [60] proposed an "adrenergic-cholinergic" hypothesis of affective disorder. In this model, depression is associated with adrenergic underactivity and cholinergic overactivity, while mania is associated with adrenergic overactivity and cholinergic underactivity. Cholinergic overactivity would lead to an increase in acetylcholine. The authors suggest that the increased Cho:Cr ratio found in elderly depressed subjects pretherapy may be due to increased acetylcholine, although acetylcholine contributes very little signal to the Cho ^{1}H MRS signal. Following successful therapy, the Cho:Cr ratio would decrease to normal values. Additionally, it should be noted that morphometric MRI studies have indicated that caudate and putamen volumes are decreased in volume in elderly depressed subjects in comparison with matched control subjects [61]. This would lead to different proportions of gray and white matter within the VOI and, thereby, potentially confound ^{1}H MRS results as Cho has a different signal intensity in gray than in white matter [62].

The effects of medication on brain chemistry can also be determined using ^{1}H MRS. The effect of lithium on choline transport is well known. During lithium treatment of bipolar disorder, free choline within the erythrocyte has been shown to be markedly elevated [63]. Stoll et al. [64] used ^{1}H MRS STEAM spectroscopy to determine whether the Cho:Cr ratio in the parietal lobe of seven bipolar male subjects (all euythmic) was increased compared to six male controls, as might be expected from the erythrocyte studies. However, there was no significant difference in the Cho:Cr ratio in the patient group compared with the control group. Although lithium has potent effects on choline transport at therapeutic concentrations, the brain ^{1}H MRS resonance is principally derived from phosphorylcholine and glycerophosphorylcholine. Therefore, relatively large increases in the brain concentration of free choline might not be reflected in the ^{1}H MRS choline resonance.

Lithium has been shown to cause an increase in I-1-P and a reduction in Ino concentration [65] as a consequence of its inhibition of the enzyme *myo*-inositol-1-phosphatase [4,66]. Using ^{1}H MRS, it is possible to detect changes in Ino. Brühn et al. [67] used in vivo STEAM ^{1}H MRS to measure the absolute levels of Cho and Ino in the cortical gray and white matter of eight euthymic bipolar subjects on lithium treatment compared with 80 matched controls. They reported no differences in absolute Cho and Ino concentrations or in Cho:Cr and Ino:Cr ratios between patients and controls. The finding that lithium does not increase the brain ^{1}H MRS Cho resonance is in agreement with the work of Stoll et al. possibly for the same reasons.

Preece et al. [68] did a heteronuclear in vivo (8.5 T) and in vitro (11.8 T) MRS study on rats chronically treated with lithium. Using ^{31}P MRS, they measured increased PME:ATP ($\uparrow$ 52%; $n = 10$) in the brain of lithium-treated rats compared to rats given saline. The magnitude of the PME:ATP increase correlated with brain lithium levels in the rats, as measured by ^{7}Li

MRS. In vivo ¹H MRS detected no changes in the Ino levels. However, in vitro ¹H MRS of perchloric acid extracts of rat brain did detect decreased Ino:Cr levels in the lithium-treated rats compared with the controls (↓ 19%; $n = 5$). This result would suggest that there is a decrease in Ino in the brain as a result of lithium treatment, but the magnetic fields typically used for in vivo studies do not provide high enough spectral resolution to measure this change. Since the ¹H MR spectra of Ino and I-1-P are similar (Fig. 4), both contributing to the in vivo resonance at 3.6 ppm, an increase in I-1-P concomitant with a decrease in Ino may not be detectable.

Another area to which ¹H MRS has been applied is in the evaluation of cerebral metabolism following electroconvulsive therapy (ECT). Animal models using combined ¹H and ³¹P MRS have shown a decrease in cerebral PCr, pH, and NTP and an increase in lactate up to 2 hours following seizures [69]. Woods et al. [70] acquired ¹H MRS spectra, at various TE values, from seven subjects with severe depression 30–36 hours before ECT, after receiving atropine anesthesia and up to a half hour after receiving either

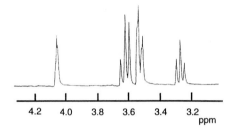

(a)

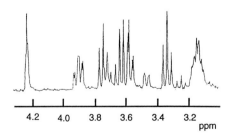

(b)

Fig. 4   8.4 T ¹H spectrum for (a) *myo*-inositol and (b) *myo*-inositol-1-phosphate.

bilateral ($n = 5$) or unilateral ($n = 2$) ECT. The region of interest was 100 cm^3 and placed in an anterior central region that included the medial frontal region of the cortex, the medial centrum semiovale, the corpus striatum, and the frontal horns. The authors noticed an increase in the lipid region of the spectra that was present up to 90 minutes after ECT but not after 32 hours. This resonance would obscure any changes in lactate if present. It should be noted that due to the rather large size of the VOI used, the possibility that the lipid signal is skull contamination cannot be excluded.

In 1993, Felber et al. [71] acquired ^{1}H and ^{31}P spectra, using STEAM (TE = 40 and 270 ms) and ISIS, respectively from a 64 ml VOI placed in a region that contained both parietal lobes and CSF from the lateral ventricles in three subjects with major depression before and up to one hour after receiving bilateral ECT. No changes were seen in either the ^{1}H or the ^{31}P spectra. The authors had anticipated an increase in lactate and decreased PCr, pH, and NTP. However, the time scale of the experiment may have been too long after the seizure for metabolite changes to have been detected.

IV. ^{19}F AND ^{7}Li MAGNETIC RESONANCE SPECTROSCOPY STUDIES

A. ^{19}F MRS Studies

Several investigators have utilized in vivo ^{19}F MRS to assess brain drug levels. Komoroski et al. [72] acquired the first in vivo spectrum of fluoxetine, a commonly used fluorinated antidepressant. A ^{19}F MR spectrum was acquired at 1.5 T, using a home-built 16-cm surface coil, from the occipital lobe of a patient receiving 40 mg/day of fluoxetine for major depression. No attempt was made to quantify the level of fluoxetine in the brain.

Animal studies indicate that the major fluorinated compounds found in brain following the administration of fluoxetine are fluoxetine and the demethylated metabolite norfluoxetine [73]. At 1.5 T, in vivo ^{19}F MRS cannot distinguish these two compounds as their chemical shifts are separated by 0.01 ppm. Throughout this section, brain fluoxetine concentration will refer to brain fluoxetine plus norfluoxetine concentration unless otherwise stated.

Having demonstrated their ability to acquire fluoxetine spectra, this same group [74] acquired ^{19}F spectra from six male subjects treated with 40 mg/day of fluoxetine. The patients studied were clinically heterogeneous with primary diagnoses of major depression ($n = 2$), bipolar disorder ($n = 1$), post-traumatic stress disorder (PTSD) ($n = 2$), and dysthymia ($n = 1$). Two subjects (with PTSD) receiving 20 mg/day fluoxetine were also studied (one was studied again on 40 mg/day).

All of the subjects receiving 40 mg/day of fluoxetine (n = 6) had a detectable ^{19}F MRS signal. The estimated brain fluoxetine concentrations ranged from 1.3 to 5.7 μg/ml. The fluoxetine brain concentrations varied according to treatment duration, with the largest signal arising from the subject who had been receiving medication the longest. No signal was obtained from subjects who received 20 mg/day of fluoxetine, possibly due to the low spectral SNR. Serum levels of fluoxetine were not measured.

Plasma levels of fluoxetine and norfluoxetine were related to brain levels of fluoxetine and norfluoxetine, as determined by ^{19}F MRS, in five subjects with major depression and three with obsessive compulsive disorder (OCD) by Renshaw et al. [75] (Table 2). All had been taking fluoxetine for a minimum of 3 months, and none had had a dose change within 4 weeks of the study. Subjects were receiving 60 mg/day (n = 4), 80 mg/day (n = 3), and 100 mg/day (n = 1). Spectra were obtained using a ^{19}F head coil on a 1.5 T system, and ^{19}F data was then acquired from the whole head.

Brain fluoxetine concentrations were 2.6 times higher ($p < 0.0008$) than plasma levels of fluoxetine and norfluoxetine. The daily dose correlated ($r = 0.82$) more closely than plasma ($r = 0.58$) levels with calculated brain levels.

In 1993 Karson et al. [39] extended their previous work to include more subjects, as well as the utilization of a ^{19}F volume coil. A total of 21 subjects were examined, including 12 adults and 9 adolescents. The subjects had diagnoses of bipolar disorder (n = 1), major depression (n = 6), dysthmia (n = 7), PTSD (n = 4), OCD (n = 1), and adjustment disorder (n = 2) and received doses of between 20 and 40 mg/day of fluoxetine.

The brain concentration of fluoxetine ranged from undetectable during the first few weeks of treatment to a maximum of 10.7 μg/ml after 27 months of treatment. These values are somewhat higher than those reported in their previous study (i.e., 1.3–5.7 μg/ml) or the values found by Renshaw et al. [75]. This may be a result of different measurement techniques or relaxation time estimates; more accurate quantitation methods need to be developed in this area. However, the brain concentration of fluoxetine appeared to increase with duration of fluoxetine treatment and correlated with daily dose of fluoxetine. At the early stages of treatment, the fluoxetine brain concentration correlated with the combined plasma concentration of fluoxetine and norfluoxetine ($r = 0.53$; $p < 0.07$; n = 6).

Two subjects had fluoxetine measured on several occasions in both the brain and plasma. The brain fluoxetine concentration was reported to be an order of magnitude greater than the plasma fluoxetine and norfluoxetine concentration ($\sim$20:1; n = 2). One subject received 30 mg/day of fluoxetine for 7 months and had a brain concentration of fluoxetine of 2.5 μg/ml. Four

Table 2   Comparison of Different Brain and Plasma Concentrations of Fluoxetine and Norfluoxetine Measured with ^{19}F MRS

Subjects	Dose	Brain concentration	Brain: Plasma (r)	Ref.
Major depression (n = 2)	40 mg/day (n = 6)	1.3–5.7 µg/mL		74
Bipolar disorder (n = 1)	20 mg/day (n = 2)			
PTSD (n = 3)				
Dysthymia (n = 1)				
Major depression (n = 5)	60 mg/day (n = 4)	~1.25–4.5 µg/mL	2.6 (0.58) (p < 0.0008)	75
OCD (n = 3)	80 mg/day (n = 3)			
	100 mg/day (n = 1)			
Bipolar disorder (n = 1)	20 mg/day (n = 10)	0–10.7 µg/mL	20 (n = 2) (0.81; p < 0.05)	39
Major depression (n = 6)	30 mg/day (n = 1)			
PTSD (n = 4)	40 mg/day (n = 10)			
Dysthymia (n = 7)				
OCD (n = 1)				
Adjustment disorder (n = 2)				
Social phobia (n = 8)	≤60 mg/ day			77
Responders (n = 5)		Responders vs nonresponders		
Nonresponders (n = 3)		Responders: 7.9 ± 5.4 µm/L Nonresponders: 1.6 ± 1.5 µm/L		

weeks after stopping fluoxetine, the brain concentration of fluoxetine was still 0.9 µg/ml. This is probably due to that fact that fluoxetine and norfluoxetine have long tissue half-lives and leave the brain slowly [73].

In vivo and in vitro spectra were acquired from postmortem brain tissue from a subject who had been treated with 40 mg/day of fluoxetine for 4.5 months prior to death. Brain tissue extracts were prepared from the frontal cortex, temporal cortex, and caudate nucleus of one hemisphere and frozen at autopsy; the other hemisphere was used for in vivo studies. High-resolution spectra were acquired from the postmortem brain tissue extracts at 7.1 T. Total fluoxetine and norfluoxetine concentrations were calculated and found to be 18.6, 12.3, and 13.4 μg/ml for the frontal cortex, temporal cortex, and caudate nucleus, respectively. These values are higher than the in vivo measurements found in previous studies, suggesting that all of the in vivo fluoxetine and/or norfluoxetine may not be visible to ^{19}F MRS. However, the effects of tissue fixation may also have influenced these results.

In order to accurately quantify any brain metabolite, it is necessary to know the T_1 value for the compound. For this reason, Komoroski et al. [76] made a preliminary effort to measure the T_1 of fluoxetine in five subjects with major depression or dysthmia (on 20 or 40 mg/day fluoxetine). They measured an average T_1 of fluoxetine in vivo to be 227 ± 72 ms (149–386 ms). T_1 was noted to increase with increasing brain concentration of fluoxetine, possibly reflecting fast exchange between bound and unbound fluoxetine.

A recent in vivo ^{19}F MRS study of social phobia [77] provided interesting preliminary results. Miner et al. measured brain fluoxetine levels in eight subjects with social phobia treated with up to 60 mg/day fluoxetine for between 8 and 20 weeks. The patients were separated into responders ($n = 5$) and nonresponders ($n = 3$) according to the Clinical Global Impression Improvement Scale. There was a trend toward higher fluoxetine levels in the responders (7.9 ± 5.4) compared with nonresponders (1.6 ± 1.5) ($\uparrow$ 80%: $p < 0.1$).

From the above studies it would appear that while ^{19}F MRS provides a means for measuring fluorinated pharmaceuticals in vivo, it is still difficult to interpret the clinical significance of the results.

B. ^{7}Li MRS Studies

Lithium salts are commonly used in the treatment of patients with bipolar disorder. However, lithium monotherapy is only effective in 50–60% patients, and many patients require additional treatment [78]. In vivo ^{7}Li MRS provides a means of determining brain lithium levels and this, in turn, may advance our understanding of the pathophysiology of bipolar disorder. Additionally, lithium treatment may result in neurotoxicity [79], and determination of the minimum lithium level required for a therapeutic response may also be estimated by in vivo ^{7}Li MRS. In turn, this might reduce the incidence of neurotoxic events by preventing treatment at supratherapeutic brain lithium levels.

The first in vivo ^{7}Li MRS was a study performed at 2 T in which rat abdomen was injected with 10 mEq/kg of LiCl and studied by ^{19}F MRS 24 hours later [6]. The lithium signal intensity measured by ^{7}Li MRS was in agreement with measurements done on tissue samples, following the MRS examination, by atomic absorption spectroscopy. This was important in demonstrating the feasibility of ^7Li MRS. This same group then went on to acquire the first in vivo measurement of lithium in human brain and calf, using a surface coil at 1.8 T, following the ingestion of Li_2CO_2 (1200 mg) for 1 week [7].

The first in vivo ^7Li spectrum from a bipolar subject was reported by Komoroski et al. [80]. They acquired localized spectra (DRESS sequence) from the occiput and calf using a 16-cm surface coil. Spectra were acquired daily over 11 days after the patient had commenced lithium therapy (900 mg/day). Serum levels of lithium were also recorded at the time of the examination. Brain lithium initially increased faster than muscle lithium, then more slowly. The lithium levels in muscle more closely matched the serum levels. A patient with schizoaffective disorder had brain lithium levels measured on multiple occasions using ^7Li MRS over a 7-month period. The serum levels varied from 0.83 to 1.25 mEq/L (0.61 ± 0.2 mEq/L), while brain levels varied from 0.45 to 0.84 mEq/L (1 ± 0.2 mEq/L) with a mean brain:serum ratio of 0.61 ± 0.14 (Table 3).

In an effort to clarify the relationship between brain, muscle, and serum lithium concentrations, Gyulai et al. [81] measured lithium levels from the calf and occipital pole of nine euthymic subjects with bipolar disorder using a 11.5-cm surface coil. All of the subjects had been receiving lithium for a minimum of 6 months and were taking no other psychotropic medications. Lithium concentrations in muscle and the occipital pole were consistently lower than serum levels (by 54 and 37%, respectively). The brain lithium concentration correlated with both the serum lithium concentration ($r = 0.71$; $p < 0.05$) and the muscle concentration ($r = 0.84$; $p < 0.005$).

Kato et al. [82] have also reported a difference between serum and brain lithium concentrations. They repeatedly measured brain lithium concentration in the frontal lobe of 10 bipolar patients using a 15-cm surface coil. In 41 examinations of 10 patients, brain lithium levels were 50–60% of the serum concentration when the latter was in the therapeutic range. Brain and serum lithium concentration were positively correlated ($r = 0.55$; $p < 0.01$) in agreement with the results of Gyulai et al. [81].

Kushnir et al. [83] reported an average brain:serum lithium ratio of 0.59 ± 0.12 in a study of eight bipolar patients who had been receiving lithium for at least a year. They measured the brain lithium concentration in vivo using a 11.5-cm square surface coil, placed over the left temporal lobe. In addition they measured the T_1 of lithium (3.5 ± 0.25 s) in five other patients using a ^7Li headcoil and used this value to quantify the lithium brain concentration.

Komoroski et al. [84] also measured the T_1 of lithium in vivo. They calculated a value of 4.6 ± 0.3 seconds in the brain of a single subject (the

Table 3 Comparison of Different Brain and Serum Lithium Concentrations Measured with ^7Li MRS

Subjects	Dose	Brain concentration	Brain: Serum (r)	T1 (n)	Ref.
Schizoaffective (n = 1) (6 examinations)	900 mg/ day	0.45–0.84 mEq/L	0.61 ± 0.14 (0.67)		80
Bipolar disorder (n = 9)	900–1500 mg/day	0.36 ± 0.1 mEq/L	0.47 ± 0.12 (0.71; $p < 0.05$)		81
Bipolar disorder (n = 10) (41 examinations)	600–1000 mg/day	~0.1–0.9 mM	0.5–0.6 (0.55; $p < 0.01$)		82
Bipolar disorder (n = 8)	450–1200 mg/day	0.46 ± 0.18 mEq/L	0.59 ± 0.12 (0.89)	3.5 ± 0.25 s (n = 5)	83
Schizoaffective (n = 1) (3 examinations)	600 mg/ day			4.6 ± 0.3 s (n = 1)	84
Bipolar disorder (n = 10)	900–1575 mg/day	0.52–0.87 mEq/L	0.77 ± 0.14 (0.9)		85
Bipolar disorder (n = 8)	600–1000 mg/day	~0.02–0.5 mM	0.45 ± 0.19 (0.66; $p < 0.001$)		86
Bipolar disorder (n = 14)	600–1000 mg/day	0.3 ± 0.16 mM	0.56 ± 0.24 (0.57; $p < 0.05$)		88
Bipolar disorder (n = 25)	N/A	0.25–0.89 mM/L	0.80 ± 0.19 (0.68; $p < 0.001$)		90

standard deviation is that of a three-parameter fit). In another subject the elimination rate of lithium from the serum, brain, and muscle was measured. This subject had been receiving 1200 mg Li_2CO_3 per day for 2 years before developing a hand tremor, which led to the discontinuation of treatment. Lithium could not be detected in serum after 3 days, in muscle after 6 days, or in brain after 10 days. The patient's hand tremor subsided over the course of one week, suggesting that lithium side effects may be more closely related to lithium brain and muscle levels than to serum levels.

González et al. [85] measured brain lithium concentration in a 60-mm slice centered 10 mm superior to the corpus callosum using a ^7Li headcoil at

1.5 T and the ISIS localization technique in 10 patients with bipolar disorder. Corrections were made for brain, muscle, and CSF contributions to the ^7Li MRS signal before calculating the brain lithium concentration. Also, the spectra were acquired with a TR of 25 seconds to eliminate T_1 effects. In this study, the brain:serum lithium ratio was 0.77 ± 0.14 mEq/L. While the plasma lithium concentration correlated well with daily dose ($r = 0.9$), brain lithium levels correlated poorly ($r = 0.56$).

Many of the previous ^7Li MRS studies compared brain and serum lithium concentration. Kato et al. [86] have also measured red blood cell (RBC) lithium concentration in order to determine if this is a better indicator of brain lithium concentration [87]. They acquired ^7Li MR spectra at 1.5 T from the frontal lobe of eight lithium-treated subjects using a 15-cm surface coil. Brain lithium concentration correlated closely with both serum concentration ($r = 0.66$; $p < 0.001$) and RBC concentration ($r = 0.44$; $p < 0.05$).

Another question of interest is the lithium brain concentration necessary to produce a therapeutic response. Kato et al. [88] measured brain and serum lithium concentration in 14 bipolar subjects 4 weeks after commencing lithium treatment (600–1000 mg/day) for mania or hypomania (12 bipolar I disorder; 2 bipolar II disorder) using in vivo ^7Li MRS. The patients were assessed using the Japanese version of the Petterson Mania Rating Scale (PMRS). The lithium brain concentration (0.3 ± 0.16 mM) and serum concentrations (0.55 ± 0.16 mM) were significantly correlated ($r = 0.57$; $p < 0.05$), the mean ratio being 0.56 ± 0.24, which is within the range seen by other workers. The brain lithium concentration was significantly correlated with a reduction in the PMRS ($r = 0.65$; $p < 0.05$), but the serum concentration was not. The authors draw the conclusion that in the nonresponders, either lithium uptake in the brain is less efficient or it is eliminated faster. This is an important result, suggesting that the clinical response to lithium therapy may depend upon brain lithium levels.

In 1994, Plenge et al. [89] measured brain lithium concentration in two normal subjects every 2 hours over a 24-hour period and 48 hours later to determine the extent to which lithium brain and serum concentration vary throughout the day. Two normal subjects took 1000 and 1200 mg Li_2CO_3 daily, respectively, for 7 days to establish a steady state. The 12-hour serum lithium concentrations were 0.9 and 0.7 mM/L, respectively. On day 8, ^7Li MR spectra were acquired every 2 hours for 24 hours from a 40-mm DRESS axial slice above the lateral ventricles and then again 48 hours later. Serum lithium levels were also acquired. The brain lithium concentration varied from 0.45 to 0.93 mM/L over the 24-hour period and brain:serum lithium ratios varied from 0.5 to 1, maximizing at 1.2 after 48 hours; the ratio was independent of the serum lithium concentration (~0.4–1.4 mM/L). These results may explain the variations seen in brain lithium concentrations as measured by other workers.

Sachs et al. [90] measured brain lithium concentration in 25 bipolar subjects. Lithium levels ranged from 0.25 to 1.16 mM/L in the serum and from 0.25 to 0.89 mM/L in the brain with a mean brain:serum ratio of 0.80 $\pm$ 0.19. This ratio is high but is similar to that reported by González et al. [85], who used a similar measurement technique. Overall, serum lithium concentration correlated well with brain lithium concentration ($r = 0.68$; $p < 0.001$). However, in 18 subjects where the serum concentration of lithium was within the therapeutic range (0.6–1 mM/L), brain levels varied from 0.29 to 0.88 mM/L and the correlation between serum and brain lithium levels was less robust ($r = 0.39$). These results suggest that a substantial number of patients maintained with therapeutic serum lithium levels may have subtherapeutic brain levels.

V. CONCLUSION

In vivo MRS is a valuable tool in the evaluation of cerebral metabolism in subjects with affective disorders. ^{31}P MRS demonstrates alterations in the phosphosmonoester resonances in bipolar disorder, as well as alterations in the high-energy phosphates in bipolar disorder and unipolar depression. Although fewer studies have utilized in vivo ^{1}H MRS, the studies that have been performed are of great value particularly in considering patient response to medication and the effects of medication on the Cho and Ino resonances.

In vivo MRS is unique as an noninvasive method of determining brain drug concentrations, as has been demonstrated by the in vivo ^{19}F and ^{7}Li MRS studies described here. In vivo ^{19}F MRS studies have been used successfully to determine brain fluoxetine concentration, comparing these concentrations to plasma levels and treatment response. In vivo ^{7}Li MRS has proved successful in determining brain lithium concentrations. Brain lithium concentrations did not always correlate with serum lithium levels, which may explain why some bipolar subjects do not respond to lithium treatment despite having therapeutic serum lithium levels.

In conclusion, in vivo MRS is an important research tool in the assessment of affective disorders and, with the development of more accurate measurement and quanitation techniques, should give valuable insight into the etiology of affective disorders.

REFERENCES

1. E. B. Cady, *Clinical Magnetic Resonance Spectroscopy*, Plenum Press, New York, 1990.

2. D. L. Rothman, E. J. Novotny, G. I. Shulman, A. M. Howesman, O. A. C. Petroff, G. Mason, T. Nixon, C. C. Hanstock, J. W. Prichard, and R. G. Shulman, 1H-[13C] NMR measurements of [4-13C] glutamate turnover in human brain, *Proc. Natl. Acad. Sci. 89*:9603 (1992).

3. D. Fiat, J. Dolinsek, J. Hankiewicz, M. Dujovny, and J. Ausman, Determination of regional cerebral oxygen consumption in the human: ^{17}O natural abundance cerebral magnetic resonance imaging and spectroscopy in a whole body system, *Neurol. Res. 15*(4):237 (1993).

4. M. J. Berridge, C. P. Downes and M. R. Hanley, Neural and developmental actions of lithium: a unifying hypothesis, *Cell 59*:411 (1989).

5. D. T. Wong, F. P. Bymaster, and E. A. Engleman, Prozac (fluoxetine, Lilly 110140), the first selective serotonin uptake inhibitor and an antidepressant drug: twenty years since its first publication, *Life Sci. 57*(5):411 (1995).

6. P. F. Renshaw, J. C. Haselgrove, J. S. Leigh, and B. Chance, In vivo nuclear magnetic resonance imaging of lithium, *Magn. Res. Med. 2*:512 (1985).

7. P. F. Renshaw, J. C. Haselgrove, L. Bolinger, B. Chance, and J. S. Leigh, Relaxation and imaging of lithium in vivo, *Magn. Res. Imaging* 4:193 (1986).

8. K. Albert, H. Rembold, G. Kruppa, E. Bayer, M. Bartels, and G. Schmalzing, In vivo ^{19}F nuclear magnetic resonance spectroscopy of trifluorinated neuroleptics in the rat, *NMR Biomed. 3*(3):120 (1990).

9. J. J. Ackerman, T. H. Grove, G. G. Wong, D. G. Gadian, and G. K. Radda, Mapping of metabolites in whole animals by ^{31}P NMR using surface coils, *Nature 283*(5743):167 (1980).

10. P. A. Bottomley, T. B. Foster, and R. D. Darrow, Depth-resolved surface-coil spectroscopy (DRESS) for in vivo ^1H, ^{31}P and ^{13}C NMR, *J. Magn. Res. 59*:338 (1984).

11. R. J. Ordidge, A. Connelly, and J. A. H. Lohman, Image selective in vivo spectroscopy (ISIS). A new technique for spatially selective NMR spectroscopy, *J. Magn. Res. 60*:283 (1986).

12. R. S. Lara, G. B. Matson, J. W. Hugg, A. A. Maudsley, and M. W. Weiner, Quantitation of in vivo phosphorus metabolites in human brain with magnetic resonance spectroscopic imaging (MRSI), *Magn. Res. Imaging 11*:271 (1993).

13. W. -I. Jung, S. Widmaier, M. Bunse, U. Seeger, K. Straubinger, F. Schick, K. Küper, G. Dietze, and O. Lutz, ^{31}P transverse relaxation times of ATP in human brain in vivo, *Magn. Res. Med. 30*:741 (1993).

14. T. R. Brown, B. M. Kincaid, and K. Ugrubil, NMR chemical shift imaging in three dimensions, *Proc. Natl. Acad. Sci. 79*:3523 (1982).

15. R. Buchli, C. O. Duc, E. Martin, and P. Boesiger, Assessment of absolute metabolite concentrations in human tissue by ^{31}P MRS in vivo. Part I: Cerebrum, cerebellum, cerebral gray and white matter, *Magn. Res. Med. 32*:447 (1994).

16. J. W. Pettegrew, M. S. Keshaven, K. Panchalingam, S. Strychor. D. B. Kaplan, M. G. Tretta, and M. Allen, Alterations in brain high-energy phosphate and membrane phospholipid metabolism in first-episode, drug-naive schizophrenics, *Arch. Gen. Psychiatry 48*:563 (1991).

17. L. Gyulai, L. Bolinger, J. S. Leigh, C. Barlow, and B. Chance, Phosphorylethanolamine: the major constituent of the phosphomonoester peak observed by P-31 NMR in developing dog brain, *FEBS Lett.* *178*:137 (1984).
18. P. M. Kilby, N. M. Bolas, and G. K. Radda, ^{31}P-NMR study of brain phospholipid structures in vivo, *Biochim. Biophys. Acta* *1085*:257 (1991).
19. G. J. Tortora and N. P. Anagnostakos: *Principles of Anatomy and Physiology*, Harper & Row, New York, 1987.
20. A. L. Leninger, *Biochemistry*, Worth Publishers, Inc., New York, 1978.
21. R. L. Veech, J. W. R. Lawson, N. W. Cornell, and H. A. Krebs, Cytosolic phosphorylation potential, *J. Biol. Chem.* *254*(14):6538 (1979).
22. O. A. C. Petroff, J. W. Prichard, K. S. Behar, J. R. Alger, J. A. den Hollander, and R. G. Schulman, Cerebral intra-cellular pH by ^{31}P nuclear magnetic resonance spectroscopy, *Neurology* *35*:781 (1985).
23. S. R. Dager and R. G. Steen, Applications of magnetic resonance spectroscopy to the investigation of neuropsychiatric disorders, *Neuropsychopharmacology* *64*:249 (1992).
24. J. Frahm, H. Brühn, M. L. Glyngell, K.-D. Merboldt, W. Hänicke, and R. Sauter, Localized high resolution NMR spectroscopy using stimulated echoes: initial applications to human brain in vivo, *Magn. Res. Med.* *9*:79 (1989).
25. P. A. Bottomley, U. S. Patent 4,480,228 (1984).
26. C. T. Moonen, M. von Kienlin, P. C. van Zijl, J. Cohen, J. Gillen, and P. Daly, Comparison of single-shot localization methods (STEAM and PRESS) for in vivo proton NMR spectroscopy, *NMR Biomed.* *2*:201 (1989).
27. D. L. Birken and W. H. Oldendorf, N-acetyl-L-aspartic acid: a literature review of a compound prominent in ^{1}H-NMR spectroscopic studies of brain, *Neurosci. Biobehav. Rev.* *13*:23 (1989).
28. G. Tsai and J. Coyle, N-Acetylaspartate in neuropsychiatric disorders, *Prog. Neurobiol.* *46*:531 (1995).
29. O. A. C. Petroff, D. D. Spencer, J. R. Alger, and J. W. Prichard, High-field proton magnetic resonance spectroscopy of human cerebrum obtained during surgery for epilepsy, *Neurology* *39*:1197 (1989).
30. S. H. Zeisel, Choline phospholipids: signal transduction and carcinogenesis. *FASEB J.* *7*:551 (1993).
31. B. L. Miller, A review of chemical issues in ^{1}H NMR spectroscopy: N-acetyl-aspartate, creatine and choline, *NMR. Biomed.* *4*:47 (1991).
32. T. Michaelis, K. -D. Merboldt, W. Hänicke, M. L. Glyngell, H. Brühn, and J. Frahm, On the identification of cerebral metabolites in localized ^{1}H NMR spectra of human brain in vivo, *NMR Biomed.* *1*:90 (1991).
33. H. C. Charles, F. Lazeyras, K. R. R. Krishnan, O. B. Boyko, M. Payne, and D. Moore, Brain choline in depression: In vivo detection of potential pharmacodynamic effects of antidepressant therapy using hydrogen localized spectroscopy, *Prog. Neuropsychopharmacol. Biol. Psychiatry* *18*:1121 (1994).
34. A. L. Stoll, P. F. Renshaw, E. De Micheli, R. Wurtman, S. S. Pillay, and B. M. Cohen, Choline ingestion increases the resonance of choline-containing compounds in human brain: an in vivo proton magnetic resonance study, *Biol. Psychiatry* *37*:170 (1995).

35. T. Shonk and B. D. Ross, Role of increased cerebral myo-inositol in the dementia of Down syndrome, *Magn. Res. Med. 33*:858 (1995).
36. K. L. Behar and T. Ogino, Assignment of resonances in the ¹H spectrum of rat brain by two-dimensional shift correlated and J-resolved NMR spectroscopy, *Magn. Res. Med. 17*:285 (1991).
37. G. D. Tollefson, A. H. Rampey, J. H. Potvin, M. A. Jenike, A. J. Rush, R. A. Dominiquez, L. M. Koran, M. K. Shear, W. Goodman, and L. A. Genduso, A multicenter investigation of fixed-dose fluoxetine in the treatment of obsessive-compulsive disorder, *Arch. Gen. Psychiatry 51*:559 (1994).
38. M. S. Wallin and A. M. Rissanen, Food and mood: relationship between food, serotonin and affective disorders, *Acta. Psychiatr. Scand. Suppl. 377*:36 (1994).
39. C. N. Karson, J. E. O. Newton, R. Livingston, J. B. Jolly, T. B. Cooper, J. Sprigg, and R. A. Komoroski, Human brain fluoxetine concentrations, *J. Neuropsychiatry Clin. Neuorsci. 5*:322 (1993).
40. T. Kato, T. Shioiri, S. Takahashi, and T. Inubushi, Measurement of brain phosphoinositide metabolism in bipolar patients using in vivo ³¹P-MRS, *J. Affect. Disord. 22*:185 (1991).
41. J. H. Allison, M. E. Blisner, W. H. Holland, P. P. Hipps, and W. R. Sherman, Increased brain myo-inositol-1-phosphate in lithium-treated rats, *Biochem. Biophys. Res. Commun. 71*:664 (1976).
42. P. F. Renshaw, M. D. Schnall, and J. S. Leigh Jr., In vivo P-31 NMR spectroscopy of agonist-stimulated phosphatidylinositol metabolism in cat brain, *Mag. Res. Med. 4*:221 (1987).
43. A. J. Prange, I. C. Wilson, C. W. Lynn, L. B. Alltop, and R. A. Stikeleather, L-Trytophan in mania. Contribution to a permissive hypotheses of affective disorder. *Arch. Gen. Psychiatry 30*:56, 1974.
44. T. Kato, S. Takahashi, T. Shioiri, and T. Inubushi, Brain phosphorus metabolism in depressive disorders detected by phosphorus-31 magnetic resonance spectroscopy, *J. Affect. Disord. 26*:223 (1992).
45. M. S. Buchsbaum, J. Wu, L. E. DeLisi, H. Holcomb, R. Kessler, J. Johnson, A. C. King, E. Hazlett, K. Langston, and R. M. Post, Frontal cortex and basal ganglia metabolic rates assessed by positron emission tomography with [¹⁸F]2-deoxyglucose in affective illness, *J. Affect. Disord. 10*:137 (1986).
46. H. S. Mayberg, P. J. Lewis, W. Regenold, and H. N. Wagner Jr., Paralimbic hypoperfusion in unipolar depression, *J. Nucl Med. 35*:929 (1994).
47. S. Schlegel, J. B. Aldenhoff, D. Eissner, P. Linder, and O. Nickel, Regional cerebral blood flow in depression: associations with psychopathology, *J. Affect. Disord. 17*:211 (1989).
48. T. Kato, S. Takahashi, T. Shioiri, and T. Inubushi, Alterations in brain phosphorous metabolism in bipolar depression detected by in vivo ³¹P and ⁷Li magnetic resonance spectroscopy, *J. Affect. Disord. 27*:53 (1993).
49. T. Kato, S. Takahashi, T. Shioiri, J. Murashita, H. Hamakawa, and T. Inubushi, Reduction of brain phosphocreatine in bipolar II disorder detected by phosphorus-31 magnetic resonance spectroscopy, *J. Affect. Disord. 31*:125 (1994).
50. T. Kato, T. Shioiri, J. Murashita, H. Hamakawa, T. Inubushi, and S. Takahashi,

Phosphorus-31 magnetic resonance spectroscopy and ventricular enlargement in bipolar disorder, *Psychiatry Res. 55*:41 (1994).

51. V. Swayze II, N. C. Andreasen, R. Alliger, J. C. Ehrhardt, and W. T. C. Yuh, Structural brain abnormalities in bipolar affective disorder: ventricular enlargement and focal hyperintensities, *Arch. Gen. Psychiatry 47*:1054 (1990).

52. R. F. Deicken, G. Fein, and M. W. Weiner, Abnormal frontal lobe phosphorus metabolism in bipolar disorder, *Am. J. Psychiatry 152*(6):915 (1995).

53. R. F. Deicken, G. Fein, and M. W. Weiner, Decreased temporal lobe phosphomonoesters in bipolar disorder, *J. Affect. Disord. 33*:195 (1995).

54. P. Williamson, D. Drost, J. Stanley, T. Carr, S. Morrison, and H. Merskey, Localized phosphorus-31 magnetic resonance spectroscopy in chronic schizophrenic patients and normal controls, *Arch. Gen. Psychiatry 48*:578 (1991) L.

55. C. M. Moore, J. D. Christensen, B. Lafer. M. Fava, and P. F. Renshaw, Phosphorus-31 magnetic resonance spectroscopy of the basal ganglia in depressed subjects, Proceedings of the Society of Biological Psychiatry, New York, 1996.

56. R. F. Deicken, G. Calabrase, E. L. Merrin, G. Fein and M. W. Weiner, Basal ganglia phosphorus metabolism in chronic schizophrenia, *Am. J. Psychiatry 152*(1):126 (1995).

57. B. V. Siegel Jr., M. S. Buchsbaum, W. E. Bunny Jr., L. A. Gottschalk, R. J. Haier, J. B. Lohr, S. Lottenberg, A. Najafi, K. H. Nuechterlein, S. G. Potkin, et al., Cortical-striatal-thalmic circuits and brain glucose metabolic activity in 70 unmedicated male schizophrenic patients, *Am. J. Psychiatry 150*:1325 (1993).

58. R. Sharma., P. N. Venkatasubramanian, M. Bárány, and J. M. Davis, Proton magnetic resonance spectroscopy of the brain in schizophrenic and affective patients, *Schizophr. Res. 8*:43 (1992).

59. H. Breer and M. Kipper, Regulation of high affinity choline uptake, *J. Neurobiol. 21*(2):269 (1990).

60. D. S. Janowsky, M. K. El Yousef, J. M. Dario, and H. J. Sekerke, A cholinergic adrenergic hypothesis of mania and depression, *Lancet 2*(778):632 (1972).

61. K. R. Krishnan, W. M. Mc Donald, P. M. Doraiswamy, L. A. Tupler, M. Husain, O. B. Boyko, G. S. Figiel, and E. H. Ellinwood Jr., Neuroanatomical substrates of depression in the elderly, *Eur. Arch. Psychiatry Clin. Neurosci. 243*(1):41 (1993).

62. G. Tedeschi, A. Bertolino, A. Righini, G. Campbell, R. Raman, J. H. Duyn, C. T. Moonen, J. R. Alger, and G. Di Chiro, Brain regional distribution pattern of metabolite signal intensities in young adults by proton magnetic resonance spectroscopic imaging, *Neurology 45*(7):1384 (1995).

63. A. L. Stoll, B. M. Cohen, and I. Hanin, Erythrocyte choline concentrations in psychiatric disorders, *Biol. Psychiatry 29*:309 (1991).

64. A. L. Stoll, P. F. Renshaw, G. S. Sachs, A. R. Guimarães, C. Miller, B. M. Cohen, B. Lafer, and R. G. Gonzáles, The human brain resonance of cholinecontaining compounds is similar in patients receiving lithium treatment and controls: an in vivo proton magnetic resonance spectroscopy study, *Biol. Psychiatry 32*:944 (1992).

65. W. R. Sherman, L. Y. Munsell, B. G. Gish, and M. P. Honchar, Effects of

systematically administered lithium in phosphoinositide metabolism in rat brain, kidney, and testis, *J. Neurochem.* *44*(3):798 (1985).

66. J. R. Atack, H. B. Broughton, and S. J. Pollack, Structure and mechanism of inositol monophosphate, *FEBS Lett.* *361*:1 (1995).

67. H. Brühn, G. Stoppe, J. Staedt, K. D. Merboldt, W. Hänike, and J. Frahm, Quantitative proton MRS in vivo shows cerebral myo-inositol and cholines to be unchanged in manic-depressive patients treated with lithium, Proceedings of Society of Magnetic Resonance in Medicine, New York, 1993, p. 1543.

68. N. E. Preece, D. G. Gadian, J. Houseman, and S. R. Williams, Modulation of cerebral inositol phosphate metabolism by lithium, Proceedings of the Society of Magnetic Resonance in Medicine, San Francisco, 1991, p. 428.

69. O. A. C. Petroff, J. W. Prichard, T. Ogino, M. Avison, J. R. Alger, and R. G. Schulman, Combined ^{1}H and ^{31}P nucleur magnetic resonance spectroscopic studies of bicuculline-induced seizures in-vivo, *Ann. Neurol. 20*:185 (1986).

70. B. T. Woods and T-K. Chiu, In vivo ^{1}H spectroscopy of the human brain following electroconvulsive therapy, *Ann. Neurol. 28*:745 (1990).

71. S. R. Felber, R. Pycha, M. Hummer, F. T. Aichner, and W. W. Fleischhacker, Localized proton and phosphorous magnetic resonance spectroscopy following electroconvulsive therapy, *Biol. Psychiatry 33*:651 (1993).

72. R. A. Komoroski, J. E. O. Newton, C. Karson, D. Cardwell, and J. Sprigg, Detection of psychoactive drugs in vivo in humans using ^{19}F NMR spectroscopy, *Biol. Psychiatry 29*:711 (1991).

73. L. Lemberger, R. F. Bergstorm, R. L. Wolen, N. A. Farid, G. G. Enas, and G. R. Aronoff, Fluoxetine: clinical pharmacology and physiologic disposition, *J. Clin. Psychiatry 46*:14 (1985).

74. C. N. Karson, J. E. O. Newton, P. Mohanakrishnan, J. Sprigg, and R. A. Komoroski, Fluoxetine and trifluoperazine in human brain: a ^{19}F-nuclear magnetic resonance spectroscopy study, *Psychiatry Res. 45*:95 (1992).

75. P. F. Renshaw, A. R. Guimarães, M. Fava, J. F. Rosenbaum, J. D. Pearlman, J. G. Flood, P. R. Puopolo, K. Clancy, and R. G. Gonzáles, Accumulation of fluoxetine and norfluoxetine in human brain during therapeutic administration, *Am. J. Psychiatry 149*(11):1592 (1992).

76. R. A. Komoroski, J. E. O. Newton, D. Cardwell, J. Sprigg, J. Pearce, and C. N. Karson, In vivo ^{19}F spin relaxation and localized spectroscopy of fluoxetine in human brain, *Magn. Res. Med. 31*:204 (1994).

77. C. M. Miner, J. R. T. Davidson, N. L. S. Potts, L. A. Tupler, H. C. Charles, and K. R. R. Krishnan, Brain fluoxetine measurements using fluorine magnetic resonance spectroscopy in patients with social phobia, *Biol. Psychiatry 38*:696 (1995).

78. P. P. Roy-Byrne, R. T. Joffe, T. W. Uhde, and R. M. Post, Approaches to the evaluation and treatment of rapid-cycling affective illness, *Br. J. Psychiatry 145*:543 (1984).

79. H. E. Hansen and A. Amidsen, Lithium intoxication (report of 23 cases and review of 100 cases from the literature), *Q. J. Med. 47*:123 (1978).

80. R. A. Komoroski, J. E. O. Newton, E. Walker, D. Cardwell, N. R. Jagannathan,

S. Ramaprasad, and J. A. Sprigg, In vivo NMR spectroscopy of lithium-7 in humans, *Magn. Res. Med. 15*:347 (1990).

81. L. Gyulai, S. W. Wicklund, R. Greenstein. M. S. Bauer, P. Ciccione, P. C. Whybrow, J. Zimmerman, G. Kovachich, and W. Alves, Measurement of tissue lithium concentration by lithium magnetic resonance spectroscopy in patients with bipolar disorder, *Biol. Psychiatry 29*:1161 (1991).

82. T. Kato, S. Takahashi, and T. Inubushi, Brain lithium concentration by ^{7}Li and ^{1}H-magnetic resonance spectroscopy in bipolar disorder, *Psychiatry Res. 45*: 53 (1992).

83. T. Kushnir, Y. Itzchak, A Valevski, M. Lask, I. Modai, and G. Navon, Relaxation times and concentrations of ^{7}Li in the brain of patients receiving lithium therapy, *NMR Biomed. 6*:39 (1993).

84. R. A. Komoroski, J. E. O. Newton, J. A. Sprigg, D. Cardwell, P. Mohanakrishnan, and C. N. Karson, In vivo ^{7}Li nuclear magnetic resonance study of lithium pharmacokinetics and chemical shift imaging in psychiatric disorders, *Psychiatry Res. 50*:67 (1993).

85. R. G. Gonzáles, A. R. Guimarães, G. S. Sachs, J. F. Rosenbaum, M. Garwood, and P. F. Renshaw, Measurement of human brain lithium in vivo by MR spectroscopy, *Am. J. Neuroradiol. 14*:1027 (1993).

86. T. Kato, T. Shioiri, T. Inubushi, and S. Takahashi, Brain lithium concentrations measured with lithium-7 magnetic resonance spectroscopy in patients with affective disorders: relationship to erythrocyte and serum concentrations, *Biol. Psychiatry 33*:147 (1993).

87. A. Frazer, J. Mendels. S. K. Secunda, C. M. Cochrane, and P. Bianchi, The prediction of brain lithium concentrations from plasma or erythrocyte measures, *J. Psychiatr. Res. 10*:1 (1973).

88. T. Kato, T. Inubushi, and S. Takahashi, Relationship of lithium concentration in the brain measured by lithium-7 magnetic resonance spectroscopy to treatment response in mania, *J. Clin. Psychopharmac. 14*(5):330 (1994).

89. P. Plenge, A. Stensgaard, H. V. Jensen, C. Thomsen, E. T. Mellrup, and O. Henriksen, 24-hour lithium concentration in human brain studied by lithium-7 magnetic resonance spectroscopy, *Biol. Psychiatry 26*:511 (1994).

90. G. S. Sachs, P. F. Renshaw, B. Lafer, A. L. Stoll, A. R. Guimarães, J. F. Rosenbaum, and G. R. Gonzáles, Variability of brain lithium levels during maintenance treatment: a magnetic resonance spectroscopy study, *Biol. Psychiatry 38*:422 (1995).

9

PET Studies in Mood Disorders

Anand Kumar
University of Pennsylvania School of Medicine, Philadelphia, Pennsylvania

I. INTRODUCTION

The application of in vivo imaging techniques such as positron emission tomography (PET) and magnetic resonance imaging (MRI) to the clinical neurosciences has opened unlimited possibilities to elucidate the neuroanatomical, physiological, and neurochemical underpinnings of major psychiatric disorders [1–4]. The use of these high-resolution techniques has made it possible for investigators not only to cross-sectionally describe the physiological and biochemical changes occurring in subjects with major mental disorders, but also to follow these changes with treatment over an extended period of time. PET, functional MRI (fMRI), and magnetic resonance spectroscopy (MRS) often overlap in scope, thereby obscuring historical distinctions between anatomical abnormalities and physiological perturbations [5–7]. Recent advances using fMRI and the application of MR neuroanatomical methods to the analysis of PET brain images have made it possible to concurrently examine neuroanatomical and neurophysiological abnormalities in subjects with psychiatric disturbances in the nonactivated "resting" state and during specific cognitive and behavioral challenges.

Despite the remarkable potential of these technologies to elucidate the biological underpinnings of major mental disorders, several methodological and clinical limitations have, to some degree, limited the conclusions that could be drawn from these neuroimaging studies. Technical issues such as partial volume effect, variance in resting physiological measures (such as rCMRglc and rCBF), differences in ambient scanning conditions, and diverse methods of image analysis across research groups have contributed to the apparent inconsistencies in the physiological findings in subjects with mood disorders [2–4]. In addition to these technical issues, marked differences in clinical populations such as unipolar versus bipolar depressives, psychotic versus nonpsychotic subgroups, and winter versus summer seasonal affective disorders have also resulted in discrepancies across studies [2,8]. Despite these limitations, it is possible to look back on approximately a decade and a half of PET studies in mood disorders and draw some definitive conclusions [9]. Increasingly sophisticated PET scanners, together with improved methods of image analysis and the utilization of more specific radioligands, have opened the door for more systematic and focused studies that may further clarify the biological basis of mental illness.

The primary objective of this chapter is to critically review the clinical studies in mood disorders using PET. We will first review the PET studies in primary depression (defined as idiopathic major depressive disorder, for which there is no obvious medical or neurological cause) in adults and elderly subjects [10]. Resting 18 fluoro-2-deoxy-D-glucose (18 FDG) and regional cerebral blood flow (rCBF) studies using PET in the resting and activated states are discussed, together with their strengths and limitations. This is followed by a description of the salient findings of PET studies in depression secondary to specific neurological disorders and their neurobiological implications. We conclude by discussing some of the preliminary results from neuroreceptor studies and the potential offered by specific radioligands designed to examine the neurochemical basis of mental disorders.

II. RESTING 18 FDG STUDIES IN PRIMARY DEPRESSION

Glucose metabolism estimated using 18 FDG PET is a reliable and valid method that is widely used to examine neuronal function in vivo in subjects with mood disorders and other psychiatric disturbances [11–13]. Most of the information currently available on in vivo brain imaging in psychiatric disorders has been obtained from resting FDG studies of specific clinical populations. In a preliminary study of resting glucose metabolism using 18 FDG in subjects with unipolar depression, bipolar depression, mixed bipolar state, and controls, Baxter et al. [14] reported that subjects with unipolar depression showed a significantly lower normalized metabolic rate for the caudate nucleus when compared with controls and patients with bipolar depression. Subjects with bipolar depression and mixed states showed a global reduction in glucose metabolism that increased when they cycled to the euthymic or manic state. These early results were interpreted as providing evidence for reductions in neuronal function in subjects with major depressive disorder. Additionally, they provided some evidence for the role of the caudate nucleus in unipolar depression. In an influential study [15] exploring the role of the prefrontal cortex in depression, Baxter et al. reported that the resting glucose metabolism in the anterolateral prefrontal cortex (ALPFC rCMRglc normalized to the ipsilateral hemispheric metabolism) was lower in subjects with unipolar depression, bipolar depression, and obsessive-compulsive disorder with depression when compared with controls. The hypometabolism in the ALPFC correlated significantly with the Hamilton Rating Scale for Depression (HRSD) scores and "normalized" when the depression was successfully treated. These data not only provided support for the role of the prefrontal cortex in depression, but also indicated that neuronal function, quantified using rCMRglc as an index, normalized after effective pharmacotherapy. A report by Martinot et al. [16] on resting CMRglc in 10 severely depressed subjects before and after treatment demonstrated significant right-left prefrontal metabolic asymmetry and whole-cortex hypometabolism in the depressives when compared with controls. While the prefrontal asymmetry normalized with treatment, the hypometabolism persisted, suggesting that some of the metabolic abnormalities seen in the depressed state do not resolve with successful treatment of depression.

Not all reports corroborate the earlier finding of reduced prefrontal glucose metabolism in depression. In a resting 18 FDG study of six major depression subjects who were chronically ill with poor response to antidepressant medications, Kling et al. [17] found no differences in their global or regional glucose metabolism when compared with nondepressed controls. Post et al. [18] reported that their sample of 13 affectively ill patients showed hypometabolism in the right temporal lobe (with a similar tread in the left) when compared with controls. In a report comparing rCMR glc in subjects with affective disorders and schizophrenia, Cohen et al. [19] found no global differences in glucose metabolism between controls and those with affective disorders (both unipolar and bipolar depressives). However, patients with affective disorders, like those with schizophrenia, had low metabolic rates in the midprefrontal cortex while performing an auditory discrimination task. Other brain regions did not show comparable hypometabolism. Cohen et al. [20], in an 18 FDG study of subjects with winter seasonal affective disorder (SAD), demonstrated a reduction in the metabolic rate for glucose globally and in the superior medial frontal cortex. In addition, subjects with winter SAD had lower glucose metabolism in the basal ganglia than nondepressed controls. The global hypometabolism did not normalize with light treatment for SAD. In a later resting 18 FDG study from the same group, subjects with summer SAD [21] presented with a decrease in global CMRglc associated with an increase in normalized rCMRglc in the orbital frontal region when compared with nondepressed controls. Hurwitz et al. [22] in a resting 18 FDG study on six subjects with unipolar depression reported significant reductions in glucose metabolism in the anterior and right frontal cortex when compared with normal controls. The hypometabolism appeared to be lateralized and more striking in the right nondominant hemisphere. No changes in metabolism were noted with imipramine treatment.

The aforementioned studies dealt almost exclusively with young adults in the 20- to 60-year age range. In a study examining resting glucose metabolism in a small sample of subjects with late life major depression (LLD), Kumar et al. [2] demonstrated widespread hypometabolism (in neocortical and subcortical regions) in the LLD group when compared with controls. The hypometabolism seen in the LLD group was comparable to that observed in subjects with probable dementia of the Alzheimer type (DAT) (Fig. 1). These findings are consistent with Sackheim et al.'s rCBF studies using Xenon 133 [23] in which widespread, profound decreases in neocortical blood flow were demonstrated in subjects with LLD when compared with controls. The observation that the physiological perturbations in LLD are widespread and comparable in magnitude to similar measures in subjects with DAT suggests that the pathophysiology of depression occurring in late life may differ from the more classical forms of depression observed in younger adults.

Results of studies reporting changes in rCMRglc with successful treatment of depression vary across groups. While some investigators [14,16,24–27] report "normalization" of metabolic asymmetries and focal hypometabolism with successful treatment of depression, others report no change in metabolism with treatment and resolution of symptoms [20,22]. Normalization is more often reported in relation to circumscribed, focal deficits than more widespread metabolic abnormalities [14–16,20,25–27] (Fig.

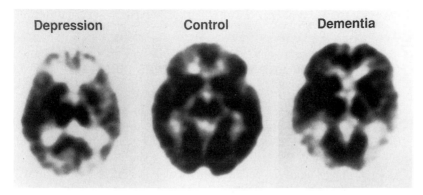

Fig. 1   The widespread decline in rCMRglc in subjects with late life major depression (comparable to Alzheimer's disease) compared to controls.

2). The treatment modalities examined varied considerably across studies, and few attempts were made to compare different treatment approaches in a systematic manner [14,20,27]. Therefore, while some studies report a return of glucose metabolic rates to normal levels, others suggest that glucose hypo-

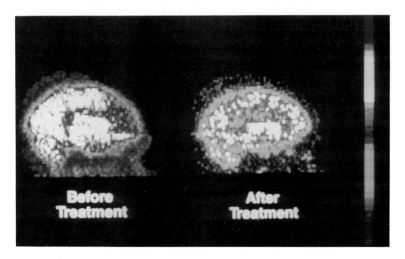

Fig. 2   The apparent normalization in rCMRglc in the prefrontal cortex in unipolar depression with successful treatment. (Courtesy of Lewis Baxter, University of Alabama, Birmingham, Alabama.)

metabolism is more of a trait than a state marker persisting across different mood states [20].

III. H₂¹⁵O BLOOD FLOW AND VOLUME STUDIES USING PET

Several studies have applied PET methodology using $H_2^{15}O$ water to examine cerebral blood flow (rCBF) in the resting state in patients with major depressive disorder. Bench and collaborators [28], in a study examining rCBF in the resting state in patients with primary depression with and without cognitive impairment and nondepressed controls, used a relatively unique method of PET image analysis called Statistical Parametric Maps (SPM). Using the SPM technique, they reported that the depressed group as a whole showed a reduction in rCBF in the left anterior cingulate and left dorsolateral prefrontal cortex (DLPFC) when compared with controls [28]. The investigators argue that the prefrontal and limbic areas constitute an anatomical network that may be functionally abnormal in major depression. When depressed subjects with and without cognitive impairment were compared, the cognitively impaired group showed reductions in rCBF in the left medial frontal gyrus and increased rCBF in the cerebellar vermis when compared with the cognitively intact group [29]. In an additional analysis examining the relationship between focal measures of rCBF and clinical symptomatology, the same group [30] found significant correlations between decreased perfusion in the DLPFC and left angular gyrus and certain clinical features of depression. In a study designed to examine cerebral blood flow, blood volume (CBV), and local cerebral metabolic rate for oxygen ($CMRO_2$), Raichle et al. reported a decrease in rCBF and $CMRO_2$ in their sample of five depressed subjects when compared with controls [31]. Drevets et al. [32], in a study of resting rCBF using PET in a relatively homogeneous subgroup diagnosed with familial pure depressive disorder (FPDD), reported increased rCBF in an area extending from the left ventrolateral prefrontal cortex onto the medial prefrontal cortical surface. In addition, they reported an increase in rCBF in the left amygdala in the FPDD group when compared with controls. In the same study, the investigators examined rCBF in 10 subjects who had met criteria for FPDD in the past but were asymptomatic and unmedicated at the time of the scan. These subjects had normal blood flow in the prefrontal cortex but demonstrated an increase in the rCBF in the left amygdala. The increased rCBF in the left amygdala was interpreted as representing more of a trait marker for FPDD than a state marker for depression (32). In a study from NIMH, Ketter and colleagues [33] compared nine mood disordered subjects to 18 healthy controls using $H_2^{15}O$ PET. The depressed subjects showed a decrease in rCBF in the prefrontal cortices, superior temporal and supramarginal gyri, mesial temporal lobe, and anterior cingulate gyrus. The left mesial temporal area, which includes the amygdala, was the region that showed the most marked reduction in rCBF.

Despite the apparent discrepancy in resting FDG studies of glucose metabolism in subjects with major depressive disorder, there is an emerging consensus that in the "depressed state" subjects (with both unipolar and bipolar disorders and seasonal affective disorders) exhibit a reduction in resting glucose metabolism when compared with nondepressed controls. The extent of the hypometabolism, however, is unclear and varies across studies. Reductions in both global and regional metabolism have been reported [2,14–24]. Reports range from hypometabolism in discrete frontal lobe regions to widespread decline in rCMglc involving subcortical regions and the cerebellum [2,14–24]. Several methodological and clinical differences between these different reports need to be considered. While all of them claim to have studied people in the "resting state," the resting state utilized varies across studies [2,14,15,20,21]. Another caveat that should be borne in mind is that subjective emotional experiences during the uptake period that could additionally alter metabolism/flow were not controlled for during these studies. Certain investigators had their subjects performing an auditory discrimination task during the uptake period [19–21]; others had subjects lie in a room with their eyes either closed or open [2,14,15]. The extent of room noise also provided an additional source of variance during the uptake period [2,3]. Methods of image analysis also varied across studies, and none of the aforementioned studies utilized an MR facilitated co-registration method of analysis [2,14–23]. In addition, absolute metabolic rates for glucose and metabolic ratios (using different denominators) have been reported [2,3,14–24]. Some earlier studies [34] compared an anterior-posterior metabolic gradient, from the frontal to the occipital lobes, between groups—a method of analysis not commonly utilized at present. In a widely cited study by Baxter et al., rCMRglc was reported only in the ALPFC, thereby precluding any comment on the role of other brain regions in the pathophysiology of depression [15,24]. Further, reports of focal increases in rCMRglc or rCBF occurring in the context of global reductions in CMRglc or CBF may not represent true biological increases in metabolism or flow and may be conceptually misleading [2,21,32].

In addition to these obvious methodological differences between studies, several studies examined relatively small numbers of subjects [2,14,15,17,22]. This compromises the degree to which their findings may be generalized to larger patient groups. Although all patients were studied in a "depressed state," the primary psychiatric diagnosis varied across studies [8]. Subjects with unipolar depression, bipolar depression, SAD, mixed states, and FPDD were all studied, which may partly explain the variability seen in these reports [14–24,28–32]. While all investigators made special

Table 1 Results of Selected Resting FDG and rCBF Studies in Major Depression

Study	Clinical group	Method	Findings compared to controls	Ref.
Baxter et al., 1985	UD (n = 11), BP (n = 5), MS (n = 3), drug-free	Resting 18 FDG	Up—reduction in normalized caudate rCMRglc; BP&MS—global reduction in CMRglc	14
Baxter et al., 1989	UD (n = 10), BP (n = 10), OCD with Dep (n = 10), Drug-free	Resting 18 FDG	Reduction in normalized ALPFC rCMRglc	15
Post et al., 1986	Primary depression (n = 5) ethymic/minor depression, (n = 7) Drug-Free	Resting FDG (somatosensory stimulation)	Reduction in temporal lobe normalized rCMRglc	18
Martinot et al., 1990	UD (n = 3), BD (n = 7), medicated	Resting FDG	Prefrontal asymmetry and global hypometabolism	16
Cohen et al., 1989	BD (n = 10), UD (n = 5), no/o substance abuse, some were medicated	18 FDG-Auditory discriminating task during uptake	Decrease in midprefrontal cortex and increase in parietal cortex	19
Cohen et al., 1992	SAD (n = 7), drug-free	18 FDG-Auditory discriminating task	Decrease in global CMRglc	20
Hurwitz et al., 1990	UD (n = 6), on oxazepam	Resting FDG	Frontal hypometabolism	22
Kumar et al., 1993	LLD (n = 8), drug-free	Resting FDG	Widespread hypometabolism—neocortical, subcortical, and limbic regions	2
Mayberg et al., 1990	PD with depression (n = 5), on L-dopa	Resting FDG	Reduction in normalized caudate and orbital frontal lobes compared to PD nondepressed	59
Mayberg et al., 1992	HD with depression (n = 5), drug-free	Resting FDG	Paralimbic hypometabolism compared to HD without depression	60
Bench et al., 1992	Primary major depression (n = 33), 19 of 33 were medicated	Resting rCBF	Decreased rCBF in left anterior cingulate and left DLPFC	7
Drevets et al., 1992	FPDD (n = 13), drug-free	Resting rCBF	Increased rCBF in left prefrontal cortex and left amygdala	32
Ketter et al., 1994	UD (n = 9)	Resting rCBF	Decrease in neocortical and limbic region	47

UD = Unipolar depression; BD = bipolar depression; OCD = obsessive-compulsive disorder; PD = Parkinson's disease; HD = Huntington's disease; FPDD = familial pure depressive disorder; MS = mixed states.

efforts to keep subjects drug-free at the time of the study, the extent of drug-free periods varied across patients [2,14–24]. Differences in age, sex, and treatment refractoriness of subjects were also common across study groups [2,14–24]. Despite these substantial differences, all of the major studies that examined rCBF and resting FDG using PET in major depression demonstrated either focal or widespread reductions in rCMRglc and rCBF in the resting state in depressed subjects when compared with controls [2,14–24,28–31]. The Drevets et al. report stands out as perhaps the only methodologically well-performed PET study of rCBF reporting an increase in rCBF in depressed subjects when compared with controls [32]. The clinical subgroup studied was extremely homogeneous and perhaps biologically unique, which may explain the finding of rCBF increase in FPDD. Therefore, while resting FDG studies, almost without exception, show a decrease in glucose metabolism in depressed subjects in the resting state, results from rCBF tends to be less consistent.

The normalization of metabolism most commonly observed with treatment is largely restricted to metabolic asymmetries and other focal abnormalities while more global hypometabolism, sometimes observed in depression, appears to persist. Studies examining treatment effects on metabolism tend to be "naturalistic," and the need to compare different interventions in a longitudinal design is evident. Table 1 summarizes the main features of the resting FDG and rCBF studies using PET in major depression.

IV. ACTIVATION STUDIES IN MOOD DISORDERS USING PET

While resting studies (perhaps more accurately referred to as nonactivation studies) give us some baseline information on neural function, activation paradigms have been used to further probe neuronal function and its physiological responses in mental disorders [35–37]. Several cognitive tasks have been used to map brain function in healthy adult subjects without neurological or psychiatric disturbances. These studies have provided us with extremely valuable information regarding focal brain activation and neural circuits that may be involved in processing language, memory, spatial, and other behavioral information specifically designed to activate the limbic and neocortical circuits [37–41]. By using such sophisticated methods we expect to examine and compare the different strategies that the brain utilizes in performing these complex tasks, in both the normal as well as pathological states [42–53]. These paradigms could also provide additional information on the effect of treatment on neuronal circuitry and processing.

A study using Xenon 133 reported that subjects with mood disorders, in contrast to subjects with schizophrenia, activated the left DLPFC while performing the Wisconsin Card Sort (WCS), thereby suggesting that in tasks requiring executive functions, subjects with depression do not show the same "failure to activate" when compared with subjects with schizophrenia [53]. However, in an $H_2{}^{15}O$ PET study examining neuronal response to a spatial task, George et al. [52] reported that compared to nondepressed controls, mood disordered subjects activated a broader portion of the temporal/parietal cortex and failed to activate the left medial prefrontal cortex. In an activation paradigm specifically designed to challenge the limbic system—The Stroop Interference Task, in which a subject is asked to read a color word and pronounce not the word, but instead the color in which it was printed—subjects with mood disorders failed to activate the cingulate during the task, but instead activated the DLPFC [51]. During another task challenging limbic function—an activation task involving recognizing aspects of facial emotion—depressed subjects failed to activate the right insula when compared with controls [50]. Such challenge paradigms and the failure of depressed subjects to activate comparable brain regions have been interpreted as evidence of a selective defect in processing emotional stimuli when compared with nondepressed controls [50]. It has also been suggested, based on these data, that subjects with major depression show more striking neuronal compromise during tasks requiring limbic system involvement as opposed to purely neocortically mediated tasks [53].

Caution is required in interpreting data obtained from these activation studies. There is still no clear understanding of the exact relationship between specific mental effort and rCBF [53]. While failure to activate comparable regions of the brain as nondepressed controls or a blunting of the "limbic response" to challenge tasks may reflect alternate brain strategies being used by subjects with depression, they may not represent specific neuronal deficits [53]. In addition, no studies have examined neuronal activation after successful treatment of depression. It is therefore unclear whether these alternative processing channels are state- or trait-related and what specific biological abnormalities they represent. Despite these limitations, these studies do provide interesting descriptive data on neuronal processing and cerebral blood flow activation in subjects with mood disorders when compared with nondepressed controls.

V. PET STUDIES IN DEPRESSION SECONDARY TO NEUROLOGICAL DISEASE (SECONDARY DEPRESSION)

While most cases of clinically diagnosed major depression tend to be idiopathic in nature with no clear-cut anatomical or physiological antecedents, major depression has been commonly reported in specific neurological conditions where there is focal insult to the central nervous system [54–56]. These emotional sequelae to the specific CNS insults, together with primate and clinical studies of patients with specific head injuries, have provided useful models with neuroanatomical pathways that serve as a basis for exploring the biological basis of primary depression [57,58]. Depression is frequently seen in conditions with both neocortical and basal ganglia damage [54–62]. Depression secondary to cerebrovascular accidents, especially of the left hemisphere, has been widely reported [55,56]. Diseases of the basal ganglia such as Parkinson's disease (PD) and Huntington's disease (HD) are also frequently associated with depression and provide useful models to concurrently probe the physiological and anatomical basis of depression that accompanies these disorders [54,59–61] (Fig. 3).

PD is frequently associated with behavioral disturbances, of which depression is the most common [54]. The prevalence of depression (both major and minor) in PD ranges from 20 to 90% [54]. While the cause of depression in PD is unknown, disruption to specific mesocortical and mesolimbic dopaminergic and monoaminergic connections has been implicated

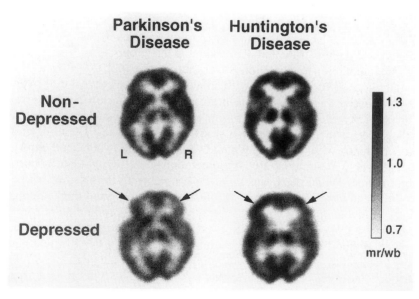

Fig. 3 The decline in rCMRglc in the orbitofrontal regions in subjects with PD and HD with depression when compared to subjects without depression. (Courtesy of Helen Mayberg, University of Texas Health Sciences Center, San Antonio, Texas.)

[54,61]. No specific neuroanatomical differences have been identified between PD subjects with and without depression [59,61]. Using resting FDG PET, focal as well as global decrements in glucose metabolism have been reported in subjects with PD [59,61]. However, until recently the physiological concomitants of mood disturbance in PD have remained elusive [59,61]. Physiological studies using FDG PET and blood flow have identified abnormalities in specific brain regions that may have implications for the pathophysiology of depression [59,61]. In a resting FDG study examining glucose metabolism in subjects with PD with and without major depression, Mayberg et al. [59,61] demonstrated hypometabolism in the caudate and orbital inferior frontal region in PD depressed subjects when compared with PD nondepressed subjects. In addition, the magnitude of the metabolic decrement in the inferior orbital frontal lobe correlated significantly with the severity of depression quantified using the HRSD [59]. These data provide support for the role of the orbital frontal region in the development of depression in PD.

HD is a genetic disorder in which motor changes frequently coexist with behavioral and emotional perturbations [60,61]. Resting FDG studies in subjects with HD with and without depression reveal that the orbital frontal-inferior prefrontal cortex is hypometabolic in HD patients with depression when compared with those without depression [60]. Comparable resting 18 FDG studies in subjects with complex partial seizures with and without depression also demonstrate that depression, in this group, is associated with glucose hypometabolism in the inferior frontal cortex [62].

Metabolic studies in patients with subcortical strokes reveal that hypometabolism in the limbic regions of interest—orbital inferior frontal cortex and temporal cortex—is commonly seen when mood disturbances accompany the subcortical stroke [55]. In a study reporting on 18 FDG utilization in three patients who developed manic episodes following head injury, Starkstein et al. [63] demonstrated hypometabolism in the right lateral basotemporal region. While there was no comparison group in this study of patients with head injury without mania, the authors interpreted their findings to reflect involvement of the basotemporal region in the production of manic symptoms [63]. Collectively, these studies indicate that the paralimbic cortex is involved in mood regulation independent of the primary CNS insult. This regional localization matches known pathways of basal ganglia frontal lobe connections and the basotemporal limbic circuits that link the orbital cortex with the temporal lobe [57,58]. While the specific biological mechanisms involved in altered mood states remain unknown, PET studies consistently showing paralimbic involvement in mood disturbances provide additional evidence that this region has an important role in the regulation of affect across diverse clinical states.

VI. NEURORECEPTOR IMAGING USING PET: TECHNICAL AND METHODOLOGICAL CONSIDERATIONS

The initial application of PET focused on its ability to map glucose metabolism and blood flow in the brain both in the nonactivated state and during specific cognitive and sensory challenges. While these studies have provided us with useful information about brain function, the larger promise of PET is to extend these preliminary studies to the examination of specific receptors and synaptic processes in the brain using radioligands that help image neurotransmitter systems such as the opiate, serotonin, muscarinic cholinergic, and dopamine systems [64–88]. Another focus of interest is extending neuroimaging beyond the receptor to examine presynaptic neurotransmitter reuptake sites and secondary messenger systems in the brain [4].

While the potential of neuroreceptor and neurochemical imaging remains considerable, its application to the study of psychiatric disorders has been slower than initially anticipated and has yet to yield a cohesive set of findings elucidating the biochemical basis of major psychiatric disorders including depression. While several radiotracers now exist for imaging and quantifying neuroreceptors, several technical and methodological obstacles needed to be worked out before neuroreceptor imaging could be used in a systematic and incremental fashion to the study of major mood disorders [4,64–66,79,89]. Several promising in vitro studies using radioligands were not followed by their rapid application to the study of clinical brain disorders [4,64]. The complexities involving human neuroreceptor imaging are numerous [4]. Limitations of radiosynthesis using short-lived positron-emitting isotopes have now been largely overcome [4]. However, other issues such as blood-brain permeability, metabolic stability, and nonspecific binding and dependence of tracer binding on blood flow have all complicated human neuroreceptor studies [4,64–66,69,71,79]. In addition, the presence of metabolites in the blood and brain and the role of endogenous ligands in neuroreceptor binding studies have had a sobering impact on clinical studies using PET [4] (see Table 2).

Early neuroreceptor studies in psychiatry largely centered around estimating the Bmax of dopamine 2 (D2) receptors in the striatum of patients diagnosed with schizophrenia [66–73]. Controversies surrounding the specificity of radioligands, together with differences in clinical groups examined, confused interpretation of the early results [66–73]. However, more recent studies indicate that the Bmax of striatal D2 receptors is increased not only in subjects with schizophrenia but also in subjects with psychotic depression and mania associated with psychosis [66–73]. These results collectively suggest that the dopamine system is involved in psychosis across clinical entities

Table 2 Positron Emission Tomography and Single-Photon Emission Computed Tomography (Courtesy Dr. J. J. Frost, Johns Hopkins Hospital, Baltimore, MD)

	Labeled drug	
Neuroreceptor	Positron-emitting	Single photon–emitting
Opiate	C-11 carfentanil (μm)	
	C-11 diprenorphine (μ,δ,κ)	
	F-18 acetylcyclofoxy ($\mu,\kappa K$)	
	C-11 buprenorphine ($\nu,\delta,\kappa K$)	
	Dopamine D2 and 5-HT2	
	F-18 spiperone	I-123-N-iodoallyspiperone
	F-18 fluoroethylspiperone	
	Br-76 bromospiperone	
	C-11 methylbenperidol	
Dopamine D2	C-11 raclopride	I-123 iodopride
		I-123 benzamide
Dopamine D1	Br-76 bromo SCH 23390	
	C-11 SCH 23390	
5-HT2	C-11 ketanserin	I-123 methyl iodo LSD
	C-11 methylketanserin	I-123 ethyl iodo LSD
	F-18 fluoroethylketanserin	
	C-11 methylbromo LSD	
Muscarinic	C-11 dexetimide	I-123 iodo-QNB
	F-18 fluorodexetimide	I-123 iododexetimide
	C-11 QNB	
	C-11 scopolomine	
Benzodiazepine	C-11 Ro 15–1788	I-123 iomazenil
	C-11 suriclone	
Histamine H-1	C-11 pyrilamine	
	C-11 doxepin	

and is not specific for any single disease category. The serotonin system has been implicated in the pathophysiology of mood disorders [1,74,75]. In a PET study of cortical S2 serotonin receptors after stroke, Mayberg et al. [76] demonstrated that higher S2 serotonin receptor binding occurred in the uninjured regions of the right parietal and temporal cortex [76]. The ratio of binding in the ipsilateral to contralateral cortex showed a significant negative correlation with severity of depression scores [76]. Changes in serotonin 2 receptors have been demonstrated in healthy nondepressed controls using other ligands such as 18F-Altanserin [82]. PET studies of mu opiate receptor binding also report an increase in binding measured using C-11 carfentenil in subjects with major depression [4,77,80]. These findings are not inconsistent with regional increases in mu opiate receptor density demonstrated in autoradiographic studies of brains of suicide victims [78]. Other investigators have focused on neurotransmitter precursor uptake sites in specific brain regions using PET [85,86]. Studies aimed at quantifying presynaptic Serotonin reuptake sites using both PET and SPECT have been done in primates and have broadened to include healthy human subjects [85]. Preliminary studies in subjects with major depression demonstrate an alteration in the transport of serotonin precursors into the brain when compared with controls [85]. There are isolated studies that demonstrate a reduction in dopamine 1 receptor binding potentials in the frontal cortex in bipolar depressives and reductions in the cortical amino acid pool in unipolar depressives when compared with controls [86,87]. These preliminary studies were performed on small numbers of subjects and clearly need to be replicated using larger samples before definitive conclusions can be drawn. Therefore, while neuroreceptor imaging has resulted in several intriguing findings related to mood disorders, it has yet to yeild a cohesive and consistent picture of the neurochemical underpinnings of major mood disturbances. Neurochemical imaging is clearly very complex and studies on subjects with psychiatric disorders need to be based on methodologically sound preliminary work performed on primates and healthy subjects that may then be systematically applied to well-defined clinical populations [88,89].

Despite its complexities and ongoing technical challenges, PET has contributed enormously to our understanding of brain function [88,90]. Major technical developments over the last several years, both in terms of improved scanners and more sophisticated methods of image analysis, have provided us with more precise and detailed information about neurophysiology, both at rest and in the activated state. Novel challenge paradigms, designed to stimulate neocortical and limbic areas, have provided us with glimpses of neuronal circuitry and how it may be altered in different psychiatric disorders. Neurochemical studies using PET have begun to answer questions about specific neurotransmitter systems and their role in psychiatric disturbances. The biological issues surrounding mental disorders including mood disturbances are complex, and no single technology is likely to provide all the answers. PET and fMRI together with MRS should be considered complementary imaging modalities that can be used in the systematic study of the human brain and its perturbations. Such a synergistic approach is more likely to be rewarding in our attempts to unravel the major issues in clinical neuroscience.

REFERENCES

1. H. A. Sackeim and I. Prohovnik, Brain imaging studies of depressive disorders, *Biology of Depressive Disorders, Part A: A Systems Perspective* (J. Mann and D. J. Kupfer, eds.), Plenum Press, New York, 1993, pp. 205–258.

2. A. Kumar, A. Newburg, A. Alavi, et al., Regional cerebral glucose metabolism in late life depression and Alzheimer's disease: a preliminary PET study, *Proc. Natl. Acad. Sci. USA 90*:7019 (1993).

3. A. Kumar, M. B. Shapiro, C. Grady, et al., High-resolution PET studies in Alzheimer's disease, *Neuropsychopharmacology 4*:35 (1991).

4. J. J. Frost, Receptor imaging by positron emission tomography and single-photon emission computed tomography, *Invest. Radiol. 27 (suppl)*:s54 (1992).

5. M. E. Moseley and G. H. Glover, Functional MR imaging, capabilities and limitations, *Functional Neuroimaging 5*:161 (1995).

6. S. Ogawa, D. Tank, R. Menon, et al., Intrinsic signal changes accompanying sensory stimulation: functional brain mapping with MRI, *Proc. Natl. Acad. Sci. USA 89*:5951 (1992).

7. C. J. Bench, K. J. Friston, R. G. Brown, L. C. Scott, R. S. J. Frackowiak, and R. J. Dolan, The anatomy of melancholia—focal abnormalities of cerebral blood flow in major depression, *Psychol. Med. 22*:607 (1992).

8. J. M. Schwartz, L. R. Baxter, J. C. Maziotta, R. H. Gerner, and M. E. Phelps, The differential diagnosis of depression: relevance of positron emission tomography studies of cerebral glucose metabolism to the bipolar-unipolar dichotomy, *JAMA 258*:1368 (1987).

9. A. Kumar, Functional brain imaging in late-life depression and dementia, *J. Clin. Psychiatry 54*:21 (1993).

10. *Diagnostic and Statistical Manual of Mental Disorders*, 4th ed., American Psychiatric Association, Washington, DC, 1994.

11. L. Sokoloff, M. Reivich, C. Kennedy, et al., The [^{14}C]deoxyglucose method for measurement of local cerebral glucose utilization: theory, procedure, and normal values in the conscious and anesthetized albino rat, *J. Neurochem. 28*: 897 (1977).

12. M. Reivich, D. E. Kuhl, A. Wolf, et al., The ^{18}F-fluorodeoxyglucose method for the measurement of local cerebral glucose utilization in man, *Circ. Res. 44*: 127 (1979).

13. M. E. Phelps, S. C. Huang, E. J. Hoffman, et al., Tomographic measurement of local cerebral glucose metabolic rate in humans with (F-18)-2-deoxy-D-glucose: validation of method, *Ann. Neurol. 6*:371 (1979).

14. L. R. Baxter, M. E. Phelps, J. C. Maziotta, J. M. Schwartz, R. H. Gerner, C. E. Selin, and R. M. Sumida, Cerebral metabolic rates for glucose in mood disorders, *Arch. Gen. Psychiatry 42*:441 (1985).

15. L. R. Baxter, J. M. Schwartz, M. E. Phelps, J. C. Maziotta, B. H. Guze, C. E. Selin, R. H. Gerner, and R. M. Sumida, Reduction of prefrontal cortex glucose metabolism common to three types of depression, *Arch. Gen. Psychiatry 46*:243 (1989).

16. J. L. Martinot, P. Hardy, A. Feline, J. D. Huret, B. Mazoyer, D. Attar-Levy, S. Pappata, and A. Syrota, Left prefrontal glucose hypometabolism in the depressed state: a confirmation, *Am. J. Psychiatry 147*:1313 (1990).
17. A. S. Kling, E. J. Metter, W. H. Riege, and K. Kuhl, Comparison of PET measurement of local brain glucose metabolism and CAT measurement of brain atrophy in chronic schizophrenia and depression, *Am. J. Psychiatry 143*:175 (1986).
18. R. M. Post, L. E. DeLisi, H. H. Holcomb, T. W. Uhde, R. Cohen, and M. S. Buchsbaum, Glucose utilization in the temporal cortex of affectively ill patients: positron emission tomography, *Biol. Psychiatry 22*:545 (1987).
19. R. M. Cohen, W. E. Semple, M. Gross, T. E. Nordahl, A. C. King, D. Pickar, and R. M. Post, Evidence for common alterations in cerebral glucose metabolism in major affective disorders and schizophrenia, *Neuropsychopharmacology 2*:241 (1989).
20. R. Cohen, M. Gross, T. Nordahl, W. E. Semple, D. A. Oren, and N. Rosenthal, Preliminary data on the metabolic brain pattern of patients with winter seasonal affective disorder, *Arch. Gen. Psychiatry 49*:545 (1992).
21. P. F. Goyer, P. M. Schulz, W. E. Semple, M. Gross, T. E. Nordahl, A. C. King, T. A. Wehr, and R. M. Cohen, Cerebral glucose metabolism in patients with summer seasonal affective disorder, *Neuropsychopharmacology 7*:233 (1992).
22. T. A. Hurwitz, C. Clark, E. Murphy, H. Klonoff, W. R. W. Martin, and B. D. Pate, Regional cerebral glucose metabolism in major depressive disorder, *Can. J. Psychiatry 135*:684 (1990).
23. H. A. Sackeim, I. Prohovnik, J. R. Moeller, R. P. Brown, S. Apter, J. Prudic, D. P. Devanand, and S. Mukherjee, Regional cerebral blood flow in mood disorders, *Arch. Gen. Psychiatry 47*:60 (1990).
24. L. R. Baxter, PET studies of cerebral function in major depression and obsessive-compulsive disorder: the emerging prefrontal cortex consensus, *Ann. Clin. Psychiatry 3*:103 (1991).
25. J. C. Wu, J. C. Gillin, M. S. Buchsbaum, T. Hershey, J. C. Johnson, and W. E. Bunney, Jr., Effect of sleep deprivation on brain metabolism of depressed patients, *Am. J. Psychiatry 149*:538 (1992).
26. M. S. Nobler, H. A. Sackeim, I. Prohovnik, J. R. Moeller, S. Mukherjee, D. B. Schnur, J. Prudic, and D. P. Devanand, Regional cerebral blood flow in mood disorders, III, *Arch. Gen. Psychiatry 51*:884 (1994).
27. E. Rubin, H. A. Sackeim, M. S. Nobler, and J. R. Moeller, Brain imaging studies of antidepressant treatments, *Psychiatr. Ann. 24*:653 (1994).
28. C. J. Bench, L. C. Scott, R. G. Brown, K. J. Friston, R. S. J. Frackowiak, and R. J. Dolan, Regional cerebral blood flow in depression determined by positron emission tomography, *J. Cereb. Blood Flow Metab. 11 (suppl 2)*:S654 (1991).
29. R. J. Dolan, C. J. Bench, R. G. Brown, L. C. Scott, K. J. Friston, and R. S. J. Frackowiak, Regional cerebral blood flow in depressed patients with cognitive impairment, *J. Neurol. Neurosurg. Psychiatry 55*:768 (1992).

30. C. J. Bench, K. J. Friston, R. G. Brown, R. S. J. Frackowiak, and R. J. Dolan, Regional cerebral blood flow in depression measured by positron emission tomography: the relationship with clinical dimensions, *Psychol. Med. 23*:579 (1993).
31. M. E. Raichle, J. R. Taylor, P. Herscovitch, et al., Brain circulation and metabolism and depression, *The Metabolism of the Human Brain Studied with Positron Emission Tomography* (T. Greitz, D. H. Ingvar, and L. Widen, eds.), Raven Press, New York, 1985, pp. 453–456.
32. W. C. Drevets, T. O. Videen, J. L. Price, S. H. Preskorn, S. T. Carmichael, and M. E. Raichle, A functional anatomical study of unipolar depression, *J. Neurosci. 12*:3628 (1992).
33. M. S. George, T. A. Ketter, and R. M. Post, SPECT and PET imaging in mood disorders, *J. Clin. Psychiatry 54 (suppl)*:6 (1993).
34. M. S. Buchsbaum, J. C. Wu, L. E. DeLisi, H. H. Holcomb, R. Kessler, J. Johnson, A. C. King, E. Hazlett, K. Langston, and R. M. Post, Frontal cortex and basal ganglia metabolic rates assessed by positron emission tomography with F-18 2-deoxyglucose in affective illness, *J. Affect. Disord. 10*:137 (1986).
35. J. V. Pardo, P. J. Pardo, K. W. Janer, and M. E. Raichle, The anterior cingulate cortex mediates processing selection in the Stroop attention conflict paradigm, *Proc. Natl. Acad. Sci. USA 87*:256 (1990).
36. J. V. Pardo, P. J. Pardo, and M. E. Raichle, Neural correlates of self-induced dysphoria, *Am. J. Psychiatry 150*:713 (1993).
37. M. S. George, T. Huggins, W. McDermut, P. I. Parekh, D. Rubinow, and R. M. Post, Abnormal facial emotion recognition in depression: serial testing in an ultra-rapid cycling patient, *Behav. Modif.* (in press).
38. D. R. Rubinow and R. M. Post, Impaired recognition of affect in facial expression in depressed patients, *Biol. Psychiatry 31*:947 (1992).
39. P. T. Fox and M. A. Mintun, Noninvasive functional brain mapping by change distribution analysis of averaged PET images of H_2 ^{15}O tissue activity, *J. Nucl. Med. 30*:141 (1989).
40. P. T. Fox, H. Burton, and M. E. Raichle, Mapping human somatosensory cortex with positron emission tomography, *J. Neurosurg. 67*:34 (1987).
41. P. T. Fox, M. E. Raichle, M. A. Mintun, and C. Dence, Nonoxidative glucose consumption during food physiologic neural activity, *Science 241*:462 (1988).
42. M. S. George, T. A. Ketter, D. Gill, L. B. Marangell, P. J. Pazzaglia, and R. M. Post, Blunted CBF with emotion recognition in depression, 146th Annual Meeting of the American Psychiatric Association, San Francisco, May 22–27, 1993, Abstract NR114.
43. M. S. George, T. Kimbrell, P. I. Parekh, et al., Actively depressed subjects have difficulty inducing, and blunted limbic rCBF during, transient sadness, 148th Annual Meeting of the American Psychiatric Association, Miami, May 20–25, 1995, Abstract NR167.
44. T. A. Ketter, P. J. Andreason, M. S. George, P. J. Pazzaglia, L. B. Marangell, and R. M. Post, Blunted CBF response to procaine in mood disorders, 146th Annual Meeting of the American Psychiatric Association, San Francisco, May 22–27, 1993, Abstract NR297.

45. T. A. Ketter, M. S. George, P. J. Anderson, et al., rCMR in unipolar versus bipolar depression. 147th Annual Meeting of the American Psychiatric Association, Philadelphia, May 21–26, 1994, Abstract NR444.

46. T. A. Ketter, P. J. Andreason, M. S. George, et al., Reduced resting frontal lobe cerebral blood flow in mood disorders, 146th Annual Meeting of the American Psychiatric Association, San Francisco, May 22–27, 1993, Abstract NR298.

47. T. A. Ketter, M. S. George, H. A. Ring, P. Pazzaglia, L. Marangell, T. A. Kimbrell, and R. M. Post, Primary mood disorders: structural and resting functional studies, *Psychiatr. Ann. 24*:637 (1994).

48. M. S. George, T. A. Ketter, P. I. Parekh, B. Horwitz, P. Herscovitch, and R. M. Post, Brain Activity during transient sadness and happiness in healthy women. *Am. J. Psychiatry 152*:341 (1995).

49. T. A. Ketter, P. J. Andreason, MS. George, P Herscovitch, and R. M. Post, Paralimbic rCBF increases during procaine-induced psychosensory and emotional experiences (abstr), *Biol. Psychiatry 33*:66A#107 (1993).

50. M. S. George, T. A. Ketter, D. Gill, et al., Brain regions involved in recognizing facial emotion or identity: an 015 PET study, *J. Neuropsychiatry Clin. Neurosci. 5*:384 (1993).

51. M. S. George, T. A. Ketter, P. I. Parekh, et al., Regional brain activity when selecting a response despite interference: an H2150 PET study of the Stroop and an emotional Stroop. *Human Brain Mapping 1*:194 (1994).

52. M. S. George, T. A. Ketter, P. I. Parekh, et al., Spatial ability in affective illness: differences in regional brain activation during a spatial matching task (H2150 PET), *Neuropsychiatry, Neuropsychol. Behav. Neurol. 7*:143 (1994).

53. M. S. George, T. A. Ketter, and R. M. Post, Activation studies in mood disorders, *Psychiatr. Ann. 24*:648 (1994).

54. R. Mayeux, Y. Stern, J. Rosen, and J. Leventhal, Depression, intellectual impairment, and Parkinson's disease, *Neurology 31*:645 (1981).

55. S. E. Starkstein, R. G. Robinson, and T. R. Price, Comparison of cortical and subcortical lesions in the production of poststroke mood disorders, *Brain 110*: 1045 (1987).

56. R. G. Robinson, K. L. Kubos, L. B. Starr, et al., Mood disorders in stroke patients: importance of location of lesion, *Brain 107*:81 (1984).

57. M. M. Mesulam, Patterns in behavioral neuroanatomy: association areas, the limbic system, and hemispheric specialization, *Principles for Behavioral Neurology* (M. M. Mesulam, ed.), FA Davis, Philadelphia, 1985, pp. 1–70.

58. G. E. Alexander, M. D. Crutcher, and M. R. De Long, Basal gangliathalamocortical circuits: parallel substrates for motor, oculomotor, 'prefrontal' and 'limbic' functions, *Prog. Brain Res. 85*:119 (1990).

59. H. S. Mayberg, S. E. Sarkenstein, B. Sazdot, T. Preziosi, P. L. Andrezejewski, R. F. Dannals, H. N. Wagner, Jr., and R. G. Robinson, Selective hypometabolism in the inferior frontal lobe in depressed patients with Parkinson's disease, *Ann. Neurol. 28*:57 (1990).

60. H. S. Mayberg, S. E. Starkstein, C. E. Peyser, J. Brandt, R. F. Dannals, and S. E. Folstein, Paralimbic frontal lobe hypometabolism in depression associated with Huntington's disease, *Neurology 42*:1791 (1992).

61. H. S. Mayberg, Functional imaging studies in secondary depression, *Psychiatr. Ann. 24*:643 (1994).

62. E. B. Bromfield, L. Altshuler, D. B. Leiderman, M. Balish, T. A. Ketter, O. Devinsky, R. M. Post, and W. H. Theodore, Cerebral metabolism and depression in patients with complex partial seizures, *Arch. Neurol. 49*:617 (1992).

63. S. E. Starkstein, H. S. Mayberg, M. L. Berthier, P. Fedoroff, T. R. Price, R. F. Dannals, H. N. Wagner, R. Leiguarda, and R. G. Robinson, Mania after brain injury: neuroradiological and metabolic findings, *Ann. Neurol. 27*:652 (1990).

64. G. Sedvall, L. Farde, A. Persson, and F. A. Wiesel, Imaging of neurotransmitter receptors in the living human brain, *Arch. Gen. Psychiatry 43*:995 (1986).

65. R. B. Innis, Neuroreceptor imaging with SPECT, *J. Clin. Psychiatry 11(suppl)*: 29 (1992).

66. D. F. Wong, H. N. Wagner, L. E. Tune, R. F. Dannals, G. D. Pearlson, J. M. Links, C. A. Tamanga, E. P. Broussole, H. T. Ravert, A. A. Wilson, T. J. K. Toung, J. Malat, J. A. Williams, L. A. O'Tuama, S. H. Snyder, M. J. Kuhar, and A. Gjedde, Positron emission tomography reveals elevated D_2 dopamine receptors in drug-naive schizophrenics, *Science 234*:1158 (1986).

67. L. E. Tune, D. F. Wong, G. D. Pearlson, M. E. Strauss, T. Young, E. K. Shaya, R. F. Dannals, A. Wilson, H. T. Ravert, J. Sapp, T. Cooper, G. A. Chase, and H. N. Wagner, Jr., Dopamine D_2 receptor density estimates in schizophrenia: a positron emission tomography study with ^{11}C-methylspiperone, *Psychiatry Res. 49*:219 (1993).

68. D. F. Wong, G. D. Pearlson, L. T. Young, H. Singer, V. Villemagne, L. Tune, C. Ross, R. F. Dannals, J. M. Links, B. Chan, A. A. Wilson, H. T. Ravert, H. N. Wagner Jr., and A. Gjedde, D_2 dopamine receptors are elevated in neuropsychiatric disorders other than schizophrenia, *J. Cereb. Blood Flow Metab. 9(suppl)*:s593 (1989).

69. D. F. Wong, A. Gjedde, H. N. Wagner Jr., R. F. Dannals, K. H. Douglass, J. M. Links, and M. J. Kuhar, Quantification of neuroreceptors in the living human brain, II: assessment of receptor density and affinity using inhibition studies, *J. Cereb. Blood Flow Metab. 6*:147 (1986).

70. D. F. Wong, A. Gjedde, and H. N. Wagner Jr., Quantification of neuro-receptors in the living human brain, I: association rate of irreversibly bound ligands, *J. Cereb. Blood Flow Metab. 6*:137 (1986).

71. D. F. Wong, H. N. Wagner Jr., P. F. Dannals, J. M. Links, J. J. Frost, H. T. Ravert, A. A. Wilson, A. E. Rosenbaum, M. F. Folstein, J. D. Petronis, K. H. Douglas, J. K. T. Toung, and M. J. Kuhar, Effects of age on dopamine and serotonin receptors measured by positron tomography in the living human brain, *Science 226*:1393 (1984).

72. L. Farde, F. A. Wiesel, H. Hall, C. Halldin, S. Stone-Elander, and G. Sedvall, No D_2 receptor increase in PET study of schizophrenia, *Arch. Gen. Psychiatry 44*:671 (1987).

73. G. D. Pearlson, D. F. Wong, L. Tune, C. A. Ross, G. Chase, J. M. Links, R. F. Dannals, A. A. Wilson, H. T. Ravert, H. N. Wagner Jr., and J. R. DePaulo, In vivo D_2 dopamine receptor density in psychotic and nonpsychotic patients with bipolar disorder, *Arch. Gen. Psychiatry 52*:471 (1995).

74. D. G. Grahame-Smith, Serotonin function in affective disorders, *Acta Psych. Scand.* *89*:7 (1989).
75. G. Curzon, Transmitter amines in depression, *Psychol. Med.* *12*:465 (1982).
76. H. S. Mayberg, R. G. Robinson, D. F. Wong, R. Parikh, P. Bolduc, S. E. Sarkenstein, T. Price, R. F. Dannals, J. M. Links, A. A. Wilson, H. T. Ravert, and H. N. Wagner, PET imaging of cortical S2 serotonin receptors after stroke: lateralized changes and relationship to depression, *Am. J. Psychiatry 145*:937 (1988).
77. H. S. Mayberg, R. F. Dannals, C. A. Ross, A. A. Wilson, H. T. Ravert, and J. J. Frost, Mu opiate receptor binding is increased in depressed patients measured by PET and C-11-carfentanil, ACNP 1991, Abstract P61.
78. R. Gross-Iseroff, K. A. M. Dillon, and A. Bigeon, Regionally selective increases in m opiod receptor density in the brains of suicide victims, *Brain Res. 530*:312 (1990).
79. K. A. Frey, V. A. Holthoff, R. A. Koeppe, D. M. Jewett, M. R. Kilbourn, and D. E. Kuhl, Parametric in vivo imaging of benzodiazepine receptor distribution in human brain, *Ann. Neurol. 30*:663 (1991).
80. J. J. Frost, K. H. Douglas, H. S. Mayberg, et al., Multicompartmental analysis of [^{11}C]-carfentanil binding to opiate receptors in humans measured by positron emission tomography, *J. Cereb. Blood Flow Metab. 9*:398 (1989).
81. P. Barenstein and M. Koepp, Bezodiazepine receptor imaging with positron emission tomography and single photon emission tomography, *Nervenarzt 66*: 412 (1995).
82. B. Sadzot, C. Lemaire, P. Maquet, E. Salmon, A. Plenevaux, C. Cegueldre, J. P. Hermanne, M. Guillaume, R. Cantineau, D. Comar, et al., Serotonin 5HT2 receptor imaging in the human brain using positron emission tomography and a new radioligand, [18F] altanserin: results in young normal controls, *J. Cereb. Blood Flow Metab. 15*:787 (1995).
83. T. Brucke, S. Wenger, S. Asenbaum, E. Fertl, N. Pfafflmeyer, C. Muller, I. Podreka, and P. Angelberger, Dopamine D$_2$ receptor imaging and measurement with SPECT, *Adv. Neurol. 60*:494 (1993).
84. L. Farde, H. Hall, E. Ehrin, and G. Sedvall, Quantitative analysis of D2 dopamine receptor binding in the living human brain by PET, *Science 231*:258 (1985).
85. H. Ågren, L. Reibring, R. Hartvig, J. Tedroff, P. Bjurling, H. Lundgvist, and B. Långström, Monoamine Metabolism in human prefrontal cortex and basal ganglia, PET studies using [β-^{11}C] L-dopa in healthy volunteers and patients with unipolar major depression, *Depression 1*:71 (1993).
86. H. Kishimoto, O. Takazu, S. Ohno, T. Yamaguchi, H. Fujita, H. Kuwahara, T. Ishii, M. Matsushita, S. Yokoi, and M. Lio, ^{11}C-Glucose metabolism in manic and depressed patients, *Psychiatry Res. 22*:81 (1987).
87. T. Suhara, K. Nakayama, O. Inoue, H. Fukuda, M. Shimizu, A. Mori, and Y. Tateno, Dopamine 1 receptor binding in mood disorders measured by positron emission tomography, *Psychopharmacology 106*:14 (1992).
88. B. H. Guze, L. R. Baxter, M. P. Szuba, and J. M. Schwartz, Positron emission

tomography and mood disorders, *Brain Imaging in Affective Disorders* (P. Hauser, ed.), American Psychiatric Press, Washington, DC, pp. 63–87 (1991).

89. G. Pawlik, C. Beil, I. Hebold, K. Weinhard, and W. D. Heiss, Positron emission tomography in depression research: principles-results-perspectives, *Psychopathology 19 (suppl 2)*:85 (1986).

90. M. E. Phelps, J. C. Mazziotta, L. R. Baxter, and R. Gerner, Positron emission tomographic studies of affective disorders: problems and strategies, *Ann. Neurol. 15 (suppl)*:149 (1984).

10

Brain SPECT in Mood Disorders

Madhukar H. Trivedi and Mustafa M. Husain
University of Texas Southwestern Medical Center,
Dallas, Texas

I. INTRODUCTION

Medical models of disorders have traditionally been based on a thorough understanding of the pathophysiology of various disease entities. Major psychiatric disorders have clear biological underpinnings, as evidenced by genetic, family, biochemical, electrophysiological, and treatment studies. However, even with recent advances in diagnostic methods and antidepressant and antimanic treatments, descriptively defined disorder groupings still appear to encompass heterogeneous populations. New functional brain imaging techniques afford us the opportunity to examine the active human brain during various stages of chronic, episodic, and debilitating mood disorders. Additionally, these techniques allow us to identify major psychiatric disorders even in the absence of measurable structural brain abnormalities.

In theory, functional neuroimaging should fulfill one or more of the following clinical and/or research objectives: (a) assist in diagnosis, (b) improve the identification of disorder subtypes, especially based on pathophysiology, (c) aid in identifying prognostic and prescriptive predictors of treatment response, (d) aid in predicting relapse and recurrence of the disease, (e) assist in identifying those at risk for the development of the disorder prior to its expression, and (f) identify specific neurofunctional networks that participate in psychopathological states or in the response to cognitive, emotional, or pharmacological challenge(s) or activation(s).

Recent emphasis on the understanding of brain dysfunction in mood disorders has resulted in the pursuit of objective and reliable measures of hypothesized brain abnormalities. Single photon computed emission tomography (SPECT) and positron emission tomography (PET) are yielding a picture of depression and mania (both primary and secondary) as disorders associated with dysfunction of specific brain regions. The complex interaction of structural and functional systems in the central nervous system (CNS) makes it unlikely that single sites are responsible for such disorders, or even that single systems are abnormal in isolation. The brain processes and regions that together may be associated with a particular cognitive process or behavior may be seen as a functional unit or neural circuit. The same function may be performed by different combinations of neural circuit(s) at different times and under different conditions.

Global cerebral hypoactivity (metabolism or perfusion), accompanied by regional hypoactivity in the anterior dorso-lateral frontal lobes and the limbic circuit, appears to be a common pathway for both primary and secondary depressions. Extrafrontal regional abnormalities, associated with depressive disorders, are found in the anterior temporal lobes, the amygdala, the cingulate gyrus, and the caudate nuclei. Frontal hypometabolism has been correlated with the severity of the symptomatic state and appears to normalize with successful remission of symptoms. Which abnormalities are state dependent and which are trait related or scars of the disorder is unclear at the present time. Further characterization of these differences will advance our understanding of the pathophysiology of depression as well as provide improvements in treatment guidelines. Additionally, this information may provide the clinician with data on the predictive value of treatment response, predict relapse and recurrence in the chronic and episodic subgroups of the disorder, and be utilized in developing better pharmacological interventions for unipolar and bipolar mood disorders. Findings implicate the left hemisphere in the control of negative emotions, whereas positive emotions appear to to be under the control of the right hemisphere.

II. NEUROANATOMY OF MOOD DISORDERS

Because of the problems outlined above, researchers must integrate information from multiple conceptual levels in order to understand and explain the psychiatric disorders being studied. The distinction between overt brain structural abnormalities and brain dysfunction is critical in conceptualizing mood disorders. As noted by Jackson [1], marked abnormal brain function is not always associated with aberrant brain structure. He observed in his studies of epilepsy that problems in function or behavior could exist despite grossly normal brain structure. In primary mood disorders, visually apparent structural abnormalities are absent in most individuals, although studies of large groups of mood disorder patients have revealed some subtle structural differences. The neuropathology seen in secondary mood disorders is of interest for the following reasons. First, associations exist between organic brain lesions (e.g., Parkinson's disease, Huntington's disease, poststroke depression) and the symptoms of affective disorders, including mood, cognitive, psychomotor, behavioral, and physiological manifestations. Interestingly, the secondary mood syndrome can be episodic, despite the presence of fixed structural lesions (e.g., multiple sclerosis). Second, antidepressant medications provide symptomatic relief for comorbid mood disruptions without altering the primary neuropathological abnormality. Finally, it is also conceivable that secondary mood disorders may be accompanied by specific neurochemical changes induced by the primary structural damage. Understanding the relationship between the primary brain lesion and the consequent neurochemical alterations may also help clarify the underlying pathophysiology of primary mood disorders. The complex interaction of structural and functional systems in the CNS makes it unlikely that single sites are responsible for disorders, or even that single systems are abnormal in isolation. New functional imaging tools, such as SPECT, PET, and functional magnetic resonance imaging (fMRI), can reveal abnormal brain function despite generally normal brain structure.

A. Neurofunctional Substrates in Mood Disorders

Most researchers have concluded that coordinated regional brain systems or networks participate in regulating emotion in both health and disease [2–7]. There are extremely complex interconnections of the limbic system and the cortex, the monoamine pathways, as well as detailed subcortical projections. The limbic system, first described by Papez, has remained a primary focus for research in this area. The Papez circuit's depiction of the limbic system consists of a circle on the medial aspect of both hemispheres involving the amygdala and extending to the insula, orbitofrontal cortex, and anterior temporal lobes [8]. The frontal convexity initiates a pathway directly along the cortex of the cingulate gyrus. The dorsolateral prefrontal cortex also has interconnections with the cingulate, the hippocampus, and the septo-hypothalamic region, allowing for direct prefrontal input into neuroendocrine pathways. In addition to efferent projections from the prefrontal lobe to key limbic regions, the prefrontal cortex has afferent input directly from the amygdala and indirectly from the hypothalamus and mamillary bodies through the anterior thalamus. Additionally, many limbic regions are linked to the prefrontal cortex through the medial dorsal thalamus[9]. This neural circuit has been postulated to be consistent with a mood-processing system that can gather higher-order sensory information, integrate it with past emotional experiences, and endow it with emotional significance yielding behavioral and emotional responses from the individual.

Similarly, Nauta [10] has suggested three components of the limbic systems: (a) the *cortical limbic lobe* consisting of the cingulate and parahippocampal gyri, hippocampus, and amygdala, (b) a *subcortical system* including the limbic midbrain (septo-hypothalamo-mesencephalic continuum), which receives afferents from amygdala, hippocampus, spinal cord, and lower brainstem and sends efferents to the thalamus, visceral motor system, and hypophyseal complex, and (c) a *visceroendocrine pathway* consisting of visceral-sensory fibers ascending from the spinal cord and medulla oblongata. The frontal lobe has the greatest variety of connections to these three limbic systems. Dorsal and medial components send fibers dorsally along the cortex of the cingulate gyrus giving off a variety of collaterals. Finally, Livingston [11] has proposed two limbic circuits: medial and basolateral. The medial limbic system is composed of hippocampal gyrus, fornix, cingulate gyrus, anterior thalamic nuclei, septal nuclei, and mammillary bodies. The basolateral limbic circuit is composed of the orbital frontal cortex, dorsal medial thalamic nucleus, amygdala, and anterior temporal cortex. Livingston hypothesized that the frontal lobe plays a dominant role in modulating these two circuits and that normal behavior is reflected as a balance between the activities of these two circuits.

The limbic system has rich innervations from fibers of the monoamine systems. Dopamine, serotonin, and norepinephrine systems ascend and descend through the brain to the limbic and prefrontal cortex as well as to striatum and other cortical areas. There are extensive projections from the cingulate gyrus to the medial, lateral, and basal surfaces of the cerebral hemispheres and extensive connections between striatal components and cortical components, and between the thalamic nuclei and the limbic system. Moreover, the monoamine receptors are distributed in the striatum, cortex, and limbic system, and this extensive network is involved in feedback and modulation among regions.

Evidence for limbic system dysregulation in mood disorders comes from neuropsychological, brain imaging, CNS lesion, and neural stimulation studies in human beings as well as other species [12–14]. However, numerous researchers have argued that it is important to also take into account MacLean's description of the triune brain (with its attendant developmentally hierarchical components) in addition to the Papez circuit in understanding complex human emotional systems. The triune brain consists of three concentric brain systems, physically layered on top of each other, with each successive layer representing an evolutionary advance, allowing for the introduction of new behaviors while recapitulating older ones. The brain structures that regulate affect are represented in all three components of the triune brain. Direct damage to some primitive brain structure, such as the caudate, may be associated with defects in emotion, recognition or mood regulation. Damage to the developmentally early limbic brain would be more likely to disrupt affective regulation, whereas direct damage to the neocortex might lead to mood disruption through interruption of frontal cortical regulation of the limbic circuit. Therefore, research focusing exclusively on the role of the limbic structures in regulating mood (e.g., the subjective internal state of emotion) and affect (the external displays of mood) does not entirely explain the presentation of depression secondary to lesions or injuries to the cortex. It is theorized that regions in the prefrontal lobes may regulate the more primitive unmodulated behaviors ingrained in subcortical structures and the limbic system, and removal of this highest level of integrative function may then release the more primitive, limbic-mediated behaviors. Recent functional brain-imaging studies that document changes in neocortical functioning during depression appear to confirm the role of all the interconnections. The triune brain model, with its assumption of multiple, layered, interacting systems, provides a theoretical framework for understanding much of the brain-imaging, stimulation, and CNS injury data in mood disorder research. This model also can be used to explain some of the discrepant findings from brain-imaging research.

Another way to conceptualize the neurofunctional aspects of clinical depression involves understanding the interconnections of the subcortical structures linked to emotion modulation with the cortex, especially the prefrontal cortex. The prefrontal cortex projects to numerous areas in the brainstem (e.g., ventral midbrain, raphe nucleus, and locus ceruleus) and appears to be essential in regulating the general state of arousal and tone [15]. Similarly, brainstem areas project back to the prefrontal lobes, providing noradrenergic, dopaminergic, and serotonergic input. One would hypothesize that dorsal lateral prefrontal, medial prefrontal, and orbital frontal cortex, mesial and lateral temporal cortex (including amygdala and hippocampus) should have a major role in mood control. Subcortically, the cingulate gyrus, thalamus, and anterior caudate (and other striatal tissues) should be affected.

Conceptualized in this manner, certain clinical syndromes could result from damage at any point in the circuit—at the level of the frontal lobes or subcortically in the basal ganglia or thalamus. For example, damage at the orbitofrontal circuit results in disinhibition, irritability, and decreased sensitivity to social clues as seen in mania. Anterior cingulate (medial frontal) damage produces apathy and reduced motivation, behaviors commonly associated with depression. Dorsolateral prefrontal damage results in a dementia syndrome with problems in set-shifting and word-list generation. Some investigators have established additional links between dorsolateral prefrontal damage and patients with schizophrenia [16,17]. Many of the symptoms and phenomenology of clinical depression can thus be loosely mapped onto these circuits; in fact, one might infer that the lateral frontal, the anterior cingulate, and, to a lesser extent, the dorsolateral prefrontal circuits are involved in clinical depression [18].

B. Structural Correlates of Mood Disorders

In addition to the systems approach discussed in the previous section, several distinct brain structural regions appear to be important in regulating mood, health, and disease. Three of these regions are described below.

1. Prefrontal Cortex

The prefrontal cortex is unique within the CNS for its strong connections with virtually all other regions of the brain—it is thus uniquely situated to simultaneously control motor behavior, interpret the significance of sensory input from several modalities, and then set the internal state of arousal and tone through connections with limbic and neuroendocrine regions. However, it is difficult to localize behaviors to specific subregions of the frontal lobes because these regions often participate together in producing or modulating behavior through the basal ganglia-thalamic-cortical loops.

2. Lesion Studies

A variety of approaches have been utilized to demonstrate the effects of discrete damage to the frontal lobes. In general, the literature in this area is inconsistent. It does appear, however, in some cases, that specific behavioral sequelae result from frontal lobe damage. The particular responses are dependent on which specific regions of the frontal lobes are damaged and whether or not there is premorbid brain damage [19]. For example, orbito-frontal leukotomies were often reported to produce euphoria and disinhibition, and were therefore used in the treatment of catatonically depressed patients [20]. More anterior leukotomies, involving the frontal convexity, were found to produce flattening of affect and were used in the treatment of agitated or manic patients [21]. It appears that damage to the prefrontal lobes may be necessary to produce distinct behavioral syndromes, but damage does not invariably produce consistent mood changes. A variety of other factors, including the frontal lobes' governance over or interconnection with limbic structures, may also be instrumental in producing specific behaviors. It is generally believed that the premorbid personality coarsens after prefrontal lobe damage. [22] If a patient is initially fretful and anxious, prefrontal lobe damage often intensifies this tendency, while a jocular individual may become disinhibited and intrusive after frontal lobe damage.

3. Structural Imaging Studies

Historically, studies of the structural anatomy of patients with affective illness have been largely inconclusive. Recently, however, well-designed studies employing advanced imaging techniques have found differences in the prefrontal lobes and neighboring regions between depressed subjects and controls. Several investigators have found an increase in ventricular size in patients with recurrent mood disorders compared to age-matched controls [23,24]. Recent work by Coffey and colleagues [25], using magnetic resonance imaging (MRI) revealed a 7% smaller mean total frontal lobe volume in 48 inpatients with severe depression compared to 76 healthy controls.

Structural MRI has been used in at least two other studies implicating frontal lobe dysfunction in depression. Rangel-Guerra and colleagues [26], using MRI to examine bipolar affective disorder (BPAD) subjects, found increased T_1 values in frontal and temporal white matter, which normalized with lithium therapy. This increase in T_1 values may reflect shifts in water distribution, which may in turn represent changes in metabolism. Dolan and colleagues [27] examined 14 medicated patients with BPAD, medicated patients with unipolar depression, and 10 controls. They also found increases in T_1 signal intensity in the frontal white matter, but only for the unipolar depressed subjects as compared with controls. It remains unclear whether these findings represent a change in brain structure, or function, or both.

4. Cingulate

The cingulate gyrus is an extension of the limbic system present in mammals; it appears to play a significant role in certain uniquely mammalian behaviors, such as mating, pair-bonding, parenting, and play [28,29]. In addition, it appears to play an important part in regulating attentional mechanisms and selecting an appropriate response in the presence of distractions or competing responses [30–32]. Stimulation of the anterior cingulate leads to decreased spontaneous movements, inhibition and facilitation of cortically induced reflex movements such as chewing, licking, and swallowing. On the other hand, stimulation of the posterior cingulate induces grooming and sexual as well as other pleasurable reactions.

Some studies of depressed subjects have found increased cingulate activity at rest, and three studies have shown that patients with baseline cingulate hyperactivity selectively respond to a night of sleep deprivation, i.e., sleep deprivation reverses the hyperactivity in conjunction with an improvement in mood [30,33,34]. These studies suggest that limbic hyperactivity may be associated with depression and that an antidepressant response to sleep deprivation occurs in association with a normalization of limbic tone.

5. Amygdala

The amygdala is a collection of nuclei situated within the mesial temporal lobes with important afferent and efferent connections throughout the rest of the limbic system, as well as the cortex [36,37]. Historically, the findings of Kluver and Bucy [38] indicated that bilateral removal of the temporal lobe (including the amygdala) in rhesus monkeys resulted in docile animals exhibiting no fear and little emotion, constantly examining all objects in their environment and engaging in indiscriminate eating and sexual activity. Because of the amygdala's unique input from multiple sensory areas and direct connections back out to all levels of cortex, it appears to function as a quick response route for determining the affective significance of external stimuli and acts as another valuable, noncortical route for evaluating the external world [39]. Drevets et al. [71] have reported hyperactivity of the amygdalar function in their studies on depressed patients.

III. NEURAL BASES OF MOOD STATE

As discussed in the previous sections, the limbic system plays a crucial role in the regulation of mood [40–42]. The limbic system is strategically organized to receive complex sensory information, process it with information from past experiences, imbue it with affective significance, and produce appropriate behavioral responses. Anterior paralimbic and related structures have been particularly implicated in the mediation of both physiological and pathological emotional experience. In healthy controls, self-induction of transient emotions (e.g., sadness, happiness, anger, and anxiety) has been associated with changes in paralimbic function [43,44]. Anterior paralimbic activation patterns have been observed in conjunction with the induction of acute affective changes by neuropsychological (self-induced sadness) and pharmacological (acute intravenous procaine) methods in healthy volunteers from a series of studies at the National Institute of Mental Health (NIMH). This concordance extended to regional correlational relationships, i.e., left amygdala activation correlated with negative affective shifts (self-induced sadness and procaine-induced dysphoria), while deactivation correlated with positive affective shifts (self-induced happiness and procaine-induced euphoria).

Neuropsychological studies have also explored components of affective processing. For example, facial expression matching has been associated with anterior paralimbic (right anterior cingulate and inferior frontal) activation, which does not occur with facial identity matching or spatial object relationship matching [45]. Likewise, understanding the emotional content of spoken language activates the bilateral prefrontal cortex, while emotional tonal comprehension (prosody) activates right prefrontal and anterior temporal structures [46].

IV. SPECT STUDIES IN MOOD DISORDERS

Functional brain-imaging studies of mood disorders have demonstrated broad agreement, as well as some variability of findings. Variability may arise from a number of sources, including:

1. Variability in image acquisition and analysis methodology.
2. Heterogeneity of mood disorders - unipolar vs. bipolar, nonpsychotic vs. psychotic, seasonal vs. nonseasonal, familial vs. nonfamilial, pure (no comorbidity) vs. complicated (comorbid anxiety, substance abuse or other disorders), episodic vs. chronic, mild vs. severe, and melancholic (anoretic, insomniac, agitated) vs. atypical (hyperphagic, hypersomnic, retarded) subtypes, as well as state vs. trait differences, and various treatment effects.

The following sections will examine current studies in mood disorders utilizing a variety of methodologies.

A. Primary Depression

1. Resting Studies

Numerous investigators, using PET and SPECT, have demonstrated that depressed patients have decreased metabolism or regional cerebral blood flow (rCBF) in the prefrontal lobes, particularly in the left anterolateral prefrontal cortex (Table 1) [47–57].

Curran et al. [58] studied 20 elderly patients with unipolar depression, 30 age-matched normal volunteers, and 20 Alzheimer's patients utilizing technetium-99-hexamethylpropyleneamine oxime (^{99m}Tc-HMPAO) SPECT and found no difference in patients with onset of illness before age 60 compared to patients with onset after 60. They also reported a slightly better outcome in patients with higher tracer uptake in subcortical areas and in right parietal and posterior cingulate cortex.

Murphy [59] studied four patients with seasonal affective disorders (SAD) and four age- and gender-matched controls using Xenon-133 (^{133}Xe) probes. They found no difference in the resting study. However, they did report a significantly different percentage change following 2 hours of 1500 lux artificial daylight, with normals showing significant reduction while three of the four SAD patients showed no change.

Austin et al. [60] evaluated 40 unipolar, depressed patients and 20 age- and gender-matched controls with ^{99m}Tc-HMPAO SPECT. Twenty of the 40 patients had endogenous depressive disorder, and 10 of the 40 had psychotic symptoms; no hemispheric differences were identified between patients and controls in their CBF. Patients with depression showed reduced rCBF in temporal, inferior frontal, and parietal cortices as well as in the basal ganglia and thalamus. Interestingly, positive correlations were found between rCBF and the interior and posterior cingulate cortices (predominantly more on the right) as well as the superior frontal and parietal areas. This indicates that while reduced rCBF is seen in major depressive disorder, endogenous illness is associated with relatively greater rCBF in the cingulate and frontal cortex compared to the nonendogenous subgroup.

Philpot et al. [61] studied 10 elderly patients with major depressive disorder and nine normal controls at rest and during a cognitive challenge designed to assess frontal lobe function (through a verbal fluency task) using ^{99m}Tc-HMPAO SPECT. Depressed patients showed significant rCBF reductions in the right and left parietal, left temporal, and left occipital regions. Interestingly, during the cognitive challenge, patients exhibited an increase in rCBF such that the differences between patients and normals disappeared, except

Table 1 SPECT Studies in Depression

Subjects	Depressed	Controls	Method	HRS-D	Meds	Findings	Ref.
N	13	13	Xe^{133}	25 ± 11	Off	↓ L hem rCBF (trend	47
Age	30 ± 7	"Matched"	probes			on the right)	
M/F	4/9	4/9				Corr w/HRS-D bilateral	
						hem	
N	20	20	Xe^{133}	NR	Off	6/20 bipolars	48
Age	19–69	NR	SPECT			↓ global rCBF in	
M/F	NR	NR				unipolar, normal in	
						bipolar, rCBF ↑ with	
						Rx	
N	24	20	Xe^{133}	28 ± 7	Off	8/24 bipolars	49
Age	2 ± 12	41 ± 11	probes			↑ L front & ↓ R post	
M/F	5/19	8/12				rCBF ratio in	
						unipolar; bipolars	
						normal	
N	14	25	Xe^{133}	27 ± 3	On	Normal rCBF	50
Age	31 ± 9	28 ± 11	probes				
M/F	8/6	11/14					
N	44	29	Xe^{133}	24 ± 10	Off	13/44 bipolars	51
Age	40 ± 12	33 ± 11	SPECT			↓ R par & temp rCBF	
M/F	17/27	10/19				in unipolar; ↑ L hem,	
						par & temp in bipolar;	
						normal A/P gradient	
N	21	21	Au^{195}	24 ± 10	Off	↓ global rCBF, R > L;	52
Age	46 ± 13	31 ± 8	"probe"			corr w/symptoms,	
M/F	11/10	12/9				BPRS and HRS-D.	
N	24	31	Xe^{133}	NR	Mixed	2/24 bipolars	53
Age	61 ± 13	"Matched"	probes			Normal rCBF, but	
M/F	NR	"Matched"				values corr with	
						symptom clusters	
N	38	8	Xe^{133}	18 ± NR	18 On	4/38 bipolars	54
Age	59 ± NR	58 ± 10	SPECT	20	Off	↑ R frontal rCBF and	
M/F	14/24	6/2				↑ R A/P gradient	
N	24	6	^{123}IMP	23 ± 10	On	2/24 bipolars	55
Age	55 ± 15	53 ± 21	SPECT			↓ cerebrum/cerebellum	
M/F	14/10	5/1				for cortical & striate	
						regions. Corr w/HRS-	
						D	
N	41	40	Xe^{133}	32 ± 8	Off	25/41 bipolars	56
Age	60 ± 12	61 ± 11	probes			↓ global flow; network	
M/F	12/29	12/28				of ↓ regions that corr	
						w/age and HRS-D.	
N	38	16	Xe^{133}	27 ± 6	Off	8/38 bipolars	57
Age	39 ± 13	44 ± 24	SPECT			↓ L cortical rCBF in	
M/F	17/21	8/8				bipolar and in	
						endogenous patients.	

(continued)

Table 1 (*continued*)

Subjects	Depressed	Controls	Method	HRS-D	Meds	Findings	Ref.
N	10	8	Tc-99m	28 ± 8		↓ L ALPFC lower part	76
Age	39 ± 9	42 ± 10	HMPAO	MDD		slp dep responders @	
M/F	5/5	4/4	SPECT	Only		baseline: ↑ R, L orb front ↑ R hippocamp, para hippocamp, amygdala, ↑ R, L inf temp	
N	40	20	Tc-99m	22 ± 6	15 On	↓ A/P gradient ↓ temp,	
Age	46 ± 14	47 ± 15	HMPAO			inf front, parietal +	
M/F	18/22	9/11	SPECT			corr bet newcastle and cing, frontal - corr bet HRSD & ant uptake	
N	14	10	Tc-99m	23 ± 15	Off	↓ rCBF bilat temp ↓	62
Age	34 ± 3	33 ± 3	HMPAO			L/R prefrontal ratio	
M/F	3/11	NR	SPECT			HRSD neg corr w/ant frontal and L prefrontal	
N	30	30	133 Xe	33 ± 8	Off	30 Alzeimer's pts	56
Age	66 ± 7	64 ± 9	Probes			additional controls	
M/F	11/19	10/20				↓ Global CBF SSM: distinct patterns for MDD and Alzeimer's	
N	16	12	Tc-99m	22 ± 7	4 on	12 remitted depressed	
Age	43 ± 14		HMPAO	to	12 off	served as controls	
M/F	10/6		SPECT	3 ± 3		recovery leads to 1 bilat ant cing & basal ganglia	
N	13	11	Tc-99m	22 ± 5		↓ prefrontal bilat., ↓	67
Age	42 ± 11	35 ± 13	HMPAO			ant. temp ↓ ant cing.	
M/F	3/10	9/2	SPECT			↓ caudate	
N	14		Tc-99m	NR	on	Controls: 45 pts w/CFS	
Age	70 ± 13		HMPAO			& 27 pts w/AIDS	
M/F	5/9		SPECT			temporal & frontal lobe defects Dep & CFS > Normals	
N	68	N/A	Xe133	31 ± 7	Off	Study assessed acute &	74
Age	57 ± 14		Probes			short term effects of	
M/F	26/42					ECT on CBF further ↓ gCBF & ant cortical ↓ corr w/ outcome	

(*continued*)

Table 1 (*continued*)

Subjects	Depressed	Controls	Method	HRS-D	Meds	Findings	Ref.
N	26	NA	Xe[133]	24 ± 3	off	Off meds at baseline, on	106
Age	63 ± 5		Probes			antidep at end of Rx	
M/F	11/15					baseline: ↓ L > R	
						frontol on Rx: ↑ L	
						frontal	
N	11	11	Xe[133]	30 ± 7	off	11 manic pts also	35
Age	30 ± 12	30 ± 13	probes			studied	
M/F	3/8	4/7				↓ A/P gradient in both	
						patient groups	
						↓ L inf front in MDDs	

Hem = hemisphere; corr = correlation; Rx = treatment; front = frontal; post = posterior; par = parietal; temp = temporal; slp dep = sleep deprived; orb = orbital; inf = inferior; ant = anterior; cing = cingulate; dep = depressed.

in the right parietal cortex. Again, rCBF correlated positively with severity of psychotic symptoms, but negatively with somatic symptoms and anxiety.

Yazici et al. [62] investigated 14 patients with endogenous major depressive disorder and 10 normal controls with the help of ^{99m}TC-HMPAO; 3 of the 14 patients also exhibited psychotic symptoms. Patients showed a significant reduction in rCBF in bilateral temporal lobes and a reduced right/ left prefrontal region ratio. The Hamilton Rating Scale for Depression (HRS-D) score was negatively correlated with anterofrontal and left prefrontal cortices.

Thomas et al. [63] examined 42 patients with depression—21 with major depression and 21 with dysthymia and major depression (double depression)—using ^{99m}Tc-HMPAO SPECT. Interestingly, the authors found significantly lower rCBF in all regions for patients with major depression compared to patients with double depression, but found no correlation between severity of the illness and rCBF. This latter finding is intriguing in that rCBF may be a better correlate of either disease subtype, or perhaps more likely the duration of the illness.

Lesser et al. [64] investigated 39 elderly patients with major depression and 20 healthy control subjects using both ^{133}Xe and ^{99m}Tc-HMPAO SPECT. They reported reduced rCBF right hemisphere, orbitofrontal, and inferior temporal rCBF in patients compared to normal controls—male gender also predicted reduction in CBF.

Amsterdam and Mozley [65] reported temporal lobe asymmetry in patients with major depression utilizing iodine-123-isopropyliodoamphetamine (^{123}I-IMP) SPECT. However, the main finding appears to be significantly greater IMP uptake in the right temporal lobes of depressed responders compared to medical controls, once again demonstrating preliminary evidence of prognostic predictor value.

Sackeim et al. [56] compared 41 patients with major depression and 40 matched normal controls using ^{133}Xe inhalation technique during the resting state; they reported a marked reduction in global cerebral blood flow. They also applied a scaled subprofile method of analysis and identified topographical abnormalities in patients with major depression. This analysis revealed a flow reduction in frontal, superior temporal, and anterior parietal regions. Such fixed voxel-based analyses are increasingly used to begin to identify whole neural circuits associated with mood and other disorders.

Mayberg et al. [67] examined 13 severe, treatment-resistant unipolar depressed patients and 11 age-matched normal volunteers (not gender-matched) utilizing ^{99m}Tc-HMPAO SPECT; all patients were on medications at the time of the study. They also reported significant reduction bilaterally in frontal cortex, anterior temporal cortex, anterior cingulate gyrus, and caudate regions in depressed patients compared to normal volunteers. One interesting finding in this study was the negative correlation between rCBF and psychomotor slowing.

Baxter and colleagues [68] used fluorodeoxyglucose-18 (^{18}F) PET to study patients with unipolar depression, bipolar depression, obsessive-compulsive disorder (OCD) with secondary depression, and normal controls. Glucose metabolism in the left ALPFC was significantly lower for all depressed patients than in controls or nondepressed OCD subjects. In addition, they found a significant negative correlation between HRS-D ratings and left prefrontal cortex metabolism; in other words, the more severe the depression, the lower the left frontal cortex metabolism. Baxter et al. [68] also found that left frontal hypermetabolism normalized in responders after drug therapy.

Bench and colleagues [69] used oxygen-15 (^{15}O) PET to study 33 patients with primary depression and 23 age-matched controls. The results showed that the depressed group had reduced blood flow in the left anterior cingulate and the left anterolateral prefrontal cortex (ALPFC). In a subgroup analysis of this study, it was discovered that depressed subjects with cognitive impairments had decreased activity in the left anteromedial frontal cortex and increased activity in the cerebellar vermis when compared with non–cognitively impaired subjects. These results suggest that depressed subjects with cognitive impairments show additional deficits in the more medial areas of the frontal lobes. This same group has now expanded their work with 40 depressed patients to determine whether depression subtype (psychomotorically slow, anxious, or cognitively impaired) affects brain regions and which of those regions are most impacted. Their results indicate the following: (a) psychomotor slowing is highly correlated with decreased flow in the left ALPFC, (b) cognitive impairment involved decreased activity in the left medial prefrontal region, and (c) anxiety in depression is associated with increased activity in the right posterior cingulate and bilateral inferior parietal regions.

Ketter and colleagues' study [70] revealed that depressed subjects compared to healthy controls had significantly lower resting blood flow in the ALPFC (particularly left ALPFC), left mesial temporal lobe, right anterior cingulate gyrus, and bilateral supramarginal gyrus.

One of the few studies in this field with discordant results was conducted by Drevets and colleagues [71]. Although they did find abnormalities in the left ALPFC, their research using ^{15}O PET to study 23 patients with familial pure depressive disorder (FPDD) compared to 33 controls revealed *increased* blood flow to the left ALPFC. The authors speculate that the increased left frontal activity may be due to the particular subgroup utilized or the fact that subjects were actively ruminating about sad thoughts during the scan. They also discovered that worsening depression correlated with a drop in left frontal activity, similar to findings of other studies.

2. *Treatment Studies*

  a. *Antidepressant Medications* There have been two antidepressant studies utilizing SPECT for patients with depressive disorders. Goodwin et al. [66] reported an increase in rCBF to bilateral anterior cingulate and putamen, as well as an increase in the right posterior cingulate and thalamus in 16 remitted depressed patients following treatment. Reischies et al. [84] studied 20 patients in the symptomatic and remitted states with ^{133}Xe-SPECT, but found only a left central flow decrease at the end of treatment. It is important to point out that their pretreatment had shown increased rCBF in the right frontal cortex.

Several functional brain-imaging studies have examined how successful antidepressant treatments influence rCBF or metabolism. Although there are undoubtedly some nonspecific treatment effects reflected in functional images of the brain, this technology offers an opportunity to correlate treatment effects with clinical improvement. In examining the effects of antidepressant medications on rCBF and metabolism, the literature reveals widely divergent findings. Inconsistencies may result from several factors: use of off-on study paradigms (patients are scanned at baseline; again on medication), as well as on-on and off-off; small sample sizes; heterogeneous medication regimens, including the use of different classes of medications; and variations in the time points selected for brain scans both within and between studies.

Given the variability in research design and small sample sizes, it is not surprising that consistent results are elusive. The most common point of agreement, which still remains tentative, is that successful pharmacological treatment of depression may be associated with increased blood flow or metabolism in the basal ganglia, prefrontal cortex, and/or cingulate cortex [72].

    b. Electroconvulsive Therapy There is more information regarding the effects of electroconvulsive therapy (ECT) on rCBF and metabolism than any other psychiatric treatment because ECT's effects on rCBF have contributed to the development of a model of epilepsy. Nobler et al. [73], using a planar view ^{133}Xe inhalation technique, found that global flow decreased 50–60 minutes following treatment compared to 30 minutes before treatment. In addition to the global effects, they demonstrated that patients receiving right unilateral ECT showed no acute change in flow in the left hemisphere; all of the blood flow effects (marked reductions) pertained to the right hemisphere. However, with bilateral ECT, the reductions were symmetrical.

    A second area of interest was Nobler et al.'s observation that the degree of rCBF reduction predicted the patient's ultimate response to ECT. Nonresponders showed essentially no changes in rCBF in this network acutely following ECT. In contrast, patients who eventually responded to ECT showed a significant acute change in rCBF in this network, actually exaggerating the hypoperfusion already evident in frontal regions. This finding is significant because these patients entered ECT showing profound regional deficits in rCBF, particularly in the prefrontal cortex, as well as a global flow deficit about 15% below that of healthy controls. Yet successful ECT treatment, at least acutely, appeared to exaggerate these abnormalities in conjunction with clinical recovery.

    In order to better understand these results, Nobler et al. carried out parallel studies using antidepressant medications, as opposed to ECT, as the treatment modality [74]. During the study, the subjects received either nortriptyline or sertraline in a double-blind manner. Subjects were scanned at baseline and again after 4–6 weeks of treatment. Following treatment, global flow *increased* significantly across the sample as a whole, as opposed to decreasing with ECT. However, further analysis revealed that the increased flow for the group was produced by those patients who ultimately did not get well; responders showed essentially no change in global flow. In fact, responders showed increased hypofrontality similar to that observed in the ECT study. Thus, as with ECT, antidepressants may be further affecting regions that were abnormal at baseline—not as may be expected in the direction of normalization, but toward accentuated abnormality.

    c. Sleep Deprivation Studies of other treatments for depression have produced mixed results, often confounded by small sample sizes. Four studies have used PET or SPECT to examine the regional brain changes that occur following sleep deprivation in depressed patients [75–78]. In general, those depressed subjects who responded positively (i.e., showed clinical improvement) to sleep deprivation showed higher baseline levels of rCBF or metabolism in limbic structures, particularly the right anterior cingulate gyrus and also bilateral fronto-orbital cortex [76], compared to controls; after sleep deprivation, responders showed normalized activity in these limbic structures. The same researchers have also noted a significant decrease of relative basal ganglia D_2 receptor occupancy among responders to total sleep deprivation compared to nonresponders [77]. It is intriguing that normal controls showed no consistent effects of sleep deprivation, in spite of the fact that a number of behavioral and psychological effects have been attributed to sleep deprivation in normal subjects.

    d. Light Therapy Some preliminary work has been done with imaging studies and light therapy for SAD. Cohen et al. [79] examined six patients with SAD using PET. Global metabolism in these patients was reduced both before and after successful light treatment. Regional function prior to treatment revealed a mixture of hypometabolic and hypermetabolic areas in the frontal cortex, which largely disappeared with treatment. Another preliminary study using the planar ^{133}Xe CBF method in four patients with SAD found no acute effect of light therapy (following 2 hours of 1500 lux artificial light) [80].

3. Challenge/Probe Studies

In order to develop a complete picture of the neuroanatomy of depression, researchers have begun to study subjects performing specific tasks or experiencing emotions that are in some way related to clinical depression. To date, these studies have been predominantly conducted with PET. Results from these studies are still preliminary, but generally consistent. Depressed mood disorder patients display decreased regional brain activation in tasks that involve a large limbic or paralimbic component. In contrast, there are no large differences between mood disorder patients and healthy controls in tasks that largely involve cortical activity.

    Several studies [81,82] have utilized intravenous procaine, a pharmacological limbic probe, to assess mood disordered patients' limbic response: these studies have found that mood disordered patients do not activate key regions to the same degree as controls. In studies involving selective attention, such as the Stroop Interference Task [32,83,85], mood disorder subjects fail to activate the cingulate and instead activate the DLPFC. In other words, they fail to activate a limbic area and instead activate a more cortical area during performance of the task. Thus, in depressed patients with mood disorders, there is blunted paralimbic activation during a task with a compensatory cortical activation.

Another example of limbic blunting emerges from activation studies involving recognition of aspects of human faces—facial emotion or identity. Depressed patients have a selective deficit in matching faces for their emotional content, a task that normally activates limbic and paralimbic regions including the anterior temporal lobes and prefrontal cortex [86,87]. In fact, depressed patients perform similarly to patients who have sustained damage to their right hemisphere. A PET scan revealed that depressed subjects failed to activate the right insula during this task when compared to controls [88]. A SPECT study using a similar mood induction paradigm [89] found left frontal rCBF to be higher during sad and lower during happy mood induction (relative to right frontal rCBF).

In general, activation studies of mood disorder patients performing tasks mediated through the cortex have found little difference from control groups. Berman et al. [90] found that mood disorder subjects activated the left DLPFC to the same degree as controls, while patients with schizophrenia had blunted activation. This finding is especially interesting, since many depressed patients have decreased DLPFC activity at rest and it appears that they can activate this area normally when performing a task that specifically brings this area on line. In another task involving cortical areas, there was no difference detected in rCBF activation between depressed patients and controls during a spatial matching task [91].

B. Primary Mania

There are very few functional imaging studies of manic patients, primarily because of the difficulties involved in obtaining the necessary levels of cooperation required for scans from acutely manic patients. In addition, acutely manic patients are generally involved in a treatment program including acute pharmacotherapy, making medication-free studies impractical. The few studies of rCBF and metabolism that have been conducted with manic patients have had variable and often conflicting results.

A study conducted at UCLA noted that global cerebral metabolism in medication-free hypomanic or euthymic bipolars did not differ from normal controls, but was increased compared to bipolars in depressed or mixed states [92]. Kishimota and colleagues [93] noted significant increases in ^{11}C-glucose uptake in three medication-free manic patients compared to controls, in contrast to widespread decreases in nine unipolar depressed patients. O'Connell and colleagues [94] reported that 11 manic patients had increased temporal lobe rCBF compared to controls and similar to patients with schizophrenia and atypical psychosis. Additionally, they noted decreased normalized frontal and basal ganglia rCBF in both manic and schizophrenic patients compared to controls. Across mixed subjects (schizophrenia, mania, and controls), mania ratings had positive correlations with caudate and right temporal CBF.

There have been few studies of manic patients using more biochemically specific imaging methods. O'Connell's study [94] reported increased caudate D_2 receptors in psychotic, but not nonpsychotic, bipolar patients.

C. Secondary Mood Disorders

Depression is common in a number of neurological diseases, and is often indistinguishable from mood symptoms characteristic of primary affective illness. The association of depression with diseases involving the basal ganglia (e.g., Parkinson's disease, Huntington's disease, and strokes involving the basal ganglia) is particularly strong—depression occurs with a mean frequency of about 40% in these patient groups. Brain-imaging studies of patients with depression secondary to these and other neurological and medical disorders have consistently found frontal and anterior hypoactivity compared to either healthy controls or controls matched for the primary illness. Additionally, the degree of anterior hypoactivity has often correlated with the severity of rated depression. These findings are consistent with the majority of studies of primary depression, leading to the tentative conclusion that prefrontal hypoactivity may represent one common pathway/neural substrate of the depressive syndrome independent of illness etiology.

Mayberg's studies in this area include a series of consecutive experiments utilizing ^{18}F PET scans of patients with Parkinson's disease, Huntington's disease, and chronic stroke lesions of the basal ganglia [95–98]. Depressed and nondepressed patients in each group were matched for age, illness duration, disease stage, and neurological disability. When the three groups were compared, it was apparent that the pattern of cortical metabolism failed to discriminate patients by disease group. In contrast, however, paralimbic frontal and temporal cortex hypometabolism did differentiate the depressed from the nondepressed patients, independent of disease etiology.

Additional work in this area has been conducted by Bromfield and colleagues [99], who scanned 23 patients with complex partial seizures, 6 of whom were depressed. Compared to five nondepressed epilepsy patients with similar seizure foci, depressed epilepsy subjects displayed bilaterally decreased inferior frontal cortical metabolism. Similar findings of decreased left prefrontal function have also been found in depressed subjects with bulimia nervosa [100] and human immunodeficiency virus (HIV) dementia [101].

There are very few functional imaging studies in secondary mania. Starkstein and colleagues [102] reported right temporal lobe hypometabolism in three patients with mania secondary to stroke. Again, these findings are consistent with other clinical and structural imaging data, indicating that left-sided lesions may be associated with secondary depression and right-sided lesions with secondary mania.

D. Receptor Imaging Studies in Mood Disorders

Mayberg et al. [103] found that patients after right-sided but not left-sided strokes had greater ipsilateral than contralateral asymmetry in serotonin ($5HT_2$) receptors in undamaged temporal and parietal regions. Additionally, in subjects with left-sided strokes, the ipsilateral/contralateral temporal lobe $5HT_2$ receptor ratio correlated inversely with depression scores, suggesting that a failure to upregulate ipsilateral $5HT_2$ receptors after left-sided strokes could be related to the development of secondary depression.

D'haenen et al. [104], utilizing $2\text{-}^{123}I$-ketanserin as a $5HT_2$ receptor ligand with SPECT, reported a higher uptake of the tracer in the parietal cortex of patients with depression. They also noted asymmetry (right greater than left) in the infero-frontal region in depressed subjects and not in that of control subjects, indicating a $5HT_2$ receptor change in major depression. Finally, D'haenen and Bossuyt [105], utilizing ^{123}I-iodobenzanide, a D_2 receptor ligand with SPECT, found an increase in D_2 receptor in depression.

In summary, despite the lack of receptor imaging studies in the area of secondary mood disorders, the existing data is consistent with other clinical and structural imaging evidence that left-sided lesions appear to be associated with secondary depression, while right-sided lesions may be associated with secondary mania.

V. CONCLUSIONS

In spite of some descrepancies, consistent findings are emerging from the functional brain-imaging literature outlined above. There is evolving a strong indication of reduced global cerebral blood flow or metabolism, particularly in the unipolar population, and possibly reduced basal ganglia flow/metabolism in both bipolar and unipolar populations. Most recent work (except the work of Drevets et al. [71]) has reported reduced dorso-lateral frontal rCBF or regional cerebral glucose metabolism (rCGM) in major depressive disorder, usually worse on the left. Also, interestingly, there has been reported a correlation between the degree of prefrontal hypoperfusion and symptom severity. Thus, there is an overall impression of reduced global metabolism, possible basal ganglia involvement, some distinction among subjects along the bipolar/unipolar dichotomy, reduced left frontal function, and a relationship between alterations in "resting" flow or metabolism and symptomatology. Additionally, treatment studies have also showed correlation with symptomatic improvement, except in the studies utilizing ECT as a treatment modality.

A. Neuroanatomical Model of Mood Disorders

Based on the findings from brain-imaging studies as well as other neuroscience approaches, various investigators have attempted to describe a neuroanatomic model for mood disorders. A comprehensive neuroanatomical model of mood disorders must integrate information from multiple levels of the neurobehavioral spectrum. At the neurochemical level there is evidence of alterations in the integrative function of the monoamine neurotransmitters, dopamine, norepinephrine, and serotonin. At the level of gene transcription, there are clear vulnerabilities, particularly in the bipolar forms of mood disorders, as well as the impact of stress and environmental factors on gene expression. Disorders of mood regulation, while based in the brain, have effects throughout the body; similarly, medical conditions such as endocrinopathies involving thyroid or cortisol can cause depression with associated regional brain dysfunction. Secondary mood disorders resulting from structural insults to the brain also provide clues to the function of various parts of the brain in generating mood disorders.

In attempting to integrate these discrete pieces of information, two areas of the brain must serve as the focus: the limbic system and the prefrontal cortex. The limbic system, generally defined to include the amygdala and hippocampus, septum, cingulate and anterior thalamus, functions as a critical generator and modulator of normal and pathological degrees of emotion. It appears that right limbic activity is associated with negative emotions such as anger, anxiety, and sadness, while left limbic activity is predominantly linked to positive emotions such as happiness and euphoria.

The prefrontal cortex is presumed to serve a modulating and governing role over more primitive limbic activity with corresponding areas of emotional dominance. For example, in healthy subjects, during periods of transient sadness, there would be increased activity in the anterior limbic system and the prefrontal cortex, with left frontal activity representing a brake on left limbic activity, permitting the emotion of sadness. Depressive disorders would occur if the governing role of the prefrontal cortex was lost due to stroke, tumor, or prolonged and unresolved grief reaction resulting in regulatory dysfunction. Depressive disorders might also result if the limbic affective drive were intrinsically stronger than the ipsilateral governing prefrontal cortex; depression could occur after a period of prolonged limbic hyperactivity leading to compensatory blunting in some limbic circuits. The exact nature of inhibition/release of inhibition from one hemisphere to the other accounting for these changes has just begun to be elucidated. In mania, for example, there might be a relative loss of right cortical oversight, leaving right-sided limbic activity unchecked.

It appears that the prefrontal lobes permit complex, flexible, and environmentally contingent cognitions, while limbic cognitions may be more primitive, preprogrammed, and autonomous. If negative biases toward the self or the world were laid down in primitive limbic memories on the basis of childhood experience, they may come to predominate with a decrease or breakdown in prefrontal activity, resulting in clinical depression with prominent "automatic" thoughts. Cognitive and interpersonal therapy may be a way of rehabilitating or temporarily substituting for normal prefrontal governance of limbic tone, allowing more refined rational responses to modulate primitive automatic thoughts. The extent of the prefrontal dysfunction also appears to be correlated with the severity of the symptomatic expression and may be related to the state marker of the disorder, whereas some of the subcortical changes may be related to trait markers of the disorder.

B. Future Directions

There is clearly much work to be done before a true neuroanatomy of mood disorders can be established. Several key areas must be addressed in order to provide the information and understanding essential to the development of such a model:

1. Perform more large-scale studies of depressed patients to assess the frequency and severity of prefrontal changes for various types of mood disorders.
2. Perform serial scans throughout an individual's lifetime to determine which brain changes are part of the state of depression and which may represent vulnerability factors.
3. Integrate regional brain activity data with knowledge of underlying pharmacological mechanisms.
4. Expand the role of imaging technology in treatment, including the analysis of differential treatment responses.
5. Perform brain activation studies with different pharmacological or cognitive probes in order to utilize subjects as their own controls and also improve our ability to identify neural networks in a challenge environment.

Acknowledgments

This review was supported in part by a grant from NARSAD, The National Alliance for Research in Schizophrenia and Depression (Dr. Trivedi), and

NIMH grants MH-41115 (Dr. Rush) and MH-52870 (Dr. Trivedi). Acknowledgments go to Dr. A. John Rush, Betty Jo Hay Distinguished Chair in Mental Health, Dr. Kenneth Z. Altshuler, Stanton Sharp Distinguished Chair, Professor and Chairman, Department of Psychiatry, and Dr. Devous, Nuclear Medicine Center, for administrative support.

REFERENCES

1. J. H. Jackson, On temporary mental disorders after epileptic paroxysms. *W. Riding Lu. Asylum Med. Rep. 5*:103 (1874).
2. H. A. Sackeim, E. Putz, W. Vingiano, et al., Lateralization in the processing of emotionally laden information. I. Normal functioning, *Neuropsychiatr. Neuropsychol. Behav. Neurol. 1*:97 (1988).
3. H. A. Sackeim, I. Prohovnik J. R. Moeller, et al., Regional cerebral blood flow in mood disorders. I Comparison of major depressives and normal controls at rest, *Arch. Gen. Psychiatry 47*:60 (1990).
4. H. A. Sackeim and I. Prohovnik, Brain imaging studies of depressive disorders, *The Biology of Depressive Disorders. Part A: A Systems Perspective* (J. J. Mann and D. J. Kupfer, eds.), Plenum, New York, 1993, p. 205.
5. J. M. Schwartz, L. R. Baxter, J. C. Mazziota, et al., The differential diagnosis of depression. Relevance of positron emission tomography studies of cerebral glucose metabolism to the bipolar-unipolar dichotomy, *JAMA 258*:1368 (1987).
6. L. R. Baxter Jr., J. M. Schwartz, M. E. Phelps, et al., Reduction of prefrontal cortex glucose metabolism common to three types of depression, *Arch. Gen. Psychiatry 46*:243 (1989).
7. L. R. Baxter, M. E. Phelps, J. C. Mazziotta, et al., Cerebral metabolic rates for glucose in mood disorders: Studies with PET and FDG, *Arch. Gen. Psychiatry 42*:441 (1985).
8. J. W. Papez, A proposed mechanism of emotion, *Arch. Neural Psychiatry 38*: 725 (1937).
9. P. D. MacLean, *The Triune Brain in Evolution: Role in Paleocerebral Functions*, Plenum Press, New York, 1990.
10. W. J. H. Nauta, The problem of the frontal lobe: a reinterpretation, *J. Psychiat. Res. 8*:167 (1971).
11. K. E. Livingston, Limbic system dysfunction induced by "kindling": its significance for psychiatry, *Neurosurgical Treatment in Psychiatry, Pain and Epilepsy*, (W. H. Sweet, S. Obrador, and J. G. Martin-Rodriguez, eds.), University Park Press, Baltimore, 1977, p. 63.
12. J. R. Stevens, V. H. Mark, F. Ervin, et al., Deep temporal stimulation in man, *Arch. Neurol. 21*:157, (1969).
13. E. Halgren, R. D. Walter, D. G. Cherlow, et al., Mental phenomena evoked by electrical stimulation of the human hippocampal formation and amygdala, *Brain 101*:83 (1978).
14. R. G. Heath, Pleasure response of human subjects to direct stimulation of the

brain: physiologic and psychodynamic considerations, *The Role of Pleasure in Behavior* (R. G. Heath, ed.), Hoeber, New York, 1964, p. 219.

15. M. S. George, R. M. Post, T. A. Ketter, et al., Neural mechanisms of mood disorders, *Current Review of Mood Disorders, Vol. 2: Neurobiology of Mood and Anxiety Disorders* (A. John Rush, ed.), Current Medicine Philadelphia (in press).

16. D. R. Weinberger, K. F. Berman, and R. F. Zec, Physiologic dysfunction of dorsolateral prefrontal cortex in schizophrenia. I. Regional cerebral blood flow evidence, *Arch. Gen. Psychiatry 43*:114 (1986).

17. D. R. Weinberger, R. F. Berman, and B. P. Illowsky, Physiological dysfunction of dorsolateral prefrontal cortex in schizophrenia. III. A new cohort and evidence for a monoaminergic mechanism, *Arch. Gen. Psychiatry 45*:609 (1988).

18. T. A. Ketter, M. S. George, H. A. Ring, et al., Primary mood disorders: structural and resting functional studies, *Psychiatr. Ann. 24*:637 (1994).

19. D. T. Stuss and D. F. Benson, *The Frontal Lobes*, Raven Press, New York, 1986.

20. T. Mclardy and A. Meyer, Anatomical correlates of improvement after leucotomy, *J. Men. Sci. 95*:182 (1949).

21. F. Reitman, Orbital cortex syndrome following leucotomy, *Am. J. Psychiatry 103*:238 (1946).

22. R. D. Adams and M. Victor, *Principles of Neurology*, 3rd ed., McGraw-Hill, New York, 1985.

23. C. H. Kellner, D. R. Rubinow, and R. M. Post, Cerebral ventricular size and cognitive impairment in depression, *J. Affect. Disor. 10*:215 (1986).

24. L. L. Altshuler, A. Conrad, P. Hauser, et al., Reduction of temporal lobe volume in bipolar disorder: a preliminary report of magnetic resonance imaging [letter to the editor], *Arch. Gen. Psychiatry 48*:482 (1991).

25. C. E. Coffey, W. E. Wilkinson, R. D. Weiner, et al., Quantitative cerebral anatomy in depression: a controlled magnetic resonance imaging study, *Arch. Gen. Psychiatry 50*:7 (1993).

26. R. A. Rangel-Guerra, H. Perez-Payan, L. Minkoff, et al., Nuclear magnetic resonance in bipolar affective disorders, *AJNR 4*:229 (1983).

27. P. J. Dolan, A. M. Poynton, P. K. Bridges, et al., Altered magnetic resonance white-matter TI values in patients with affective disorders, *Br. J. Psychiatry 157*:107 (1990).

28. B. M. Slotnick, Disturbances of maternal behavior in the rat following lesions of the cingulate cortex, *Behaviour 29*:204 (1967).

29. F. C. Beyer, L. Agnuiano, and J. Mena, Oxytocin release in response to stimulation of cingulate gyrus, *Am. J. Physiol. 200*:625 (1961).

30. J. V. Pardo, P. J. Pardo, K. W. Janer, et al., The anterior cingulate cortex mediates processing selection in the Stroop attentional conflict paradigm, *Proc. Natl. Acad. Sci. USA 87*:256 (1990).

31. T. Paus, M. Petrides, A. C. Evans, et al., Role of the human anterior cingulate cortex in the control of oculomotor, manual and speech responses: A positron emission tomography study, *J. Neurophysiol. 70*:453 (1993).

32. C. J. Bench, C. D. Frith, P. M. Grasby, et al., Investigations of the functional anatomy of attention using the Stroop test, *Neuropsychologia 31*:907 (1993).

33. J. C. Wu, J. C. Gillin, M. S. Buchsbaum, et al., Effects of sleep deprivation on brain metabolism of depressed patients, *Am. J. Psychiatry 149*:538 (1992).

34. D. Ebert, H. Feistel, and A. Barocka, Effects of sleep deprivation on the limbic system and the frontal lobes in affective disorders: a study with Tc-99m-HMPAO SPECT *Psychiatry Res. 40*:247 (1991).

35. E. Rubin, H. A. Sackeim, I. Prohovnik I, et al., Regional cerebral blood flow in mood disorders: IV. Comparison of mania and depression, *Psychiatry Res. 61*:1 (1995).

36. J. P. Aggleton, ed., *The Amygdala*, Wiley-Liss, New York, 1992.

37. D. G. Amaral, J. L. Price, A. Pitkanen, et al., Anatomical organization of the primate amygdaloid complex, *The Amygdala: Neurobiological Aspects of Emotion, Memory and Mental Dysfunction* (J. P. Aggleton, ed.), Wiley-Liss, New York, 1992, p. 1.

38. H. Kluver, and P. C. Bucy, Preliminary analysis of functions of the temporal lobes in monkeys, *Arch. Neurol. 42*:979 (1939).

39. E. T. Rolls, A theory of emotion and consciousness, and its application to understanding the neural basis of emotion, *The Cognitive Neurosciences* (M. S. Gazzaniga, ed.), MIT Press, Cambridge, MA, 1995, p. 1091.

40. J. W. Papez, A proposed mechanism of emotion, *Arch. Neurol. Psychiatry 38*:725 (1937).

41. P. MacLean, Some psychiatric implications of physiological studies on fronto-temporal portion of limbic system (visceral brain), *Electroencephalogr. Clin. Neurophysiol. 4*:407 (1952).

42. R. M. Post, Does limbic system dysfunction play a role in affective illness? *The Limbic System: Functional Organization and Clinical Disorders* (B. K. Doane and K. E. Livingston, eds.), Raven Press, New York, 1986, p. 229.

43. M. S. George, T. A. Ketter, P. I. Parekh, et al., Brain activity during transient sadness and happiness in healthy women, *Am. J. Psychiatry 152*:341 (1995).

44. T. A. Kimbrell, M. S. George, P. I. Parekh, et al., Regional brain activity during self-induced anger and anxiety, *Biol. Psychiatry 37*(9):617 (1995).

45. M. S. George, T. A. Ketter, D. S. Gill, et al., Brain regions involved in recognizing facial emotion or identity: an oxygen-15 PET study, *J. Neuropsychiatry Clin. Neurosci. 5*:384 (1993).

46. M. S. George, P. I. Parekh, N. Rosinsky, et al., Understanding emotional prosody activates right hemisphere regions, *Arch. Neurol.* (in press).

47. R. J. Mathew, J. S. Meyer, D. J. Francis, K. M. Semchuk, K. Mortel, and J. L. Claghorn, Cerebral blood flow in depression, *Am. J. Psychiatry 137*:1449 (1980).

48. A. J. Rush, M. A. Schlesser, E. Stokely, F. R. Bonte, and K. Z. Altshuler, Cerebral blood flow in depression and mania, *Psychopharmacol. Bull. 18*(3):6 (1982).

49. P. Uytdenhoef, P. Portelange, J. Jacquy, G. Charles, P. Linkowski, and J. Mendlewicz, Regional cerebral blood flow and lateralized hemispheric dysfunction in depression, *Br. J. Psychiatry 143*:128 (1983).

50. R. E. Gur, B. E. Skolnick, R. C. Gur, S. Caroff, W. Rieger, W. D. Obrist, D. Younkin, and M. Reivich, Brain function in psychiatric disorders: II. Regional cerebral blood flow in medicated unipolar depressives, *Arch. Gen. Psychiatry* *41*:695 (1984).

51. M. D. Devous, A. J. Rush, M. A. Schlesser, et al., Single-photon tomographic determination of regional cerebral blood flow in psychiatric disorders, *J. Nucl. Med. 25*:P57 (1984).

52. S. Schlegel, J. B. Aldenhoff, D. Eissner, P. Lindner, and O. Nickel, Regional cerebral blood flow in depression: associations with psychopathology, *J. Affec. Disord. 17*:211 (1989).

53. P. Silfverskiold and J. Risberg, Regional cerebral blood flow in depression and mania, *Arch. Gen. Psychiatry 46*:253 (1989).

54. F. M. Reischies, J. P. Hedde, and R. Drochner, Clinical correlates of cerebral blood flow in depression, *Psychiatry Res. 29*:323 (1989).

55. R. A. O'Connell, R. L. VanHeerthum, S. B. Billick, A. R. Holt, A. Gonzalez, H. Notardonato, D. Luck, and L. N. King, Single photon emission computed tomography (SPECT) with [^{123}I] IMP in the differential diagnosis of psychiatric disorders, *J. Neuropsychiatry 1*(2):145 (1989).

56. H. A. Sackeim, I. Prohovnik, J. R. Moeller, R. Mayeux, Y. Stern, and D. P. Devanand, Regional cerebral blood flow in mood disorders II. Comparison of major depression and Alzheimer's disease, *J. Nucl. Med. 34*(7):1090 (1993).

57. V. Delvenne, F. Delecluse, P. Hubain, A. Schoutens, V. DeMaertelaer, and J. Mendlewicz, Regional cerebral blood flow in patients with affective disorders, *Br. J. Psychiatry 157*:359 (1990).

58. S. M. Curran, C. M. Murray, M. VanBeck, N. Dougall, R. E. O'Carroll, M.-P. Austin, K. P. Ebmeier, and G. M. Goodwin, A single photon emission computerized tomography study of regional brain function in elderly patients with major depression and with Alzheimer-type dementia, *Br. J. Psychiatry 163*:155 (1993).

59. D. G. M. Murphy, D. M. Murphy, M. Abbas, E. Palazidou, C. Binnie, J. Arendt, D. Campos Costa, and S. A. Checkley, Seasonal affective disorder: response to light as measured by electroencephalogram, melatonin suppression, and cerebral blood flow, *Br. J. Psychiatry 163*:327 (1993).

60. M.-P. Austin, N. Dougall, M. Ross, C. Murray, R. E. O'Carroll, A. Moffott, K. P. Ebmeier, and G. M. Goodwin, Single photon emission tomography with ^{99m}Tc-exametazime in major depression and the pattern of brain activity underlying the psychotic/neurotic continuum, *J. Affect. Disord. 26*:31 (1992).

61. M. P. Philpot, S. Banerjee, H. Meedham-Bennett, D. C. Costa, and P. J. Ell, ^{99m}Tc-HMPAO single photon emission tomography in late life depression: a pilot study of regional cerebral blood flow at rest and during a verbal fluency task, *J. Affect. Disord. 28*:233 (1993).

62. K. M. Yazici, O. Kapucu, B. Erbas, E. Varoglu, C. Gulec, and C. F. Bekdik, Assessment of changes in regional cerebral blood flow in patients with major depression using the ^{99m}Tc-HMPAO single photon emission tomography method, *Eur. J. Nucl. Med. 19*:1038 (1992).

63. P. Thomas, G. Vaiva, E. Samaille, M. Maron, C. Alaix, M. Steinling, and M. Goudemand, Cerebral blood flow in major depression and dysthymia, *J. Affect. Disord. 29*:235 (1993).
64. I. M. Lesser, I. Mena, K. B. Boone, B. L. Miller, C. M. Mehringer, and M. Wohl, Reduction of cerebral blood flow in older depressed patients, *Arch. Gen. Psychiatry 51*:677 (1994).
65. J. D. Amsterdam and P. D. Mozley, Temporal lobe asymmetry with iofetamine (Imp) SPECT imaging in patients with minor depression, *J. Affect. Disord. 24*:43 (1992).
66. G. M. Goodwin, M. P. Austin, N. Dougall, et al., State changes in brain activity shown by the uptake of ^{99m}Tc-exametazime with single photon emission tomography in major depression before and after treatment, *J. Affect. Disor. 29*:243 (1993).
67. N. S. Mayberg, P. J. Lewis, W. Regenold, and H. N. Wagner, Paralimbic Hypoperfusion in Mayberg Unipolar Depression. *J. Nucl. Med. 35*:929 (1994).
68. L. R. Baxter, J. M. Schwartz, M. E. Phelps, et al., Reduction of prefrontal glucose metabolism common to three types of depression, *Arch. Gen. Psychiatry 46*:243 (1989).
69. C. J. Bench, K. J. Friston, R. G. Brown, et al., Regional cerebral blood flow in depression measured by positron emission tomography: the relationship with clinical dimensions, *Psychol. Med. 23*:579 (1993).
70. T. A. Ketter, P. J. Andreason, M. S. George, et al., Reduced resting frontal lobe CBF in mood disorders (abstr), American Psychiatric Association Annual Meeting, New Research Program (NR297), 1993, p. 134.
71. W. C. Drevets, T. O. Videen, S. H. Preskorn, et al., A functional anatomic study of unipolar depression, *J. Neurosci. 12*:3628 (1992).
72. E. Rubin, H. Sackeim, M. S. Nobler, et al., Brain imaging studies of antidepressant treatments, *Psychiatr. Ann. 24*:653 (1994).
73. M. S. Nobler, H. A. Sackeim, I. Prohovnik, et al., Regional cerebral blood flow in mood disorders, III: treatment and clinical response. *Arch. Gen. Psychiatry 51*:884 (1994).
74. M. S. Nobler, H. A. Sackeim, I. Prohovnik, et al., Effects of antidepressant medication on rCBF in late-life depression (abstr), *Biol. Psychiatry 35*:712 (1994).
75. J. C. Wu, J. C. Gillin, M. S. Buchsbaum, et al., Effect of sleep deprivation on brain metabolism of depressed patients, *Am. J. Psychiatry 149*:538 (1992).
76. D. Ebert, H. Feistel, and A. Barocka, Effects of sleep deprivation on the limbic system and the frontal lobes in affective disorders: a study with Tc-99m-HMPAO SPECT, *Psychiatry Res. 40*:247 (1991).
77. D. Ebert, H. Feistel, A. Barocka, et al., Increased limbic flow and total sleep deprivation in major depression with melancholia, *Psychiatry Res. 55*:101 (1994).
78. S. Dube, M. A. Mintum, T. G. Nichols, et al., Brain glucose uptake changes with total sleep deprivation (SD): relationship to sleep and temperature (abstr), *Biol. Psychiatry 35*:663 (1994).

79. R. M. Cohen, M. Gross, T. E. Nordahl, et al., Preliminary data on the metabolic brain pattern of patients with winter seasonal affective disorder, *Arch. Gen. Psychiatry 49*:542 (1992).

80. D. G. Murphy, D. M. Murphy, M. Abbas, et al., Seasonal affective disorder: response to light as measured by electroencephalogram, melatonin suppression, and cerebral blood flow, *Br. J. Psychiatry 163*:327 (1993).

81. T. A. Ketter, M. S. George, H. A. Ring, et al., Primary mood disorders: structural and resting functional studies, *Psychiatr. Ann. 24*:637 (1994).

82. T. A. Ketter, P. J. Andreason, M. S. George, et al., Blunted CBF response to procain in mood disorders (abstr), American Psychiatric Association Annual Meeting, New Research Program (NR298), 1993, p. 134.

83. J. V. Pardo, J. P. Pardo, K. W. Janer, et al., The anterior cingulate cortex mediates processing selection in the Stroop attentional conflict paradigm, *Proc. Natl. Acad. Sci. USA 87*:256 (1990).

84. F. M. Reischies, J. P. Hedde, R. Drochner, Clinical correlates of cerebral blood flow in depression, *Psychiatry Res. 29*:323 (1989).

85. M. S. George, T. A. Ketter, P. I. Parekh, et al., Regional brain activity when selecting a response despite interference: an H2150 PET study of the Stroop and an emotional Stroop, *Human Brain Mapping 1*:194 (1994).

86. D. R. Rubinow and R. M. Post, Impaired recognition of affect in facial expression in depressed patients, *Biol. Psychiatry 31*:947 (1992).

87. M. S. George, T. Huggins, W. McDermut, et al., Abnormal facial emotion recognition in depression: serial testing in an ultra-rapid cycling patient, *Behav Modif.* (in press).

88. M. S. George, T. A. Ketter, D. S. Gill, et al., Blunted CBF with emotion recognition in depression, American Psychiatric Association Annual Meeting 1993, New Research #114–88, Abstract.

89. F. Schneider, R. C. Gur, J. L. Jaggie, and R. E. Gur, Differential effects of mood on cortical cerebral blood flow: a [133]xehon clearance study, *Psychiatry Res. 52*:215 (1993).

90. K. F. Berman, A. R. Doran, D. Pickar, et al., Is the mechanism of prefrontal hypofunction in depression the same as in schizophrenia? Regional cerebral blood flow during cognitive activation, *Br. J. Psychiatry 162*:183 (1993).

91. M. S. George, T. A. Ketter, P. I. Parekh, et al., Spatial ability in affective illness: differences in regional brain activation during a spatial matching task (H2150 PET), *Neuropsychiatry Neuropsychol. Behav. Neurol. 7*:143 (1994).

92. J. M. Schwartz, L. R. Baxter Jr., J. C. Mazziotta, et al., The differential diagnosis of depression. Relevance of positron emission tomography studies of cerebral glucose metabolism to the bipolar-unipolar dichotomy, *JAMA 258*: 1368 (1987).

93. H. Kishimoto, O. Takazu, S. Ohno, et al. 11C glucose metabolism in manic and depressed patients, *Psychiatry Res. 22*:81 (1987).

94. R. A. O'Connell, R. L. Van Heertum, D. Luck, et al., Single photon emission computed tomography of the brain in acute mania and schizophrenia, *J. Neuroimaging 5*:101 (1995).

95. H. S. Mayberg, S. E. Starkstein, B. Sadzot, et al., Selective hypometabolism

in the inferior frontal lobe in depressed patients with Parkinson's disease, *Ann. Neurol. 28*:57 (1990).

96. H. S. Mayberg, S. E. Starkstein, C. P. Peyser, et al., Paralimbic frontal lobe hypometabolism in depression associated with Huntington's disease, *Neurology 42*:1791 (1992).

97. H. S. Mayberg, S. E. Starkstein, P. L. Morris, et al., Remote cortical hypometabolism following focal basal ganglia injury: relationship to secondary changes in mood, *Neurology 41* (suppl):266 (1991).

98. H. S. Mayberg, Neuroimaging studies of depression in neurological disease, *Depression in Neurologic Diseases* (S. E. Starkstein and R. G. Robinson, eds.), Hopkins University Press, Baltimore, 1993, p. 186.

99. E. B. Bromfield, L. Altshuler, D. B. Leidermana DB, et al., Cerebral metabolism and depression in patients with complex partial seizures, *Arch. Neurol 49*:617 (1992).

100. P. J. Andreason, M. Altemus, A. J. Zamerkin, et al., Regional cerebral glucose metabolism in bulimia nervosa, *Am. J. Psychiatry 48*:1506 (1992).

101. P. F. Renshaw, K. A. Johnson, J. L. Worth, et al., New onset depression in patients with AIDS dementia complex (ADC) is associated with frontal lobe perfusion defects on HMPAO-SPECT scan (abstr), American College of Neuropsychopharmacology Annual Meeting, p. 94.

102. S. E. Starkstein, H. S. Mayberg, M. L. Berthier, et al. Mania after brain injury: Neuroradiological and metabolic findings, *Ann. Neurol. 27*:652 (1990).

103. H. S. Mayberg, R. G. Robinson, D. F. Wong, et al., PET Imaging of cortical S2-serotonin receptors after stroke: Lateralized changes and relationship to depression, *Am. J. Psychiatry 145*:937 (1988).

104. H. D'haenen, A. Bossuyt, J. Mertens, C. Bossuyt-Piron, M. Gijsemans, and L. Kaufman, SPECT imaging of serotonin$_2$ receptor in depression, *Psychiatry Res. Neuroimaging 45*:227 (1992).

105. H. A. D'haenen and A. Bossuyt, Dopamine D$_2$ receptors in depression measured with single photon emission computed tomography, *Biol. Psychiatry 35*: 128 (1994).

106. S. Passero, M. Nardini, N. Battistini, Regional cerebral blood flow changes following chronic administration of antidepressant drugs, *Prog. Neuro-Psychopharmacol Biol Psychiatry. 19*:627 (1995).

11

Neuroimaging in Anorexia Nervosa and Bulimia Nervosa

Kevin John Black and Kelly N. Botteron
Washington University School of Medicine,
St. Louis, Missouri

I. INTRODUCTION

Anorexia nervosa and bulimia nervosa remain several of the most important unsolved challenges of clinical medicine. Despite many advances, they are still relatively common, potentially lethal illnesses with only modestly successful current treatment. In large measure this may be attributed to a paucity of firm knowledge about the etiology and pathophysiology of eating disorders. Recent years have seen the development of new and powerful imaging tools for examining brain structure and function in vivo, and naturally there have been several attempts to apply them to these important clinical conundrums.

Despite some clinical similarities, anorexia and bulimia are increasingly being viewed as separate disorders. Anorexia nervosa has been described for centuries and is characterized by the core clinical feature of a fear of being fat and an incessant drive for thinness. Patients with anorexia are necessarily underweight and generally achieve this through restrictive eating habits. In some cases there is a progression that includes some purging and/or binging behavior. Bulimia nervosa is also characterized by a fear of being fat, but patients are generally of normal weight and have an irresistible urge to overeat. These binging episodes are followed by self-induced vomiting or other purging behaviors. In addition to a differentiation of the disorders by clinical features and longitudinal course, there appears to be differences in genetic loading, and recent twin studies have suggested relatively high heritability in anorexia, but much lower heritability in bulimia [1].

Although eating disorders have often been explained with a psychodynamic and family systems emphasis, increasing research evidence over the past decade highlights the importance of neurobiological factors. These neurobiological investigations have largely focused on neuroendocrine and neurochemical dysfunction [2] but have included a relatively small number of structural and functional neuroimaging studies. Although it is clear that malnutrition and starvation may initiate or exaggerate many of the differences reported, it is also established that the physiological response to starvation alters the normal regulation of eating behaviors, potentially perpetuating the disorder. Given clear genetic vulnerability to eating disorders, it is apparent that some neurobiological variables must predate and predispose individuals to anorexia and bulimia. Unlike many other psychiatric disorders the clear impact of the disordered behavior (eating) on neurobiological variables complicates research efforts and the interpretation of results. In this chapter, we critically review available imaging studies of eating disorders and discuss the potential for future studies in these populations. Additionally, we review certain methodological issues which are clearly evident and critical to investigations in this population, but which also pertain to imaging studies of other psychiatric illnesses.

II. SCIENTIFIC QUESTIONS OF INTEREST

Given the clinical importance of eating disorders and the number of important questions that remain unanswered, there is a clear need for new research techniques which may reveal insights into the cause or treatment of these illnesses. Modern imaging techniques would seem to be an obvious candidate. However, the existence of serious methodological concerns in this population (see next section) leads one to wonder whether useful imaging studies of eating disorders are even possible. Thus, before considering how to interpret or perform such studies, we should clearly understand the scientific questions of interest, and decide whether even flawless imaging studies can answer the questions. As the saying goes, "anything not worth doing well is not worth doing."

A. Etiology

Knowledge of the causes of anorexia nervosa or bulimia could be immensely valuable. However, epidemiological and genetic studies may be more obvious potential sources of knowledge about etiology. Imaging studies can unfortunately reflect either causes or consequences of the illness. In order for imaging studies to strongly suggest etiology, they would have to either (a) detect abnormalities prior to any clinical evidence of illness or (b) demonstrate pathology not attributable to effects of the illness itself. In either case, etiology could only be established if the observed pathology could be associated with a known cause or mechanism of injury (degenerative, infectious, vascular, etc.). In fact, demonstration of neuroimaging differences may not narrow the etiology to being primarily "biological," since psychosocial manipulations can cause significant changes in brain function and possibly structure.

Absent a high-risk group identifiable prior to onset of any clinical symptoms, the first type of study is nearly impossible. The second type of study is conceivable, but it can be difficult to demonstrate that changes in the brain are primary, not secondary to the eating disorder or its metabolic consequences.

B. Pathophysiology

The motivation for studies of pathophysiology is clear: even if specific etiologies are not discovered, much could be gained from knowing which brain regions and functions are involved in mediating specific symptoms and signs, such as the abnormal self-concept or the changes in eating behavior. Within-group comparisons of the currently affected to the remitted state might be expected to help answer these questions. However, complete remissions are less common than temporary normalization of weight and eating behavior.

Also, some brain changes secondary to starvation or its secondary effects may persist even after prolonged clinical remission. Another strategy to show which brain changes in patients can be attributed to secondary effects of the illness would be to study patients with exogenous starvation prior to and during starvation with follow-up exams at intervals after refeeding. However, such a study raises obvious practical and ethical difficulties. Furthermore, the effects of the illness on brain imaging may extend beyond those mediated by starvation and may include direct effects of cognition and conation on brain activity.

C. Other Potential Goals of Imaging Studies

Even if imaging studies are difficult to interpret vis-à-vis etiology and physiology, they may provide valuable exploratory observations which can refine hypotheses to be tested with other tools, such as animal models or pharmacological challenge models. Furthermore, the frequency in eating disordered patients of depressive symptoms, compulsive behavior, and distorted perceptions and cognitions suggests the possibility of studying these symptoms in this population. For instance, activity of a particular nucleus in the brain could be compared in patients with a given symptom and in those with the same eating disorder but without that symptom. Finally, although probably of little relevance to psychiatry, imaging studies in patients with eating disorders may be a valuable source of information about the cerebral consequences of starvation.

In summary, modern neuroimaging methods have tremendous potential to help define the causes and physiology of eating disorders. However, because of clear secondary effects of starvation on brain structure and function, deriving useful information regarding these questions from imaging studies requires exceptionally careful experimental design.

III. METHODOLOGICAL PROBLEMS IN THIS POPULATION

A. Structural Imaging Studies

1. Effects of Starvation on Structural Imaging

The effects of significant weight loss and starvation on the structure of the brain is a potentially major confounding variable in the investigation of the pathophysiology of eating disorders. It appears clear that starvation alone has major effects on overall brain size and CSF spaces, however, there is little work examining specific regional changes that may be pertinent to regional investigations of eating disordered subjects. There have been almost no MRI studies examining the effects of starvation in non–eating disordered populations. One MRI investigation examined children with kwashiorkor (protein-energy malnutrition) and reported that children with acute kwashiorkor demonstrate significant cerebral atrophy as evidenced by widened cortical sulci, enlarged ventricles, widened interhemispheric fissure, and cerebellar folia [3]. Gray and white matter were qualitatively thought to be equally affected. The atrophic changes appeared to resolve quickly over a 30- to 90-day period of refeeding. This study was not quantitative, and no specific regional differences were examined or reported. Given this limited knowledge base regarding the direct effects of starvation, it can be difficult to separate the effect of starvation from other potential pathophysiological mechanisms in eating disordered populations.

2. Differences in Overall Brain Size

Because overall cerebral volume and ventricular volume appear to be clearly altered in eating disordered subjects, any specific regional investigations need to correct for overall differences in brain size. Most of the studies reported have attempted to do this by examining ratio measures with specific structures examined as a relative proportion of overall brain size. Although this may be a reasonable approach for studies with small numbers, ratio estimates have potential disadvantages and can lead to spurious conclusions [4,5]. For example, similar ventricular size in a subject and a control would result in an increased ventricular-to-brain ratio (VBR) in the subject when the subject has decreased brain volume. However, the reported increased VBR may not reflect any expansion of ventricular volume. Multivariate statistical methods can address this issue more effectively by partialling out effects of overall differences in brain volume, however, larger subject populations are generally necessary.

3. Problems with Image Analysis Methods

Most studies of eating disordered subjects have relied on qualitative ratings of images or simple area measures. Both of these have numerous potential limitations for examining structural differences, because of their insensitivity as estimators of structural volumes and problems with interscan and interrater reliability. In addition, area measures are sensitive to differences in head positioning, slice thickness, partial volume effects, and other variables [6], as discussed in detail in earlier chapters. It is important to keep these limitations in mind when reviewing the available literature.

4. Choice of Controls

The choice of control subjects has emerged as an important issue in all neuroimaging research and is certainly pertinent to this population as well. The majority of reported studies have included suboptimal control populations, including (a) individuals scanned for clinical indications, such as headaches, seizures, or other neurological symptoms whose scans were interpreted as normal, or (b) individuals with other psychiatric disorders. Often the psychiatric status and demographic characteristics of the first population are unknown, and the second population is undesirable because of potential structural alterations associated with other psychiatric disorders.

B. Functional Imaging Studies

A number of methodological questions arise in patients with anorexia or bulimia. Although perhaps more obvious in eating disordered patients, these considerations are no less pertinent to imaging studies in other psychiatric illnesses. According to Brodie [7]:

> Many isolated but seemingly attractive findings have resulted in speculative musings, rather than the construction of a significant, testable hypothesis and validation with an independent sample. . . . Functional imaging with PET and SPECT is based on complex technology, which is easy to misuse. . . . [If] rigorous scientific (as well as statistical) standards are not met, then it is possible to easily mislead even the sophisticated reader. . . . It would be extremely difficult for the most intelligent but unspecialized reader to recognize the scientific issues that could compromise the conclusions drawn by the authors.

1. Effects on Functional Imaging of Pseudoatrophy

As discussed below, symptomatic patients with eating disorders have on average less brain tissue than normals, and this abnormality can persist even after normalization of weight. This so-called pseudoatrophy leads to two significant difficulties in interpreting functional imaging studies, since volumetric abnormalities can cause either partial volume errors or localization errors.

First, pseudoatrophy can be expected to cause partial volume errors. This is because functional imaging methods generally compute a value such as regional cerebral blood flow (rCBF) over a given region of space, without complete knowledge of the anatomical contents of that region. If a given region in one subject or condition contains 20% less brain than an identically sized region in another subject, one might expect the computed rCBF to be 20% less even if the average true blood flow per gram of brain tissue remains perfectly constant. In reality, the situation is more complex, as the relationship between volume and apparent rCBF need not be linear. Partial volume errors should be suspect in any comparison between groups with different diagnoses or treatment status.

On the face of it, pseudoatrophy could be ignored if a study finds regions of *higher* activity in patients than in normal controls. However, this may not be true, depending on study methods and interpretation. Assume, for instance, that some region (say putamen) has relatively little pseudoatrophy, while cortex is more affected. Assume also that to eliminate global shifts in activity, comparisons of regional metabolism are only performed after first normalizing regional activity by dividing by global activity. Then even if the true metabolic rate per gram of gray matter is identical between patients and normals, a comparison of patients to normals will show a spurious "hot spot" in the putamen of patients, simply due to a "denominator effect" of lower global activity in the patients.

Ideally, one would like to correct *post hoc* for potential partial volume errors. However, this is not trivial. The simple fix of showing that volume does not differ between groups is only defensible if the methods used to determine volume are known to be at least as sensitive to error as the methods used to determine rCBF. More sophisticated approaches, however, may be adequate [8].

Second, pseudoatrophy may affect the anatomical interpretation of functional imaging data. To give one simple example, imagine a study comparing blood flow between patients and normals. Suppose that anatomical regions of interest are identified in a brain atlas and then transferred to each subject's image as follows: an algorithm matches the "edges" of the blood flow image to the edges of the atlas, with the image edges defined by a high spatial gradient. This approach may show adequate accuracy when used for comparing normal subjects to each other. However, suppose patients have marked cortical atrophy but little if any subcortical atrophy. Such a pattern of atrophy might "shrink" the apparent edges of the brain, while leaving subcortical gray matter relatively stationary. Then our hypothetical stereotactic method would give incorrect anatomical locations for many points in the brain by "stretching" subcortical structures too far laterally. This would probably lead to regions of spuriously elevated or depressed rCBF in any group comparison between patients and normal controls. Other methods of identifying anatomical locations of points in functional images may similarly produce spurious group differences; it may be necessary to validate one's methods across a range of disease severity.

A related concern arises when regions of interest are traced on the image itself. The effects of atrophy or of global changes in metabolism can be expected to change the visual appearance of the "edge" one detects either visually or using computer-aided visual techniques. This may result in systematic biases in ROI composition between groups. (This concern applies to structural as well as functional imaging studies).

These considerations may seem obvious in eating disorders, where there are known volumetric differences across diagnoses and across treatment states. However, volumetric abnormalities have been reported in many illnesses, ranging from schizophrenia to major depression to Parkinson's disease, and correction for partial volume effects may be needed in any functional imaging study across different clinical states.

2. Global Effects

As mentioned in the discussion of partial volume effects, patients may have very different average activity than normals. For instance, we cannot assume that patients have similar global cerebral blood flow to normal controls. However, when searching for regional differences in activity between patients and controls, functional imaging data is often normalized to a standard global flow or metabolic value. Such normalization may be reasonable in experiments within samples from a single population, but in comparisons across diagnostic groups, it can not only lose important data but may also cause artifactual regional findings. Such problems can be avoided entirely only by performing quantitative, rather than qualitative, studies.

3. Effects on Functional Imaging from Starvation

Patients with anorexia or bulimia can show numerous abnormalities of metabolism, some of which persist even when their weight is normal [9,10]. Many of these changes are probably secondary to chronic or repeated self-starvation, rather than a primary part of the psychiatric illness. Unfortunately, many of these changes are potentially very relevant to interpreting functional imaging studies, even though they may be of little relevance to disease etiology. Since there is little data on the magnitude of such effects on imaging results, we will only enumerate them, with brief comments on their potential relevance to functional imaging.

Bone density is often abnormal in patients with anorexia or bulimia. Frank osteopenia with pathological fractures has been reported in a few eating disordered patients, while more modest abnormalities are very common [11–13]. PET and SPECT studies must correct counts measured outside the head for having been attenuated by the skull. Some groups do this using an individually acquired transmission image, which allows precise correction. However, what many researchers do instead is reconstruct brain activity identically for each subject by assuming a constant thickness of skull or using a geometric phantom. This shortcut may produce artifactual increases in activity in eating disordered patients.

A common PET technique for measuring brain metabolism uses ^{18}F-fluorodeoxyglucose (FDG) as a radioactive tracer for glucose. However, this technique depends on assumptions that may not be valid across patient groups. Tracer kinetic models assume that the radioactive tracer behaves biologically in the same way as the biological compound of interest, or at least in a consistently different way, which can be accounted for in the model used to interpret the data. In the case of FDG imaging, a "lumped constant" (LC) accounts for differences between the brain's utilization of FDG and glucose. Unfortunately, the LC is not actually constant, and in fact varies with a number of factors, including blood glucose (which can be easily monitored during the study). It is reasonable to assume that chronic or recurrent *starvation might affect utilization of glucose* and FDG differently, and hence change the LC. To our knowledge, there is no proof that the LC derived from studies of normal controls is unchanged in well-fed patients with eating disorders, much less in patients with starvation. One way of avoiding such difficulties may be to use a radioligand such as 1-^{11}C-glucose, which is physiologically indistinguishable from unlabeled glucose [14]. A similar criticism applies to other "constants" used in FDG PET studies (rate constants representing the speed of glucose or metabolite movement between compartments), although these can sometimes be directly estimated from the imaging data.

There are other, *miscellaneous* metabolic effects of eating disorders that could potentially affect functional brain imaging studies. These include metabolic alkalosis (and compensatory respiratory changes in pCO_2) in bulimic patients with frequent vomiting, anemia, elevated levels of ketones (metabolized differently in different brain regions [15]), bradycardia, and secondary changes in steroid hormones. In addition to secondary metabolic changes, interpretation of imaging studies in patients with eating disorders must take into account *differences in mental state*, including secondary or comorbid psychiatric syndromes. Sadness, anxiety, and obsessions are all common in these patients and are associated in other populations with physiological changes, which can affect interpretation of functional imaging data, including not only changes in regional brain activity, but also changes in pCO_2 or activity of the temporalis and masseter muscles.

The take-home message of these first three methodological questions is simply that *patients may be different from normals!* When comparing patients to normal controls, one must skeptically review any assumptions inherent in study methods.

4. How Normal Are the Controls?

In addition to adequate imaging methods *per se*, all psychiatric research must include careful clinical ascertainment. In eating disorders research, the high prevalence of subclinical binging or purging in the normal population [16] mandates careful assessment of "normal" volunteers as well as of patient volunteers. Also, the clinical observation that some patients have features of both bulimia and anorexia nervosa, perhaps at different times, suggests careful attention to psychiatric history as well as current psychiatric status. Finally, as mentioned above, state differences in anxiety, depression, or obsessions must be carefully assessed at the time of each study.

5. *Fishing or Science?*

Statistical questions are very important in interpreting any imaging study. The presentation of data in the form of a picture tends to obscure the number of measurements being reported. A typical PET image involves the acquisition of millions of data points; a single functional MRI study can involve gigabytes of data. Analyzing such data for significant differences between groups is challenging and raises questions beyond the scope of this chapter. However, a few points should be kept in mind as a guide to the literature.

Studies that test a specific *a priori* hypothesis are very powerful. On the other hand, studies that "fish" for any difference between images of patients and normals are very worrisome for Type 1 errors. Although a number of statistical techniques have been described that purport to winnow out true differences from chance findings, replication with separate data remains the gold standard. If one must search for any possible difference between groups, then using half one's data to generate anatomically specific hypotheses and the other half to replicate these hypotheses combines the strengths of these two approaches.

Other aspects of experimental design are also important. For instance, if one suspects a group difference in physiological responses to a given stimuli, testing a complex stimulus (such as the sight and smell of food) may most closely reflect observed clinical differences. However, any resulting between-group differences would be very difficult to interpret. More definite conclusions could be drawn from an experiment that found group differences using a more well-characterized stimulus (such as visual presentation of pictures of high-calorie food versus visual presentation of pictures of low-calorie food).

IV. CT AND MRI MORPHOLOGICAL STUDIES

Multiple studies have demonstrated dramatic morphological differences in subjects with eating disorders in comparison to controls, and remarkably some of these global changes seem to resolve or attenuate with treatment and resolution of clinical symptoms. Postmortem examinations prior to the advent of current neuroimaging modalities reported that cachetic patients who died from anorexia nervosa demonstrated cerebral atrophy [17]. Numerous reports have been published describing the qualitative observations of cerebral atrophy and ventricular enlargement demonstrated by CT in individuals with anorexia and bulimia nervosa. More than 10 controlled studies (Table 1) have reported that patients with anorexia and bulimia demonstrate cerebral atrophy as represented by widened cortical sulci, a widened interhemispheric fissure, and dilatation of the lateral ventricles.

A. Cerebral Atrophy and Ventricular Enlargement

1. CT and MRI Investigations

Cerebral atrophy has been variously defined by different authors. Some authors have relied on qualitative measures such as blind clinical impressions [18] or structured rating scales [19]. Other authors have operationalized the definition based on linear measures of sulcal widths or a compilation of measures. For example, Krieg et al. [20,21] in their studies defined atrophy based on measures of cortical sulci width and the width of the interhemispheric fissure on three specified axial CT slices. Atrophy was defined as a width of 3 mm or greater on at least six sulci, the insular cisterns and the interhemispheric fissure. However, irrespective of how atrophy was defined or which control group was used for comparison, all studies found that subjects with current anorexia and bulimia had increased levels of cortical atrophy [18,19,21–27].

Assessment of ventricular size in studies of eating disordered patients reported to date has generally been based on traditional ventricular brain ratio (VBR) measures: (ventricular area/cerebral area) × 100. VBR is measured based on a single axial CT image that demonstrates the ventricles at their largest [28]. Some reports have also been based on qualitative ratings based on blind clinical ratings or structured rating scales. Although most investigators have reported that ventricular size was increased in both anorectics and bulimics [19,21–25,29–32], a few investigators have found no significant differences [18,26,27].

2. Potential Reversibility of Atrophic Changes

Several longitudinal studies have reported that the atrophic changes noted decrease in severity or resolve with weight increase in anorectics [22–24,33,34]. Some studies have reported that cortical atrophy was more reversible than noted ventricular changes [19,33]. Because many authors have noted reversibility of the structural findings, some have suggested that the term atrophy may be inappropriate and have advocated the terms "pseudoatrophy" or cerebral "dystrophy." Artmann et al. [34] examined several subjects at multiple time points and noted that the reversal of atrophy was delayed relative to the regaining of weight and concluded that a minimum of 2 months or more is necessary to observe changes. Younger subjects were noted to have more robust resolution of structural changes.

Table 1 Ventricular Findings in Anorexia and Bulimia Nervosa

Source	Imaging method	Eating disorder subjects	Control subjects	Matching variables	Group differences	Clinical correlates	Ref.
Kohlmeyer et al., 1983	CT, ratings, linear measures	23 AN	0			+ length of illness; atrophy reversible with weight gain	33
Artmann et al., 1985	CT, rating scale, sulcal widths	35 AN	0			atrophy: + degree of underweight; decr. atrophy with weight gain	34
Lankenau et al., 1985	CT, VBR	16 AN 5 BN	14 P	Age, sex	AN > P	+ degree underweight	29
Datlof et al., 1986	CT, regional VBR	14 AN	7 N	Age, sex	3rd ventricle and frontal horn in AN > N increased cerebral area in AN	None	30
Dolan et al., 1988	CT, VBR, sulcal ratings	25 AN	17 C	Age, sex, education	VBR and sulcal widening, AN > C	sulcal widening + related to age of onset; widening decreased with weight gain	19
Kreig et al., 1986, 1988	CT, VBR, sulcal widths	50 AN	50 P	Age, sex	VBR and sulcal widening, AN > P	VBR: neg. relation to weight, age, T3; sulcal widening: neg. relation to weight, + relation to cortisol	21,27
Hoffman et al., 1989	MRI, VBR	10 AN	10 HA	Age	Vomiting, AN > HA	None	26
Hoffman et al., 1989	MRI, VBR, cerebral/ cranium	8 BN	8 HA	Age	Cortical atrophy in BN > HA	None	25,26
Krieg et al., 1989	CT, VBR, sulcal widths	50 AN 50 BN	50 P	Age, sex	VBR and atrophy, AN > BN > P	Negative correlation with triiodothyronine	21
Laessle et al., 1989	CT, VBR	17 AN 22 BN	22 C		AN and BN > C	Positive relation, lower body mass index	31
Kiriike et al., 1990	CT, VBR	17 BN	21 NS	Age	BN > NS	None	32
Palazidou et al., 1990	CT, linear and area measures	17 AN 3 BN	9 C	Age, sex, education	No difference in VBR or ventricular measures cortical atrophy, greater in AN vs. C	None	27

Table 1 (*continued*)

Source	Imaging method	Eating disorder subjects	Control subjects	Matching variables	Group differences	Clinical correlates	Ref.
Kornreich et al., 1991	CT—linear measures, MRI—ratings	13 AN	15 sinusitis		Sulci wider, AN > C	None	18

AN, Anorexia nervosa; BN, bulimia nervosa; C, screened normal control; N, neurological control; NS, neurological control, screened; P, psychiatric control; HA, headache control.

Most investigators believe that the changes are not completely reversible, however, this has not been well addressed because of methodological limitations. Measures to date of atrophy and ventricular dilatation have been based on linear or area measures, and these measures have somewhat poor reproducibility for a single individual from scan to scan because of variations in head position and slice positioning. Volumetric measures from thin slice MRI images of total cerebral volume and total ventricular volume could avoid some of these methodological problems but have not yet been reported in eating disordered populations.

3. Correlates of cerebral Atrophy and VBR

a. Clinical Characteristics Anorectic patients with increased VBR have been reported by most authors to have lower body mass indices [22,24,31] or greater amounts of weight loss [29,34]. A similar relationship has been reported between estimates of cortical atrophy and lower weight [22,34]. However, a few investigators have not found this association [18,19,25,27,30]. Some investigators have reported a positive relationship between age of onset of illness and widening of cortical sulci [19], whereas others have not found an association between age of onset or length of illness and measures of atrophy or ventricular enlargement [18,22,23,25,26,31, 32,34]. No groups have demonstrated a relationship between severity of illness as assessed by structured rating scale [22,25,35].

Very few specific clinical symptoms have been found to have a significant relationship to ventricular size. Lankenau et al. [29] did report a negative relationship between ventricular size and vomiting and laxative abuse, and a relationship with vomiting was also reported by Hoffman et al. [25].

Some patients with bulimia have a history of earlier anorexia nervosa, raising the possibility that the observed atrophy and ventricular enlargement may be secondary to the earlier anorexia. Studies examining the possibility have found no difference between bulimia patients with or without a history of anorexia [20,35].

b. Cognitive Performance   Only a few investigations have examined for a potential relationship between neuropsychological performance and atrophy or ventricular enlargement. There is no reported association with IQ scores [29,32]. Laessle et al. [31] did not observe any relationship between impaired performance on vigilance tasks and increased VBR (examined as a dichotomous variable) in a mixed population of anorectics and bulimics. The subjects with anorexia and bulimia were significantly impaired on these vigilance tasks in comparison to normal controls. Kohlmeyer et al. [33] reported that perceptual speed and concentration improved in parallel to resolution of cerebral atrophy and ventricular enlargement in anorectic patients studied longitudinally.

In general, these studies have not found a clear relationship between gross structural brain changes and neuropsychological performance in eating disordered subjects. Although this seems counterintuitive, there may be several factors contributing to the lack of findings. First, the studies have had a relatively small number of subjects. Second, some have included mixed populations of subjects with anorexia and bulimia, thereby potentially increasing the variability in neuropsychological performance and structural brain measures and possibly obscuring any real differences. Also, the brain measures examined are relatively nonspecific; specific regional measures may be more likely to demonstrate significant relationships. This phenomenon has been demonstrated in several other psychiatric disorders such as schizophrenia, where global structural measures did not correlate with performance but specific regional measures did. A good example is the demonstration that superior temporal gyrus volume significantly correlates with measures of thought disorder [36].

c. Neuroendocrine and Metabolic Correlates   Individuals with anorexia and bulimia demonstrate significant alterations in endocrine and metabolic indices. Metabolic abnormalities are observed in some normal-weight bulimics (who intermittently go on restrictive diets) as well as anorectics and seem to best be characterized as adaptations to conditions of starvation. Patients with anorexia and bulimia both demonstrate increased levels of β-hydroxybutyric acid and cortisol, decreased norepinephrine response to orthostatic challenge, and decreased levels of T3 [2,10]. These alterations resolve with different time frames once patients are successfully treated. β-Hydroxybutyric acid normalizes quickly with adequate caloric intake, norepinephrine response normalizes within a week or two, and T3 and cortisol changes normalize slowly over a period of weeks after increased weight gain . [37].

Some investigators have examined for potential relationships between gross structural changes and endocrine and metabolic measures. Bulimic and anorectic patients have demonstrated a significant relationship between increased VBR and plasma levels of triidothyronine [23,35], although negative results have also been reported [32]. Increased cortisol levels have been associated with increased sulcal width in anorectic patients [22]. However, this has not been replicated in patients with bulimia [32,35]. Other indices of starvation including increased levels of β-hydroxybutyric acid and norepinephrine are hypothesized as potentially related to signs of cerebral atrophy, although a significant correlation has not been reported [22,24,35]. These findings support the hypothesis that the structural changes observed in patients with anorexia and bulimia may be secondary to metabolic and endocrine dyscontrol whether or not there is substantial weight loss.

3. Significance of Cortical Atrophy and Ventricular Enlargement

Although many studies seem to report both increased ventricular size and cortical atrophy, several have noted only one measure to be abnormal in eating disordered patients. In fact VBR and measures of cortical atrophy are not necessarily closely related and have been reported by some to have no significant correlation [26]. Processes that effect cortical gray volume may demonstrate cortical atrophy, while processes that effect subcortical structures such as the basal ganglia or white matter may demonstrate ventricular enlargement. However, the fact that most studies have demonstrated that both measures are abnormal suggests that a generalized process or combination of effects may be responsible for the morphometric changes. Clearly, studies that examine specific regional volumes and relative changes in gray matter, white matter, and CSF would help to elucidate these issues.

Early theories suggested that structural brain alterations in anorectic patients were simply related to the degree of weight loss and that reversibility was solely dependent upon weight gain. However, since similar findings have been demonstrated in a subgroup of normal-weight patients with bulimia, this explanation is inadequate. Several alternative hypotheses related to secondary metabolic and endocrine effects of starvation are frequently cited. First, some investigators suggest that malnutrition leads to a decrease in serum proteins with a subsequent decline in colloid osmotic pressure and shift of fluids out of intravascular spaces, however, most eating disordered patients in fact do not demonstrate decreased plasma protein or albumin levels [22,33]. Second, a change in vascular permeability secondary to increased vasopressin has been proposed [23,38]. Third, neuronal loss secondary to malnutrition is a possibility, and neuronal loss with gliosis had been reported in a previous postmortem study [39]. Fourth, some hypothesize that associated hypercortisolemia may result in cortical atrophy as it has been demonstrated that patients with Cushing's disease may have similar reversible changes [40]. Finally, it may be that the gross structural changes noted are secondary to other metabolic and endocrine reactions to starvation, such as alterations in thyroid hormones.

Despite the robustness of the findings of ventricular enlargement and cerebral atrophy, these changes are nonspecific findings, which have been reported in other disorders as well such as Cushing's disease, alcohol dependence, schizophrenia, and other psychiatric disorders. In other disorders, such as schizophrenia, more specific regional explorations have resulted in positive findings that correlate with clinical and functional variables and appear to be more disorder specific. Such specific regional investigations may also be relevant and productive in eating disordered subjects, however, very little has yet been reported for this population.

B. The Pituitary in Eating Disorders

One prospective systematic investigation examining the pituitary was reported by Doraiswamy et al. [41]. Eighteen women with anorexia nervosa and bulimia were systematically assessed and examined on sagittal MRI and reported to have smaller pituitary area and smaller pituitary height in comparison to systematically assessed normal controls matched for age and gender. Both anorectics and bulimics were significantly different from controls and not significantly different from each other. There was no gross hypothalamic or pituitary pathology in any subject with an eating disorder. There was a trend for pituitary area to be negatively correlated with length of illness. This study examined a small group of anorectic and bulimic patients, which could have obscured potential differences between the groups. Additionally, although attempts were made to standardize the subject's head position, the sagittal MRI scans were 5 mm thick, and area, not volumetric, measures were reported. Midsagittal area measures have been reported to have some problems with reliability secondary to sensitivity to substantial measurement changes with small variations in midsagittal slice sampling [42,43].

Subsequently this subject group was further expanded to 26 patients—12 bulimics and 14 anorectics—and further linear and volumetric estimates of the pituitary were completed [44]. Controls were 14 normal volunteers who were screened for psychiatric illness. Volumetric estimates were based on pituitary height and length measures from sagittal images and width measures from coronal images using the following formula: volume = $0.5 \times$ height $\times$ length $\times$ width. These estimates were calculated in seven control subjects and four anorectics who had the appropriate scanning sequences. Anorectics and bulimics had significantly smaller pituitary heights and greater pituitary-optic chiasma distances in comparison to controls. Anorectics had significantly smaller pituitary volumes. Duration of illness was negatively correlated with pituitary height and area. Kornreich et al. [18] also reported decreased pituitary height in anorectic patients. They noted that the anorectic adolescent patients frequently had a concave upper border in comparison to the usual convex pituitary border observed in normal adolescent girls. They found no clinical correlations to pituitary height.

On MR images of the normal pituitary there is generally noted an area of high signal intensity in the posterior pituitary lobe, which has been called the posterior pituitary high signal [45]. This area of hyperintensity is thought to reflect storage of neurohypophyseal hormones such as vasopressin and antidiuretic hormone (ADH). Several authors have reported the lack of this area of hyperintensity in some anorectic patients [41,45], however, group comparisons have failed to demonstrate any significant difference from controls [41].

Although differences in pituitary morphology have been consistently reported by several investigators in patients with eating disorders, it is unclear what the significance of this change is to the pathophysiology of eating disorders. It is known that extreme changes in diet and weight can lead to changes in pituitary size. Starvation has been associated with a reduction in relative pituitary size [46], and conversely pregnancy has been associated with increased pituitary size [47]. Additionally, neuroendocrine disorders have been associated with changes in the neuromorphology of the pituitary [48], and individuals with eating disorders demonstrate significant neuroendocrine dysfunction [2]. Thus, the changes in eating disordered patients may be a secondary phenomenon, potentially unrelated to the pathophysiology that may underly or initiate the disorder. However, they may also represent changes that are important in the initiation and/or maintenance of eating disordered behaviors.

C. Other Brain Regions

The scope of other specific published regional investigations is limited to one additional MRI study of midsagittal anatomy in 24 women with eating disorders (12 anorectics, 12 bulimics) in comparison to 11 systematically assessed age-matched normal controls. In this study Husain et al. [49] examined measures of the corpus callosum (length, width, and area), overall cerebral cortex (area), septum pellucidum (area), thalamus (area), fourth ventricle (area), and midbrain and pons (areas). Area measures were completed by computer assisted manual planimetric tracing. Areas of the thalamus and midbrain were significantly smaller in the patients with anorexia than in controls, and these differences persisted when corrected for potential differences in overall brain size. No significant differences were demonstrated for patients with bulimia. This report further supports the idea that regional structural differences may be present in patients with eating disorders.

V. FUNCTIONAL IMAGING STUDIES

A. Functional Studies by Investigator Group

1. Munich

Investigators at the Max Planck Institute of Psychiatry have reported incrementally on a number of imaging studies with eating disorder patients. In addition to their structural imaging studies (reviewed above), they have performed functional imaging experiments in this population.

First, they performed a 133Xe SPECT inhalation study of regional cerebral blood flow in 12 young female patients who met Washington University [50] and DSM-III-R criteria for anorexia nervosa [21]. Patients were examined both in the anorectic state (although without ketosis) and again after weight gain and normalization of thyroid, cortisol, and norepinephrine. The scans were done in the eyes-closed-rest state. Eleven of the 12 patients had normal flow with this technique (compared to control values from a mixed-gender normal population), and there were no significant hemispheric or regional abnormalities. These patients also had undergone transmission CT, and there was significantly lower global "cerebral blood flow" in patients with larger CSF spaces, consistent with a partial-volume effect. A strength of this early study was the careful clinical and laboratory characterization of the patients and the insistence that all patients have normal levels of β-OH-butyric acid (a marker of starvation) at the time of the first scan.

These researchers also performed FDG PET studies with seven anorectic women, five of whom were rescanned after weight gain, and in nine female patients with bulimia [51]. (Importantly, four of the seven patients with anorexia also reported binge eating and vomiting.) Scans were done in the eyes-closed-rest state. The scans were done using a PET scanner with a 7-mm center-to-center slice distance. Rate constants (used in calculating the glucose metabolic rates) were adjusted to fit measured tissue activity, but treatment of the lumped constant was not reported. Regions of interest were drawn on each image by inspecting the data from that image with the aid of an interactive computer program.

In a before-after comparison of five anorectic patients [52], the salient finding was of an increased global metabolic rate (about 110% of a comparison group of young men), which normalized after weight gain. The authors also compared regional CMRGlu between conditions in 30 regions of interest and reported that the increased global rate reached local significance in the caudate, (left) lentiform nucleus, and temporal cortex. However, there is no correction for multiple comparisons. The conservative Bonferroni correction would require a significance level of $p = 0.05/30 < 0.0017$, whereas the most significant region attained a p-value of only 0.02. Additionally, the biological meaning of these possible local increases is questionable, since they roughly parallel the overall global change in rCMRGlu.

The authors then compared the data from all seven patients with anorexia (before weight gain) to that of their nine patients with bulimia [51]. The anorectic patients had a lower mean global CMRGlu than either the bulimic patients or a (different) control group of young men, although this difference was not statistically significant ($p = 0.22$). (This is difficult to interpret given that the mean global flow in this control group is 10% higher than that of the control group referenced in the previous study.) In this study Krieg et al. report relative regional rates by dividing each region's CMRGlu by that patient's global CMRGlu. They report this data after combining regions of interest from the left and right hemispheres and find that the untreated anorectic patients have significantly higher *relative* caudate metabolism than bulimics or controls, which survives a test for multiple comparisons (apparently using 15 as the number of regions compared, rather than 30 for separate measurements of left and right hemisphere regions). However, the biological significance of this finding is uncertain, since after reconstructing the *absolute* caudate CMRGlu from the data reported, the three groups are indistinguishable. The authors prudently remain "reserved . . . in interpreting the differences in caudate activity" as being biologically significant "until future studies have clarified this issue" [51]. They also remind the reader that there is no *a priori* reason to implicate this state abnormality in the caudate in the pathogenesis of the psychological disturbance of anorexia nervosa.

2. UC-Irvine

Wu and colleagues [53] performed FDG PET studies on eight women with DSM-III-R bulimia (with no prior anorexia) and eight matched normal control subjects. Patients reported a weekly average of 14 episodes each of bingeing and vomiting, but "had been eating normally on the day before the scan." Notably, the mean Hamilton depression rating scale score for patients was 20.8. Patients otherwise were in good health and had normal "laboratory screening tests," including normal plasma glucose levels during the experiment. Tests for peripheral indicators of starvation such as circulating ketones are not specifically mentioned. FDG was administered while patients performing the Continuous Performance Test (without feedback) in a darkened room. One-hour PET scans were then performed at rest, with slices taken parallel to the canthomeatal line (which approximates the plane containing the anterior and posterior commissures). The center-to-center slice separation was 10 mm, and the scanner resolution is reported as 7.6 mm in plane and 9.9 mm axially (presumably this is also the resolution of the images used in the glucose utilization model). Scans were reconstructed using a calculated (not measured) attenuation factor. Glucose utilization was computed using published values (i.e., from a different population) for the kinetic constants and the lumped constant and using venous blood (from an arm wrapped in a heating pad) to estimate the arterial FDG concentration. Glucose use was computed for each of 24 regions of cortex. These regions were defined by drawing a constant-thickness band on each of three PET slices using an automated edge-detection algorithm and dividing the band on each slice radially into eight sections in an automated way. The slices were chosen blindly as those that by visual inspection most nearly matched target slices from a standard photographic brain atlas. Then the authors examined an additional 20 subcortical regions, defined by automated proportional measurements from the "edge" of the brain, on the PET slice most nearly corresponding to one of two slices in a standard atlas. Data were analyzed by a repeated measures ANOVA (i.e., different regions within each patient).

Although Krieg et al. tested the caudate region before other subcortical regions due to the *a priori* expectation of caudate hypermetabolism [51], this difference did not reach statistical significance. They also report statistically significant interactions (at the 0.05 level) in the comparison of left versus right metabolic rates. The bulimic patient group had higher absolute and relative metabolism on the left than on the right, as opposed to the opposite laterality in control subjects. The results did not change after exclusion of a few left-handed subjects.

This study is interesting but is somewhat difficult to interpret. Methodological concerns include the possibility of residual metabolic effects of chronically poor nutrition despite one day of good eating, the assumption of similar bone attenuation between groups, the assumption of patients handle glucose and FDG in the same way as normal controls, the use of the image itself to define the anatomical regions of interest, and the comparison of data from 44 regions in only 16 subjects. The authors appropriately caution the reader that the small sample mandates a replication study. In summary, the authors tested one *a priori* hypothesis, which was not replicated, and they performed exploratory analyses that provide useful hypotheses for testing in a subsequent study. The lack of relative caudate hypometabolism, seen in several other groups with significant depressive symptoms, is intriguing.

Following up on this point, Hagman et al. [54] compared these data to those of eight additional female patients, who met DSM-III-R criteria for major depression. As noted, the bulimic patient group also had substantial depressive symptoms, and most met criteria for either major depression or dysthymia. Twenty-eight regions (defined somewhat differently than those discussed above) were compared across the three groups. In the 16 "cortical peel'' regions, there was a significant ($p = 0.0001$) lobe-by-hemisphere-by-group interaction, indicating regional differences between diagnostic groups in the amount and direction of left-right asymmetry. Each group (especially controls) differed from the other two on post hoc ANOVAs. An analysis of medial frontal and subcortical regions showed a similar difference ($p = 0.03$), with post hoc tests suggesting differences of each patient group versus normals. A cluster analysis using subcortical areas to classify patients led to one cluster with largely normal subjects, a second cluster with almost all the depressed patients, and bulimic patients being scattered among the second or a third cluster or remaining unclassified. Finally, the authors presented exploratory hypothesis-generating data correlating the activity in specific regions with binge and purge frequency or the score on an Eating Attitudes Test [55]. Each clinical measure had different areas of correlation on the PET data, with the only overlap being that both binge and vomiting frequency were correlated positively with activity in the right posterior thalamus.

The authors summarize this data as follows [54]: "Normal women have higher right than left cortical metabolic rates and active basal ganglia. Bulimics lose the normal right activation in some areas but maintain basal ganglia metabolic activity. Depressives retain right hemisphere activation, but show decreases in basal ganglia metabolism. This suggests that (despite substantial depressive features) the pathophysiologic basis of bulimia differs from that of major affective disorder." This study shows significant differences in FDG activation among these three diagnostic groups and offers important hypotheses for validation in a separate sample. As discussed above, some methodological assumptions limit our ability to relate the group differences to the pathophysiology of bulimia.

3. NIMH/NIAAA

Andreason et al. [56] studied 11 bulimic women on an inpatient unit. Each patient met DSM-III-R criteria for bulimia nervosa and appropriate exclusionary criteria were used, although anorexia nervosa was not specifically excluded. Patients were scanned after 3–5 weeks of documented abstinence from bingeing and purging, at normal body weights. They were compared to 18 normal, age- and education-matched female volunteers "screened for a history of psychiatric, neurological, and medical illness." PET scans were done at a consistent time after a meal. Seven slices of PET data (center-to-center slice separation 14 mm) were acquired parallel to the canthomeatal line, with an in-plane resolution of about 5 mm and an axial resolution of about 10 mm. Data were reconstructed using a measured attenuation correction from a transmission scan. The PET scans were acquired after subjects performed a continuous discrimination task for 30 minutes after FDG administration, and subjects in all three groups performed the task similarly. Four scans were acquired over the next 30 minutes, with the subjects' eyes covered. Glucose utilization rates were computed using published values for kinetic constants and the lumped constant. Sixty regions of interest were drawn on each image by raters blind to diagnosis, based on a template keyed to a standard brain atlas. Finally, the authors analyzed the data for three a priori hypotheses, and also reported data from all other regions for hypothesis-generating value.

There was no difference in global metabolic rates between patients and normals. The authors did replicate in part the reversed (left-predominant) hemispheric asymmetry of FDG metabolism reported by Wu et al. [53]. This reached statistical significance in only three of the regions tested. Contrary to the authors' second hypothesis that orbitofrontal regions would be hyperactive, especially in patients with higher measures of obsessive-compulsive behavior, two of the regions tested had significantly lower metabolic activity in patients than in controls. However, their third hypothesis, that depressed bulimic patients would have lower left dorsolateral prefrontal cortex metabolism, was substantiated.

This study was very carefully done in many respects in both clinical and imaging domains. The use of published values for the constants used in the metabolic rate computation is suspect, though probably less so in this normal weight group known to have been eating normally eating for 3 weeks. The placement of regions by visual inspection of the image may theoretically bias the absolute metabolic rates in the cortex if there are significant group differences either in true global metabolic rate or in brain volume. However, this would probably not affect left-right comparisons. Finally, the left-right comparisons (at least) were not corrected for the (unclear) number of areas compared, rendering suspect the reported replication of altered left-right asymmetry. However, one such comparison reached a significance of $P = 0.003$, which would survive a Bonferroni correction for 16 regions. On the whole, this study tends to support the findings of Wu et al., and the inverse correlation of left dorsolateral prefrontal cortex activity with severity of depression is consistent with the results of several other studies [57].

4. Kagoshima University

Nozoe and colleagues reported on SPECT studies of women with eating disorders [58]. Their 1993 publication compares seven young (average age 19) patients who met DSM-III-R criteria for anorexia nervosa with five "healthy female volunteers." A 1995 report compared five women with bulimia, eight with anorexia, and nine normals [59], presumably including the subjects from the previous report; in this case patients were scanned while symptomatic. Their work represents an intriguing study design but has important methodological flaws.

In the first study, patients were scanned while symptomatic and again an average of 70 days later, after treatment (degree of clinical response is not stated). In the second report, patients were scanned while symptomatic. No exclusion for bulimic symptoms in anorexia, or vice versa, was stated. All subjects were right-handed. Subjects were scanned using ^{99m}Tc-HMPAO while at rest (eyes closed) and then again 15 minutes later after a second injection of ^{99m}Tc-HMPAO while eating a 96 kcal piece of cake "within 3 min, using their left hand and keeping their eyes closed." Hematocrit, which affects blood flow, did not differ between groups. Scans acquired parallel to the canthomeatal plane with a gamma camera were reconstructed with no attenuation correction. Only qualitative images were obtained and were reported as the ratio of counts in each cortical region to counts in a cerebellar region, transformed by the function $2x/(3 + x)$. Ten cortical regions of interest were examined, defined by rectangular regions of interest placed manually on two slices chosen to best match template slices in a brain atlas. Data were analyzed by ANOVA and post hoc tests, without correction for multiple comparisons.

In the first report, the authors report a difference in scaled temporal lobe counts between controls and treated patients and a greater activation with eating in one region in untreated patients than in controls. In the second paper, patients with bulimia had higher relative activity than other diagnostic groups in inferior frontal and left temporal regions. (However, they also had somewhat higher global cortical activity.) They also had a left hemisphere predominance of activity in temporal lobe, whereas controls have a right predominance. The sparse clinical state data, the short time between "before" and "after" scans compared to ^{99m}Tc's 6-hour half-life, the lack of correction for multiple comparisons, the extremely complex nature of the activating stimulus, and the nonquantitative nature of the study combine to make interpretation of these results difficult.

5. Brussels

Delvenne et al. [60] performed FDG PET scans on 20 girls and women with anorexia nervosa diagnosed by a structured interview. Seven had episodes of binge eating, and three had concurrent major depression. They compared the results to scans of 10 female volunteers without a history of psychiatric illness.

Patients were scanned after one week of hospitalization, during which bingeing and purging were prevented and patients ate at least 1500 kcal per day. Serum protein, thyroid function, and serum glucose were normal at the time of the scan, and urine was negative for ketones, though patients remained under 85% of ideal body weight. Fifteen PET slices parallel to the canthomeatal line were obtained in the eyes-closed-rest state. Attenuation correction was done with a measured transmission scan, arterial sampling was done for glucose and FDG determinations, and immobility during the scan was checked using lines drawn on the subject's face and laser beams mounted on the scanner. The cerebral metabolic rate for glucose (CMRGlu) was computed using calculated rate constants but assuming an equivalent lumped constant between groups. A number of irregular regions of interest were drawn directly on the PET slices (blindedness is not stated) by comparison with a standard atlas. Weighted averages of these regions were used to create 16 larger regions of interest, which were then compared between groups using a multivariate analysis of variance (MANOVA).

The salient finding of this study was a significantly lower global CMRGlu in patients compared to normals. When corrected for hemispheric CMRGlu, there was no significant regionally selective difference in relative CMRGlu between patients and controls, though on post hoc t-tests, relative CMRGlu was significantly lower in patients in the superior frontal and parietal cortical regions ($p < 0.002$).

This study was carefully done, though a few comments regarding methodology are in order. Clinically, a separation of patients with and without bulimic features could perhaps have produced more homogeneous samples. The use of a constant for the lumped constant again may be inaccurate. Also, drawing regions of interest by direct inspection of the data may bias the results as patients may have a visually apparent "edge" at a different anatomical location than normals. However, a significant problem in clinical interpretation of this study is the possibility that these underweight patients, whom we might expect to show pseudoatrophy, may have only an apparent decline in global activity due to pseudoatrophy, rather than a real difference in metabolic rate per gram of brain.

B.   Summary of Functional Imaging Studies

These early functional imaging studies of eating disorders help point out the need for thorough understanding of the assumptions implicit in published functional imaging methods, which may not be tenable when a patient group is compared to a group of normal volunteers. Although other interpretations of the data are plausible, in our opinion there are no clearly replicated specific functional imaging abnormalities demonstrated thus far in patients with eating disorders, except perhaps for the loss of right greater than left cortical asymmetry in CMRGlu in bulimic patients compared to normals. However, several suggestive regional differences are mentioned in these reports which might be examined in future studies.

VI. CONCLUSION AND SUGGESTIONS FOR FUTURE RESEARCH

Neuroimaging research in eating disordered populations is clearly still in its infancy. Relatively few studies have been completed, but almost all suggest the potential for significant neuromorphometric and functional differences from control populations. Recent advances in image analytic techniques, especially MRI, allow for highly detailed, regionally specific, and reliable measures of many specific brain regions. These techniques, however, appear to be sparsely applied, if at all, to these populations.

However, it is important to acknowledge that several difficulties complicate research with eating disordered patients. First, there is the problem of secondary effects from starvation alone. It is difficult if not impossible to begin prospective studies prior to the secondary effects of starvation, and it is not feasible to have a control group of equally starved individuals who could be matched on other variables as well. However, samples of less severely affected outpatient subjects in combination with longitudinal studies of more severely affected but recovered patients may help to differentiate these effects. Second, there is symptomatic clinical overlap between subjects with anorexia and bulimia but increasing evidence that they may be distinct disorders with different etiologies and pathophysiologies. Thus, it will be important for future clinical samples to be well characterized and as homogeneous as possible to avoid obscuring real differences by increased variability inherent in mixed subject populations [57]. Third, the interpretation of functional imaging studies in these patients is hampered by the clear demonstration of gross structural differences in these populations combined with our lack of knowledge regarding the specific neurmorphometric parameters of the regions of interest. This points to a clear need for further specific neuromorphometric investigations using state-of-the-art, thin-slice, high-resolution MRI in combination with highly reliable specific regional image analysis.

Future structural and functional studies that can build on the knowledge of previous studies reviewed here and address methodological issues discussed in detail in this chapter will add significantly to our understanding of the pathophysiology of eating disorders. These traditional MRI and PET investigations in combination with newer techniques such as pharmacological challenge PET, functional MRI, and magnetic resonance spectroscopy will add to our understanding and treatment of these important and challenging disorders.

REFERENCES

1. J. Treasure and A. Holland, Genetic vulnerability to eating disorders: evidence from twin and family studies, *Anorexia Nervosa* (S. M. H. Remschmidt, ed.), Hogrefe & Huber, Toronto, 1990, pp. 59–68.

2. K. A. Halmi, S. Ackerman, J. Gibbs, and G. Smith, Basic biological overview of the eating disorders, in *Psychopharmacol. Third Gen. Prog.* 1987, pp. 1255–1266.
3. G. D. Gunston, D. Burkimsher, H. Malan, and A. A. Sive, Reversible cerebral shrinkage in kwashiorkor: an MRI study, *Arch. Dis. Child. 67*:1030 (1992).
4. L. M. Zatz and T. L. Jernigan, The ventricular-brain ratio on computed tomography scans: validity and proper use, *Psychiatry Res. 8*:207 (1983).
5. S. Arndt, G. Cohen, R. J. Alliger, V. W. Swayze, and N. C. Andreasen, Problems with ratio and proportion measures of imaged cerebral structures, *Psychiatry Rest. Neuroimaging 40*:79 (1991).
6. E. Plante and L. Turkstra, Sources of error in the quantitative analysis of MRI scans, *Magnetic Resonance Imaging 9*:589 (1991).
7. J. D. Brodie, Imaging for the clinical psychiatrist: facts, fantasies and other musings, *Am. J. Psychiatry 153*:145 (1996).
8. T. O. Videen, J. S. Perlmutter, M. A. Mintum, and M. E. Raichle, Regional correction of positron emission tomography data for the effect of cerebral atrophy, *J. Cereb. Blood Flow Metab. 8*: 662 (1980).
9. A. Wakeling, Neurobiological aspects of feeding disorders, *J. Psychiatr. Res. 19*:191 (1985).
10. D. W. Ploog and K. M. Pirke, Psychobiology of anorexia nervosa, *Psychol. Med. 17*:843 (1987).
11. P. J. Hay, A. Hall, J. W. Delahunt, G. Harper, A. W. Mitchell, and C. Salmond, Investigation of osteopaenia in anorexia nervosa, *Aust. N.Z.J. Psychiatry 23*: 261 (1989).
12. L. A. Verbruggen, M. Bruyland, and M. Shahabpour, Osteomalacia in a patient with anorexia nervosa, *J. Rheumatol. 20*:512 (1993).
13. B. C. VandeBerg, J. Malghem, O. Devuyst, B. E. Maldague, and M. J. Lambert, Anorexia nervosa: correlation between MR appearance of bone marrow and severity of disease, *Radiology 193*:859 (1994).
14. W. J. Powers, S. Dagogo-Jack, J. Markham, K. B. Larson, and C. S. Dence, Cerebral transport and metabolism of 1-11C-D-glucose during stepped hypoglycemia, *Ann. Neurol. 38*:599 (1995).
15. R. A. Hawkins and J. F. Biebuyck, Ketone bodies are selectively used by individual brain regions, *Science 205*:325–327 (1979).
16. D. E. Schotte and A. J. Stunkard, Bulimia vs bulimic behaviors on a college campus, *JAMA 258*:1213 (1987).
17. H. Thoma, *Anorexia nervosa*, Huber-Klett, Stuttgart, 1961.
18. L. Kornreich, A. Shapira, G. Horev, Y. Danziger, S. Tyano, and M. Mimouni, CT and MR evaluation of the brain in patients with anorexia nervosa, *AJNR 12*:1213 (1991).
19. R. J. Dolan, J. Mitchell, and A. Wakeling, Structural brain changes in patients with anorexia nervosa, *Psychol. Med. 18*:349 (1988).
20. J. C. Krieg, H. Backmund, and K. M. Pirke, Cranial computed tomography findings in bulimia, *Acta Psychiatr. Scand. 75*:144 (1987).
21. J. Krieg, C. Lauer, G. Leinsinger, J. Pahl, W. Schreiber, K. Pirke, and E. A.

Moser, Brain morphology and regional cerebral blood flow in anorexia nervosa, *Biol. Psychiatry 25*:1041 (1989).

22. J. C. Krieg, H. Backmund, and K. M. Pirke, Endocrine, metabolic, and brain morphological abnormalities in patients with eating disorders, *Int. J. Eating Disord. 5*:999 (1986).

23. J. C. Krieg, C. Lauer, and K. M. Pirke, Hormonal and metabolic mechanisms in the development of cerebral pseudoatrophy in eating disorders, *Psychother. Psychosom. 48*:176 (1987).

24. J. Krieg, K. Pirke, C. Lauer, and H. Backmund, Endocrine, metabolic and cranial computed tomographic findings in anorexia nervosa, *Biol. Psychiatry 23*:377 (1988).

25. G. W. Hoffman, E. H. Ellinwood, W. J. K. Rockwell, R. J. Herfkens, J. K. Nishita, and L. F. Guthrie, Cerebral atrophy in anorexia nervosa: a pilot study, *Biol. Psychiatry 26*:321 (1989).

26. G. W. Hoffman, E. H. Ellinwood, W. J. K. Rockwell, R. J. Herfkens, J. K. Nishita, and L. F. Guthrie, Cerebral atrophy in bulimia, *Biol. Psychiatry 25*: 894 (1989).

27. E. Palazidou, P. Robinson, and W. A. Lishman, Neuroradiological and neuropsychological assessment in anorexia nervosa, *Psychol. Med. 20*:521 (1990).

28. V. Synek and J. R. Reuben, The ventricular-brain ratio using planimetric measurement of EMI scans, *Br. J. Radiol. 49*:233 (1976).

29. H. Lankenua, M. E. Swigar, S. Bhimani, D. Luchins, and D. M. Quinlan, Cranial CT scans in eating disorder patients and controls, *Comp. Psychiatry 26*:136 (1985).

30. S. Datlof, P. D. Coleman, G. B. Forbes, and R. E. Kreipe, Ventricular dilation on CAT scans of patients with anorexia nervosa, *Am. J. Psychiatry 143*:96 (1986).

31. R. G. Laessle, J. C. Krieg, M. M. Fichter, and K. M. Pirke, Cerebral atrophy and vigilance performance in patients with anorexia nervosa and bulimia nervosa, *Neurpsychobiology 21*:187 (1989).

32. N. Kiriike, S. Nishiwaki, T. Nagata, Y. Inoue, K. Inoue, and Y. Kawakita, Ventricular enlargement in normal weight bulimia, *Acta Psychiatr. Scand. 82*: 264 (1990).

33. K. Kohimeyer, G. Lehmkuhl, and F. Poutska, Computed tomography of anorexia nervosa, *Am. J. Neuroradiol. 4*:437 (1983).

34. H. Artmann, H. Grau, M. Adelmann, and R. Schleiffer, Reversible and nonreversible enlargement of cerebrospinal fluid spaces in anorexia nervosa, *Neuroradiology 27*:304 (1985).

35. J. Krieg, C. Lauer, and K. Pirke, Structural brain abnormalities in patients with bulimia nervosa, *Psychiatry Res. 27*:39 (1989).

36. M. E. Shenton, R. Kikinis, F. A. Jolesz, S. D. Pollak, M. LeMay, C. G. Wible, H. Hokama, J. Martin, D. Metcalf, M. Coleman, and R. W. McCarley, Abnormalities of the left temporal lobe and thought disorder in schizophrenia, *N. Engl. J. Med. 327*:604 (1992).

37. J. Pahl, K. M. Pirke, U. Schweiger, M. Warnhoff, M. Gerlinghoff, W. Brink-

mann, M. Berger, and C. Krieg, Anorectic behavior, mood, and metabolic and endocrine adaptation to starvation in anorexia nervosa during inpatient treatment, *Biol. Psychiatry 20*:874 (1985).

38. J. K. Nishita, E. H. Ellinwood, W. J. K. Rockwell, C. M. Kuhn, G. W. Hoffman, W. V. McCall, and J. N. Manepalli, Abnormalities in the response of plasma arginine vasopressin during hypertonic saline infusion in patients with eating disorders, *Biol. Psychiatry 26*:73 (1988).

39. P. F. Martin, Pathologie des aspects neurologiques et psychiatriques dans quelques manifestations carenteles avec troubles digestifes et neuroendocriniens., *Helv. Med. Acta 22*:522 (1955).

40. E. R. Heinz, J. Martinez, and A. Haenggeli, Reversibility of cerebral atrophy in anorexia nervosa and Cushing's syndrome, *J. Comput. Assist. Tomogr. 1*: 415 (1977).

41. P. M. Doraiswamy, K. R. R. Krishnan, G. S. Figiel, M. M. Husain, O. B. Boyko, W. J. K. Rockwell, and E. H. Ellinwood, A brain magnetic resonance imaging study of pituitary gland morphology in anorexia nervosa and bulimia. *Biol. Psychiatry 28*:110 (1990).

42. J. A. Coffman, S. B. Schwarzkopf, S. C. Olson, and H. A. Nasrallah, Midsagittal cerebral anatomy by magnetic resonance imaging, the importance of slice position and thickness, *Schizophrenia Res. 2*:287 (1989).

43. E. H. Aylward and A. Reiss, Area and volume measurement of posterior fossa structures in MRI, *J. Psychiatr. Res. 25*:159 (1991).

44. P. M. Doraiswamy, K. R. R. Krishnan, O. B. Boyko, M. M. Husain, G. S. Figiel, V. J. Palese, P. R. Escalona, S. A. Shah, W. M. McDonald, W. J. K. Rockwell, and E. H. Ellinwood, Pituitary abnormalities in eating disorders: further evidence from MRI studies, *Prog. Neuro-Psychopharmacol. Biol. Psychiatry 15*:351 (1991).

45. N. Sato, K. Endo, H. Ishizaka, and M. Matsumoto, Serial MR intensity changes of the posterior pituitary in a patient with anorexia nervosa, high serum ADH, and oliguria, *J. Comp. Assisted Tomography 17*:658 (1993).

46. M. G. Mulinos and L. Pomerantz, Pseudo-hypophysectomy: a condition resembling hypophysectomy produced by malnutrition, *J. Nutr. 19*:493 (1940).

47. J. G. Gonzales, G. Elizondo, D. Saldivar, H. Nanex, L. E. Todd, and J. Z. Villareal, Pituitary gland growth during normal pregnancy: An in vivo study using magnetic resonance imaging, *Am. J. Med. 85*:217 (1988).

48. D. W. Chakeres, A. Curtin, and G. Ford, Magnetic resonance imaging of pituitary and parasellar abnormalities, *Radiol. Clin. North Am. 27*:265 (1989).

49. M. M. Husain, K. J. Black, P. M. Doraswamy, S. A. Shah, W. J. K. Rockwell, E. H. Ellinwood, and K. R. R. Krishnan, Subcortical brain anatomy in anorexia and bulimia, *Biol. Psychiatry 31*:735 (1992).

50. J. P. Feighner, E. Robins, S. B. Guze, R. A. Woodruff, G. Winokur, and R. Munoz, Diagnostic criteria for use in psychiatric research, *Arch. Gen. Psychiatry 26*:57 (1972).

51. J.-C. Krieg, V. Holthoff, W. Schreiber, K. M. Pirke, and K. Herholz, Glucose metabolism in the caudate nuclei of patients with eating disorders, measured by PET, *Eur. Arch. Psychiatry Clin. Neurosci. 240*:331 (1991).

52. K. Herholz, J. C. Krieg, H. M. Emrich, G. Pawlik, C. Beil, K. M. Pirke, J. J. Pahl, R. Wagner, K. Wienhard, D. Ploog, and W. D. Heiss, Regional cerebral glucose metabolism in anorexia nervosa measured by positron emission tomography, *Biol. Psychiatry 22*:43 (1987).

53. J. C. Wu, J. Hagman, M. S. Buchsbaum, B. Blinder, M. Derrfler, W. Y. Tai, E. Hazlett, and N. Sicotte, Greater left cerebral hemispheric metabolism in bulimia assessed by positron emission tomography, *Am. J. Psychiatry 147*:309 (1990).

54. J. O. Hagman, M. S. Buchsbaum, J. C. Wu, S. J. Rao, C. A. Reynolds, and B. J. Blinder, Comparison of regional brain metabolism in bulimia nervosa and affective disorder assessed with positron emission tomography, *J. Affective Disord. 19*:153 (1990).

55. D. M. Garner and P. E. Garfinkel, The eating attitudes test: an index of the symptoms of anorexia nervosa, *Psychol. Med. 9*:273 (1979).

56. P. J. Andreason, M. Altemus, A. J. Zametkin, A. C. King, J. Lucinio, and R. M. Cohen, Regional cerebral glucose metabolism in bulimia nervosa, *Am. J. Psychiatry 149*:1506 (1992).

57. W. C. Drevets and M. E. Raichle, Positron emission tomographic imaging studies of human emotional disorders, *The Cognitive Neurosciences* (M. Gazzaniga, ed.), MIT Press, Cambridge, MA, 1995, pp. 1153–1164.

58. S. Nozoe, T. Naruo, Y. Nakabeppu, Y. Soejima, M. Nakajo, and H. Tanaka, Changes in regional cerebral blood flow in patients with anorexia nervosa detected through single photon emission tomography imaging, *Biol. Psychiatry 34*:578 (1993).

59. S. Nozoe, T. Naruo, R. Yonekura, Y. Nakabeppu, Y. Soejima, N. Nagai, M. Nakajo, and H. Tanaka, Comparison of regional cerebral blood flow in patients with eating disorders, *Brain Res. Bull. 36*:251 (1995).

60. V. Delvenne, F. Lotstra, S. Goldman, F. Biver, V. DeMaertelaer, J. Appelboom-Fondu, A. Schoutens, L. M. Bidaut, A. Luxen, and J. Mendelwicz, Brain hypometabolism of glucose in anorexia nervosa: a PET scan study, *Biol. Psychiatry 37*:161 (1995).

12

A Review of Magnetic Resonance Imaging Studies of Brain Abnormalities in Schizophrenia

Martha E. Shenton, Cynthia G. Wible, and Robert W. McCarley
Harvard Medical School, Boston; Brockton Veterans Affairs Medical Center, Brockton; Massachusetts Mental Health Center, Boston; and McLean Hospital, Belmont, Massachusetts

---

Part of Table 1, and parts of the introduction were adapted from M. E. Shenton, Temporal lobe structural abnormalities in schizophrenia: A selective review and presentation of new MR findings, *Psychopathology: The Evolving Science of Mental Disorders* (S. Matthysse, D. Levy, J. Kagan, and F. M. Benes, eds.), Cambridge University Press, New York, 1996, p. 51.

297

I. INTRODUCTION

A. Early Evidence Suggesting Brain Abnormalities in Schizophrenia

Schizophrenia is a major public health problem that affects close to 1% of the general population and is extremely costly to the patient, the patient's family, and the larger community. Currently there is no clear understanding of the pathology, and for this reason schizophrenia is categorized as a "functional" psychosis rather than an "organic" psychosis.

That schizophrenia has an organic basis, however, has been suspected since Kraepelin [1] and Bleuler [2] first delineated the syndrome(s). Kraepelin [1], in fact, believed that the symptoms of schizophrenia, which he called "dementia praecox," or early dementia, originated from abnormalities in both the frontal and temporal lobes. He believed that abnormalities in the frontal lobe were responsible for a disturbance in reasoning, while abnormalities in the temporal lobe were responsible for hallucinations and delusions. Bleuler [2] focused more on the symptoms of schizophrenia as the sine qua non of this disorder, and he coined the term "schizophrenia" both to describe and to highlight the observed separation between thought and affect in these patients. Bleuler [2] did not, however, agree with Kraepelin [1] that the course of schizophrenia was always progressive. Instead, he noted that some patients did not show a progressive deterioration. Like Kraepelin [1], however, he too believed that schizophrenia would ultimately be linked to abnormalities in the brain.

Other workers at the end of the nineteenth century, such as Crichton-Browne [3], as well as Alzheimer [4], Kahlbaum [5], and Hecker [6], also believed that to understand the etiology of schizophrenia, an understanding of the brain and its functions was necessary. Consequently, the end of the nineteenth century was a period in schizophrenia research marked by intense activity in both the classification of schizophrenia as well as in the investigation of neuroanatomical abnormalities in schizophrenia. During this time period the first real evidence in support of an organic basis for schizophrenia came from qualitative studies of postmortem brains. These studies showed enlarged lateral ventricles (e.g., Ref. 6) and widespread changes in the neocortex of schizophrenic patient, which were not associated with gliosis (e.g., Ref. 4). Later findings from autopsy and pneumoencephalography studies also suggested enlarged lateral ventricles in schizophrenia (e.g., Refs. 7–10) as well as tissue loss in the region of the superior temporal gyrus of the temporal lobe [8]. Moreover, the work of Jacobi and Winkler [9] was particularly influential because it supported Kraepelin's [1] speculation that schizophrenia was the result of damage to both the temporal and frontal lobes. These investigators, in fact, were the first to show a link between hallucinosis and temporal lobe damage and between intellectual deficits and frontal lobe damage.

More methodologically controlled postmortem studies, however, frequently led to negative findings (e.g., Refs. 11–14), and the interpretation of results became more tentative as concerns were raised about possible methodological artifacts. (See Seidman [15], and Kirch and Weinberger [16] for a more comprehensive review of the early postmortem studies in schizophrenia.) Such concerns led to further skepticism about the role of brain dysfunction in schizophrenia, and Dunlap [11,12], an important figure in american psychiatry during the early part of the twentieth century, concluded that there were no abnormalities observed in the postmortem studies of schizophrenic patients that could not also be observed in normal controls. Plum [17] meted the final blow when he stated that "schizophrenia is the graveyard of neuropathologists." Further investigations of brain abnormalities in schizophrenia were thus abandoned, and conclusions drawn from better controlled studies led to the conviction that neurological changes were not confirmed in the brains of schizophrenic patients.

While some researchers continued to believe that brain abnormalities were implicated in schizophrenia (e.g., Refs. 18–21), it was not until 1976, with the emerging technology of computed tomography (CT), that interest was rekindled by the first CT study of schizophrenia by Johnstone and coworkers [22]. In this study, enlarged lateral ventricles were reported in schizophrenic patients, thus confirming earlier pneumoencephalography studies (e.g., Refs. 9–10). This one study, using a new technology to view the brain, has now led to more than 100 CT studies investigating brain abnormalities in schizophrenia (see review by Shelton and Weinberger [23]). Most of these studies (75%) have reported enlarged lateral ventricles even though fewer than 10% of the CT scans have been interpreted as abnormal by a clinical neuroradiologist. That fewer than 10% of the scans have been interpreted as abnormal further emphasizes the subtlety of the changes noted in schizophrenia.

B. Current Interest in Brain Abnormalities in Schizophrenia

The current proliferation of studies investigating brain abnormalities in schizophrenia has continued both with the more recent postmortem studies (beginning with Scheibel and Kovelman [24,25]) and with the newer technology of magnetic resonance (MR) imaging (the first schizophrenia study was conducted by Smith and coworkers [26]). These newer studies, based on more reliably diagnosed patients (e.g., using DSM-III and DSM-III-R criteria [27,28]) and on more advanced quantitative measurement techniques, have fostered a renewed interest in investigating neuroanatomical abnormalities in the brains of schizophrenic patients. For the first time it now seems likely that major advances in schizophrenia research are at hand and that brain abnormalities will be delineated.

The first new findings, from postmortem studies, have shown a strong convergence of morphometric and neurohistological abnormalities in limbic and temporal lobe structures, which include the amygdala-hippocampal complex, and parahippocampal gyrus, as well as increases in the temporal horn of the lateral ventricle [29–38]. Many of these findings have been lateralized to the left temporal lobe, leading to speculation that schizophrenia may be an anomaly in the development of cerebral asymmetry (e.g., Ref. 33). Other postmortem findings, though less consistent across studies, have reported smaller overall brain size (e.g., Ref. 39) and abnormalities in the cingulate gyrus (e.g., Refs. 40, 41) and in the basal ganglia (e.g., Ref. 31). (For comprehensive reviews see Benes [42], Chua and McKenna [43], and Bogerts et al. [44].) These findings have had a powerful influence on the direction of MRI studies in schizophrenia.

This chapter reviews MRI findings in schizophrenia. MRI technology represents an advance in medical imaging that makes it possible to examine previously unmeasurable small brain structures in schizophrenic patients (for a more complete description of the principles of MRI and advances in MRI imaging, see Chapter 1). We here review MRI studies in schizophrenia, beginning with findings from whole brain and ventricular studies, followed by a review of temporal, frontal, parietal, and occipital lobe findings. This is followed by a section reviewing basal ganglia, thalamus, corpus callosum, cerebellum, and septi pellucidi studies.

Our own research in schizophrenia has focused primarily on the temporal lobe, a region of the brain that we think is importantly linked to schizophrenic pathology. We do not suggest, however, that temporal lobe abnormalities evinced in schizophrenia are isolated and not linked to other brain abnormalities. Instead, we recognize that the temporal lobe is highly connected with other brain areas, including the frontal lobe (e.g., Refs. 45–52), that brain function depends upon such interconnectivity, and that a finding of temporal or medial temporal lobe abnormalities does not imply that other brain areas, such as the frontal and parietal lobes, are not also critically involved in schizophrenic pathology. Accordingly, we suggest that abnormalities in one part of the brain, such as the temporal lobe, may be related to and may, indeed, be reflected by abnormalities in an interconnected network that is not proximal but nonetheless importantly linked.

It is within this context that we present a review of MRI findings in schizophrenia. For heuristic purposes, and because many MRI studies in schizophrenia have focused on specific structures within the temporal, frontal, parietal, and occipital lobes, we group the studies in this chapter by lobe.

We also include an extensive table (Table 1) listing 67 MRI studies. These studies are listed chronologically, from 1988 to the present, and they are listed alphabetically within each year. A reference number is also included so that the reader can more easily locate studies in the table that correspond to reference citations in the text and in the chapter references. No abstracts are included in the table because we wanted to include only studies that had received the scrutiny of peer-reviewed journals. We selected 1988 as the cut-off date because most MRI studies prior to this date were from first-generation MRI scanners, where the quality of the images was poorer than from second-generation MRI scanners (post-1988).* We also chose to pare down the size of the table by excluding studies that (a) had fewer than 10 subjects (e.g., Refs. 26,53), (b) focused primarily upon relaxation times, or qualitative ratings, rather than on area or volume measures (e.g., Refs. 54–58), (c) focused primarily on other modes of imaging such as cerebral blood flow (e.g., Ref. 59), (d) had subject groups too complicated to describe briefly [60], (e) did not include a control group and/or focused on family members (e.g., Refs. 61–64), or (f) focused solely on the corpus callosum, where measures were limited to one dimension (e.g., Refs. 65–71). In the interest of conserving space, we also chose to exclude from the table all MRI studies focusing solely on other MRI findings in schizophrenia, including basal ganglia, thalamus, corpus callosum, cerebellum, and septi pellucidi MRI studies in schizophrenia. These studies are nonetheless reviewed in the text (see Sec. II. F).

In addition to Table 1, we also include a summary table (Table 2) indicating the percent positive and negative findings for the MRI studies listed in Table 1. Here, as in the text of this chapter, we counted data sets only once. Thus, MRI studies that reported data from the same subjects in different studies that included, for example, a slightly different analysis such as adding a clinical correlate, were still counted only once, even if the data set was presented in more than one study listed in Table 1. We begin with a review of whole brain and ventricular MRI findings in schizophrenia.

II. REVIEW OF MRI FINDINGS IN SCHIZOPHRENIA

A. MRI Whole Brain and Ventricle Findings

1. Whole Brain

The role of brain size and its relation to mental illness can be traced as far back as Pinel [72]. Some investigators have even proposed that brain size is related to socioeconomic status, IQ, and, or, to cognitive defects [72–73],

---

* We note, however, that by selecting 1988 as the cut-off, we are excluding several early seminal studies such as Andreasen et al.'s 1986 MRI study [122].

Table 1 MR Imaging Studies in Schizophrenia

Author and ref.	WB	V	TL	FL	PL	OL	BG	O	Subject characteristics	Imaging parameters	Measurements	Findings
DeLisi et al., 1988 [152]			+						24 SZ, age 32, 10 F, 11 sets/sibs +2 unrelated 18 NCL, age 35, 7 F (families ≥ 2 SZ)	0.5 T; 1-cm thick contig. coronal slices (12)	Planimetric measurements on 2 slices: HIPP, AMYG, PHG	Bilat. ↓ AMYG-HIPP and PHG; (trend: ↓ L AMYG-HIPP, R PHG)
Kelsoe et al., 1988 [89]	*	+	–	–				–	27 SZ, age 29, 5 F, 2 LH, duration = 8.4 YR 14 NCL, age 31, 4 F, 1 LH	0.5 T; 1-cm thick contig. coronal slices (12–13)	Area/volume measures (not blind to diagnosis): cerebrum, prefrontal, TL, CC AMYG-HIPP, LAT VENT, caudate, globus pallidus/putamen	62% ↑ LAT VENT (esp. L), 73% ↑ 3rd VENT. No other differences
Rossi et al., 1988 [126]		+	+	+				+	12 SZ (chronic), age 32, 4 F, all RH, duration = 7.9 YR 12 NCL, age 31, 4 F, all RH (Ss matched: age, sex, & handedness)	0.5 T; 10-mm thick axial slice (1); 5-mm thick midsagittal slice (1)	Area measures: CC (midsagittal slice); 4th VENT & VBR (axial slice). Image intensity measures: TL and FL	↑ VBR & ↓ CC. Intensity differences prefrontal WM & ant. L TL on 1 pulse sequence, but not on other. No difference 4th VENT
Johnstone et al., 1989 [109]	*	+	+						21 SZ, age 36, 6 F, duration = ≥ 5 YR 20 Bipolars (12 M, age 35; 8 F, age 43)	0.15 T; 8-mm thick coronal slices (6–10) (1-cm gap)	Slice with largest area: total brain area (coronal surface), TL, LAT VENT	SZ: L TL < R (more than for NCL & BP). M SZ: ↑ LAT VENT esp. TH, and esp. in poor outcome SZ. F ↓ brain area than M

Study				Subjects	Scan parameters	Measures	Findings
Rossi et al., 1989 [149]		+		15 SZ, age 27, all M, all RH, duration = 4.26 YR; 11 NCL, age 28, all M, all RH; 21 NCL (16 M, age 33; 5 F, age 39) (Ss not matched SES)	0.5 T; 8-mm thick contig. coronal slices (7–8)	Linear area measurements by a radiologist on slice showing largest extent: TL	SZ: ↓ L TL. R TL > L TL in both SZ & NCL
Stratta et al., 1989 [127]	+	+	+	+ 20 (chronic) SZ, age 33, 5 F, all RH, educ = 11.85, duration = 8.23 YR; 20 NCL, age 32, 5 F (hosp. staff), all RH, educ = 17.1 YR (groups differ: educ)	0.5 T; 10-mm thick axial slices (8); 5-mm midsagittal scan (1)	Linear area measures: corpus callosum (CC) (midsagittal), 4th VENT, CC-to-brain ratio, asymmetry of hemispheres, & VBR	↑ VBR. No difference 4th VENT. Wider R frontal than L in SZ, but not in NCL (also > R frontal protuberance than NCL). NCL: ↑ CC brain ratio
Suddath et al., 1989 [128]	+	+	−	17 SZ (chronic), age 31, 7 F; 17 NCL, age 33, 7 F (Ss matched: age & sex)	0.5 T; 1-cm thick contig. coronal slices (12)	Volumes from computerized area measures: 3–4 slices for prefrontal lobe (total, GM & WM); 6–8 for TL (total/GM-anterior, central, posterior & WM), LATVENT	Ss overlap with Kelso et al. (1988) study. R TL > L TL, all Ss. 20% ↓ TL GM (18% ↓ R & 21% ↓ L). No ↓ TL WM, prefrontal GM or WM; ↓ L & ↓ R central TL GM 20% & 23%, corresponding to ant. HIPP region. Bilat. ↑ LATVENT 67%, related to L TL GM ↓

Table 1 (*continued*)

Author and ref.	WB	V	TL	FL	PL	OL	BG	O	Subject characteristics	Imaging parameters	Measurements	Findings
Andreasen et al., 1990 [115]	*	+		−				+	54 SZ (36 M, age 33, 18 F, age 35), 5 LH M, all F RH, educ = 13.6 M, 12.71 F, duration = > 10 YR; 47 NCL (28 M, age 33, 19 F, age 37), 3 mixed H M, 1 mixed H F, rest RH, educ = 14.57 M, 13.58 F	0.5 T; 1-cm thick contig. coronal slices (8)	Volume summed over slices: LAT VENT & 3rd VENT. Area measure: (single 1-cm slice) cranium, cerebral hemisphere, FL, & thalamus. (Ss matched: age, sex, SES, educ, ht. & wt)	M SZ: ↑ LAT VENT, ↑ cranial & ↓ thalamic, no differences 3rd VENT. Didn't replicate earlier (1986) finding of → cranial, ↓ cerebral & ↓ FL (but, differences in the Ss groups)
Barta et al., 1990 [90]	√	−	+						15 SZ, age 31, all M (living in community), 2 LH, educ = 12.3; 15 NCL, age 31, all M, 1 LH, educ = 12.8 (Ss matched: educ & PSES)	1.5 T; 3-mm thick contig. coronal slices of TL (9); 5-mm thick contig. axial slices of WB	Volumes: brain volume (GM/WM & VENT), TL (n = 9 slices), AMYG (n = 2), STG (n = 3), 3rd VENT (n = 2), & control regions (n = 1; pons & mid brain)	8.6% ↓ L AMYG, 11% ↓ L STG. (Trend for R TL & ↑ 3rd VENT). No differences in brain volume (2%) or control regions
Becker et al., 1990 [134]		+	+						10 SZ, age 26, all M, duration = 48 months. 10 NCL, age 26, all M	1.5 T; 4-mm contig. coronal slices (31)	Volumes summed over 8 slices: TL, HIPP, PHG, TH of the LAT VENT	R TL > L TL for both groups; SZ: ↓ HIPP, ↓ PHG & ↑ R TH
Bogerts et al., 1990 [75]		+	+						34 SZ (1st episode), age 25, 12 F, educ = 13.6, duration = 1.4 YR	1.0 T; 3.1-mm thick contig. coronal slices through WB (63). (WB to control for	Semiautomated computer measures: TL, HIPP/AMYG (structure, divided at mammilary	M SZ: ↓ L posterior HIPP (20%), bilat. ↓ AMYG-HIPP (9%), ↓ R TL (9%), ↑ L ant. TH

Reference	Markers	Subjects	MRI parameters	Measures	Findings
		25 NCL, age 28, 10 F (7 hosp. staff, 7 neurol with no brain abnormalities), educ = 16.7 (groups differ: ht. & educ)	overall cerebral volume)	bodies). TH of LAT VENT divided into anterior and posterior	(40%) & ↑ L total TH in both M SZ (15%) and F SZ (32%)
Dauphinais et al., 1990 [107]	* + +	12 SZ (n = 10) or SZAFF (n = 18) sib pairs & 4 Ss sibs refused, age 32, 13 F, duration = 12.8 YR 21 NCL, age 37, 9 F (NIMH staff & community volunteers)	0.5 T; 10-mm thick contig. coronal slices (12)	Area Measures: cerebrum, TL, 3rd VENT, LAT VENT (also TH), & AMYG-HIPP. A 2nd analysis used volume estimates: ROIs	No difference
Degreef et al., 1990 [129]	+	25 SZ (first episode) 17 NCL (Ss matched: sex & age)	1.0 T; 3.1-mm thick contig. coronal slices through WB	Volumes for ventricular system: LAT VENT: frontal horn (FH), occipital horn (OH), TH (anterior/posterior), plus 3rd & 4th VENTs	34% ↑ L LAT VENT: 20% ↑ FH (32% ↑ L & 20% ↑ R); 25% ↑ L OH; & 17% ↑ L TH (30% ↑ ant. part L TH). ↑ 3rd VENT
Nasrallah et al., 1990 [113]	* +	56 SZ, (41 M, age 32; 15 F, age 34), educ = 13.44 M, 13.93 F (M/F differ on educ) 35 NCL (15 M, age 27; 20 F, age 29), educ = 16.1 M, 15.1 F	1.5 T; 3-mm thick sagittal slices (8) (1-mm gap); 5-mm thick coronal slices (16–24) (5-mm gap)	Area measures: cranium, cerebrum, & frontal area. VBR, LAT VENT, & 3rd VENT (1 slice, 1-cm posterior to optic chiasm)	SZ F: (but not SZ M) ↓ craniums & ↓ brain, & ↑ LAT VENT & ↑ 3rd VENT. (Groups differ: age and educ)

Table 1 (*continued*)

Author and ref.	WB	V	TL	FL	PL	OL	BG	O	Subject characteristics	Imaging parameters	Measurements	Findings
Rossi et al., 1990 [91]	*	–	+	–				–	17 SZ, age 27, 7 F, all RH, duration = 4.4 YR (relapsing, noninstitutionalized) 13 NCL, 28, 3 F, all RH (Ss matched: educ)	0.5 T; 8-mm thick contig. coronal slices (7–8); 5-mm thick saggital slices (2)	Linear area measures by a radiologist: TL (n = 2 coronal slices); LAT VENT; (n = 1 coronal slice); cerebrum, frontal area, CC (2 saggital slices)	Ss overlap with Rossi et al. 1989 study. No differences in VBR, LAT VENT, cerebrum, CC, or frontal area, but SZ: ↓ L TL. (R TL > L TL in both groups)
Schwarzkopf et al., 1990 [135]			+						20 SZ, age 30, 9 F, duration = 9 YR 20 NCL, age 30, 9 F (Ss matched: PSES)	1.5 T; 5-mm thick coronal slices (20–30) (5-mm gap)	Volumes summed over slices: L & R LAT VENT, 3rd VENT, & cerebrum	↑ 3rd VENT but not LAT VENT. Age corr. with VENT measures in SZ, not NCL. 3rd VENT & LAT VENT cor. in SZ. No difference cerebrum
Suddath et al., 1990 [130]	+		+	–					15 SZ, twin pairs discordant for SZ, age 32, 7 F pairs, duration = 10.5 YR	1.5 T; 5-mm thick contig. coronal slices (30) (15-cm slab of brain covered)	Volume summed over slices: prefrontal & TL. n = 6 slices for: AMYG, ant. HIPP, 3rd VENT, & TH & body LAT VENT	SZ twin: ↓ L TL GM; bilat. ↓ HIPP (esp. L); No differences for L TL WM, prefrontal, or R TL (GM or WM); ↑ LAT VENT (L & R)
Blackwood et al., 1991 [92]	*	–	+	–				–	31 SZ, age 29, 7F, all RH, duration = 6 YR	0.08 T; 12-mm thick coronal slices (10)	Area measures: TL, AMYG-HIPP, PHG, head of caudate,	R TL > L TL in both groups; n.s. differences ICA or

Study	Coding	Subjects	MRI parameters	ROIs/measures	Results
	—	33 NCL, age 28, 8F, all RH (groups differed on IQ)		cingulate, frontal cortex, LAT VENT, 3rd VENT, thickness of corpus callosum. (Intracranial area [ICA] from 1 slice)	TL; L < R AMYG in NCL but not SZ. P300 latency correlated (−) with cingulate & (+) with difference between R & L AMYG in SZ. No diff. HIPP
DeLisi et al., 1991 [93]	* + − − −	30 SZ (1st episode), age 33, 7 F, all RH / 15 SZ (chronic), age 27, 6 F, 3 LH / 20 NCL (neurology Ss), age 29, 8 F, 2 LH (groups differ: PSES)	1.5 T; 5-mm thick coronal slices (30) (2-mm gap); 5-mm axial slices through WB (20) (2-mm gap)	Volume summed over slices: total brain volume (alternate slices), LAT VENT, 3rd VENT, FL, TL (missing posterior part), & AMYG-HIPP, PHG, caudate & lentiform nuclei	↑ LAT VENT (esp. L), but chr. SZ more ↑ LAT VENT than 1st episode. Only chr. SZ ↓ TL (esp. L). No difference FL, total brain volume, or other ROIs
Jernigan et al., 1991 [112]	* + + + − − +	42 SZ, age 30, 14 F, educ = 13.2, duration = 10 YR / 24 NCL, age 32, 5 F, educ = 15	1.5 T; 5-mm thick axial slices through WB (2.5-mm gap)	Volumes summed over slices: subcortical GM, VENT, & cortical GM, (n = 6 slices), cranial volume (superior & inferior divisions)	↓ AMYG, HIPP, PHG, lateral orbitofrontal regions & ↑ cortical CSF. No difference VENT. Cortical GM ↓ (not related to cranial vol.). ↓ Superior cranial volume in non–substance-abusing SZ. ↑ Lenticular nuclei, related to earlier age onset

Table 1 (*continued*)

Author and ref.	WB	V	TL	FL	PL	OL	BG	O	Subject characteristics	Imaging parameters	Measurements	Findings
Rossi et al., 1991 [148]		+							16 BP, age 47, all M, all RH 10 SZ, age 29, all M, all RH (groups differ: age)	0.5 T; 5-mm thick coronal slices (15) (2-mm gap)	Volume summed over 5 coronal slices: L & R TL. Analyses co-varied for age	Ss overlap Rossi et al. 1989/1990 studies. Bilat. ↓ TL (esp. L); TL > on R than L in both groups
Shenton et al., 1991 [136]		+							12 SZ, age 40, all M, all RH, duration = 10 YR 10 NCL, age 40, all M, all RH	1.5 T; 5-mm contig. axial slices (24) (120-mm slab of brain covered)	Computerized segmentation/ Volume of ventricular system: summed over slices	No difference LAT VENT; L > R LAT VENT in NCL. Deviation from (L > R) in SZ: related to ↑ thought disorder.
Young et al., 1991 [124]		+	+					–	31 SZ, age 29, 7 F, all RH, duration = 6 YR 33 NCL, age 28, 8 F, all RH (groups differ: IQ)	0.08 T; 12-mm thick coronal slices (10)	Tracing of digitized images: TL, AMYG-HIPP, PHG, caudate nucleus, LAT & 3rd VENT	Same Ss as Blackwood et al. (1991). R TL > L TL both groups; L AMYG < R in NCL; L PHG < R in SZ; (+) symptoms assoc. ↑ VBR; (>) symptoms assoc. with ↓ head of caudate (but n.s. from NCL)
Bornstein et al., 1992 [131]		+							72 SZ, age 33, 23 F, duration = 9 YR 31 NCL, age 29, 18 F (groups differ: age)	1.5 T; 5-mm thick coronal slices (20–30) (5-mm gap)	Volume summed over slices: L & R LAT VENT, 3rd VENT. VBR calculated for LAT VENT & 3rd VENT	↑ 3rd VENT assoc. with neuropsych attention & frontal lobe function. No such relation for LAT VENT. F SZ ↑ LAT VENT

Study	Markers	Subjects	MRI Technique	Volumes Measured	Findings
Breier et al., 1992 [95]	√ + + +	44 SZ, age 36, 15 F, 9 LH, duration = 14.7 YR; 29 NCL, age 34, 9 F, 5 LH (Ss matched: head of household SES)	2.0 T; 3-mm thick contig. coronal slices through WB	Volume summed over slices: ICV, AMYG/HIPP, prefrontal cortex (n = 13 slices), & caudate (head & body)	No differences between groups ICV; SZ bilat. ↓ AMYG; ↓ L HIPP; bilat. ↓ prefrontal WM; & ↑ L caudate. R prefrontal WM assoc. R AMYG/HIPP
Degreef et al., 1992 [132]	+	40 SZ (1st episode), age 24, 15 F, educ = 13.6; 25 NCL, age 28, 10 F, educ = 16.7 (groups differ: age, sex, & education)	1.0 T; 3.1-mm thick contig. coronal slices (63)	Volume summed over slices: frontal horn (FH), central part, occipital horn (OH), temporal horn (TH), LAT VENT, 3rd & 4th VENT assessed	Ss overlap Degreef et al. (1990) study. ↑ total ventricular volume; ↑ all parts LAT VENT (17–40%); ↑ 3rd VENT & ↑ TH. M Ss > ↑ LAT VENT & TH than F Ss
DeLisi et al., 1992 [94]	* + − −	50 Schizophreniform/acute SZAFF (1st episode, ill < 6 mo.), age 26, 18 F, 28; Schizophreniform/acute SZAFF (1st episode at 2 YR FUP), age 27, 13 F; 34 NCL (n = 20 neurol. Ss), age 28, 15 F	1.5 T; 5-mm thick axial slices through WB (2-mm gap)	Volumes summed over slices: L & R hemispheres, total brain volume, TL, FL, & LAT VENT	Ss overlap Delisi et al. (1991) study. F bilat. ↓ hemispheres. SZ: no differences in LAT VENT, total brain volume or TL. At 2 year FUP, SZ with ↑ LAT VENT at onset had poorer outcome. Of 24 at FUP, 20% ↑ LAT VENT & 20% ↓. Trend ↑ LAT VENT

Table 1 (*continued*)

Author and ref.	WB	V	TL	FL	PL	OL	BG	O	Subject characteristics	Imaging parameters	Measurements	Findings
Di Michele et al., 1992 [147]			+						25 SZ, age 28, 12 F, all RH, educ = 11.5 (living in community), duration = no > than 6 mth. contin. hospitalization. 17 NCL, age 27, 7 F (hosp. staff/rel), all RH, educ = 11.7	0.5 T; 8-mm thick contig. coronal slices (7)	Linear area measures: 2 slices used for TL. Surface of cortex measured	Bilat. ↓TL, L side < R in 1 slice. SZ divided into cognitive normal/abnormal on Luria/Nebraska Neuropsych battery. Abn. group ↑TL anomalies
Hoff et al., 1992 [78]	−		+						56 schizophreniform, age 26, 15 F, 9 LH, educ = 12.3. 57 NCL, age 29, 18 F, 9 LH, educ = 14.7 (groups differ: age & education)	1.5 T; 5-mm thick axial, coronal, & sagittal slices through WB (2-mm gap) (WB to control for cerebral volume)	Volume summed over slices: LAT VENT, TL, AMYG, HIPP, total limbic complex. Linear measure: length lateral sulcus	F SZ: < lateralization (L > R) of lateral sulcus & a correlation between < lateralization & better performance on cognitive measures
Raine et al., 1992 [145]			−	+					17 SZ, age 35, 7 F, all RH, educ = 12.6, PSES = 5.1, duration = 9.9 YR. 18 Psych. ctrls., age 36, 6 F, all RH, educ = 12.5, PSES = 5.3	0.15 T; 10-mm thick contig. coronal slices (12). Also, 10-mm thick midsaggital slice (1) & 10-mm thick axial slice (1)	Area measures: 1 coronal, 1 axial, & 1 midsaggital slice used for measuring L/R prefrontal; 1 coronal slice for L/R TL	↓L prefrontal area for coronal cut (R p < 0.065). For sagittal & axial cuts, bilat. ↓ prefrontal area. No differences: L or R TL

Study				Subjects	MRI technique	Measures	Findings
Rossi et al., 1992 [165]	+			19 NCL, age 34, 9 F, all RH, educ = 12.8, PSES = 4.7; 20 SZ (chronic/subchronic), 5 F, all RH; 12 NCL, (employees/relatives hosp. staff), all RH, (Ss matched for age [within 3 yrs.], sex, & educ [within 1 year])	0.5 T; 3-mm thick coronal slices (15)(1-mm gap) (3 SZ & 1 NCL, data no good [Ss = 17 SZ, 11 NCL])	Area measures: Planum temporale (PT), indirectly measured using length of bank of sylvian fissure	SZ: no L > R PT asymmetry, which NCL showed
Schwartz et al., 1992 [137]	+			48 SZ, age 32, 16 F, (living in community); 51 NCL, age 30, 12 F	1.5 T; 5-mm thick contig. axial slices	7 pt. rating scale adapted from Alzheimer's disease study: sylvian fissure, TL sulci, LAT VENT (TH), 3rd VENT, cerebral sulci	Sylvian fissure higher on R than L (lesser extent in NCL). > Sylvian fissure. No other differences but range of scores restricted
Shenton et al., 1992 [96]	√	+ +	−	15 SZ, age 37, all M, all RH, duration = 15.8 YR; 15 NCL, age 37, all M, all RH (Ss matched: age & sex; no difference on PSES)	1.5 T; 3-mm thick contig. axial slices through WB (54); 1.5-mm thick contig. coronal slices through WB (124)	Semiautomated segmentation & volume measures: ICV, GM, WM, CSF LAT VENT (TH), 3rd & 4th VENT, cerebral sulci, TL, AMYG-HIPP, PHG, STG, & FL (control area: superior frontal gyrus)	↓ GM: 19% ↓ L ant. AMYG-HIPP, 13% ↓ L PHG, 8% ↓ R PHG & 15% ↓ L STG. L STG ↓ assoc. ↑ TDI ($r = -0.81$). No ↓ ICV, TL, nor FL control region. Variance ↑ L LAT VENT, 180% ↑ L TH, 74% ↑ R TH

Table 1 *(continued)*

Author and ref.	WB	V	TL	FL	PL	OL	BG	O	Subject characteristics	Imaging parameters	Measurements	Findings
Swayze et al., 1992 [146]			–					+	54 SZ (36 M age 32; 18 F, age 35) 5 LH, 1 mixed 48 BP (29 M, age 33; 19 F, age 35), 5 LH, 4 mixed 47 NCL 28 M, 19 F; 4 mixed H	0.5 T; 1-cm thick coronal slices (8)	Planimetric measures on 3–4 slices, summed: TL, caudate, putamen & AMYG-HIPP (1 slice for AMYG)	R TL > L TL for all except BPs. No differences in HIPP, AMYG, or TL measures. M SZ: ↑ putamen &, to lesser extent, ↑ caudate
Zipursky et al., 1992 [108]	*	+	+	+	+	–	+		22 SZ, age 34, all M, all RH, educ = 12.5, duration = 11.3 YR 20 NCL, age 36, all M, all RH, educ = 15.5 (groups differ: educ & IQ)	1.5 T; 5-mm thick axial slices (17–20) (2.5-mm gap) (3.5-cm slab of brain covered)	Volume summed over 2–7 slices: ICV, CSF, LAT VENT, 3rd VENT, & 6 parts of cortex (prefrontal, frontal, fronto-temporal, temporo-parietal, parietal, & parietal-occipital)	↑ LAT VENT & ↑ total CSF; ICV no difference. ↓ GM in: prefrontal, frontal, fronto-temporal, temporo-parietal, & parietal-occipital areas (not parietal area). No differences in 3rd VENT
Bartley et al., 1993 [168]				+					10 MZ twins discordant for SZ, age 33, 5 F, 4 LH 10 MZ NCL twins, age 31, 4 F, 2 LH	1.5 T; 1.5-mm thick contig. coronal slices through WB (124)	Measured length & angle of sylvian fissures by tracing & measuring on 3D reconstructions: anterior, posterior, horizontal segments	L side longer than the R in RH twins. R steeper than L &, in posterior region, this more pronounced in 2nd born twins. No differences between groups

Study				Subjects	MRI Method	Volume/Area Method	Findings
Bogerts et al., 1993 [76]	+	+	+	19 (chronic) SZ, age 28, all M, duration = 7.8 YR, educ = 13; 18 NCL, age 28, all M, educ = 16.7 (groups differ: educ)	1.0 T; 3.1-mm contig. coronal slices through WB (63) (WB used to control for cerebral volume)	Volume summed over slices: AMYG-HIPP & mesiotemporal volume. Mammillary bodies used to divide AMYG/HIPP	Bilat. ↓ HIPP; ↓ total mesiotemporal (11%; L = 20%; R = 15% HIPP portion). Psychotic factor (BPRS) assoc. with ↓ L & R mesiotemporal
Buchanan et al., 1993 [97]	*	+	+	41 SZ (17 deficit [D]), age 36, 5 F, 4 LH, educ = 11.6, SES = 4.7 (24 non-deficit[ND]), age 36, 10 F, 5 LH, educ = 13.2, SES = 3.6; 30 NCL, age 34, 10 F, 5 LH, educ = 14.3, SES = 3.1	2.0 T operating at 1.5 T; 3-mm thick contig. coronal slices through WB	Volume summed over slices: ICV estimated from every other slice; L & R prefrontal, AMYG/HIPP, & caudate	No difference ICV. No difference D/ND for caudate. AMYG/HIPP. D ↑ L caudate (trend for R) & ↓ bilat. AMYG/HIPP compared to NCL. ND ↓ bilat. prefrontal WM, ↓ bilat. AMYG/HIPP & ↑ L caudate, compared to NCL. No assoc. prefrontal vol. & deficit symptoms
Colombo et al., 1993 [98]	*	–	–	18 SZ, age 28, 6 F, educ = 2 (9–13 YR); 18 NCL, age 33, 5 F, educ = 2.3 (groups differ educ)	0.5 T; 5-mm thick coronal slices (8) (1.5-mm gap)	Area measures (n = 3 slices): cerebrum, LAT & 3rd VENT, TH LAT VENT, TL, HIPP	No differences between groups on any of the measures

Table 1 (continued)

Author and ref.	WB	V	TL	FL	PL	OL	BG	O	Subject characteristics	Imaging parameters	Measurements	Findings
Harvey et al., 1993 [110]	*	+	+	+	+				48 SZ, age 31, 11 F, educ = 12, 5 LH 34 NCL, age 32, 15 F, 4 LH, educ = 13.2, (ratio of M:F > patients; Ss matched: ethnicity & PSES)	0.5 T; 5-mm thick contig, coronal slices (20); 5-mm thick contig. axial slices through WB (24)	Volume summed over slices: ICV, TL & most of FL, cortex, sulci, subcortical nuclei, AMYG/ HIPP, body & TH of LAT VENT, sylvian fissure	↓ anterior cerebrum (FL/PL, but mostly TL) assoc. ↑ cortical sulci. M/F, ethnicity & ht. related to ICV (>M); TL GM ↓ (> on R); L LAT VENT ↑ F SZ, not M SZ. Unemployment/ poor premorbid predicted ↓ cerebral & ↑ sulci. ↑ Sylvian fissure
Kawasaki et al., 1993 [99]	*	+	+					−	20 SZ, age 29, all M, all RH, educ = 14.3, duration = 6.7 YR, 10 NCL, age 30, all M, all RH, educ > 18, (groups differ: educ & SES)	1.5 T; 5-mm thick coronal slices through the TL (prefrontal & occipital areas missing); 5-mm thick axial slices (vertex missing)	Volumes summed over slices: cerebrum, prefrontal, TL, AMYG/HIPP, PHG, LAT VENT, 3rd VENT, & corpus callosum	↓ L PHG & ↑ L TH of LAT VENT & ↑ R body of LAT VENT. R TL > L TL in SZ & NCL. No other differences. Trend for (−) correlation between (+) symptoms & L TH
McCarley et al., 1993 [84]	√	+	+					−	15 SZ, age 37, all M, all RH, duration = 15.8 YR	1.5 T; 3-mm thick contig. axial slices through WB (54); 1.5-mm	Semiautomated segmentation and volume summed: ICV, GM, WM,	Same Ss as Shenton et al. (1992). ↓ L post. STG GM assoc. P300

Study					Subjects	Method	Areas	Findings
	√	+	+	−	15 NCL, age 37, all M, all RH (Ss matched: age & sex, & no difference on PSES)	thick contig. coronal slices through WB (124)	CSF (intraventricular & subarachnoidal), TL, AMYG/HIPP, PHG, STG & FL control areas: (superior frontal & cingulate gyri)	amplitude ↓ & L < R P300 topography. No assoc. with other TL or FL control areas. No correlation in NCL
Nestor et al., 1993 [85]	√	+	+	−	15 SZ, age 37, all M, all RH, duration = 15.8 YR 15 NCL, age 37, all M, all RH (Ss matched: age & sex, no difference on PSES)	1.5 T; 3-mm thick contig. axial slices through WB (54); 1.5-mm thick contig. coronal slices through WB (124)	Semiautomated segmentation and volume summed: ICV, GM, WM, CSF (intraventricular & subarachnoidal), TL, AMYG/HIPP, PHG, STG & FL control areas: (superior frontal & cingulate gyri)	Same Ss as Shenton et al. (1992). SZ correlation between ↓ scores on verbal memory, abstraction, & categorization, & ↓ TL areas, including PHG & posterior STG (L & R), suggesting a possible dysfunctional semantic system in SZ
O'Donnell et al., 1993 [86]	√	+	+	−	15 SZ, age 37, all M, all RH, duration = 15.8 YR 15 NCL, age 37, all M, all RH (Ss matched: age & sex, no difference on PSES)	1.5 T; 3-mm thick contig. axial slices through WB (54); 1.5-mm thick contig. coronal slices through WB (124)	Semiautomated segmentation and volume summed: ICV, GM, WM, CSF (intraventricular & subarachnoidal), TL, AMYG/HIPP, PHG, STG & FL control areas: (superior frontal & cingulate gyri)	Same Ss as Shenton et al. (1992). N2 amplitude ↓ assoc. ↓ L STG GM, ↓ bilat. medial TL structures, & to chronicity. P3 amplitude ↓ assoc. with ↓ L post. STG, & delusions/ thought disorder

Table 1 (continued)

Author and ref.	WB	V	TL	FL	PL	OL	BG	O	Subject characteristics	Imaging parameters	Measurements	Findings
Andreasen et al., 1994 [111]	√	+	+	+	+	+		+	52 SZ, age 30, 16 F, duration = > 10 YR, PSES = 13.3 YR 90 NCL, age 27, 42 F, PSES = 13 YR	1.5 T; 1.5-mm thick contig. coronal slices through WB (124)	Volume summed over slices: ICV, CSF, FL, TL, PL, OL, cerebellum, VENT (intraventricular CSF)	36 M SZ/all NCL part of Andreasen et al. (1994) study. SZ M: ↓ ICV, ↑ total CSF/↑ VENT, & ↓ FL, ↓ TL, ↓ PL, ↓ OL & ↑ CSF/all lobes. F SZ: ↑ total CSF, ↑ CSF FL/TL, & ↓ FL & ↓ cerebellum
Bilder et al., 1994 [100]	*	–			+	+		+	70 (1st episode SZ/ SZ AFF), age 26, 31 F, educ = part college 51 NCL, age 28, 22 F, educ = college grad (groups differed: ht., ethnicity, & educ; no difference: PSES or handedness)	1.0 T; 3.1-mm thick contig. coronal slices through WB (63) [Some slices missing (due to artifact), so Ss "n" varied for ROIs]	Volume summed over slices: cortical GM & hemispheric WM but not subcortical structures. This included: occipitoparietal (OL/ PL), sensorimotor, premotor, prefrontal & TL regions	M > F OL/PL & TL. NCL:L hemisphere > R for OL/PL & sensorimotor areas; R hemisphere > L in premotor, prefrontal, & TL areas. SZ n.s. in regional or hemispheric volume but ↓ asymmetry than NCL-significant in OL/PL, premotor, & prefrontal

Study				Subjects	Imaging	Measures	Findings
DeLisi et al., 1994 [167]	+			85 SZ/SZ AFF/ Schizophreniform (1st episode), age 27, 35 F (7 M & 4 F LH), PSES = 3.4 (1 = highest, 5 = lowest) 40 NCL, age 27, 16 F, (2 M & 4 F LH), PSES = 2.8	1.5 T; 5-mm thick coronal slices (30)(2-mm gap)	Linear area measures: Each slice containing sylvian fissure used to measure length of planum temporale (PT) (@ 11 slices). Volume of STG measured (Total area of PT > than that reported in other studies)	No difference SZ/ NCL total PT. NCL: length of sylvian fissure longer on R side ant., but longer on L side post. (corresponding to PT). SZ: less R > L asymmetry ant., & F SZ showed a trend for less L > R asymmetry post. (n = 2 slices). No differences ant. STG volume
Egan et al., 1994 [133]	+	+	— —	16 SZ, age 30, 3 F, all RH, educ = 12.6, duration = 9.1 YR 16 NCL, age 31, 3 F, all RH, educ = 13.7 (Ss matched: age, sex, educ)	0.5 T; 1-cm thick contig. coronal slices (12)	Area and volume measures summed across slices: TL GM & WM (5 1-cm slices); HIPP & AMYG (1 slice), FL GM & WM (5 slices), total volume (12 slices), PL (1 slice). 3rd VENT & LAT VENT (2 slices)	Ss overlap with Suddath et al. (1989) study. No differences FL GM or WM or in PL. SZ: ↑ LAT VENT & ↑ 3rd VENT. Total TL ↓, TL GM ↓, TL WM ↓, bilat. ↓ AMYG & HIPP (esp. on L). Correlations between HIPP & N200 & between R HIPP & visual P300

Table 1 (*continued*)

Author and ref.	WB	V	TL	FL	PL	OL	BG	O	Subject characteristics	Imaging parameters	Measurements	Findings
Goldberg et al., 1994 [125]	+	+	+						15 MZ twin pairs discordant for SZ, age 32, 7 F pairs, duration = 10.5 YR	1.5 T; 5-mm thick contig. slices (30) (15-cm of brain covered). [10 of twins also rCBF study (6 M/4 F)]	Volume summed over slices: HIPP, 3rd VENT, large section of LAT VENT	Ss same as Suddath et al. (1990). ↓ L HIPP assoc. ↑ (+) symptoms & logical memory. (↓ prefrontal rCBF assoc. ↑ (−) symptoms & to persev. on WCST)
Gur et al., 1994 [114]	√	+							81 SZ (50 M, age 30; 31 F, age 32), all RH, educ = 13, duration = ≤2 YR 81 NCL (50 M, age 28; 31 F, age 30), all RH, educ = 14.6 (groups differ: educ, not PSES)	1.4 T; 5-mm thick contig. slices through WB	Volume summed over slices: brain, ventricular & sulcal CSF. Also: VBR = (ventricular CSF/ brain volume * 100) & SBR = (sulcal CSF/brain volume * 100)	Gender: M ↑ brain volume, M ↑ CSF volume, F ↑ VBR; SZ: ↓ brain volume, ↑ VBR; F SZ ↑ SBR. (−) symptom SZ ↑ VENT CSF but *not* ↓ brain volume, whereas (+) symptom SZ ↓ brain volume but *not* ↑ VENT CSF
Kleinschmidt et al., 1994 [79]								−	26 SZ (1st episode), age 30, 13 F, all RH, educ = 14.3 26 NCL (med or psych students), age 25, 13 F, all RH, educ ≥ 15 (groups differ: age, educ, SES)	1.5 T; 1.17-mm thick contig. sagittal slices through WB (128)	Linear area measures on tracings: Steinmetz et al. (1990) PT criteria used. Manual tracings on GM provided curved length measures	No differences between groups were found

Study				Subjects	MRI Method	Measurement	Findings
Kikinis et al., 1994 [169]	+	−		15 SZ, age 37, all M, all RH, duration = 15.8 YR; 15 NCL, age 37, all M, all RH (Ss matched: age & sex, no difference on PSES)	1.5 T; 3-mm thick contig. axial slices through WB (54); 1.5-mm thick contig. coronal slices through WB (124)	3D surface renderings of L & R TL & FL to make qualitative ratings: sulcal gyral pattern (> horizontal or vertical) & quantitative ratings based on geometry limited diffusion	Ss same as Shenton et al. (1992). SZ: qualitative rating: ↑ vertical sulci in the L TL. NCL: showed ↑ horizontal sulci. Quantitative rating: ↑ TL sulci (>L) in SZ. No differences FL
Marsh et al., 1994 [105]	*	+	+	33 SZ, age 31, 8 F, duration = 11.5 YR; 41 NCL, age 33, 14 F (hosp. Staff or community volunteer)	0.5 T; 10-mm thick contig. coronal slices (12)	Volume summed over 2 consecutive coronal slices: cerebrum, 3rd VENT, LAT VENT. 1 anterior/1 posterior slice: AMYG-HIPP	M > cerebrum F (R hemisphere); SZ: bilat. ↓ AMYG, ↓ HIPP, & ↓ AMYG-HIPP; ↑ 3rd VENT; ↑ LAT VENT (28.6%)
Rossi et al., 1994 [101]	*	+	+	19 SZ, age 33, all M, living in community, all RH, educ = 10.4, duration = 11.57 YR; 14 NCL, age 31, all M, RH, educ = within 3 YR of SZ	0.25 T; 5-mm thick coronal slices through WB (1-mm gap)	Volume summed over slices: brain volume, LAT VENT, & 3rd VENT, (3 slices). Caudate, lenticular nucleus, putamen, nucleus accumbens, AMYG/HIPP (2 slices on average)	↓ AMYG-HIPP (>L); ↑ 3rd VENT; & trend for ↓ BG (L putamen & L lenticular nuclei), & trend for ↓ ↑ VBR ratio & ↓ limbic structures. No differences: brain volumes

Table 1 (continued)

Author and ref.	WB	V	TL	FL	PL	OL	BG	O	Subject characteristics	Imaging parameters	Measurements	Findings
Rossi et al., 1994 [166]	+								22 SZ, age 30, 9 F, all RH, duration = 7.1 YR. 23 NCL, age 32, 10 F, all RH (nurses & employees med. center)	0.5 T; 2-mm thick contig. axial slices (29)	Linear area measures: Used Steinmetz et al. (1991) criteria to assess planum temporale (PT) on 1 slice	Ss overlap with Rossi et al. (1992). L PT > R PT both groups. SZ split into (+) thought disorder (−) thought disorder groups. ↑ thought disorder assoc. with ↓ PT asymmetry
Schlaepfer et al., 1994 [105]	*		+	+	+			−	46 SZ, age 32, 14 F, educ = 12. 60 NCL, age 32, 17 F, educ = 14.3. 27 BP, age 35, 11 F, educ = 14.3 (SZ differ: race & educ)	1.5 T; 5-mm thick contig. axial slices through WB	Volume summed over slices for 5 regions: dorsolateral prefrontal, inferior parietal, STG, sensory & motor areas, & OL. [10 slices used to measure the cortical "rim" for these regions & for estimate of WB]	↓ prefrontal, ↓ inferior parietal, & ↓ STG (heteromodal assoc. areas); no differences: control GM (sensory motor or OL), total GM, or CSF%. Trend for SZ ↓ brain volume ($p < 0.07$)
Zipursky et al., 1994 [88]	*		+	+	+				22 SZ (n = 3 SZAFF), age 34, all M, all RH, duration = 11.3 YR, educ = 12.5. 20 NCL, age 36, all M, all RH, educ	1.5 T; 3-mm thick contig. coronal slices (22); 5-mm thick axial slices used to estimate WB (2.5-mm gap)	Volume summed over slices: TL, STG, HIPP, LAT VENT (TH & body), 3rd VENT, frontal-parietal reference (FPRA), &	Ss same as in Zipursky et al. (1992). No diff. ICV; SZ ↑ CSF in TL sulci compared to FPRA (L & R); also ↑ CSF in TL

Study				Subjects	Measures	Findings
				= 15.5 (groups differ: educ & IQ)	intracranial volume (ICV) estimate	sulci & FPRA (L & R) compared to NCL. SZ ↓ GM STG (L & R), ↓ GM TL, & ↓ GM FPRA; ↑ LAT VENT & ↑ 3rd VENT. No diff. HIPP volume
Corey-Bloom et al., 1995 [77]	+	–	–	16 SZ (onset > 45 yr.), age 59, 5 F, 2 LH, educ = 12; 14 SZ (onset < 45 yr.), age 59, 4 F, all RH, educ = 13.1; 28 NCL, age 61, 15 F, 3 LH, educ = 13.2 (no differences: age, sex, educ or handedness)	1.5 T; 5-mm thick axial slices through WB (2.5-mm gap)	Volume summed over slices: cortical fluid, LAT VENT, caudate, lenticular nucleus, thalamus, dorsal frontal cortical GM, mesial TL GM, & cerebral WM; SZ with late onset SZ ↑ LAT VENT compared to NCL & early onset SZ. No differences among groups in any other measures
Flaum et al., 1995 [102]	*	+	+	102 SZ, age 32, 32 F, educ = 12.6, duration = 17.4 months; 87 NCLS, age 30, 42 F, educ = 14.8 [groups differ: ht. (M & F NCLs taller), educ, IQ, & ratio M/F]	1.5 T; 5-mm thick axial slices through WB (2.5-mm gap); 3-mm thick coronal slices thru central 2/3rds of brain for smaller cortical structures (1.5-mm gap)	Volume summed over slices: ICV, cerebrum, cerebellum, TL, LAT VENT (TH), STG, 3rd VENT, HIPP, caudate, thalamus, AMYG, putamen, & globus pallidus; ↑ LAT VENT & ↑ 3rd VENT; ↓ thalamus, ↓ STG, ↓ HIPP. No difference ICV, cerebellum, TL, TH, or caudate. No difference: L/R TL. All groups L > R for LAT VENT & thalamus; R > L for TH, STG, & caudate

Table 1 (*continued*)

Author and ref.	WB	V	TL	FL	PL	OL	BG	O	Subject characteristics	Imaging parameters	Measurements	Findings
Kulynych et al., 1995 [80]	−								12 SZ, age 30, all M, all RH; 12 NCL, age 26, all M, all RH	1.5 T; 1.5-mm thick contig. sagittal slices through WB (124)	Linear area measures 3D surface renderings to assess surface planum temporale (PT) & Heschl's gyrus	L PT > R PT in both groups. No difference between groups for Heschl's gyrus
Nopoulos et al., 1995 [103]	√	+	−	+			−	−	24 SZ/SZAFF (n = 2) (1st episode), age 23, 12 F, duration = 14 weeks; 24 NCL, age 24, 12 F, (Ss matched: PSES & and parents education)	1.5 T; 1.5-mm thick contig. coronal slices through WB (124)	Volume summed over slices: ICV, total brain tissue, TL, FL, PL, OL, & total CSF (including ventricular CSF & surface/intersulcal CSF)	Ss overlap with Andreasen et al. (1994) study. No difference: total brain volume/ICV, but SZ ↑ CSF (total ventricular & surface/intersulcal CSF). SZ: ↓ FL. No other differences
O'Donnell et al., 1995 [81]		+							47 SZ, age 40, all M, all RH, (15 MRI scans), duration = 17.2 YR; 47 NCL, age 40, all M, all RH (Ss matched: age & sex, no difference on PSES)	1.5 T; 1.5-mm thick contig. coronal slices through WB (124)	Volume summed over slices: STG, AMYG/HIPP, TL, PHG	Overlap in Ss with Shenton et al. (1992) study. SZ: P300 latency ↑ with age (not so in NCL), suggesting neurodegeneration. Also, ↓ L post. STG GM ↑ with age in SZ

Reference				Subjects	Method	Measures	Findings
Petty et al., 1995 [82]		+		14 SZ, age 37, 5 F, all RH; 14 NCL, age 37, 5 F, all RH (Ss matched: PSES)	1.5 T; 1.5-mm thick contig. coronal slices through WB (124)	Linear area measures: Length of PT: Steinmetz et al., 1989 criteria. Also, 3D reconstructions of PT to tesselate surface with triangles	NCL: L > R PT. In SZ there was a reversal (R > L PT in 13/15 SZ). SZ with ↑ thought disorder showed ↑ reversed asymmetry
Vita et al., 1995 [104]	*	+ −	−	19 (6 chronic, 13 subchronic), age 26, 7 F, educ = 9.8, duration = 1.6 YR; 15 NCL, age 29, 6 F (10 community & 5 Ss minor head trauma seen in emergency room), educ = 12.9	0.5 T; 5-mm thick coronal slices (2-mm gaps)	Volume summed over slices: Total cranial volume (?), prefrontal, TL, STG, LAT VENT (FH, TH, OH). (GM & WM combined)	No difference cranial volume, prefrontal or TL. STG also n.s. (but GM & WM combined); ↑ LAT VENT (> body & OH); [↑ thought disorder assoc. with ↓ prefrontal & ↓ L STG, but ↑ R STG]
Wible et al., 1995 [83]		+	−	14 SZ, age 37, all M, all RH; 15 NCL, age 37, all M, all RH (Ss matched: age & sex, no differences: PSES)	1.5 T; 1.5-mm thick contig. coronal slices through WB (124)	Volume summed over slices: average of n = 36 slices for prefrontal GM, n = 25 for prefrontal WM. (Correlations with TL measures from Shenton et al., 1992 study)	Ss same as Shenton et al., (1992) study. No differences prefrontal WM/GM, but L prefrontal GM assoc. with L STG, L PHG, & L AMYG-HIPP. (−) symptoms assoc. (−) with L prefrontal WM

Table 1 (*continued*)

Author and ref.	WB	V	TL	FL	PL	OL	BG	O	Subject characteristics	Imaging parameters	Measurements	Findings
Kulynych et al., 1996 [157]	+								12 SZ, age 26, all M, all RH 12 NCL, age 30, all M, all RH	1.5 T; 1.5-mm thick contig. coronal slices through WB (124)	Volume summed over slices: ICV. ICV & STG also from 3D surface renderings	Ss same as in Kulynych et al. (1995) study. L > R whole STG (GM & WM) for both groups. This asymmetry significant only for NCL. No differences L/R whole STG. GM of STG not reported
Sullivan et al., 1996 [87]	*	+	+	+	+		–	+	34 SZ, age 37, all M, all RH, educ = 12.8 47 NCL, age 38, all M, all RH, educ = 16.3 (Ss	1.5 T; 5-mm thick axial slices (17–20) (2.5-mm gaps) (3.5-cm slab of brain covered)	Volume summed over 2–7 slices: ICV, GM, WM, & CSF, 3rd & LAT VENT, & 6 parts of cortex (prefrontal, frontal,	SZ same as in Zipursky et al., (1992) study. ↓ cortical GM, but no ↑ cortical sulci or WM. Total

matched: age & handedness)

fronto-temporal, temporoparietal, parietal, & parietal-occipital)

neuropsych correlated (+) with cortical GM & (−) with cortical sulci. No difference ICV

In the column "Subject Characteristics", #subjects, mean age, sex, handedness (#LH, #mixed, #all RH), education, duration of illness, SES/PSES (and any matching/differences) are listed if they were reported in the study. When the table does not specify "whole brain" (/), whole brain was not measured, but instead was estimated (∗) based on either a few slices, and/or interpolated over slices with gaps between them; "+" in ROI column indicates abnormal finding, "−" indicates no abnormality noted; numbers in parentheses in the Imaging Parameters column indicate the number of slices. When a "slab" of brain was imaged, and is described in the study, this is also listed in parentheses in the Imaging Parameters column. KEY for Abbreviations: SZ, schizophrenic; NCL, normal control; SZAFF, schizoaffective disorder; BP, bipolar; M, male; F, female; L, left; R, right; age, mean age; duration, mean duration of illness; educ, mean education level; SES, socioeconomic status; PSES, parental socioeconomic status; WB, whole brain; V, or VENT, ventricles; TL, temporal lobe; FL, frontal lobe; PL, parietal lobe; OL, occipital lobe; BG, basal ganglia; CC, corpus callosum; PT, Planum temporale; CaSept, cavities of septum pelucidum; Thal, thalamus; GM, gray matter; WM, white matter; AMYG, amygdala; HIPP, hippocampus; AMYG-HIPP, amygdala-hippocampal complex; PHG, parahippocampal gyrus; VBR, ventricular brain ratio; STG, superior temporal gyrus; CSF, cerebrospinal fluid; FPRA, frontal-parietal reference area; ICA, intracranial volume; ICV, intracranial area; LAT VENT, lateral ventricles (TH, temporal horn; FH, frontal horn; OH, occipital horn).

Source: Parts of table adapted from M. E. Shenton, Temporal lobe structural abnormalities in schizophrenia: a selective review and presentation of new MR findings, *Psychopathology: The Evolving Science of Mental Disorders* (S. Matthysse, D. Levy, J. Kagan, F. M. Benes, eds.), Cambridge University Press, New York, 1996, p. 51.

Table 2 Summary of MRI Studies Reporting Positive and Negative Findings in Schizophrenia

Brain region	%+	%−	N Total	+	−	Refs. +	−
Whole brain	19	81	27	5	22	89–104, 105–110	111–115
Lateral ventricles	73	27	37	27	10	75[a],77,89,93–94, 99,102–105, 107–111, 113–115, 126–134[a]	78,91–92,96,98, 101,112, 135–137
Third ventricles	58	42	19	11	8	89,101–102,105, 107,113,129, 131–133,135	90,93,96,98,108, 115,130,137
Fourth ventricles	0	100	3	0	3		96,126–127
Temporal lobe (TL)	76	24	50	38	12		
Whole TL	55	45	31	17	14	75,90,91,93, 107–112,126, 128,130,133, 147–149	78,89,92,94,96, 98–100[b], 102–104,134, 145–146
Medial TL	75	25	24	18	6	75–76,90,92[b], 95–97,99, 101–102,105, 107,112,128, 130,133–134, 152	77,88,93,98, 110,146
STG (gray matter)	100	0	3	3	0	88,96,106	
STG (GM & WM)	50	50	4	2	2	90,102	104,157
PT	50	50	6	3	3	82,165,167	166,79,80
Frontal lobe	46	54	28	13	15	88,95,97,100[b], 103,106,108, 110–112, 126–127,145	77,83,89,91–93, 96,99,104, 113,115,128, 130,133,169[b]
Parietal lobe	56	44	9	5	4	88,100[b],108,111–112	103,108,112,133
Occipital lobe	50	50	6	3	3	100[b],108,111	103,106,112
Generalized (G) vs. Local (L)	L	G ?	?	L	G		
Gray matter	66.7	16.7 16.7	1	4	1	L: 96,106,112,130;?:95;G:108	
Gray and white matter (combined)	25	50 25	1	1	2	L:103;?:100;G:97,111	
Other:			51	33	18		
Basal ganglia	60	40	15	9	6	95,97,112,146, 177,179–182	77,89,92[b]–93, 101–102
Thalamus	80	20	5	4	1	102,115,189–190	77
Corpus callosum	60	40	15	9	6	65,69–71, 126–127, 193–195	67–68,89, 91–92,99
Cerebellum	29	71	7	2	5	95,111	102,197–200
Cavum septi pellucidi	100	0	8	8	0	199[b],203[b]–204,207[b]–212[b]	

[a] Temporal horn only.
[b] Finding (+/−) not based on area, length, or volume.

although there are no confirmatory data to support these assumptions. Overall brain size is of interest to schizophrenia research because such anomalies might be related to perinatal complications, or to neurodevelopmental abnormalities, or to both. The interpretation and meaning of such differences, however, remain far from clear, and controversy surrounding this issue continues as noted in a recent series of letters to the editor (e.g., [74]).

Here, we summarize MRI studies of brain size in schizophrenia. (For a review of gray matter volume reduction, see Sec. II. E.) The 27 studies* listed in Table 1 either measured whole brain volume from contiguous slices through the entire brain (n = 6) or, more commonly, included an estimate of brain volume based on one or more slices. When brain volume included gray matter, white matter, and cerebrospinal fluid (CSF), it is listed as intracranial volume (ICV) cranium (Table 1). When brain volume was limited to gray and white matter, excluding CSF, and excluding cerebellum, it is listed as "cerebrum," or "brain volume." When the brain measure was an area measure, based on one or a small number of slices that included gray matter, white, matter, and CSF, it is listed intracranial area (ICA).

The 27 MRI studies varied considerably in MRI methodology, including slice thickness (ranging from 1 cm to 1.5 mm), contiguous versus gaps between slices, and MR scans of the entire brain versus part of the brain for estimates of brain volume. Given these differences in methodology, it is surprising that there is such consistency among the findings. More specifically, of the 27 studies, 18 did not report differences in cerebral volume/intracranial volume between schizophrenics and control subjects [89–106]. One other study by Dauphinais et al. [107] showed no differences between groups until after the temporal lobe was subtracted from the rest of the brain volume. Moreover, a study by Zipursky et al. [108] reported no differences in intracranial volume between schizophrenic patients and control subjects, but did report a decrease in overall cortical gray matter in schizophrenic patients. Two other studies showed an increase in the overall brain size of males compared to females, but no differences between schizophrenics and controls [109,110]. Thus, if we count the latter four studies as essentially negative findings, 22 of 27 MRI studies (81%) showed no differences in overall brain volume between schizophrenics and control subjects (see Tables 1 and 2).

Of the five positive findings, four studies showed a decrease in overall brain size in patients [111–114] and one study showed an increase [115]. However, in one of these studies brain volume was less only when non-

---

* Not included are studies from data sets reported elsewhere in Table 1 [83–88]. Also not included are studies that measured whole brain to control for smaller ROIs, but which did not report data for whole brain (e.g., Refs. 75–82).

substance abuse schizophrenics were separated. Then and only then was there a reduction in the superior portion of cranial volume in non-substance abusing schizophrenics [112]. In two other studies, decreased brain volume was related to gender [111,113]. More specifically, Andreasen and coworkers [111] reported no differences between groups until gender was assessed, whereupon male schizophrenics had smaller intracranial brain volume than male controls. In contrast, Nasrallah et al. [113] noted a reduction in brain volume in female schizophrenics, but not male schizophrenics, compared to sex-matched controls.

In a fourth study, Gur et al. [114] reported brain volume reduction in schizophrenics compared to controls. These investigators further reported a correlation between patients with negative symptoms and increased intraventricular CSF, but these patients demonstrated no reduction in brain volume. In contrast, they reported a different correlation for patients with positive symptoms: reduced brain volume but no increase in intraventricular CSF. These investigators speculated that patients with negative symptoms may show atrophic changes that occur over time, while patients with positive symptoms may show a more dysgenic pathophysiological process. An association between negative symptoms and increased ventricular CSF is consistent with early CT studies [23] and with some more recent MRI studies (e.g., Refs. 53,94,109). The finding of a correlation between brain volume and positive symptoms is of interest and will need to be confirmed in future studies.

Of note, in the six studies that used contiguous, thin slices through the brain, four reported no differences in brain volume between schizophrenics and controls [90,95,96,103]. Of the two that reported differences, both came from large studies [111,114], where small differences between groups, if they are present, are more likely to be detected than in small sample studies.

These MRI studies, taken together, lean heavily towards negative findings (81%), although it is premature to conclude that small differences in brain volume are inconsequential. For example, that small differences in brain volume are important is suggested by a recent study by Jacobsen and coworkers [116]. These investigators reported smaller brain volume in patients with childhood-onset schizophrenia (by age 12), compared with age-matched controls. These findings suggest that small decreases in brain volume "might reflect a more severe genetic and/or environmental neurodevelopmental insult, leading to earlier onset" [116]. They also suggest that homogeneous patient groups may lead to the detection and clarification of small differences in brain volume.

Thus, to conclude, there is enormous individual variation in head/brain size, and many methodological problems in the MRI studies herein reviewed could have easily obscured small but important differences. Some possible methodological artifacts include differences in control groups, such as the use of neurology cases (e.g., Ref. 93), lack of a being blind to group membership [89], differences in age (e.g., Ref. 113), and using a small number of slices to estimate whole brain (e.g., Refs. 71,92). All of these possible confounds suggest that further research is needed before definitive conclusions can be drawn concerning the importance and meaning of small differences in brain size between schizophrenics and controls.

2. Corrections for Head/Brain Size

The observed individual variation in head/brain size has led many investigators to speculate about what the appropriate correction factor is for this variable (e.g., Refs. 117–121). The general assumption is that large variations in normal head/brain size need to be taken into account when looking at smaller areas within the brain. Otherwise, a person with a small head might be mistakenly categorized as having, for example, a small cingulate gyrus, when, in fact, if head size was taken into account, no such mistake would be made. As research efforts continue to focus more on regional, or small, differences in the brain, the problem of measuring brain volume and of how to correct for individual variations require further clarification before data from studies of regional differences between groups can be interpreted (see Gur et al. [114] for a more complete discussion).

Among the most commonly employed methods to correct for head/brain size variations are ratio measures. One such ratio measure is ventricle-brain ratio (VBR), long used as an index of ventricular enlargement relative to total brain. Analogous corrections have also been based on proportional measures, including region of interest (ROI), divided by an estimate of brain size [e.g., intracranial cavity (ICC)], and then multiplied by 100. Other corrections, such as regression analyses, have also been used to partial out those aspects of measurement thought to be attributable to head/brain size variations, including height, weight, gender, and age (e.g., Refs. 88,108,111,115,119,121–123). Our own laboratory reports both corrected and uncorrected ROI comparisons, and many of the MRI studies reviewed in this chapter use one or more forms of correction. In reviewing MRI findings it is, nonetheless, important to keep in mind that overall head/brain size shows enormous variability, that it is affected by many variables such as gender and age, and that at this time it is not known to what extent brain size is effected in schizophrenia, nor is it known what the implications of such differences might be. It is also not clear which of several correction factors should be used to evaluate smaller ROIs within the brain. These questions can only be addressed by further research.

3. Ventricular Findings

Interest in assessing lateral ventricles in schizophrenia began with measurements of casts made from postmortem brains and continued with pneumoencephalographic studies (e.g., Refs. 7–10) and with early CT studies [23]. CT technology was a major breakthrough because it afforded a less invasive and more accurate assessment of the lateral ventricles. The most robust finding from the CT literature, in fact, has been enlarged lateral ventricles in schizophrenia, which have often been associated with cognitive impairments, negative symptoms, or poor premorbid functioning (for a review, see Shelton and Weinberger [23]). Enlarged lateral ventricles are not, however, specific to schizophrenia as there are many other disorders such as Alzheimer's disease and Huntington's chorea that can result in enlarged lateral ventricles as can treatments such as chemotherapy and steroid therapy. Nonetheless, lateral ventricular enlargement may indicate tissue loss in surrounding brain areas or failure of development, and for this reason it is of interest to schizophrenia research.

In general, as detailed below, lateral ventricular enlargement in schizophrenia, reported in 75% of CT studies [23], has been replicated in recent MRI studies of schizophrenia (73%). MRI studies of third and fourth ventricles in schizophrenia have also been conducted, although the findings are less consistent across studies.

For illustrative purposes, Fig. 1 shows a three-dimensional (3D) reconstruction of the ventricular system, including lateral, third, and fourth ventricles, from an in vivo MRI scan of a normal control subject. Table 1* lists 37 MRI studies that evaluated the lateral ventricles (see also Table 2). Of these, 25 showed enlarged lateral ventricles in schizophrenic patients compared to controls [75,77,89,93,99,102–105,107–111,113,115,126–134]. One other study reported no differences between first-episode patients and controls on lateral ventricular size, but did report that patients with enlarged lateral ventricles had a worse outcome at follow-up than patients who did not show enlarged lateral ventricles at baseline [94]. Another study reported an increase in intraventricular CSF and VBR in schizophrenic patients compared to controls [114]. Thus, of the 37 MRI studies reviewed, 27, or 73%, reported lateral ventricular enlargement in schizophrenia. Only 10 MRI studies reported negative findings [78,91,92,96,98,101,112,135–137].

We list our two studies [96,136] among those that did not report lateral ventricular enlargement in schizophrenia. The earlier study [136] we discuss

---

* There are 45 MRI studies listed in Table 1 that have evaluated lateral ventricles, parts of the lateral ventricle, third ventricle, and/or fourth ventricle in schizophrenic patients. Seven of these studies were from data sets reported elsewhere in the table, and they are therefore not counted twice [84–88, 124–125], and one study did not measure lateral ventricles but is included here because it measured the third ventricle. Excluding these eight studies in the tabulation, 37 MRI studies reported findings for part or all of the lateral ventricles. (Included in the latter count are two studies that measured *only* the temporal horn of the lateral ventricles [75,134].)

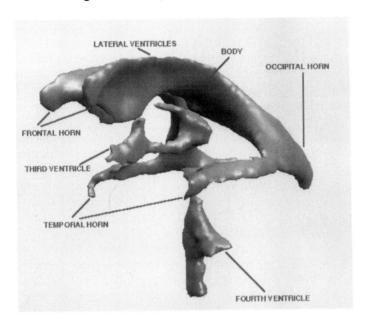

Fig. 1 This image of the ventricle system of the human brain was derived from 1.5-mm contiguous in vivo MR images that were segmented to define the ventricles, after which a three-dimensional surface-rendering program was used to visualize them (see Ref. 96 for more details). These ependymal-lined cavities lie in the center of the brain and contain cerebrospinal fluid. Note the component parts of the ventricular system: lateral ventricles (body, temporal horn, frontal horn, and occipital horn), third and fourth ventricles.

below. In the more recent study [96], while we reported no mean differences between groups in lateral ventricular volume, we did report a statistically significant increase in the variance of left lateral ventricles in schizophrenic patients as well as a statistically significant 180% increase in the left temporal horn of the lateral ventricle and a 74% increase in the right temporal horn in schizophrenics compared to controls.

An increase in the temporal horns of the lateral ventricles, especially on the left, has also been reported in several other MRI studies (e.g., Refs. 75,93,99,107,109,129). This increase in CSF in the temporal horn region of the brain is consistent with postmortem studies of tissue loss in the surrounding limbic system structures, including the amygdala-hippocampal complex and parahippocampal gyrus [31–39]. It is also consistent with recent MRI studies investigating medial-temporal lobe structures in schizophrenia—see Sec. II.B.3. Only one study reported a proportional increase in the body and occipital horns of the lateral ventricles [104]. One other study reported an increase in all regions of the lateral ventricle in first episode patients [132]. Suddath and coworkers [128] also reported a correlation between lateral ventricular enlargement and reduced left temporal lobe gray matter, again suggesting that tissue surrounding the lateral ventricles, particularly temporal lobe structures lying along the temporal horn, may be implicated in schizophrenia.

In four studies gender effects were noted. Bornstein et al. [131] reported no differences between schizophrenics and controls on lateral ventricular size until males and females were analyzed separately, whereupon female schizophrenics showed larger lateral ventricle size than female control subjects. Harvey et al. [110] also noted an effect only for female schizophrenics, while Andreasen and coworkers [111,115] noted an increase in lateral ventricles only in male schizophrenic patients.

The picture becomes more complex when we move from CT studies to MRI studies in terms of evaluating correlations between the lateral ventricles and clinical symptoms. While some studies report correlations with negative symptoms, others have reported correlations with positive symptoms. More specifically, Johnstone and coworkers [109] reported a correlation between enlarged lateral ventricles and poor outcome in schizophrenia reminiscent of early CT findings. Similarly, DeLisi et al. [93] reported enlarged lateral ventricles in chronic schizophrenic patients compared to first-episode patients as well as a correlation between enlarged lateral ventricles and poor outcome [94]. Additionally, Corey-Bloom et al. [77] reported a higher correlation between late-onset schizophrenic patients and enlarged lateral ventricles compared to early-onset schizophrenic patients.

Gur et al. [114], however, as noted previously, observed a more complex pattern of clinical correlations: negative symptoms were correlated with increased ventricular CSF but not a reduction in brain volume, while positive symptoms were correlated with a reduction in brain volume but not with increased ventricular CSF. In contrast, two other research groups reported a correlation between positive symptoms and enlarged lateral ventricles [99,124]. And finally, one study from our laboratory reported a correlation between thought disorder and deviations from the observed normal left > right lateral ventricle size in male chronic schizophrenics [136]. The observed fluctuation in positive versus negative symptoms and their correlation with ventricular enlargement may be a function of what the increase in CSF reflects, i.e., tissue loss in temporal or limbic system structures or perhaps loss in prefrontal lobe structures.

Of the 10 negative findings, 6 were from studies with 20 or fewer subjects in each group [91,96,98,101,135,136], one used a relatively weak magnet (0.08T) with 12-mm-thick slices [92], and one used a seven-point rating scale developed for Alzheimer's disease studies, which may have been too restrictive a range of scores for differentiating schizophrenic patients from controls [137]. Hoff et al. [78], who also reported a negative finding, used a slightly older control group than patient group, which may have contributed to not finding a difference between groups in the volume of the lateral ventricles, since there is strong evidence to suggest that CSF spaces increase with age (e.g., Ref. 138). The last negative finding, by Jernigan and coworkers [112], used a measure of intraventricular CSF that included third, fourth, and lateral ventricles, which may possibly have obscured differences between groups.

The third ventricle has also been reported to be enlarged in schizophrenic patients. Nineteen MRI studies of third ventricle in schizophrenia are listed in Table 1, which includes lateral ventricle findings. Of these, 11 studies reported an increase in third ventricle in schizophrenia [89,101,102,105,107, 113,129,131–133,135], 1 study reported a trend for an increase in third ventricle [90], and 7 studies reported no differences between groups [93,96,98,108,115,130,137]. Thus, 58% of the MRI studies reported an increase in third ventricle in schizophrenic patients. Of the three studies that evaluated the fourth ventricle, none reported differences between control subjects and schizophrenic patients [96,126,127].

In summary, these findings suggest that particular features of abnormal brain morphology, such as enlarged lateral and third ventricles, may be present in a subgroup of schizophrenic patients. The most robust, consistent finding across studies was enlarged lateral ventricles. Methodological differences, as discussed above, may be responsible for the small number of studies reporting negative findings, although there is also the possibility that a small subset of patients does not show such enlargement (e.g., Ref. 114).

B. MRI Temporal and Medial-Temporal Lobe Findings

1. Introduction

Since 1988 there have been 50 MRI studies* investigating temporal lobe abnormalities in schizophrenia. Of these, 38, or 76%, reported abnormalities [75,76,78,81,82,88,90–92,95,97,99,101,102,105–112,126,128,130,133,134, 147–149,152,157,165–169], while 12 did not [77,79,80,89,93,94,98,100,103, 104,145,146]. These are thus among the most robust findings in the MRI literature (see also Tables 1 and 2).

---

* Fifty-seven MRI studies investigating temporal lobe abnormalities in schizophrenia are listed in Table 1. Seven of these studies include data presented elsewhere in the table, and they are therefore not counted twice [83–87,124–125]. Of the final 50 MRI studies, we include as a positive finding two studies that did not use area, length, or volume measures but instead reported differential based on asymmetry [92,100].

Below we review these findings, beginning with a review of total temporal lobe size differences, where the data are the least consistent across studies. This is followed by a review of medial-temporal lobe volume findings, which includes the amygdala-hippocampal complex and the parahippocampal gyrus. The evidence here is quite strong with 75% of MRI studies reporting medial-temporal lobe abnormalities in schizophrenia. These findings are also consistent with findings from postmortem studies (e.g., Refs. 29–39). Finally, we review superior temporal gyrus (STG) and planum temporale (PT) findings in schizophrenia. The latter structure, PT, is thought to be an important biological substrate of language [139–144], and thus perhaps relevant to both language and thought disturbances observed in schizophrenia.

The temporal lobe itself can be seen in Fig. 2, which depicts a lateral view of the human brain. The temporal lobe has three main gyri: the STG, which lies closest to the Sylvian fissure, followed by two successive parallel gyri, the middle and inferior temporal gyri (see Fig. 2). The transverse gyri of Heschl and PT are located on the superior surface of the temporal lobe (not visible in Fig. 2). The medial temporal lobe structures, in the medial inferior portion of the temporal lobe, run along the longitudinal or parallel

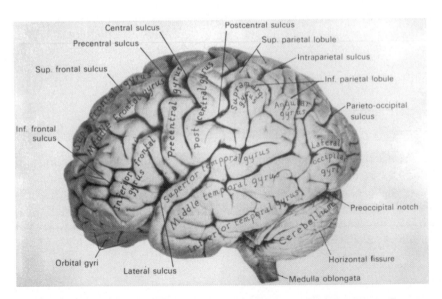

Fig. 2 Photograph of the lateral view of the human brain. (From Carpenter and Sutin, *Human Neuroanatomy*, 1983, courtesy of Williams & Wilkins, New York, New York.)

axis and include both the hippocampus and the adjacent amygdala (the para-hippocampal gyrus lies medial and lateral to these structures) (see also Chapter 4). Below we review the MRI findings in schizophrenia for these regions of interest (ROI).

2. Whole Temporal Lobe Findings

Table 1 lists 31 MRI studies that evaluated the size of the temporal lobe in schizophrenic patients and normal controls (see also Table 2). Seventeen (55%) of these studies reported differences between groups [75,90,91,93,107–112,126,128,130,133,147–149], while 14 (45%) of these studies reported no difference between groups [78,89,92,94,96,98–100, 102–104,134,145–146]. Figure 3 depicts an outline of the temporal lobe, manually drawn on a 1.5-mm coronal MR image (viewer's left is the subject's right).

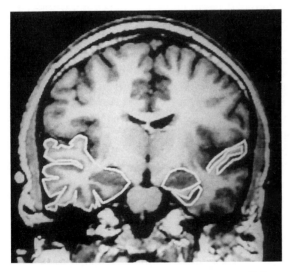

Fig. 3 Coronal 1.5-mm slice showing medial temporal and neocortical structures. The region bordering the Sylvian fissure is the superior temporal gyrus (left side of images are right side for viewer). The almond-shaped region in the medial portion of the temporal lobe is the amygdala, and the region demarcated beneath is the parahippocampal gyrus. The whole temporal lobe is also outlined. [Reprinted by permission of *The New England Journal of Medicine*, Shenton ME, Kikinis R, Jolesz FA, Pollak SD, LeMay M, Wible CG, Hokama H, Martin J, Metcalf D, Coleman M, McCarley RW, 327, 606, 1992, Copyright (1992), *Massachusetts Medical Society*.]

Of the 17 MRI studies reporting differences in temporal lobe volume, one study reported a reduction in the right temporal lobe in first-episode male patients (9% reduction) [75], and another showed a trend for a reduction in schizophrenic patients in the right temporal lobe [90]. Jernigan and co-workers [112] also reported a reduction in the area of the temporal lobe that included medial temporal lobe, but left versus right was unspecified. Eight other studies showed a bilateral reduction in the temporal lobe in schizophrenic patients [107,108,110,111,128,133,147,148], although three of these studies showed a greater reduction on the left [128,147,148], while one study showed a greater reduction on the right [110]. Six other studies reported a reduction in volume in the left temporal lobe in schizophrenic patients compared to controls [91,93,109,126,130,149] (one of these studies compared differences between schizophrenic and nonschizophrenic twins [130]). Suddath and coworkers [128], as noted previously, also reported a correlation between lateral ventricular enlargement and reduced left temporal lobe gray matter in schizophrenic patients compared to controls.

Of the 11 studies that examined asymmetry in the temporal lobe, all reported right > left temporal lobe in both normal controls and in schizophrenic patients [91,92,99,100,109,124,128,134,146,148,149]. For example, Suddath and coworkers [128] reported right > left temporal lobe in 13 out of 15 controls and in 14 out of 15 schizophrenic patients. This finding is consonant with reports of right > left temporal lobes from data on normal controls, including infants and children, where the Sylvian fissure extends farther back on the left, but is steeper on the right due to the posterior vertical ramus, which is reflected in a larger area [141,150,151].

To summarize, the data on temporal lobe volume differences, taken together, are equivocal, although when differences were reported, they most often involved the left temporal lobe being smaller in schizophrenic patients. This lack of consistency in findings across studies may be due to several methodological differences. First, some studies relied upon only a small number of slices to estimate temporal lobe size (e.g., Refs. 89,91,98,133,145–148), while others used a much larger number (e.g., Refs. 75,96,99,103,110,111). Using a small number of slices is analogous to limiting the data or sampling points which, if the effect size is small, would reduce the likelihood of detecting differences when small differences between groups may be present. Our own study, however, does not support this as we reported no differences between groups and we used a large number of slices [96]. Second, the boundaries for defining the anterior and posterior extent of the temporal lobe have been inconsistent across studies. Third, some studies used thick slices through the temporal lobe (e.g., Refs. 89,91,92,109,133,145,146), while other studies used relatively thin slices (e.g., Refs. 75,96,100,103,111,134). And finally, most studies interpolated volumes over gaps between slices (e.g.,

Refs. 78,93,94,98,102,104,108,109,112,148), while only a few studies summed volume over slices with no gaps between them (e.g., Refs. 75,90,96,99,103,110,111). All of these differences likely contributed to the lack of consensus in findings across studies.

Differences in temporal lobe volume may, however, be far less informative than volume differences in specific structures within the temporal lobe. It is important to keep in mind that the division of the brain into separate lobes is based on gross structure, not function. An investigation of specific structures within the temporal lobe are reviewed below.

3. Medial-Temporal Lobe Findings

Medial-Temporal lobe structures include the amygdala-hippocampal complex and the parahippocampal gyrus. Figure 3 provides an illustration of the spatial location of these structures and their proximity to STG. An outline of the amygdala can be seen as the almond-shaped object on the viewer's right (subject's left) (see Fig. 3). Below the amygdala, and also on the viewer's right, the parahippocampal gyrus is outlined. Towards the outside of the image, again on the viewer's right, the STG is outlined (see also Chapter 4).

Table 1 lists 24 MRI studies, not counting data sets reported elsewhere in the table [81,84–86,125], that have evaluated medial-temporal lobe structures in schizophrenia. Of the 24 studies, 17 reported volume reductions in the amygdala-hippocampal complex, the parahippocampal gyrus, or both [75,76,90,95–97,99,101,102,105,107,112,128,130,133,134,152] and one [92] reported a left < right asymmetry in normal controls that was not observed in schizophrenic patients. Thus 18, or 75%, of the MRI studies reported abnormalities in medial-temporal lobe structures in schizophrenia (see Table 2). These findings are, as previously noted, in general agreement with postmortem findings (e.g., Refs. 24–39).

Most of these studies reported a more prominent volume reduction in the anterior portion of the amygdala-hippocampal complex in schizophrenic patients (see Table 1). There were three exceptions: two studies by Bogerts and coworkers [75,76] and one by Flaum and coworkers [102], which reported a more prominent volume reduction in the posterior portion of the hippocampus. Also, most but not all of these studies reported medial temporal lobe volume reduction that was more prominent on the left and more commonly observed in male schizophrenics (e.g., Refs. 75,76,90,96,99, 101,134). Additionally, as noted above, one study by Blackwood and coworkers [92] did not report volume reduction in medial temporal lobe structures but instead reported a left < right asymmetry in normal controls that was not observed in schizophrenic patients. Another study, by Dauphinais and coworkers [107], reported a reduction in amygdala-hippocampal volume when volume measures were used but not when area measures were used. The latter finding emphasizes the point that volume measures, derived from multiple slices over a given area, are more precise than area measures, which are derived from only one or a few slices.

Of the six negative findings [77,88,93,98,110,146], two studies used only three to four slices to estimate the volume of mesial temporal lobe structures [98,146], one study did not include portions of the posterior temporal lobe [93], one study included a sample of patients and controls that differed in the proportion of males and females [110], and still another study evaluated mesial temporal lobe gray matter but did not separate this into the amygdala-hippocampal complex and the parahippocampal gyrus [77]. And, finally, the sixth negative finding study [88] evaluated only a portion of the hippocampus and did not include the amygdala. Sampling problems thus may have led to these studies not finding differences between normal controls and schizophrenic patients.

With respect to *correlations with other brain areas*, it is of interest to note that reduced volume in the hippocampus, amygdala, and parahippocampal gyrus was often accompanied by an increase in CSF in the lateral ventricles, particularly in the temporal horn region (e.g., Refs. 75,76,90,96,99, 107,134). These findings suggest that when mesial temporal lobe structures are reduced in schizophrenic patients, there is a concomitant increase in CSF in the surrounding area of tissue loss, and this is most evident in temporal horn CSF.

The volume of medial temporal lobe structures has been shown to be correlated with prefrontal cortex volume. Two separate studies [95,97] have reported a correlation between reduced amygdala-hippocampal volume and *prefrontal white matter* volume. Additionally, Weinberger and coworkers [59] reported an association between left hippocampal volume reduction in the affected twin of monozygotic twins discordant for schizophrenia and decreased regional cerebral blood flow (rCBF) in the dorsolateral prefrontal cortex during the Wisconsin Card Sorting Test (same subjects as listed in Table 1 [125,130]). And, finally, Wible et al. [83], from our laboratory, reported a correlation between left prefrontal *gray matter* and reduced gray matter volume in left parahippocampal gyrus, left amygdala-hippocampal gyrus, and left superior temporal gyrus. These findings are of interest because there are, as noted earlier, both direct and indirect neural connections between prefrontal cortex and medial temporal lobe structures which may be affected in schizophrenia, and this may be evinced in the correlational patterns observed in schizophrenic patients that are not evinced in normal control subjects.

Several *correlations between reductions in medial temporal lobe structures and clinical symptoms* have also been reported. For example, Bogerts et al. [76] reported a correlation between bilateral reduction in medial temporal lobe structures as a whole and the psychotic factor on the BPRS (Brief Psychiatric Rating Scale). Moreover, Goldberg et al. [125], in an evaluation of monozygotic twin pairs discordant for schizophrenia, reported a correlation between reduced volume in the left hippocampus and an increase in positive symptoms as well as a disruption in logical memory in schizophrenic twins compared to nonschizophrenic twins. The amygdala, hippocampus, and parahippocampal gyrus are functionally important for associative links in memory, and such a correlation is consonant with what is known about both the structure and function of these brain areas (e.g., Refs. 153,154). These investigators also reported a different pattern of correlations for reduced prefrontal cerebral blood flow, which was associated with an increase in negative symptoms and with perseveration on the Wisconsin Card Sorting Test [59].

Nestor et al. [85], from our laboratory, also investigated clinical correlates of mesial temporal lobe reduction. In this study we reported an association between poor scores on verbal memory, abstraction, and categorization, and reduced volume (bilaterally) in both the parahippocampal gyrus and posterior STG. Again, these associations are consonant with what we know about the structure and function of these brain areas and their role in associative links in memory, particularly verbal memory. Nestor et al. [85], in fact, interpreted these data as possibly related to a dysfunctional semantic system in schizophrenia.

O'Donnell et al. [86], also from our laboratory, reported an association between reduced mesial temporal lobe volume (as a whole), reduced left posterior STG, and reduced N200 amplitude, an event related potential important to the categorization of objects and events in the world. Additionally, Egan et al. [133] noted a correlation between reduced volume in the amygdala-hippocampal complex, especially on the left, and reduced N200 amplitude. These investigators also reported an association between right hippocampal volume reduction and reduced visual P300 amplitude, an event related potential important to evaluating novel, highly relevant, or discrepant events in the environment.

In summary, initial interest in MRI studies of mesial temporal lobe structures was fueled by postmortem investigations of morphometric abnormalities, which showed a selectivity for temporal and medial temporal lobe structures, especially in the left temporal lobe (e.g., Refs. 24–39). A review of the MRI studies of medial temporal lobe structures in schizophrenia have also shown reduced volumes in schizophrenic patients, which are more prominent on the left and more commonly observed in male patients (see Tables 1 and 2). These findings are among the most consistent and robust of all MRI findings. They also appear to be importantly related to disturbances in associative links in memory. (See Chapter 4 for a more detailed discussion of possible neural circuitry abnormalities related to disturbances in associative links in memory observed in schizophrenic patients).

4. Superior Temporal Gyrus and Planum Temporale Findings

Heschl's transverse gyri, located on the superior surface of STG, contains primary auditory cortex. More posteriorly in STG is Wernicke's area (Brodmann's area 41 and 42), which includes PT and is thought to be a neural substrate of language (e.g., Refs. 139,140). Electrical stimulation studies of posterior STG have reported disordered thinking (e.g., Ref. 144), while stimulation of more anterior STG results in auditory hallucinations as well as complex auditory hallucinations such as the experience of "memories" of voices and/or complex sounds such as songs [140]. These findings are reminiscent of the verbal memory deficits, disordered thinking, and auditory hallucinations that are hallmark symptoms of schizophrenia, and thus make this brain region of particular interest to schizophrenia researchers.

Seven MRI studies have evaluated the STG in schizophrenic patients (see Tables 1 and 2). Five of these studies reported STG volume reduction in schizophrenic patients [88,90,96,102,106], while two studies did not [104,157].

The first two MRI studies investigating STG abnormalities in schizophrenia both reported left STG volume reduction in schizophrenic patients. The first study, by Barta and coworkers [90], reported an 11% reduction in tissue in left STG, thus confirming Southard's [7,8] early anecdotal reports of "suprasylvian atrophy" and a "withering away" of left STG in the postmortem brains of schizophrenic patients. These investigators further related volume reduction in left anterior STG with auditory hallucinations, again confirming Southard's early observation of a link between auditory hallucinations and left STG tissue loss. The second study, by our research group [96], also reported a reduction in volume in left STG (15%). In addition, we reported a high correlation between volume reduction in left posterior STG and increased thought disorder, as measured by the Thought Disorder Index (TDI [155,156]). And, as previously noted, we reported correlations between reduced N200 amplitude and volume reduction in left posterior STG [86]. We also reported correlations between reduced P300 amplitude and volume reduction in left posterior STG [84], as well as between volume reduction in posterior STG (bilaterally) and deficits in verbal associative memory [85].

These two MRI studies [90,96] thus relate left STG volume reduction to occurrences of auditory hallucinations and thought disorder—both cardinal symptoms of schizophrenia. Figure 4 illustrates the negative correlation ($r = 0.81$) between left posterior STG volume (mL) reduction and increased thought disorder (Fig. 4A). This figure also illustrates the individual volumes

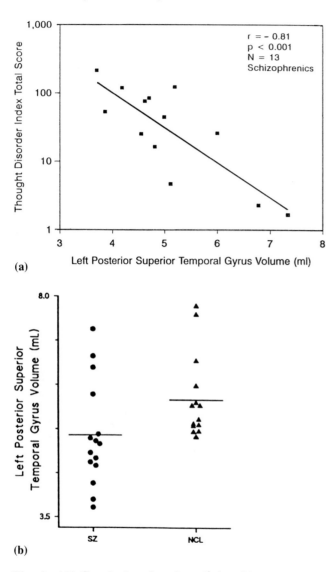

(a)

(b)

Fig. 4 (A) Graph showing the relationship between left posterior STG and thought disorder in schizophrenic patients. (B) Graph showing the volume in mL for the left posterior superior temporal gyrus (STG) for normal controls and schizophrenic patients. [Adapted from Shenton et al., *N. Engl. J. Med.* 327:609 (1992).]

(mL) for left posterior STG in both normal controls and schizophrenic patients (Fig. 4B). And, finally, Fig. 5 depicts the appearance of volume reduction in both medial and neocortical areas of the brain in an in vivo MR 1.5-mm image of a schizophrenic patient (Fig. 5A) contrasted with a normal control subject (Fig. 5B). Note the enlarged lateral ventricles, the increased CSF in the temporal horn region of the lateral ventricles (see arrow on viewer's right, subject's left), and the reduction in volume, seen as tissue loss, in the amygdala, STG, and parahippocampal gyrus in the schizophrenic patient.

More recently, five additional MRI studies have evaluated the STG in schizophrenic patients. Three of these studies reported differences in volume between schizophrenics and controls [88,102,106], while two did not [104,157]. Of the positive findings, Schlaepfer and coworkers [106], from the same laboratory as Barta et al. [90], reported gray matter volume reduction in STG as well as in prefrontal and parietal lobe regions, leading them to

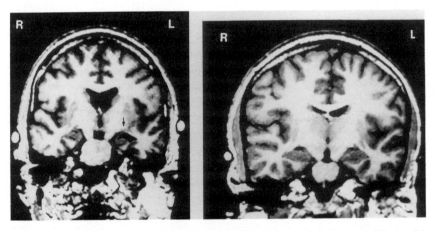

Fig. 5 Coronal 1.5-mm slice of (A) a normal control (left) and (B) a schizophrenic patient (right). Note the increased CSF (black) in the left Sylvian fissure in the patient image (viewer's right), as well as tissue loss in the left superior temporal gyrus, and a black CSF-filled region within the left amygdala. The lateral ventricles are also enlarged as can be seen in the black CSF regions in the center of the image. This is in contrast to the slice at approximately the same anatomical level for the normal control (left). [Reprinted by permission of *The New England Journal of Medicine*, Shenton ME, Kikinis R, Jolesz FA, Pollak SD, LeMay M, Wible CG, Hokama H, Martin J, Metcalf D, Coleman M, McCarley RW, 327, 606, 1992, Copyright (1992), *Massachusetts Medical Society*.]

speculate that heteromodal areas of the neocortex may be implicated in schizophrenic pathology. Zipursky et al. [88] also reported volume reduction in the gray matter of STG, bilaterally, in schizophrenic patients. Similarly, Flaum et al. [102] reported volume reduction in STG (gray and white matter combined) in schizophrenic patients compared to control subjects.

Of the two negative findings [104,157], both of these studies combined gray and white matter in their analyses and may therefore have inadvertently obscured possible differences between groups. Moreover, in one of these studies, increased thought disorder was associated with left STG volume reduction and increased right STG volume [104].* And finally, in the second study [157], while there were no differences between groups, there was a left > right STG for both groups that was statistically significant only for normal controls, suggesting a possible anomalous asymmetry in schizophrenic patients. Thus, while more studies need to be done, those reviewed strongly suggest that STG abnormalities are evident in schizophrenic patients.

Given the excitement generated by the STG findings in schizophrenia, seven new studies were presented at conference proceedings during 1995. Six abstracts reported volume reduction in STG in schizophrenic patients compared to controls [158–163], especially in male schizophrenics, and one abstract reported no differences between groups [164]. The latter study, however, did not separate gray and white matter in their analysis of STG.

These new findings further suggest that in areas of the brain that are asymmetrical in the normal human brain, such as STG and PT, it is important to control for gender effects in analyzing differences between normal controls and schizophrenic patients. It is also of interest to note that in the one study that evaluated gray and white matter separately for STG [160], there were no differences reported between groups in the white matter of STG, only in the gray matter, again emphasizing the importance of evaluating the gray and white matter separately.

Six MRI studies have evaluated the *planum temporale* in schizophrenia (see Tables 1 and 2). The methods for measuring PT, however, have varied (see Table 1), and such differences likely account for a lack of consistency among the findings. For example, Rossi et al. [165] used the bank of the Sylvian fissure to estimate the PT, as well as an area measure of the PT [166], whereas DeLisi et al. [167] measured the length of the PT on images that included the Sylvian fissure, and Petty et al. [82] used both length measures of the PT as well as a novel and sophisticated method that tesselated surfaces with triangles on 3D reconstructions.

---

* This finding suggests that had gray and white matter been separated, volume differences may have been detected.

Of the six studies reported in the literature, three reported differences in PT asymmetry [82,165,167], one reported no differences between groups in PT asymmetry but instead noted a correlation between high thought disorder and reduced normal left > right PT asymmetry [166], and two studies reported no differences between groups in PT asymmetry [79,80].

Other studies evaluating differences in the temporal lobe have included an analysis of the Sylvian fissure (e.g., Refs. 78,168) and an analysis of the sulco-gyral pattern [169]. Hoff and coworkers [78], for example, noted that there was less lateralization of left > right asymmetry for the lateral sulcus in female schizophrenics, which was correlated with better cognitive performance. DeLisi and coworkers [167], from the same laboratory, reported a longer length for the Sylvian fissure on the right side in controls anteriorly, but longer on the left side posteriorly, corresponding to PT. In schizophrenic patients, in contrast, there was less right > left asymmetry anteriorly, and female schizophrenics showed a trend for less left > right asymmetry posteriorly. Bartley et al. [168], who also evaluated the Sylvian fissure, noted that the left side was longer than the right in right-handed twins and that the right side was steeper than the left, although no differences were reported between controls and schizophrenics. Schwartz et al. [137] noted that the Sylvian fissure was larger on the right than the left, and that schizophrenic patients showed an increase in Sylvian fissure size compared to controls. These findings of asymmetry in the length of the Sylvian fissure, an indirect assessment of temporal lobe length, are consonant with reports by LeMay and coworkers on the asymmetry of cerebral hemispheres in normal brains [150,151].

Kikinis et al. [169], from our research group, evaluated the sulco-gyral pattern in the temporal and frontal lobe and reported an increase in the number of sulco-gyral lines in the temporal lobe in schizophrenic patients compared to controls. The latter finding was interpreted as suggestive of neurodevelopmental differences since the sulco-gyral pattern is set very early in fetal development (e.g., Refs. 36,39).

In summary, these findings suggest that the STG and PT are abnormal in schizophrenia. More work is, however, needed to both better define and measure these structures. Moreover, care needs to be taken in carefully defining homogeneous patient groups so that differences in small regions of the brain can be more profitably explored. As these are among the more interesting findings in the MR literature, there will likely be further interest in investigating abnormalities in these structures in order to understand the role they play in schizophrenic pathology.

C. MRI Frontal Lobe Findings

The prefrontal cortex is one of the most complex, highly evolved neocortical areas of the human brain. It comprises close to 30% of neocortex and it has both afferent and efferent connections to all other areas of cortex, as well as to limbic and basal ganglia structures. Moreover, given its modulatory role in all aspects of human functioning, it is a logical candidate for studies investigating brain abnormalities in schizophrenia. This region of the brain has been assessed in schizophrenia by cerebral blood flow and glucose utilization studies, as well as by xenon 133 and single positron emission computed tomography studies (e.g., Refs. 59,170–172). The findings, however, have been inconsistent, with some studies reporting hypofrontality, some not, and at least one study reporting hyperfrontality in schizophrenic patients (e.g., Ref. 173) (for reviews, see Andreasen et al. [172] and Wible et al. [83]). MRI studies, herein reviewed, have also led to conflicting findings.

Twenty-eight studies listed in Table 1* evaluated the frontal lobe (see also Table 2). Of these, 13, or 46%, reported frontal lobe abnormalities in schizophrenic patients compared to controls [88,95,97,100,103,106,108, 110–112,126,127,145], while 15, or 54%, did not [77,83,89,91–93,96,99,104, 113,115,128,130,133,169].

In reviewing the 13 positive findings, 3 of these studies did not measure volume per se but instead assessed image intensity differences [126], width of frontal area [127], and decreased asymmetry compared to controls in occipital, parietal, premotor, and prefrontal regions of the brain [100]. In addition, one study reported a bilateral decrease in prefrontal lobe white matter in nondeficit schizophrenic patients compared to controls, but not in deficit patients [97], and another study [110] reported a decrease in the anterior cerebrum which included parietal and temporal lobe in addition to prefrontal lobe.

The remaining 8 positive finding studies reported reduced volume, or reduced area, in the frontal lobe in schizophrenia and included (a) Jernigan et al.'s [112] report of reduced volume in lateral orbitofrontal gray matter, (b) Brier et al.'s [95] report of reduced volume in bilateral prefrontal white matter, but not gray matter, (c) Raine et al.'s [145] report of reduced left prefrontal area derived from one coronal slice, but bilateral reduction when area was derived from one sagittal or one axial slice, (d) Zipursky et al.'s [108] report of reduced gray matter volume in all but parietal lobe, (e) Andreasen et al.'s [111] report of reduced volume in frontal, temporal, parietal, and occipital lobe in male schizophrenics, but only reduced frontal lobe and cerebellar volume in female schizophrenics, (f) Schlaepfer et al.'s [106], report of reduced gray matter volume in heteromodal areas (i.e., prefrontal cortex, inferior parietal lobe, and STG), (g) Zipursky et al.'s [88] report of reduced gray

---

* Thirty-two MRI studies evaluated the frontal lobe in schizophrenia. Of these, 4 are not included because data sets from these studies are reported in studies elsewhere in the table [84–86,87], thus leaving 28 MRI studies of the frontal lobe.

matter volume in a frontal-parietal reference area (used as a contrast area for temporal lobe measures), and (h) Nopoulos et al.'s [103] report of reduced volume in the frontal lobe in first episode schizophrenics, but not in temporal, parietal, or occipital lobes. Of these positive finding studies, the Brier et al. study [95] and the Nopoulos et al. study [103] included the largest number of slices to estimate prefrontal lobe volume.

Of the 15 negative findings, 5 used only a small number of slices [91,92,115,128,133]. Using only a small number of slices reduces the number of data points and, accordingly, leads to less precise measurement, which could obscure small differences between groups. Additionally, one negative finding came from a study that evaluated the sulco-gyral pattern of the frontal and temporal lobes [169] and not volume per se, where it was determined that the temporal lobe, but not the frontal lobe, showed sulco-gyral abnormalities.

Particularly noteworthy among the negative findings is the study by Wible et al. from our laboratory [83]. This study evaluated 1.5-mm slices that included an average of 36 slices per subject for the assessment of gray matter and 25 slices per subject for an estimate of white matter in the prefrontal lobe. No differences were reported between controls and schizophrenic patients on either prefrontal gray matter or white matter. However, there was an interesting correlation between left prefrontal gray matter in the prefrontal cortex and gray matter of the left STG, left parahippocampal gyrus, and left amygdala-hippocampus. These correlations were only noted for the patient group. Moreover, there was a negative correlation between negative symptoms and left prefrontal gray matter. These findings suggest that differences in the prefrontal cortex, in at least a subgroup of patients, may be too small to detect even with state-of-the-art images, but which are nonetheless correlated with reductions in areas of the temporal lobe that are neuroanatomically and functionally related. Brier et al. [95] also noted correlations between prefrontal and temporal lobe regions. Their measure of right prefrontal white matter was correlated with right amygdala-hippocampus in schizophrenic patients, which they interpreted as supporting the hypothesis of abnormal limbic-cortical connections in schizophrenia. This finding thus further supports the importance of connections between prefrontal and limbic structures in the brain.

In summary, some MRI studies have reported frontal lobe abnormalities in schizophrenia while others have not. It is difficult to reconcile these conflicting results. Methodological differences in these studies could account for some of the differences, as many studies have used only a small number of slices to assess prefrontal cortex. Also, this area is large in comparison to other structures in the brain and the fact that most studies only use a small number of slices to estimate frontal lobe is reminiscent of the approach used to estimate temporal lobe size. That is, the studies vary tremendously in how much of the frontal lobe they include.

The one study that has included an extensive number of slices through the entire extent of the prefrontal cortex, parcellating both gray and white matter, reported no differences in volume [83]. This study, however, investigated male chronic schizophrenics with predominantly positive symptoms, thereby raising the question of whether the lack of consistency among MRI findings of frontal lobe involvement in schizophrenia might not also be due to differences in patient populations. Our study included a very homogeneous patient group, which, as discussed earlier, may show a selectivity to temporal lobe abnormalities in the brain rather than to frontal lobe abnormalities. And finally, our study, like all of the MRI studies reviewed, did not delineate parts of prefrontal cortex, which need to be investigated in future studies. Future studies are needed to address these issues.

D. MRI Parietal and Occipital Lobe Findings

A review of the parietal and occipital lobe MRI findings in schizophrenia is necessarily brief given the fact that few studies have evaluated these brain regions in schizophrenia. These areas have generally been included as control or comparison regions or as part of the entire cortex. Nine MRI studies have evaluated the parietal lobe [88,100,103,106,108,110–112,133], and six have evaluated the occipital lobe [100,103,106,108,110,111] (see Tables 1 and 2).

The findings for the occipital lobe are equivocal, with three studies reporting differences between groups [100,108,111] and three reporting no differences [103,106,112]. This lack of consistency in findings is true also for the parietal lobe. Here, five studies have reported differences between groups [88,100,106,110,111], while four studies have not [103,108,112,133].

Of the four parietal lobe studies reporting negative findings, Egan et al. [133] used only a 1-cm thick slice to evaluate the parietal lobe, and thus it is not surprising that no differences were detected. Three studies, however, using multiple thin MR slices, also did not report differences between groups [103,108,112]. Of particular note, Nopoulos et al. [103] used 1.5-mm contiguous coronal slices and only reported frontal lobe volume reduction in schizophrenic patients. Additionally, Zipursky et al. [108] measured gray matter in frontal, temporal, parietal, and occipital lobe, and these investigators reported a reduction in gray matter in all lobes except the parietal lobe in schizophrenic patients.

Of the five parietal lobe studies reporting differences between groups, two combined measures of parietal lobe with other brain areas [88,110], and one reported asymmetry differences rather than volume differences [100]. Thus, only two studies reporting volume differences between groups actually evaluated the parietal lobe separately [106,111]. The first study, by Andreasen and coworkers [111], reported MR volume reductions in the frontal, temporal, parietal, and occipital lobes of male schizophrenics. In contrast, female schizophrenics showed volume reductions in only the frontal lobe and in the cerebellum. The second study, by Schlaepfer and coworkers [106], evaluated heteromodal association areas of cortex, which included gray matter of the dorsolateral prefrontal cortex (DLPC), inferior parietal lobe (IPL), and STG. Results from this study showed that all three areas were reduced in schizophrenic patients compared to controls.

The meaning and implication of parietal lobe anomalies in schizophrenia have been speculated upon by these same investigators in an extensive review [174]. Here, Pearlson and coworkers observe that heteromodal brain regions, and their interconnections, are important for mediating complex cognitive tasks, including language, attention, working memory, oculomotor smooth pursuit eye movements, as well as for the focusing and execution of attention—all of which have been noted to be impaired in schizophrenic patients. Additionally, these researchers suggest that another reason these brain regions may be particularly relevant to schizophrenia is because they undergo myelination and reorganization of synaptic connections (pruning) late in human development, during adolescence and early adulthood, at a time when the incidence of schizophrenia is observed to increase. Moreover, these investigators point out that heteromodal brain areas are among the most highly asymmetrical in the human brain and that this asymmetry is observed in fetal development. Such observations are consonant with general hypotheses that hemispheric asymmetry abnormalities may represent a fundamental genetic and/or neurodevelopmental abnormality in schizophrenia (e.g., Refs. 3,7,8,33). Such speculations are reminiscent of Crichton-Browne's 1879 thoughts on this subject [3]: "It seemed not improbable that cortical centres which are last organized, which are the most highly evolved and voluntary and which are supposed to be localized in the left side of the brain, might suffer first in insanity."

In our own laboratory we have recently presented data from an MRI study where we parcellated the parietal lobe into postcentral gyrus, superior parietal gyrus, and IPL [175]. In addition, we further parcellated the IPL into the supramarginal gyrus and the angular gyrus. All of these regions of interest were delineated on 1.5-mm coronal slices that extended through the entire extent of the parietal lobe in a group of 15 chronic male schizophrenics and 15 age- and gender-matched normal controls. We found no volume differences between groups, but we did observe a reversal of the normal controls' left > right asymmetry for the total parietal lobe, which was largely due to a reversal of asymmetry in the IPL. The IPL is functionally important for the focusing of attention, and for smooth pursuit eye movements, as well as for spatial working memory—all of which are impaired in schizophrenia (see review in Pearlson et al. [174]). We plan to follow up on this work in a larger sample and to extend it to first-episode patients.

In summary, MRI studies of the parietal and occipital lobe have been few, although the data from the parietal lobe studies look most promising. More studies are needed, however, that specifically evaluate these areas of the brain before we can determine conclusively the role that they play in the pathophysiology of schizophrenia.

E. Generalized Versus Localized Findings

At the end of the nineteenth century, Alzheimer [4] described schizophrenia as a disease of the neocortex. Around this same time, Crichton-Browne [3] described insanity as a specific malady of the left hemisphere. A major issue today, as in the time of Alzheimer and Crichton-Browne, is to identify regions of the brain affected in schizophrenia and to determine whether this disorder is characterized by changes that are generalized or localized.

While the answer to this question would seem to be straightforward, it has thus far eluded researchers for several reasons. First, part of the confusion and controversy in addressing this question has to do with the definition of terms. That is, there is no general agreement or consensus concerning what is meant by "widespread," "generalized," or "localized" brain changes. For example, does "localized" refer to one brain region at the exclusion of all others? Or does "localized" mean several brain regions that are disproportionately affected, relative to other regions of the brain, but which may form an interconnected neural network, such as proposed by Pearlson and colleagues for heteromodal areas [105,174], by our laboratory for temporal and frontal brain areas [83–86,96], and by Andreasen and colleagues for frontal lobe and thalamus volume reductions [111]? Or, conversely, does the latter constellation of reduction in several interconnected brain regions fit more into the category of "widespread" changes as, for example, proposed by Zipursky et al. [88,108]? While there is no agreed-upon definition, we propose that the term "widespread" be relegated to changes in the brain that involve several brain regions with more than two lobes. In our definition, this could apply to either "generalized" or "relatively localized" changes (see below).

We propose that the term "generalized" be used for undifferentiated loss or change in a particular tissue type in a particular brain region. For example, "generalized" neocortical gray matter abnormalities would refer to changes of approximately equal magnitude in all neocortical gray matter, usually reported as volume reduction in MRI studies. How much variation in volume reduction between neocortical regions would be allowed under this definition? We would suggest 10%, but recognize that this boundary is "fuzzy." What we think important is that investigators be clear about stating the boundaries of the definition used. Finally, we note that it is important to use the correct modifier for gray matter changes, such as "cortical" including nonneocortical regions such as hippocampal, cerebellar, and primary olfactory cortex. Obviously, "gray matter" without a modifier would include both cortical and subcortical gray matter. And, finally, we propose that "localized" be used to define a predilection for abnormalities to occur in particular regions, as contrasted to generalized changes. Our definition does not exclude differences that are widespread, but rather it includes disproportionate alterations (>10–20% in some regions). "Relatively localized" may be preferred by some. This definition would, for example, apply to changes in Parkinson's disease or Alzheimer's disease.

A second problem in addressing the issue of brain changes in schizophrenia is that most investigators have focused their efforts on very specific hypotheses, relegated to specific regions of the brain, and thus areas outside specific ROIs are either not included, or they are included only as control regions. Third, most investigators do not focus on a large number of brain regions because to do so would be too labor intensive given the state of the art of current MR image processing techniques. Consequently, in our review of the MRI literature, we found only 16 studies that included more than one brain region in more than one lobe of the brain (see Table 1; e.g., Refs. 91,92,95–97,99,100,103,106,108,110–112,130,133,145). Fourth, studies evaluating brain volume have often included only an estimate of "whole brain" (see sec. II.A.1). Fifth, among studies evaluating "brain volume" or "cerebrum" from either contiguous slices or estimates based on a small number of slices, there has been enormous variability in whether or not studies measured gray matter or whether they combined gray and white matter in their analyses. And, finally, what constitutes gray matter volume and what constitutes whole brain volume has also varied across studies. For example, our laboratory's measure of overall gray matter included subcortical gray matter and cortical gray matter, as well as cerebellar gray matter [96]. More recently we reevaluated this data by subtracting subcortical gray matter, including the thalamus and basal ganglia structures, from overall gray matter, and we found once again no difference between controls and schizophrenics.

Other investigators have also used varying measures of brain volume and gray matter volume. For example, Andreasen et al. [111] used a measure of brain volume that included gray matter, white matter, and CSF, as well as a measure of brain tissue that included gray and white matter. Similarly, Flaum et al. [102], from the same laboratory, included gray matter, white matter, and cerebral sulci in their measure of cerebrum, although they excluded the red nuclei, substantia nigra, and the brainstem. In contrast, Zipursky et al. [88,108] separated cortical gray matter, but they included only seven 5-mm thick slices, with 2.5-mm gaps between slices, of 3.5 cm of the brain, thereby excluding portions of gray matter.

Consequently, it is difficult to evaluate studies that use such different measures. For this reason, we chose to evaluate the question of "generalized" or "widespread" versus "localized" volume reduction, by including only those studies that measured more than one structure in more than one lobe of the brain. Accordingly, we count 16 studies that met this criteria [91,92,95–97,99,100,103,106,108,110–112,130,133,145]. These studies are summarized in Table 1.* Of the 16 studies, 10 either combined gray and white matter (e.g., Refs. 97,100,103,111), used thick slices (e.g., Refs. 92,133), or did not use a large number of slices to estimate brain volume (e.g., Refs. 91,110,145), and one study combined slices from axial and coronal slices to estimate hemisphere volume [99]. Only six MRI studies included more than one brain region and included either separate measures of gray and white matter or a large number of slices to estimate overall gray matter [95,96,106,108,112,130]. We will first review these six studies, followed by a review of the four studies that combined gray and white matter in their analyses [97,100,103,111] and were not otherwise compromised by inadequate slice thickness or too few slices through the brain to make an accurate estimate of brain volume.

1. Gray Matter Findings

Of the six MRI studies measuring gray matter, one group of investigators interpreted their data as supporting widespread gray matter reduction [108], one group was conservative and described their findings as inconclusive on this issue [95], and four groups interpreted their data as supporting disproportionate localized neocortical gray matter reduction in schizophrenia relative to other neocortical gray matter [96,106,112,130].

More specifically, Zipursky et al. [88,108] described widespread gray matter reduction in schizophrenic patients. They measured the outer 45% of seven 5-mm MRI slices (2.5-mm gaps) in six divisions of the neocortex in controls and schizophrenics and reported a reduction in gray matter in five out of the six divisions (all but parietal lobe). They interpreted these findings as evidence for widespread gray matter reduction in schizophrenia. In evaluating the magnitude of the differences, however, we note that these reductions were smaller than those reported by other investigators for spe-

---

* Twenty-three MRI studies listed in Table 1 have compared schizophrenic patients and normal controls on more than one lobe in the brain [77,91–97,99,100,103,105,106,108,110–112,126, 128,130,133,145,169]. Of these studies, 4 showed no differences between groups on temporal or frontal lobe measures [77,93–94,105] and 3 did not measure volume reduction [100,126,169], thus leaving 16 studies that have measured volume reduction and reported at least one positive finding in schizophrenic patients compared to normal controls.

cific medial temporal lobe structures (e.g., 19% reduction in amygdala-hippocampus [96], 15 and 11% reduction in STG [96], 20% reduction in the posterior hippocampus [75]). Compared with controls, these investigators reported the following gray matter reductions in schizophrenic patients: 7% for whole gray matter, 9% for frontotemporal, 7% for temporoparietal, 8% for prefrontal, 8% for frontal, 4% for parietal, and 6% for parieto-occipital gray matter. These investigators reevaluated this same group of patients in another study where they included a frontal-parietal reference area as a control region to determine whether or not STG was disproportionately reduced in schizophrenic patients. Here they found both areas reduced [88] and concluded that gray matter reduction was generalized rather than specific to STG. However, the frontal parietal region, as discussed previously, and below, is a region of the brain that may be directly implicated in schizophrenia, and it may therefore not be the best choice of a control region.

In contrast, Brier et al. [95] reported reductions in temporal lobe structures including the amygdala and hippocampus, as well as in white matter, bilaterally, in prefrontal cortex. These latter investigators, however, were quite conservative in their interpretation of the data, and they concluded that they could not address the question of widespread versus more localized changes because they had not measured other parts of the brain.

Several other investigators have emphasized the disproportionate nature of changes in the brains of schizophrenic patients. Jernigan et al. [112], for example, noted a mild, diffuse reduction in overall white matter in schizophrenic patients as well as regional gray matter reductions that were specific to mesial temporal lobe regions and orbitofrontal regions of the brain. These findings were disproportionately greater than other cortical gray matter regions and were not related to cranial volume. Suddath et al. [130] also reported disproportionate volume reduction in left temporal lobe gray matter as well as in bilateral reductions in hippocampus, especially on the left, in schizophrenic twins compared to twin pairs discordant for schizophrenia, but they reported no differences between groups in left temporal lobe white matter or in prefrontal gray or white matter. Other gray matter regions of the brain were not, however, evaluated, although the finding of 20% volume reduction in the temporal lobe was quite compelling.

In addition, Schlaepfer et al. [106] evaluated overall gray matter, as well as gray matter in heteromodal cortical regions, which included dorsal lateral prefrontal cortex, inferior parietal lobule, and superior temporal gyrus. They reported gray matter volume reduction in the parietal lobe (inferior parietal lobule), the temporal lobe (STG), and the frontal lobe (DLPC). They concluded that these data were consistent with a reduction in specific, interconnected, heteromodal associational cortical regions of the brain in schizophrenia. Pearlson et al. [176], using the same subjects, evaluated both temporal lobe volume reductions and their specificity to schizophrenia by comparing schizophrenic patients to control subjects and to bipolar patients. Here they reported a disproportionate reduction in temporal lobe structures (i.e., amygdala, STG, and entorinal cortex) in schizophrenic patients.

Work in our own laboratory has delineated a large number of regions of interest in the same subjects. Thus far we have evaluated (a) the temporal lobe, (b) medial temporal lobe structures including the amygdala-hippocampal complex and parahippocampal gyrus, (c) STG, (d) frontal lobe gray and white matter, (e) subcortical gray matter including the basal ganglia (caudate, putamen and globus pallidus) and thalamus, (f) parietal lobe gray matter, and (g) cerebellum (gray and white matter combined). We have found no differences between groups in (a) overall gray or white matter, (b) temporal lobe gray or white matter [96], (c) prefrontal lobe gray matter or white matter [83], (d) parietal lobe gray matter [175], (e) thalamus (unpublished data), or (f) cerebellum. Instead, we found disproportionate, localized gray matter volume reductions in the temporal lobe, which included the amygdala-hippocampal complex, parahippocampal gyrus, and STG [96]. We also noted volume increases in basal ganglia structures [177]. Again, however, we want to emphasize the point that although we reported specific regions of gray matter reduction in the temporal lobe, this by no means implies that this is an exclusive site of pathology. We did, in fact, observe correlations between areas of volume reduction in temporal lobe gray matter structures and prefrontal gray matter on the left, suggesting to us that there may be an interconnected neural network that is affected in schizophrenia or that the same pathological process affects all of these structures.

2. Brain Volume (Gray and White Matter Combined) Findings

Finally, if we include studies that evaluated gray and white matter together but are not compromised by other methodological problems (see previous discussion), there were four studies that evaluated brain volume in more than one lobe [97,100,103,111]. Of these, one study reported volume reduction in all four lobes [111], one study reported volume reduction in all four lobes in first-episode patients but reported a disproportionate volume reduction in only the frontal lobe [103], and one study reported no volume reductions in any of the lobes but instead found a decreased asymmetry in schizophrenic patients compared to controls in parietal and occipital regions of the brain. We count this latter study as equivocal with respect to addressing the issue of generalized versus localized changes in brain volume. And finally, one study evaluated temporal and frontal lobe measures of the amygdala-hippocampal complex and prefrontal cortex and reported bilateral volume reduction in both brain regions [97].

In summary, these findings suggest that it is premature to draw conclusions regarding generalized versus specific localized volume reductions in the brains of schizophrenic patients. While the evidence thus far indicates that the changes are more localized (e.g., 66% of the studies evaluating gray matter showed disproportionate gray matter volume reduction in schizophrenic patients, and 50% of the studies evaluating gray and white matter combined reported disproportionate volume reduction in schizophrenic patients), there are still too few studies that have extensively evaluated a number of brain regions in the same patients. Further, there is reason to believe that even with the most sensitive, state-of-the-art imaging available, small, albeit important differences can be missed. This is suggested, for example, by our finding of no prefrontal gray matter reductions between schizophrenic and normal controls but nonetheless high correlations between left prefrontal gray matter and regions in the left temporal lobe, which showed volume reduction in schizophrenic patients. Moreover, from our review of the literature it seems likely that male schizophrenics, particularly those with more positive symptoms such as auditory hallucinations and more disorganized symptoms such as thought disorder, may show a disproportionate volume reduction in temporal lobe structures, whereas patients with more negative symptoms may show a disproportionate volume reduction in frontal lobe structures (see secs. II.B and II.C). These findings suggest that more attention should be given to delineating further subgroups of homogeneous patients as well as to focusing on several ROIs, in multiple brain regions, in the same subjects.

F. Other MRI Findings in Schizophrenia

1. Basal Ganglia Findings

Basal ganglia (BG) structures have become an important focus of attention in schizophrenia research because of (a) the extensive dopaminergic inputs into the striatum (caudate, putamen, and nucleus accumbens), (b) the therapeutic efficacy of neuroleptic medications acting on dopamine receptors (the dopamine hypothesis of schizophrenia), and (c) the importance of these structures for processing cognitive, sensory, and motor information (for a recent review see Hokama et al. [177]). The first postmortem study of the BG was conducted by Bogerts and coworkers [31], who reported no volume differences in putamen, caudate, or nucleus accumbens between controls and schizophrenics. A more recent postmortem study by Heckers et al., however, reported a bilateral increase of 9% in the volume of the striatum as well as a bilateral increase of 14% in the volume of the globus pallidus (GP) [178].

The early postmortem study by Bogerts et al. [31] was followed up by MRI studies of the BG in schizophrenia. Fifteen such studies have now been conducted evaluating area or volume measures. Ten of these studies [77,89,92,93,95,97,101,102,112,146] are listed in Table 1. The other five studies, not included in the table because they focused solely on BG, are reviewed below [177,179–182].

Of the fifteen studies, 9 reported differences between normals and schizophrenics and 6 did not (see Tables 1 and 2). More specifically, 8 studies reported an increase in some component of BG volume in schizophrenics compared to controls [95,97,112,146,177,180–182], one study reported a decrease in caudate volume in a group of patients with tardive dyskinesia compared to controls, but not in a group of patients without tardive dyskinesia [179], another study reported a trend for a decrease in caudate nuclei and lenticular nuclei [93], another reported a trend for a decrease in BG (putamen and lenticular nuclei) in male schizophrenics [101], and 4 studies reported no differences between groups [77,89,92,102]. Moreover, only one of these studies included a separate quantification of the volumes of caudate, putamen, and GP, derived from high-resolution images [177], and only 2 studies provided complete data on volumes (i.e., no gaps between slices [177,181]).

Of the four studies reporting no differences between groups, one was based on a 1-cm-thick slice [89], and one was based on an area measure of only the head of the caudate derived from 12-mm slices [92]. A third study, by Corey-Bloom and coworkers [77], used 5-mm slices with 2.5-mm gaps, which may have contributed to this negative finding. That is, partial volume effects are known to increase when thick MR slices are used, and error in measurement is also introduced when volumes are interpolated over slices. Additionally, measurement error tends to increase as the volume of the ROI decreases and as the surface area to volume area increases (see discussion in Flaum et al. [102]). Thus, in evaluating very small ROIs, such as BG structures, it is essential to use thin slices with no gaps between them in order to detect small differences between groups. And finally, the fourth study by Flaum et al. [102] also reported no differences between groups on their measures of caudate, putamen, and GP in a sample of 102 patients. These investigators also included images with gaps between slices (3-mm slices with 1.5-mm gaps), but the fact that the patients had an average duration of illness of 17 months may have been more relevant to their negative finding, since there is evidence to suggest that first-episode patients show an increase in the volume of BG structures following the introduction of neuroleptic medications (e.g., Ref. 180, and see below).

With respect to the positive findings, the study by Jernigan and coworkers [112] was the first MRI study to report an increase in the lenticular nuclei

(13%, putamen and GP). This enlargement was correlated with an earlier onset of schizophrenia, suggesting the possibility of a progressive enlargement. The caudate, however, was not affected. Since this report, Brier et al. [95] found a 10% increase in the left caudate in schizophrenic patients. Buchanan [97], using the same patients, separated the patients into deficit and nondeficit patients and reported that while there were no differences between deficit and nondeficit patients in left caudate volume, there was a trend for deficit patients to have an increase in the right caudate as well, compared to normal controls. Swayze and coworkers [146], using planimetric measurements on 1-cm slices, reported that male schizophrenics showed an increase in putamen and, to a lesser extent, in caudate.

Of the more recent studies, Elkashef et al. [181] reported an increase in left and right GP and right putamen volume in schizophrenic patients. Additionally, Hokama et al. [177], from our laboratory, using 1.5-mm contiguous slices and three-dimensional reconstruction/slicing techniques to allow comparisons of ROI definitions in multiple planes, reported a 10% increase in caudate volume, a 16% increase in putamen volume, and a 27% increase in GP volume in chronic male schizophrenic patients compared to gender- and age-matched controls.

Chakos et al. [180] evaluated first-episode patients and observed a 5.7% increase in the size of the caudate in first-episode patients from the first MRI scan to the follow-up scan 18 months later, compared to a 1.6% increase in controls. These investigators further noted that the greater the amount of neuroleptic medication received by the patients at the time of the first MR scan and the younger the age, the larger the caudate volume at follow-up 18 months later. This finding suggests that the observed increase may be an effect of neuroleptic medication. That this may be the case is further suggested by a recent abstract presented at the *International Congress of Schizophrenia Research* by Keshavan et al. [182]. These investigators evaluated caudate volume in first-episode patients at baseline and at follow-up between 6 and 24 months later, and they found an increase in caudate volume but not in prefrontal cortex or brain volume over time. This data was described more completely in their *Lancet* [183] publication, in which they reported that caudate volumes increased as much as 15% following the introduction of neuroleptic medication in first-episode, drug-naive patients with schizophrenia.

In summary, the finding of increased volume in BG structures in schizophrenic patients is consonant with recent MRI spectroscopy studies (e.g., Refs. 184,185). More research needs to be done, however, to determine whether these changes are related to neuroleptic treatment or whether they are more directly related to BG functioning or to the pathophysiology of schizophrenia. Moreover, there is evidence that BG structures show increased volume in bipolar disorder (e.g., Ref. 186), and it thus becomes important to evaluate the specificity of this finding.

2. Thalamus Findings

As schizophrenia is often considered a disorder of higher cognitive functions, including regulating internal stimuli and modulating input from the environment, it is easy to understand why the thalamus is of interest to schizophrenia researchers. This structure, made up of several nuclei, is a major relay station in the brain that modulates input from many cortical brain areas as well as input from the reticular activating system and from the limbic system (e.g., Ref. 50). The thalamus is also proposed to mediate attention and information processing, as well as to serve as a "filter" for gating the input of sensory signals to the cortex (e.g., Refs. 50,187). These functions have been suggested to evolve from elaborate connections that exist between the ventral anterior and dorsomedial nuclei of the thalamus and the prefrontal cortex and between the associational thalamo-cortico-thalamic loop of the orbitofrontal and dorsolateral prefrontal cortices, both of which involve the anterior and medial dorsal nuclei of the thalamus.

The thalamus has been evaluated in both postmortem and MRI studies. For example, Pakkenberg [188] reported 40–50% reduction in cell count in the medial dorsal nuclei of the thalamus and a 25% reduction in total volume. Measurement from MRI scans is, however, much more difficult because it is hard to outline the whole thalamus, let alone the separate nuclei of the thalamus, because this structure fades from gray into white matter with ghost like edges, even on 1.5-mm slices that provide a high contrast between gray and white matter on the MR image. It is for these reasons, in fact, that Andreasen and coworkers [102,103,189] were reluctant to overemphasize their early thalamus finding (e.g., Ref. 115), given that the interrater reliability for this structure was, understandably, lower than for other brain regions. The difficulty in measuring the thalamus on MRI scans has also likely contributed to the small number of studies undertaken.

Only five MRI studies have evaluated the thalamus in schizophrenia [77,102,115,189,190]. Three of these studies [77,102,115] are listed in Table 1. Four of these studies reported a decrease in thalamic volume in schizophrenic patients compared to controls [102,115,189,190], and one study reported an increase in the volume of the thalamus in late-onset schizophrenic patients compared to early-onset patients (or, conversely, a smaller thalamus in early-onset patients), although there were no differences observed when the patients were compared to control subjects [77] (see also Table 2).

Three of the five studies were from the same laboratory [102,115,189].

The first study by Andreasen et al. [115] reported reduced thalamus volume and enlarged lateral ventricles in male but not female schizophrenic patients, leading these investigators to speculate that the smaller thalamus might be related to periventricular injury at birth, which is more common among males. The second study by Flaum et al. [102] did not show a gender effect but instead showed a volume reduction in thalamus for both male and female patients. The third study, by Andreasen et al. [189], used a novel technique for averaging normal and schizophrenic brains and then subtracting the areas of greatest differences (+ or −) to create effect size maps. This procedure resulted in the lateral region of the thalamus and the white matter bordering the thalamus showing the greatest difference between schizophrenic and control subjects (all male). These investigators suggested that the abnormalities in image intensity observed in the thalamus in schizophrenic patients could account for most of the symptoms observed in schizophrenia.

A study by Buchsbaum et al. [190] evaluated drug-naive schizophrenics and found a decrease in metabolic activity in the right thalamus, a loss of normal right > left asymmetry, and a reduction in volume in the left anterior portion of the thalamus, when the thalamus was divided into six sections. Total thalami volume, however, was not reduced in the patient group until the thalami were subdivided. This study, therefore, leaves open the question of whether neuroleptic medication affects the volume of the thalami, since this study evaluated the thalami in drug-naive patients.

In summary, there are few MRI studies of the thalamus, although those studies that have been conducted have generally reported a reduction in volume in the thalamus in schizophrenic patients. More studies are needed to investigate the thalamus and its relation to clinical symptoms in schizophrenia.

3. Corpus Callosum Findings

The corpus callosum (CC) connects the two hemispheres of the brain; information that passes from one hemisphere to the other does so through the corpus callosum. If information flow is disrupted, this can lead to defective interhemispheric communication. Gruzelier, in fact, has hypothesized that the information-processing deficits observed in schizophrenia may be related to defective interhemispheric communication mediated by the CC [191].

One of the first CC studies in schizophrenia was a postmortem study by Rosenthal and Bigelow [192]. These investigators found a thicker CC in schizophrenic patients, which was especially pronounced in patients with an early age of onset. This study has now been followed up by CT and MRI studies of schizophrenia (see Raine et al. [70] for a review of the early studies).

We here review findings from 15 MRI studies.* Nine reported positive findings [65,69–71,126,127,193–195], while 6 reported negative findings [67,68,89,91,92,99] (see also Table 2). In reviewing the 9 positive findings, 3 by Rossi et al. [71,126,193] reported a decrease in CC area in schizophrenic patients compared to control subjects. Stratta et al. [127], from the same research group, reported an increase in CC brain ratio in normal controls compared to schizophrenic patients, and one other study reported a decrease in total CC area in schizophrenic patients compared to control subjects [194]. In contrast, Uematsu et al. [195] reported an increase in only the anterior portion of the CC in schizophrenic patients.

Hoff et al. [69], in a more recent study, reported a smaller CC area in female schizophrenic patients compared to female controls, male controls, and male schizophrenics. These investigators also noted a larger overall CC area in male subjects compared to female subjects. Raine and coworkers [70] also reported gender differences in their evaluation of CC thickness. They found that the CC was thicker in female patients but thinner in male patients, which was the reverse of that found in control subjects where male controls showed a thicker CC than female controls. Area and length measures of the CC, however, did not show differences among groups. And in a study by Casanova and coworkers [65], all 16 pairs of twins discordant for schizophrenia showed an area of overlap in CC shape that was greatest in the middle section of the CC.

It is difficult, however, to know how to reconcile these conflicting findings. This is made all the more difficult given the fact that it is hard to make comparisons across studies because different measurement techniques have been used, including (a) anterior, middle, or posterior width and/or area, (b) callosal area, (c) area of genu or area of splenium, or both, (d) callosal–to–cerebral area ratio, (e) genu–to–splenium area ratio, (f) length of CC, (g) shape of CC, and (h) density of CC.

4. Cerebellum Findings

Shelton and Weinberger [23], in their review of the CT literature, suggested that about 10% of CT scan studies reported cerebellar atrophy in schizophrenia. These early CT studies, however, were often inconsistent in their findings, and thus it is difficult to interpret them. CT scans are also not the best imaging device for visualizing and determining cerebellar atrophy because the cerebellum is difficult to visualize and to evaluate on transverse CT scans.

---

* For our review we searched for all studies that linked both MRI and corpus callosum. some studies did not, however, list MRI in either the title or in the abstract and thus our search may not have included all MRI studies of this structure.

With the advent of MRI, measuring the cerebellum became easier, although few studies have assessed this region of the brain in schizophrenic patients. In our review, we located seven MRI studies of the cerebellum in schizophrenia. Two of these reported abnormalities [111,196], and five did not [102,197–200]. These studies ranged from a single 10-mm slice for measuring the cerebellum (e.g., Refs. 198,199) to consecutive 1.5-mm slices [111]. Of note, one study that reported no differences between normal controls and schizophrenic patients did, nonetheless, report a decrease in vermal-to-brain ratio in male schizophrenic patients compared to female schizophrenic patients [200], and another study reporting negative findings found a relationship between decreased vermal-to-brain ratio and good therapeutic response to neuroleptic medication.

Of the two studies reporting positive findings, Nasrallah et al. [196], who included only male subjects in their sample, found an increase in the cerebellar structures in male schizophrenic patients compared to male controls. The second study, by Andreasen et al. [111], included 16 female schizophrenic patients and 36 male schizophrenic patients. These investigators did not report cerebellar volume reduction in male schizophrenic patients but, instead, in female schizophrenic patients. They cautioned, however, that gender comparisons from their study should be viewed as inconclusive in either direction because of the small number of female patients. Further studies are therefore needed to evaluate the cerebellum in schizophrenia. In our own laboratory we have used 1.5-mm contiguous coronal slices to evaluate the cerebellum, and we found no differences in volume between schizophrenic patients and normal controls subjects [201]. We are, however, currently delineating the cerebellum into gray and white matter and into separate lobules on contiguous 1.5-mm slices in order to determine whether or not differences will be observed using more refined units of measurement.

5. Septi Pellucidi Findings

The septum pellucidum is comprised of two laminae that form a triangular-shaped membrane, which separates the two frontal horns of the lateral ventricles. Because abnormalities generally occur as a space between the two laminae, these abnormalities are referred to as septi pellucidi. The septum pellucidum itself is bounded anteriorly by the corpus callosum and posteriorly by the fibers of the fornix. Developmental abnormalities in the formation of structures on either end of this membrane (i.e., the corpus callosum and the hippocampus) are thought to be reflected in septi pellucidi abnormalities (e.g., Ref. 202). Consequently, septi pellucidi abnormalities are of interest to schizophrenia. (For a recent review of septi pellucidi abnormalities in schizophrenia, the reader is referred to Nopoulos et al. [203,204]).

In normal development the two leaflets of the septum pellucidum include a space, or cavum, that is evident prior to birth but that generally closes at birth (80%), or a least by adulthood [205]. When this fusion process does not happen in the normal course of development, there is a cavum, or space, known as cavum septi pellucidi (CSP). No one knows what causes the bifurcated leaflets to close this space, but some have speculated that the rapid growth in fetal development of the cerebral hemispheres, and of the hippocampus and corpus callosum in particular, have a role in pushing brain areas together at the midline and fusing them (e.g., Refs. 202,203). Two types of abnormalities have been described in the literature, communicating CSP and noncommunicating CSP (e.g., see description in Shaw et al. [205] and in Lewis and Mezey [206]). Posteriorly, towards the fornix, these are referred to as noncommunicating and communicating cavum vergae pellucidi, as opposed to communicating and noncommunicating CSP. Communicating cavum disorders involve an opening to the ventricular system and are thought to be acquired abnormalities. They include trauma such as that experienced by a professional boxer (e.g., Ref. 205). Noncommunicating cavum disorders, on the other hand, are thought to be related to neurodevelopmental abnormalities (e.g., Ref. 205).

One of the first reports of an association between CSP noncommunicating septi pellucidi abnormalities and psychosis came from Lewis and Mezey [206]. This association was followed up by Mathew and colleagues [207], who conducted the first MRI study of CSP in schizophrenia, where they reported a larger CSP and a large pellucidum-to-brain ratio in schizophrenic patients compared to controls on midsagittal images.

Since this 1985 MRI study, there have been seven more MRI studies [199,203,204,208,210–212] reporting large CSP in schizophrenic patients. Findings from these studies include:

1. Larger absolute size of septum pellucidum, as well as an association between large CSP and family history of schizophrenia in schizophrenic patients [199]
2. Large CSP in 23% of first-episode patients, compared to only 2% in controls [208]
3. Large CSP in 45% of schizophrenic (likely due to using a rating scale where small and questionable CSP were included) [210]
4. Large CSP in 15% of schizophrenic patients (likely due to using 5-mm-thick slices with 5-mm gaps between slices) [211]
5. Large CSP in 25% of schizophrenics [212]
6. Large CSP in 20% of male schizophrenic patients compared to in 3% of male controls [203]
7. An association between large CSP and left temporal lobe volume

reduction in male schizophrenic patients and, compared with male controls, an association between non-CSP male schizophrenics and volume reduction in overall brain, frontal lobe, temporal lobe, and increased overall CSF (see also comments below) [204].

The studies by Degreef and coworkers [208], Jurjus and coworkers [212], and Nopoulos and coworkers [203,204] reported large CSP more frequently in males than in females. This finding suggests the importance of gender, particularly when evaluating possible prenatal or postnatal developmental abnormalities, which show a greater prevalence, in general, in males (e.g., Ref. 205).

Degreef and coworkers [209] also evaluated CSP abnormalities in postmortem brains of schizophrenic patients and normal control subjects. They reported large CSP in both first-episode patients and in chronic schizophrenic patients. In addition, their postmortem study resulted in a larger percent of reported large CSP in patients (61%) compared to controls (21%) than they reported in their MRI study, which they attributed to postmortem studies being able to evaluate differences that were smaller than 3 mm, which their MRI study could not.

And finally, the studies by Nopoulos and coworkers [203,204] deserve attention because they were the first to use 1.5-mm contiguous coronal slices to evaluate CSP in schizophrenic patients compared to controls [203]. In their first study they identified six patients with large CSP (all male) [203]. This latter group of patients, along with four new patients with large CSP, were the subject of the second study, which measured the size of the CSP in millimeters [204]. In addition to the 10 schizophrenic patients with large CSP, there were 44 schizophrenic patients without CSP and 47 control subjects. The results were quite striking. Compared with controls, the patients with no CSP showed a reduction in volume in overall brain, frontal lobe, and temporal lobe, along with an increase in overall CSF. In contrast, patients with large CSP showed a volume reduction only in the temporal lobe and only on the left. These investigators suggest that the pattern of structural abnormalities observed in large CSP schizophrenic patients may reflect a regional, localized tissue reduction, which is confined to the left temporal lobe in a subgroup of male schizophrenic patients. And although these investigators note that the sample of CSP patients is small (10 patients), the results were quite striking for localization to the left temporal lobe. Indeed, they [204] further speculate that "it may not be temporal lobe genesis that is associated with CSP but *lateralized* temporal lobe dysgenesis, as seen in this sample, that contributes to disruption of fusion of septum pellucidum leaflets. In other words, it may be that asymmetry in development of cerebral hemispheres creates diverging growth vectors, which may disrupt normal fusion."

In summary, there have been very few studies of cavum septi pellucidi in schizophrenia, although the studies that have been conducted would seem to suggest that this area of the brain may be particularly relevant to the pathogenesis of schizophrenia, at least in a subgroup of schizophrenic patients. Future studies linking these abnormalities to both clinical symptoms and to other brain areas will help to clarify their role in the pathophysiology of schizophrenia.

III. DISCUSSION

We began this chapter with a review of some of the early postmortem evidence that suggested brain abnormalities in schizophrenia. This evidence was later largely abandoned because of the many methodological artifacts in early postmortem specimens, and it was not until the advent of CT technology that there was a renewed interest in investigating brain abnormalities in schizophrenia. These studies, along with the newer postmortem studies, greatly influenced the direction of the MRI studies that followed.

The major focus of this chapter was on reviewing evidence from MRI studies for brain abnormalities in schizophrenia. This review was more extensive than two previous reviews of temporal lobe findings from our laboratory [213,214], and it was confined to MRI studies, in contrast to a recent review by Gur and Pearlson [215], which included functional imaging studies. In our review, we began with studies published in 1988, and we included findings from studies evaluating lateral ventricles, whole brain, temporal lobe, frontal lobe, parietal lobe, and occipital lobe, as well as findings relevant to "other" brain regions, including basal ganglia, thalamus, corpus callosum, cerebellum, and septi pellucidi. We included summaries at the end of each of these sections, and we will therefore not duplicate those efforts here. Instead, we will briefly summarize what we think are the salient findings from MRI studies investigating brain abnormalities in schizophrenia.

MRI studies of schizophrenia, which began only in 1984, have evolved from the use of 1-cm slices, which did not cover the whole brain, to 1.5-mm slices of the entire brain. This improvement in spatial resolution was needed in order to analyze small brain changes between normal controls and schizophrenic patients. The volume reductions observed in schizophrenia are, in fact, relatively small, on the order of 10–20% difference from controls, and thus improved measurement techniques were necessary before evidence could be accumulated to suggest small volume reductions in the brains of schizophrenic patients.

An added complication in MRI studies has been the problem of detecting and isolating small differences between groups against a background of enormous individual variation in the volume of different brain regions. We touched on this topic in our review of normal variation in head size. It is important, however, to keep in mind that the large individual variation in brain volumes, in most brain structures, makes it exceedingly difficult to isolate small volume reductions in the brains of schizophrenic patients. This difficulty is made all the more arduous when factors such as age, gender, and handedness are not carefully monitored, as these factors are known to add to the already enormous individual variation in brain regions. Such added nuisance variables, in fact, have likely contributed to both the lack of findings in some cases and to some of the differences in findings across studies. Future studies must, therefore, carefully define homogeneous patient and control groups even if this runs the risk of restricting generalizations that can be made about the larger population of patients and controls. Without such a restriction in subject populations, the added variation from nuisance variables can interfere with the ability to detect small but important differences between normal controls and schizophrenic patients and can lead to the detection of differences due to artifact or to mediating variables rather than to differences specific to the pathophysiology of schizophrenia.

Given all of the caveats, including the variability across studies in MR methodology, we are left with the difficult task of balancing the evidence that has thus far accumulated. From our review of the MRI literature, two findings stand out as the most robust—lateral ventricular enlargement (73%) and temporal and medial temporal lobe volume reduction (75%) in the brains of schizophrenic patients (see Table 2). While lateral ventricular enlargement is nonspecific, it is nonetheless suggestive of tissue loss. Moreover, the figure of 73% of MRI studies showing lateral ventricular enlargement is likely conservative, given that most of the negative finding studies came from small samples.

The second most robust findings involved temporal lobe volume reductions in medial temporal lobe structures (amygdala-hippocampal complex, parahippocampal gyrus) or STG in schizophrenic patients. These findings were most prominent in male patients, and they were frequently lateralized to the left. There was also some suggestion that such findings were correlated with more positive symptoms and with functional impairments in language, verbal memory, and other associative links in memory. The latter was particularly noted for the STG. Findings for planum temporale, however, were, less consistent across studies. These studies are more recent, and, as discussed earlier, several methodological issues need to be addressed before the data can be easily interpreted.

The findings for frontal, parietal, and occipital lobe were less consistent in reporting volume reductions in schizophrenic patients. Studies that did report frontal lobe volume reductions were more likely to report this finding in patients with negative symptoms. Far fewer studies examined the parietal and occipital lobe, although the evidence for parietal lobe abnormalities seemed the most compelling.

In evaluating other brain regions, 60% of the basal ganglia studies reported abnormalities (generally an increase in these structures), and 80% of thalamus studies reported a reduction in thalamus in schizophrenic patients compared to controls. Corpus callosum studies, based on linear and area measures, used variable methodology, and thus the findings here were harder to interpret; 60% of these studies reported abnormalities while 40% did not. For the cerebellum, 29% of these studies reported differences between controls and schizophrenics, but there have been too few studies here, and none evaluated gray and white matter separately, nor have any studies carefully evaluated the lobules within the cerebellum. And, finally, all eight MRI studies of the septi pellucidi reported abnormalities in the brains of schizophrenic patients. This brain region is of particular interest because anomalies here are likely due to neurodevelopmental anomalies, which may be related to possible growth differences in the surrounding corpus callosum and hippocampus. The pattern of structural anomalies in patients with large cavum septi pellucidi also seemed to be reflected in localized tissue reduction in the left temporal lobe in a subgroup of male patients. This finding, once again, stresses the importance of attending to gender effects which may be related to differential brain volume reduction in schizophrenia.

In summary, all of these data are exciting, particularly in light of the fact that brain imaging studies are truly in their infancy. Thus far the data favor a number of brain regions that are disproportionately affected in schizophrenia, although too few studies have investigated multiple brain regions in the same subjects in order to draw definitive conclusions. We suspect that the emerging technology of functional imaging, coupled with structural imaging, will likely lead us to a new era of studies that will help to clarify these issues as well as to chart the course of research in the coming decade. We predict that in the next 10 years we will not only gain a better understanding of which brain regions are affected (likely several different intercorrelated regions relevant to one or more subtypes of schizophrenia), but we will also learn which medications are most effective for specific alterations in the brains of schizophrenic patients. The latter may, in fact, lead to the development of specific medications that alter or arrest specific changes that seem to unfold in the brain in late adolescence or early adulthood in individuals diagnosed as suffering from schizophrenia.

ACKNOWLEDGMENTS

The authors gratefully acknowledge the technical and staff assistance of Jay Allard, Iris Fischer, Sarah Carrigan, Paola Mazzoni, Marie Fairbanks, Marianna Jakab, and Maureen Ainslie. We also thank Dr. Yoshio Hirayasu for his assistance in reanalyzing gray matter volume without subcortical gray matter and thalamus volume and Dr. Daniel Iosifescu for making critical comments and suggestions on an earlier version of this manuscript.

This work was supported, in part, by grants from the National Institute of Mental Health (MH K02 MH 01110 [MES], MH 1R29 50747 [MES], MH R01 40,799 [RWM]), and by MERIT and Schizophrenia Center Awards from the Department of Veterans Affairs (RWM).

REFERENCES

1.   E. Kraepelin, *Dementia Praecox* (E. Barclay and S. Barclay, trans.), Churchill Livingstone Inc., New York, 1919/1971.
2.   E. Bleuler, *Dementia Praecox or the Group of Schizophrenias* (H. Zinkin, trans.), International Universities Press, New York, 1911/1950.
3.   J. Crichton-Browne, On the weight of the brain and its component parts in the insane, *Brain 2*:42 (1879).
4.   A. Alzheimer, Beitrage zur pathologischen Anatomie der Hirnrinde und zur anatomischen Grundlage einiger Psychosen, *Monatsschr. Psychiatr. Neurol. 2*:82 (1897).
5.   K. Kahlbaum, *Die Katatonie oder der Spannungsirresein*, Hirshwald, Berlin, 1874.
6.   E. Hecker, Die Hebephrenic, *Arch. Pathol. Anat. Physiol. Klin. Med. 52*:394 (1871).
7.   E. E. Southard, A study of the dementia praecox group in the light of certain cases showing anomalies or scleroses in particular brain regions, *Am. J. Insanity 67*:119 (1910).
8.   E. E. Southard, On the topographic distribution of cortex lesions and anomalies in dementia praecox with some account of their functional significance, *Am. J. Insanity 71*:603 (1915).
9.   W. Jacobi and H. Winkler, Encephalographische Studien an chronisch Schizophrenen, *Archiv Psychiatrie Nervenkr. 81*:299 (1927).
10. J. O. Haug, Pneumoencephalographic studies in mental disease, *Acta Psychiatr. Scand. 38(suppl 165)*:11 (1962).
11. C. B. Dunlap, Dementia praecox: some preliminary observations on brains from carefully selected cases, and a consideration of certain sources of error, *Am. J. Psychiatry 80*:403 (1924).
12. C. B. Dunlap, Pathology of the brain in schizophrenia, *Assoc. Res. Nerv. Ment. Dis. Proc. 5*:371 (1928).
13. W. Spielmeyer, The problem of the anatomy of schizophrenia, *J. Nerv. Ment. Dis. 72*:241 (1930).
14. L. P. Rowland and F. A. Mettler, Cell concentration and laminar thickness of frontal cortex of psychotic patients, *J. Comp. Neurol. 90*:255 (1949).
15. L. J. Seidman, Schizophrenia and brain dysfunction: an integration of recent neurodiagnostic findings, *Psychol. Bull. 94*:195 (1983).

16. D. G. Kirch and D. R. Weinberger, Anatomical neuropathology in schizophrenia: post-mortem findings, *Handbook of Schizophrenia, Vol, I: The Neurology of Schizophrenia* (H. A. Nasrallah and D. R. Weinberger, eds.), Elsevier Science Publishers, New York, 1986, p. 325.

17. F. Plum, Prospects for research on schizophrenia. 3. Neuropsychology. Neuropathological findings, *Neurosc. Res. Program Bull. 10*:384 (1972).

18. P. D. Maclean, Some psychiatric implications of physiological studies on frontotemporal portion of limbic system (visceral brain), *Electroencephalogr. Clin. Neurophysiol. 4*:407 (1952).

19. S. S. Kety, Biochemical theories of schizophrenia, *Science 129*:1528 (1959).

20. J. R. Stevens, An anatomy of schizophrenia?, *Arch. Gen. Psychiatry 29*:177 (1973).

21. E. F. Torrey and M. R. Peterson, Schizophrenia and the limbic system, *Lancet 2*:942 (1974).

22. E. C. Johnstone, T. J. Crow, C. D. Frith, J. Husband, and C. Kreel, Cerebral ventricular size and cognitive impairment in chronic schizophrenia, *Lancet ii*: 924 (1976).

23. R. C. Shelton and D. R. Weinberger, X-ray computerized tomography studies in schizophrenia: a review and synthesis, *Handbook of Schizophrenia, Vol. I: The Neurology of Schizophrenia* (H. A. Nasrallah and D. R. Weinberger, eds.), Elsevier Science Publishers, New York, 1986, p. 207.

24. A. B. Scheibel and J. A. Kovelman, Dendritic disarray in the hippocampus of paranoid schizophrenia (abstract and poster session). Presented at the *Annual Meeting of the Society of Biological Psychiatry*, 1979.

25. A. B. Scheibel and J. A. Kovelman, Disorientation of the hippocampal pyramidal cell and its processes in the schizophrenic patient, *Biol. Psychiatry 16*:101 (1981).

26. R. C. Smith, M. Calderon, G. K. Ravichandran, J. Largen, G. Vroulis, A. Shvartsburd, J. Gordon, and J. C. Schoolar, Nuclear magnetic resonance in schizophrenia: a preliminary study, *Psychiatry Res. 12*:137 (1984).

27. American Psychiatric Association, Committee on Nomenclature and Statistics, *Diagnostic and Statistical Manual of Mental Disorders*, 3rd ed., American Psychiatric Association, Washington, DC, 1980.

28. American Psychiatric Association Committee on Nomenclature and Statistics, *Diagnostic and Statistical Manual of Mental Disorders*, 3rd ed., rev., American Psychiatric Association, Washington, DC, 1987.

29. F. M. Benes, I. Sorensen, and E. Bird, Reduced neuronal size in posterior hippocampus of schizophrenic patients, *Schizophr. Bull. 17*:597 (1991).

30. B. Bogerts, Zur Neuropathologie der Schizophrenien, *Fortschr. Neurol. Psychiatrie 52*:428 (1984).

31. B. Bogerts, E. Meertz, and R. Schonfledt-Bausch, Basal ganglia and limbic system pathology in schizophrenia, *Arch. Gen. Psychiatry 42*:784 (1985).

32. N. Colter, S. Battal, T. J. Crow, E. C. Johnstone, R. Brown, and C. Bruton, White matter reduction in the parahippocampal gyrus of patients with schizophrenia, *Arch. Gen. Psychiatry 44*:1023 (1987).

33. T. J. Crow, J. Ball, S. R. Bloom, R. Brown, C. J. Bruton, N. Colter, C. D. Frith, E. C. Johnstone, D. G. Owens, and G. W. Roberts, Schizophrenia as an anomaly of development of cerebral asymmetry: a postmortem study and a proposal concerning the genetic basis of the disease, *Arch. Gen. Psychiatry* 46:1145 (1989).

34. P. Falkai and B. Bogerts, Cell loss in the hippocampus of schizophrenics, *Eur. Arch. Psychiatry Neurol. Sci.* 236:154 (1986).

35. P. Falkai, B. Bogerts, and M. Rozumek, Limbic pathology in schizophrenia: the entorhinal region—a morphometric study, *Biol. Psychiatry* 24:515 (1988).

36. H. Jacob and H. Beckmann, Gross and histological criteria for developmental disorders in brains of schizophrenics, *J. R. Soc. Med.* 82:466 (1989).

37. D. V. Jeste and J. B. Lohr, Hippocampal pathologic findings in schizophrenia: a morphometric study, *Arch. Gen. Psychiatry* 46:1019 (1989).

38. J. A. Kovelman and A. B. Scheibel, A neurohistological correlate of schizophrenia, *Biol. Psychiatry* 191:1601 (1984).

39. R. Brown, N. Colter, J. A. N. Corsellis, T. J. Crow, C. D. Frith, R. Jagoe, E. C. Johnstone, and L. Marsh, Post-mortem evidence of structural brain changes in schizophrenia: differences in brain weight, temporal horn area, and parahippocampal gyrus compared with affective disorder, *Arch. Gen. Psychiatry* 43:36 (1986).

40. F. M. Benes and E. D. Bird, An analysis of the arrangement of neurons in the cingulate cortex of schizophrenic patients, *Arch. Gen. Psychiatry* 44:608 (1987).

41. F. M. Benes, G. Vincent, G. Alsterber, E. D. Bird, and J. P. San Giovanni, Increased GABA receptor binding in superficial layers of cingulate cortex in schizophrenics, *J. Neurosci.* 12(3):924 (1992).

42. F. M. Benes, Is there a neuroanatomic basis for schizophrenia? An old question revisited, *Neuroscientist* 1:104 (1995).

43. S. E. Chua and P. J. McKenna, Schizophrenia—a brain disease? A critical review of structural and functional cerebral abnormality in the disorder, *Br. J. Psychiatry* 166:563 (1995).

44. B. Bogerts, P. Falkai, B. Greve, T. Schneider, and U. Pfeiffer, The neuropathology of schizophrenia: past and present, *J. Hirnforsch.* 34:193 (1993).

45. R. F. Zec and D. R. Weinberger, Brain areas implicated in schizophrenia: a selective overview, *Handbook of Schizophrenia*: Vol. I: *The Neurology of Schizophrenia* (H. A. Nasrallah and D. R. Weinberger, eds.), Elsevier Science Publishers, New York, 1986, p. 175.

46. D. M. Pandya, G. W. Van Hoesen, and M. M. Mesulam, Efferent connections of the cingulate gyrus in the rhesus monkey, *Exp. Brain Res.* 42:319 (1981).

47. B. A. Vogt and D. N. Pandya, Cingulate cortex of the rhesus monkey: II. Cortical afferents, *J. Comp. Neurol.* 262:271 (1987).

48. B. A. Vogt, D. N. Pandya, and D. L. Rosene, Cingulate cortex of the rhesus monkey: I. Cytoarchitecture and thalamic afferents, *J. Comp. Neurol.* 262:256 (1987).

49. D. R. Weinberger, The pathogenesis: a neurodevelopmental theory, *Handbook*

of Schizophrenia: Vol. I: The Neurology of Schizophrenia (H. A. Nasrallah and D. R. Weinberger, eds.), Elsevier Science Publishers, New York, 1986, p. 397.

50. J. M. Fuster, *The Prefrontal Cortex: Anatomy, Physiology, and Neuropsychology of the Frontal Lobe*, Raven Press, New York, 1980.

51. P. S. Goldman-Rakic, L. D. Selemon, and M. L. Schwarts, Dual pathways connecting the dorsolateral prefrontal cortex with the hippocampal formation and parahippocampal cortex in the rhesus monkey, *Neuroscience 12*:719 (1984).

52. D. N. Pandya and B. Seltzer, Association areas of the cerebral cortex, *Trends Neurosci. 5*:386 (1982).

53. J. J. Levitt, M. E. Shenton, R. W. McCarley, S. F. Faux, and A. S. Ludwig, Premorbid adjustment in schizophrenia: implications for psychosocial and ventricular pathology, *Schizophr. Res. 12*:165 (1994).

54. J. A. O. Besson, F. M. Corrigan, G. R. Cherryman, and F. W. Smith, Nuclear magnetic resonance brain imaging in chronic schizophrenia, *Br. J. Psychiatry 150*:161 (1987).

55. M. K. DeMyer, R. L. Gilmor, H. C. Hendrie, W. E. DeMyer, G. T. Augustyn, and R. K. Jackson, Magnetic resonance brain images in schizophrenic and normal subjects: influences of diagnosis and education, *Schizophr. Bull. 14*: 21 (1988).

56. J. Lieberman, B. Bogerts, G. Degreef, M. Ashtari, G. Lantos, J. Alvir, Qualitative assessment of brain morphology in acute and chronic schizophrenia, *Am. J. Psychiatry 149*:784 (1992).

57. P. Williamson, D. Pelz, H. Merskey, S. Morrison, and P. Conlon, Correlation of negative symptoms in schizophrenia with frontal lobe parameters on magnetic resonance imaging, *Br. J. Pscyhiatry 165*:130 (1991).

58. P. Williamson, D. Pelz, H. Merskey, S. Morrison, S. Karlik, D. Drost, T. Carr, and P. Conlon, Frontal, temporal, and striatal proton relaxation times in schizophrenic patients and normal comparison subjects, *Am. J. Psychiatry 149*:549 (1992).

59. D. R. Weinberger, K. F. Berman, R. Suddath, and E. F. Torrey, Evidence of dysfunction of a prefrontal-limbic network in schizophrenia: a magnetic resonance imaging and regional cerebral blood flow study of discordant monozygotic twins, *Am. J. Psychiatry 149*:890 (1992).

60. M. Flaum, S. Arndt, and N. C. Andreasen, The role of gender in studies of ventricle enlargement in schizophrenia: a predominantly male effect. *Am. J. Psychiatry 147*:1327 (1990).

61. W. G. Honer, A. S. Bassett, G. N. Smith, J. S. Lapointe, and P. Falkai, Temporal lobe abnormalities in multigenerational families with schizophrenia, *Biol. Psychiatry 36*:737 (1994).

62. L. J. Seidman, D. Yurgelun-Todd, W. S. Kremen, B. T. Woods, J. M. Goldstein, S. V. Faraone, and M. T. Tsuang, Relationship of prefrontal and temporal lobe MRI measures to neuropsychological performance in chronic schizophrenia, *Biol. Psychiatry 35*:235 (1994).

63. M. C. Waldo, E. Cawthra, L. E. Adler, S. Dubester, M. Staunton, H. Naga-moto, N. Baker, A. Madison, J. Simon, A. Scherzinger, C. Drebing, G. Ger-hardt, and R. Freedman, Auditory sensory gating, hippocampal volume, and catecholamine metabolism in schizophrenics and their siblings, *Schizophr. Res. 12*:93 (1994).

64. B. A. Maher, T. C. Manschreck, B. T. Woods, D. Yurgelun-Todd, and M. T. Tsuang, Frontal brain volume and context effects in short-term recall in schizophrenia, *Biol. Psychiatry 37*:144 (1995).

65. M. F. Casanova, M. Zito, T. Goldberg, A. Abi-Dargham, R. Sanders, L. B. Bigelow, E. F. Torrey, and D. R. Weinberger, Shape distortion of the corpus callosum of monozygotic twins discordant for schizophrenia, *Schizophr. Res. 3*:155 (1990).

66. P. Conlon and M. R. Trimble, A study of the corpus callosum in epileptic psychosis using magnetic resonance imaging, *Biol. Psychiatry 24*:857 (1988).

67. W. Guenther, E. Moser, R. Petsch, J. D. Brodie, R. Steinberg, and P. Streck, Pathological cerebral blood blow and corpus callosum abnormalities in schizo-phrenia: relations to EEG mapping and PET data, *Psychiatry Res. 29*:453 (1989).

68. P. I. Hauser, D. Dauphinais, W. Berrettini, L. E. DeLisi, J. Gelernter, and R. M. Post, Corpus callosum dimensions measured by magnetic resonance imaging in bipolar affective disorder and schizophrenia, *Biol. Psychiatry 26*: 659 (1989).

69. A. L. Hoff, C. Neal, M. Kushner, and L. E. DeLisi, Gender differences in corpus callosum size in first-episode schizophrenics, *Biol. Psychiatry 35*:913 (1994).

70. A. Raine, G. N. Harrison, G. P. Reynolds, C. Sheard, J. E. Cooper, and I. Medley, Structural and functional characteristics of the corpus callosum in schizophrenics, *Arch. Gen. Psychiatry 47*:1060 (1990).

71. A. Rossi, A. Galderisi, V. Di Michele, P. Stratta, S. Ceccoli, M. Maj, and M. Casacchi, Dementia in schizophrenia: magnetic resonance and clinical corre-lates, *J. Nerv. Ment. Dis. 178*:521 (1990).

72. P. Pinel, *Traite Medico Philosophique Sur L'alienation Mentale Boulamania*, Richard Caille et Ravier, Paris, 1801.

73. E. Kretschmer, *Physique and Character*, Harcourt Brace Jovanovich Publish-ers, New York, 1925.

74. R. B. Zipursky, K. O. Lim, and A. Pfefferbaum, Brain size in schizophrenia, *Arch. Gen. Psychiatry 48*:179 (1991).

75. B. Bogerts, M. Ashtari, G. Degreef, J. M. J. Alvir, R. M. Bilder, and J. A. Lieberman, Reduced temporal limbic structure volumes on magnetic reso-nance images in first episode schizophrenia, *Psych. Res. Neuroimaging 35*(1): 1 (1990).

76. B. Bogerts, J. A. Lieberman, M. Ashtari, R. M. Bilder, G. Degreef, G. Lerner, C. Johns, and S. Masiar, Hippocampus-amygdala volumes and psychopathol-ogy in chronic schizophrenia, *Biol. Psychiatry 33*:236 (1993).

77. J. Corey-Bloom, T. Jernigan, S. Archibald, M. J. Harris, and D. V. Jeste,

Quantitative magnetic resonance imaging of the brain in late-life schizophrenia, *Am. J. Psychiatry 152*:447 (1995).

78. A. L. Hoff, H. Riordan, D. O'Donnell, P. Stritzke, C. Neale, A. Boccio, A. K. Anand, L. E. DeLisi, Anomalous lateral sulcus and cognitive function in first-episode schizophrenia, *Schizophr. Bull. 18*:257 (1992).

79. A. Kleinschmidt, P. Falkai, Y. Huang, T. Schneider, G. Furst, and H. Steinmetz, In vivo morphometry of planum temporale asymmetry in first-episode schizophrenia, *Schizophr. Res. 12*:9 (1994).

80. J. J. Kulynych, K. Vladar, B. D. Fantie, D. W. Jones, and D. R. Weinberger, Normal asymmetry of the planum temporale in patients with schizophrenia: three-dimensional cortical morphometry with MRI, *Br. J. Psychiatry 166*:742 (1995).

81. B. F. O'Donnell, S. F. Faux, R. W. McCarley, M. O. Kimble, D. F. Salisbury, P. G. Nestor, R. Kikinis, F. A. Jolesz, and M. E. Shenton, Increased rate of P300 latency prolongation with age in schizophrenia, *Arch. Gen. Psychiatry 52*:544 (1995).

82. R. G. Petty, P. E. Barta, G. D. Pearlson, I. K. McGilchrist, R. W. Lewis, Y. Tien, A. Pulver, D. D. Vaughn, M. F. Casanova, and R. E. Powers, Reversal of asymmetry of the planum temporale in schizophrenia, *Am. J. Psychiatry 152*:715 (1995).

83. C. G. Wible, M. E. Shenton, H. Hokama, R. Kikinis, F. A. Jolesz, D. Metcalf, and R. W. McCarley, Prefrontal cortex and schizophrenia: a quantitative magnetic resonance imaging study, *Arch. Gen. Psychiatry 52*:279 (1995).

84. R. W. McCarley, M. E. Shenton, B. F. O'Donnell, S. F. Faux, R. Kikinis, P. G. Nestor, and F. A. Jolesz, Auditory P300 abnormalities and left posterior superior temporal gyrus volume reduction in schizophrenia, *Arch. Gen. Psychiatry 50*:190 (1993).

85. P. G. Nestor, M. E. Shenton, R. W. McCarley, J. Haimson, R. S. Smith, B. O'Donnell, M. Kimble, R. Kikinis, and F. A. Jolesz, Neuropsychological correlates of MRI temporal lobe abnormalities in schizophrenia, *Am. J. Psychiatry 150*:1849 (1993).

86. B. F. O'Donnell, M. E. Shenton, R. W. McCarley, S. F. Faux, R. S. Smith, D. F. Salisbury, P. G. Nestor, S. D. Pollak, R. Kikinis, and F. A. Jolesz, The auditory N2 component in schizophrenia: relationship to MRI temporal lobe gray matter and to other ERP abnormalities, *Biol. Psychiatry 34*:26 (1993).

87. E. V. Sullivan, P. K. Shear, K. O. Lim, R. B. Zipursky, and A. Pfefferbaum, Cognitive and motor impairments are related to gray matter volume deficits in schizophrenia, *Biol. Psychiatry 39*:234 (1996).

88. R. B. Zipursky, L. Marsh, K. O. Lim, S. DeMent, P. K. Shear, E. V. Sullivan, G. M. Murphy, J. G. Csermansky, and A. Pfefferbaum, Volumetric MRI assessment of temporal lobe structures in schizophrenia, *Biol. Psychiatry 35*:501 (1994).

89. J. R. Kelsoe, J. L. Cadet, D. Pickar, and D. R. Weinberger, Quantitative neuroanatomy in schizophrenia: a controlled magnetic resonance imaging study, *Arch. Gen. Psychiatry 45*:533 (1988).

90. P. E. Barta, G. D. Pearlson, R. E. Powers, S. S. Richards, and L. E. Tune, Auditory hallucinations and smaller superior temporal gyral volume in schizophrenia, *Am. J. Psychiatry 147*:1457 (1990).

91. A. Rossi, P. Stratta, L. D'Albenzio, A. Tartaro, G. Schiazza, V. di Michele, F. Bolino, and M. Casacchia, Reduced temporal lobe areas in schizophrenia: preliminary evidences from a controlled multiplanar magnetic resonance imaging study, *Biol. Psychiatry 27*:61 (1990).

92. D. H. R. Blackwood, A. H. Young, J. K. McQueen, M. J. Martin, H. M. Roxborough, W. J. Muir, D. M. S. Clair, and D. M. Kean, Magnetic resonance imaging in schizophrenia: altered brain morphology associated with P300 abnormalities and eye tracking dysfunction, *Biol. Psychiatry 30*:753 (1991).

93. L. E. DeLisi, A. L. Hoff, J. E. Schwartz, G. W. Shields, S. N. Halthore, S. M. Gupta, F. A. Henn, and A. K. Anand, Brain morphology in first-episode schizophrenic-like psychotic patients: a quantitative magnetic resonance imaging study, *Biol. Psychiatry 29*:165 (1991).

94. L. E. DeLisi, P. Strizke, H. Riordan, V. Holan, A. Boccio, M. Kushner, J. McClelland, O. Van Eyle, and A. Anand, The timing of brain morphological changes in schizophrenia and their relationship to clinical outcome, *Biol. Psychiatry 31*:241 (1992).

95. A. Breier, R. W. Buchanan, A. Elkashef, R. C. Munson, B. Kirkpatrick, and F. Gellad, Brain morphology and schizophrenia: a magnetic resonance imaging study of limbic, prefrontal cortex, and caudate structures, *Arch. Gen. Psychiatry 49*:921 (1992).

96. M. E. Shenton, R. Kikinis, F. A. Jolesz, S. D. Pollak, M. LeMay, C. G. Wible, H. Hokama, J. Martin, D. Metcalf, M. Coleman, and R. W. McCarley, Abnormalities of the left temporal lobe and thought disorder in schizophrenia: a quantitative magnetic resonance imaging study, *N. Engl. J. Med. 327*:604 (1992).

97. R. W. Buchanan, A. Breier, B. Kirkpatrick, A. Elkashef, R. C. Munson, F. Gellad, and W. T. Carpenter, Structural abnormalities in deficit and nondeficit schizophrenia, *Am. J. Psychiatry 150*:59 (1993).

98. C. Colombo, M. Abbruzzese, S. Livian, G. Scotti, M. Locatelli, A. Bonfanti, and S. Scarone, Memory functions and temporal-limbic morphology in schizophrenia, *Psych. Res. Neuroimaging 50*(1):45 (1993).

99. Y. Kawasaki, Y. Maeda, K. Urata, M. Higashima, N. Yamaguchi, M. Suzuki, T. Takashima, and Y. Ide, A quantitative magnetic resonance imaging study of patients with schizophrenia, *Euro. Arch. Psych. Clin. Neurosci. 242*:268 (1993).

100. R. M. Bilder, H. Wu, B. Bogerts, G. Degreef, M. Ashtari, J. M. J. Alvir, P. J. Snyder, and J. A. Lieberman, Absence of regional hemispheric volume asymmetries in first-episode schizophrenia, *Am. J. Psychiatry 151*:1437 (1994).

101. A. Rossi, P. Stratta, F. Mancini, M. Gallucci, P. Mattei, L. Core, V. Di Michele, and M. Casacchia, Magnetic resonance imaging findings of amygdala-anterior hippocampus shrinkage in male patients with schizophrenia, *Psychiatry Res. 52*:43 (1994).

102. M. Flaum, V. W. Swayze II, D. S. O'Leary, W. T. C. Yuh, J. C. Ehrhardt, S. V. Arndt, and N. C. Andreasen, Effects of diagnosis and gender on brain morphology in schizophrenia, *Am. J. Psychiatry 152*:704 (1995).

103. P. Nopoulos, I. Torres, M. Flaum, N. C. Andreasen, J. C. Ehrhardt, and W. T. C. Yuh, Brain morphology in first-episode schizophrenia, *Am. J. Psychiatry 152*:1721 (1995).

104. A. Vita, M. Dieci, G. M. Giobbio, A. Caputo, L. Ghiringhelli, M. Comazzi, M. Garbarini, A. P. Mendini, C. Morganti, F. Tenconi, B. Cesana, and G. Invernizzi, Language and thought disorder in schizophrenia: brain morphological correlates, *Schizophr. Res. 15*:243 (1995).

105. L. Marsh, R. L. Suddath, N. Higgins, and D. R. Weinberger, Medial temporal lobe structures in schizophrenia: relationship of size to duration of illness, *Schizophr. Res. 11*:225 (1994).

106. T. E. Schlaepfer, G. J. Harris, A. Y. Tien, L. W. Peng, S. Lee, E. B. Federman, G. A. Chase, P. E. Barta, and G. D. Pearlson, Decreased regional cortical gray matter volume in schizophrenia, *Am. J. Psychiatry 151*:842 (1994).

107. D. Dauphinais, L. E. DeLisi, T. J. Crow, K. Alexandropoulos, N. Colter, I. Tuma, and E. S. Gershon, Reduction in temporal lobe size in siblings with schizophrenia: a magnetic resonance imaging study, *Psych. Res. Neuroimaging 35*:137 (1990).

108. R. B. Zipursky, D. O. Lim, E. V. Sullivan, B. W. Brown, and A. Pfefferbaum, Widespread cerebral gray matter volume deficits in schizophrenia, *Arch. Gen. Psychiatry 49*:195 (1992).

109. E. C. Johnstone, D. G. C. Owens, T. J. Crow, C. D. Frith, K. Alexandropolis, G. Bydder, and N. Colter, Temporal lobe structure as determined by nuclear magnetic resonance in schizophrenia and bipolar affective disorder, *J. Neurol. Neurosurg. Psychiatry 52*:736 (1989).

110. J. Harvey, M. A. Ron, G. D. Boulay, D. Wicks, S. W. Lewis, and R. M. Murray, Reduction of cortical volume in schizophrenia on magnetic resonance imaging, *Psychol. Med. 23*:591 (1993).

111. N. C. Andreasen, L. Flashman, M. Flaum, S. Arndt, V. W. Swayze II, D. S. O'Leary, J. C. Ehrhardt, and W. T. C. Yuh, Regional brain abnormalities in schizophrenia measured with magnetic resonance imaging, *JAMA 272*:1763 (1994).

112. T. L. Jernigan, S. Zisook, R. K. Heaton, J. T. Moranville, J. R. Hesselink, and D. L. Braff, Magnetic resonance imaging abnormalities in lenticular nuclei and cerebral cortex in schizophrenia, *Arch. Gen. Psychiatry 48*:881 (1991).

113. H. A. Nasrallah, S. B. Schwarzkopf, S. C. Olson, and J. A. Coffman, Gender differences in schizophrenia on MRI brain scans, *Schizophr. Bull. 16*:205 (1990).

114. R. E. Gur, D. Mozley, D. L. Shtasel, T. D. Cannon, F. Gallacher, B. Turetsky, R. Grossman, and R. C. Gur, Clinical subtypes of schizophrenia: differences in brain and CSF volume, *Am. J. Psychiatry 151*:343 (1994).

115. N. C. Andreasen, J. C. Ehrhardt, V. W. Swayze II, R. J. Alliger, W. T. C. Yuh, G. Cohen, and S. Ziebell, Magnetic resonance imaging of the brain in

schizophrenia: the pathophysiologic significance of structural abnormalities, *Arch. Gen. Psychiatry 47*:35 (1990).

116. L. K. Jacobsen, J. N. Giedd, A. C. Vaituzis, S. D. Hamburger, J. C. Rajapake, J. A. Frazier, D. Kaysen, M. C. Lenane, K. McKenna, C. T. Gordon, and J. L. Rapoport, Temporal lobe morphology in childhood-onset schizophrenia, *Am. J. Psychiatry 153*:355 (1996).

117. V. Synek and J. R. Reuben, The ventricular-brain ratio using planimetric measurement of EMI scans, *Br. J. Psychiatry 49*:233 (1976).

118. L. Zatz and T. L. Jernigan, The ventricular-brain ratio on computed tomography scans: validity and proper use, *Psychiatry Res. 8*:207 (1983).

119. A. Pfefferbaum, K. O. Lim, M. Rosenbloom, and R. B. Zipursky, Brain magnetic resonance imaging: approaches for investigating schizophrenia, *Schizophr. Bull. 16*:453 (1990).

120. D. H. Mathalon, E. V. Sullivan, and J. M. Rawles, A. Pfefferbaum, Correction for head size in brain-imaging measurements, *Psychiatry Res. Neuroimaging 50*:121 (1993).

121. S. Arndt, G. Cohen, R. J. Alliger, V. W. Swayze, and N. C. Andreasen, Problems with ratio and proportion measures of imaged cerebral structures, *Psychiatry Res. Neuroimaging 40*:79 (1991).

122. N. C. Andreasen, H. A. Nasrallah, V. Dunn, S. C. Olson, W. M. Grove, J. C. Ehrhardt, J. A. Coffman, and J. H. W. Crossett, Structural abnormalities in the frontal system in schizophrenia. *Arch. Gen. Psychiatry 43*:136 (1986).

123. A. Pfefferbaum, K. O. Lim, R. B. Zipursky, D. H. Mathalon, B. Lane, C. N. Ha, M. J. Rosenbloom, and E. V. Sullivan, Brain gray and white matter volume loss accelerates with aging in chronic alcoholics: a quantitative MRI study, *Alcohol. Clin. Exp. Res. 16*:1078 (1993).

124. A. H. Young, D. H. R. Blackwood, H. Roxborough, J. K. McQueen, M. J. Martin, and D. Kean, A magnetic resonance imaging study of schizophrenia: brain structure and clinical symptoms, *Br. J. Psychiatry 158*:158 (1991).

125. T. E. Goldberg, E. F. Torrey, D. F. Berman, and D. R. Weinberger, Relations between neuropsychological performance and brain morphological and physiological measures in monozygotic twins discordant for schizophrenia, *Psych. Res.: Neuroimaging 55*:51 (1993).

126. A. Rossi, P. Stratta, M. Gallucci, I. Amicarelli, R. Passariello, and M. Casacchia, Standardized magnetic resonance image intensity study in schizophrenia, *Psychiatry Res. 25*:223 (1988).

127. P. Stratta, A. Rossi, M. Gallucci, I. Amicarelli, R. Passariello, and M. Casacchia, Hemispheric asymmetries and schizophrenia: a preliminary magnetic resonance imaging study, *Biol. Psychiatry 25*:275 (1989).

128. R. L. Suddath, M. F. Casanova, T. E. Goldberg, D. G. Daniel, J. R. Kelsoe, and D. R. Weinberger, Temporal lobe pathology in schizophrenia: a quantitative magnetic resonance imaging study, *Am. J. Psychiatry 146*:464 (1989).

129. G. Degreef, B. Bogerts, M. Ashtari, and J. Lieberman, Ventricular system morphology in first episode schizophrenia: a volumetric study of ventricular subdivisions on MRI, *Schizophr. Res. 3*:18 (1990).

130. R. L. Suddath, G. W. Christison, E. F. Torrey, M. F. Casanova, and D. R. Weinberger, Anatomical abnormalities in the brains of monozygotic twins discordant for schizophrenia, *N. Engl. J. Med. 332*(12):789 (1990).

131. R. A. Bornstein, S. B. Schwarzkopf, S. C. Olson, and H. A. Nasrallah, Third-ventricle enlargement and neuropsychological deficit in schizophrenia, *Biol. Psychiatry 31*:954 (1992).

132. G. Degreef, M. Ashtari, B. Bogerts, R. M. Bilder, D. N. Jody, J. M. J. Alvir, and J. A. Lieberman, Volumes of ventricular system subdivisions measured from magnetic resonance images in first-episode schizophrenic patients, *Arch. Gen. Psychiatry 49*:531 (1992).

133. M. F. Egan, C. C. Duncan, R. L. Suddath, D. G. Kirch, A. F. Mirsky, and R. J. Wyatt, Event-related potential abnormalities correlate with structural brain alterations and clinical features in patients with chronic schizophrenia, *Schizophr. Res. 11*:259 (1994).

134. T. Becker, K. Elmer, B. Mechela, F. Schneider, S. Taubert, G. Schroth, W. Grodd, M. Bartels, and H. Beckmann, MRI findings in the medial temporal lobe structures in schizophrenia, *Eur. Neuropsychopharmacol. 1*:83 (1990).

135. S. B. Schwarzkopf, S. C. Olson, J. A. Coffman, and H. A. Nasrallah, Third and lateral ventricular volumes in schizophrenia: Support for progressive enlargement of both structures, *Psychopharmacol. Bull. 26*:385 (1990).

136. M. E. Shenton, R. Kikinis, R. W. McCarley, D. Metcalf, J. Tieman, and F. A. Jolesz, Application of automated MRI volumetric measurement techniques to the ventricular system in schizophrenics and normal controls, *Schizophr. Res. 5*:103 (1991).

137. J. M. Schwartz, E. Aylward, P. E. Barta, L. E. Tune, and G. D. Pearlson, Sylvian fissure size in schizophrenia measured with the magnetic resonance imaging rating protocol of the consortium to establish a registry for Alzheimer's disease, *Am. J. Psychiatry 149*:1195 (1992).

138. A. Pfefferbaum, D. H. Mathalon, E. V. Sullivan, J. M. Rawles, R. B. Zipursky, K. O. Lim, A quantitative magnetic resonance imaging study of changes in brain morphology from infancy to late adulthood, *Arch. Neurol. 51*(9):874 (1994).

139. C. Wernicke, *Der Aphasische Symptomenkomplex*, Cohen and Weigart, Breslau, 1874.

140. W. Penfield, L. Roberts, *Speech and Brain Mechanism*, Princeton University Press, Princeton, NJ, 1959.

141. N. Geschwind and W. Levitsky, Human brain: left-right asymmetries in temporal speech region, *Science 161*(837):186 (1968).

142. A. M. Galaburda, Anatomical asymmetry, *Cerebral Dominance: The Biological Foundations* (N. Geschwind and A. M. Galaburda, eds.), Harvard University Press, Cambridge, MA, 1984, p. 11.

143. A. M. Galaburda, J. Corsiglia, G. D. Rosen, and G. F. Sherman, Planum temporale asymmetry, reappraisal since Geschwind and Levitsky, *Neuropsychologia 25*(6):853 (1987).

144. M. M. Haglund, G. A. Ojemann, and D. W. Hochman, Optical imaging of

   epileptiform and functional activity in human cerebral cortex, *Nature*
   358(6388):668 (1992).
145. A. Raine, T. Lencz, G. P. Reynolds, G. Harrison, C. Sheard, I. Medley,
   L. M. Reynolds, and J. E. Cooper, An evaluation of structural and functional
   prefrontal deficits in schizophrenia: MRI and neuropsychological measures,
   Psych. Res. Neuroimaging 45:123 (1992).
146. V. W. Swayze II, N. C. Andreasen, R. J. Alliger, W. T. C. Yuh, and J. C.
   Ehrhardt, Subcortical and temporal structures in affective disorder and schizophrenia: a magnetic resonance imaging study, *Biol. Psychiatry 31*:221 (1992).
147. V. Di Michele, A. Rossi, P. Stratta, G. Schiazza, F. Bolino, L. Giordano, and
   M. Casacchia, Neuropsychological and clinical correlates of temporal lobe
   anatomy in schizophrenia, *ACTA Psych. Scand. 85*:484 (1992).
148. A. Rossi, P. Stratta, V. D. Michele, M. Gallucci, A. Splendiani, S. de Cataldo,
   and M. Casacchia, Temporal lobe structure by magnetic resonance in bipolar
   affective disorders and schizophrenia, *J. Affect. Dis. 21*:19 (1991).
149. A. Rossi, P. Stratta, L. D'Albenzio, A. Tartaro, G. Schiazza, V. Di Michele,
   S. Ceccoli, and M. Casacchia, Reduced temporal lobe area in schizophrenia
   by magnetic resonance imaging: preliminary evidence, *Psychiatry Res. 29*:261
   (1989).
150. M. LeMay and D. K. Kidd, Asymmetry of cerebral hemispheres on computed
   tomograms, *J. Comput. Assist. Tomogr. 2*:471 (1978).
151. M. LeMay, Left-right temporal region asymmetry in infants and children (letter), *Am. J. Neuroradiol. 7*:974 (1986).
152. L. E. DeLisi, I. D. Dauphinais, and E. S. Gershon, Perinatal complications
   and reduced size of brain limbic structures in familial schizophrenia, *Schizophr.*
   Bull. 14:185 (1988).
153. G. A. Ojemann, O. Creutzfeldt, E. Lettich, and M. Haglund, Neuronal activity
   in the human lateral temporal cortex related to short-term memory, naming,
   and reading, *Brain 111*:1383 (1988).
154. W. Penfield and P. Perot, The brain's record of auditory and visual experience:
   a final summary and discussion, *Brain 86 (Part 4)*:596 (1963).
155. M. H. Johnston and P. S. Holzman, *Assessing Schizophrenic Thinking*, Jossey-
   Bass Inc. Publishers, San Francisco, 1979.
156. M. R. Solovay, M. E. Shenton, C. Gasperetti, M. Coleman, E. Kestnbaum,
   J. T. Carpenter, P. S. Holzman, Scoring manual for the thought disorder index,
   Schizophr. Bull. 12:484 (1986).
157. J. J. Kulynych, K. Vladar, D. W. Jones, and D. R. Weinberger, Superior
   temporal gyrus volume in schizophrenia: a study using MRI morphometry
   assisted by surface rendering. *Am. J. Psychiatry 153*:50 (1996).
158. E. J. Aguilar, W. W. Bagnell, G. Haas, J. Sweeney, N. R. Schooler, J. W.
   Pettigrew, and M. S. Keshavan, Cerebral asymmetry, gender, and early schizophrenia, *Schizophr. Res. 15*:75 (1995).
159. E. R. Gautier, J. M. Kuldau, A. Weis, and C. M. Leonard, Schizophrenia and
   the temporal lobe: a replication, *American Psychiatric Association: APA New*
   Abstracts, Miami, 1995, p. 115.

160. R. R. Menon, P. E. Barta, E. H. Aylward, S. S. Richards, D. D. Vaughn, A. Y. Tien, G. J. Harris, and G. D. Pearlson, Posterior superior temporal gyrus in schizophrenia: Grey matter changes and clinical correlates, *Schizophr. Res. 15*:92 (1995).

161. N. L. Bryant, R. W. Buchanan, K. Vladar, A. Elkashef, and A. Breier, Gender differences in the temporal lobe, basal ganglia, and frontal lobe in patients with schizophrenia: an MRI volumetric study, *Schizophr. Res. 15*:77 (1995).

162. G. I. Haas, M. S. Keshavan, N. R. Schooler, W. W. Bagnell and J. W. Pettegrew, Temporal cortical volume correlates with illness duration in first episode schizophrenia, American College of Neuropsychopharmacology 34th Annual Meeting: Scientific Abstracts: San Juan, Puerto Rico, 1995, p. 112.

163. P. C. Nopoulos, M. Flaum, and N. C. Andreasen, Gender differences in schizophrenia, American College of Neuropsychopharmacology 34th Annual Meeting: Scientific Abstracts: San Juan, Puerto Rico, 1995, p. 165.

164. H. Wu, R. M. Bilder, J. Alvir, and J. A. Lieberman, Superior temporal gyrus volume and asymmetry in first-episode schizophrenia, *Biol. Psychiatry 37*:672 (1995).

165. A. Rossi, P. Stratta, P. Mattei, M. Cupillari, A. Bozzao, M. Gallucci, and M. Casacchia, Planum temporale in schizophrenia: a magnetic resonance study, *Schizophr. Res. 7*:19 (1992).

166. A. Rossi, A. Serio, P. Stratta, C. Petruzzi, G. Schiazza, F. Mancini, and M. Cassachia, Planum temporale asymmetry and thought disorder in schizophrenia, *Schizophr. Res. 12*:1 (1994).

167. L. E. DeLisi, A. L. Hoff, C. Neale, and M. Kushner, Asymmetries in the superior temporal lobe in male and female first-episode schizophrenic patients: measures of the planum temporale and superior temporal gyrus by MRI, *Schizophr. Res. 12*:19 (1994).

168. A. J. Bartley, D. W. Jones, E. F. Torrey, J. R. Zigun, and D. R. Weinberger, Sylvian fissure asymmetries in monozygotic twins: a test of laterality in schizophrenia, *Biol. Psychiatry 34*:853 (1993).

169. R. Kikinis, M. E. Shenton, G. Gerig, H. Hokama, J. Haimson, B. F. O'Donnell, C. G. Wible, R. W. McCarley, and F. A. Jolesz, Temporal lobe sulcogyral pattern anomalies in schizophrenia: an in vivo MR three-dimensional surface rendering study, *Neurosci. Lett. 182*:7 (1994).

170. M. S. Buchsbaum, R. J. Haier, S. G. Potkin, K. Nuechterlein, H. S. Bracha, M. Katz, J. Lohr, J. Wu, S. Lottenberg, P. A. Jerabek, M. Trenary, R. Tafalla, C. Reynolds, and W. E. Bunney, Frontostriatal disorder of cerebral metabolism in never-medicated schizophrenics, *Arch. Gen. Psychiatry 49*:935 (1992).

171. K. F. Berman, E. F. Torrey, and D. R. Weinberger, Regional cerebral blood flow in monozygotic twins discordant and concordant for schizophrenia, *Arch. Gen. Psychiatry 49*:927 (1992).

172. N. C. Andreasen, K. Rezai, R. Alliger, V. W. Swayze, M. Flaum, P. Kirchner, G. Cohen, and D. S. O'Leary, Hypofrontality in neuroleptic-naive patients and in patients with chronic schizophrenia: Assessment with Xenon 133 single-photon emission computed tomography and the Tower of London, *Arch. Gen. Psychiatry 49*:943 (1992).

173. J. M. Cleghorn, E. S. Garnett, C. Nahmias, G. Firnau, G. M. Brown, R. Kaplan, H. Szechtman, B. Szechtman, Increased frontal and reduced parietal glucose metabolism in acute untreated schizophrenia, *Psychiatry Res.* 28:119 (1989).

174. G. D. Pearlson, R. G. Petty, C. A. Ross, and A. Y. Tien, Schizophrenia: a disease of heteromodal association cortex? *Neuropsychopharmacology 14*(1): 1 (1996).

175. R. M. Donnino, M. E. Shenton, D. V. Iosifescu, H. Ota, R. Kikinis, R. W. McCarley, Abnormal parietal lobe asymmetry in schizophrenia, American Psychiatric Association: APA New Abstracts, New York, 1996, p. 97.

176. G. D. Pearlson, P. E. Barta, R. E. Powers, R. R. Menon, S. S. Richards, E. H. Aylward, E. B. Federman, G. A. Chase, R. G. Petty, A. Y. Tien, Medial and superior temporal gyral volume and cerebral asymmetry in schizophrenia versus bipolar disorder, *Biol. Psychiatry* (in press).

177. H. Hokama, M. E. Shenton, P. G. Nestor, R. Kikinis, J. L. Levitt, D. Metcalf, C. G. Wible, B. F. O'Donnell, F. A. Jolesz, and R. W. McCarley, Caudate, putamen, and globus pallidus volume in schizophrenia: a quantitative MRI study, *Psychiatry Res. Neuroimaging 61*:209 (1995).

178. S. Heckers, H. Heinsen, Y. Heinsen, and H. Beckman, Cortex, white matter, and basal ganglia in schizophrenia: a volumetric postmortem study, *Biol. Psychiatry 29*:556 (1991).

179. C. C. Mion, N. C. Andreasen, S. Arndt, V. W. Swayze, and G. A. Cohen, MRI abnormalities in tardive dyskinesia, *Psych. Res. Neuroimaging 40*:157 (1991).

180. M. H. Chakos, J. A. Lieberman, R. M. Bilder, M. Borenstein, G. Lerner, B. Bogerts, H. Wu, B. Kinon, and M. Ashtari, Increase in caudate nuclei volumes of first-episode schizophrenic patients taking antipsychotic drugs, *Am. J. Psychiatry 151*:1430 (1994).

181. A. M. Elkashef, R. W. Buchanan, F. Gellad, R. C. Munson, and A. Breier, Basal ganglia pathology in schizophrenia and tardive dyskinesia: an MRI quantitative study, *Am. J. Psychiatry 151*:752 (1994).

182. M. S. Keshavan, W. W. Bagwell, G. L. Hass, J. A. Sweeney, N. R. Schooler, and J. W. Pettegrew, Does caudate volume increase during follow up in first-episode psychosis?, *Schizophr. Res. 15*:87 (1995).

183. M. S. Keshavan, W. W. Bagwell, G. L. Haas, J. A. Sweeney, N. R. Schooler, and J. W. Pettegrew, Changes in caudate volume with neuroleptic treatment, *Lancet 344*:1434 (1994).

184. R. F. Deicken, G. Calabrese, E. L. Merrin, G. Fein, and M. W. Weiner, Basal ganglia phosphorous metabolism in chronic schizophrenia, *Am. J. Psychiatry 152*:126 (1995).

185. R. Sharma, P. N. Venkatasubramanian, M. Barany, and J. M. Davis, Proton magnetic resonance spectroscopy of the brain in schizophrenic and affective patients, *Schizophr. Res. 8*:43 (1992).

186. E. H. Aylward, J. V. Roberts-Twillie, P. E. Barta, A. J. Kumar, G. J. Harris, M. Geer, C. E. Peyser, and G. D. Pearlson, Basal ganglia volumes and white

matter hyperintensities in patients with bipolar disorder, *Am. J. Psychiatry* *15*:687 (1994).

187. E. G. Jones, *The Thalamus*, Plenum, New York, 1985.
188. B. Pakkenberg, Post-mortem study of chronic schizophrenic brains, *Br. J. Psychiatry 151*:744 (1987).
189. N. C. Andreasen, S. Arndt, V. W. Swayze II, T. Cizadlo, M. Flaum, D. O'Leary, J. C. Ehrhardt, and W. T. C. Yuh, Thalamic abnormalities in schizophrenia visualized through magnetic resonance image averaging, *Science 266*: 294 (1994).
190. M. S. Buchsbaum, T. Someya, C. Y. Teng, L. Abel, S. Chin, A. Najafi, R. J. Haier, J. Wu, and W. E. Bunney, PET and MRI of the thalamus in never-medicated patients with schizophrenia, *Am. J. Psychiatry 153*:191 (1996).
191. J. Gruzelier, Commentary on neuropsychological and information processing deficits in psychosis and neuro-psychophysiological syndrome relationships in schizophrenia, *Cerebral Dynamics, Laterality and Psychopathology* (R. Takahashi, P. Flor-Henry, J. Gruzelier, S. Niwa, eds.), Elsevier, Amsterdam, 1987, p. 23.
192. R. Rosenthal and L. B. Bigelow, Quantitative brain measurements in chronic schizophrenia. *Br. J. Psychiatry 21*:259 (1972).
193. A. Rossi, P. Stratta, M. Galluci, R. Passariello, and M. Casacchia, Quantification of corpus callosum and ventricles in schizophrenics with nuclear magnetic resonance imaging: a pilot study. *Am. J. Psychiatry 46*:99 (1989).
194. R. R. Lewine, L. R. Gulleu, S. C. Risch, R. Jewart, and J. L. Houpt, Sexual dimorphism, brain morphology, and schizophrenia, *Schizophr. Bull. 16*:195 (1990).
195. M. Uematsu and H. Kaiya, The morphology of the corpus callosum in schizophrenia: an MRI study, *Schizophr. Res. 1*:391 (1988).
196. H. A. Nasrallah, S. B. Schwarzkopf, S. C. Olson, and J. A. Coffman, Perinatal brain injury and cerebral vermal lobules I-X in schizophrenia, *Biol. Psychiatry 29*:567 (1991).
197. J. A. Coffman, S. B. Schwarzkopf, S. C. Olson, and H. A. Nasrallah, Midsagittal cerebral anatomy by magnetic resonance imaging: the importance of slice position and thickness, *Schizophr. Res. 2*:287 (1989).
198. R. J. Mathew and C. L. Partain, Midsagittal sections of the cerebellar vermis and fourth ventricle obtained with magnetic resonance imaging of schizophrenic patients, *Am. J. Psychiatry 142*:970 (1985).
199. M. Uematsu and H. Kaiya, Midsagittal cortical pathomorphology of schizophrenia: a magnetic resonance imaging study, *Psychiatry Res. 30*:11 (1989).
200. A. Rossi, P. Stratta, F. Mancini, S. D. Cataldo, and M. Casacchia, Cerebellar vermal size in schizophrenia: a male effect, *Biol. Psychiatry 33*:354 (1993).
201. J. J. Levitt, R. Donnino, M. E. Shenton, R. Kikinis, F. A. Jolesz, and R. W. McCarley, A quantitative volumetric MRI study of the brain stem and cerebellum in schizophrenia, *Biol. Psychiatry 39*:639 (1996).
202. P. Rakic and P. I. Yakovlev, Development of the corpus callosum and cavum septi in man, *J. Comp. Neurol. 132*:45 (1968).

203. P. Nopoulos, V. Swayze, M. Flaum, J. C. Ehrhardt, W. T. C. Yuh, and N. C. Andreasen, Cavum septi pellucidi in normals and patients with schizophrenia as detected by MRI, *Biol. Psychiatry* (in press).

204. P. Nopoulos, V. Swayze, and N. C. Andreasen, Pattern of brain morphology in patients with schizophrenia and large cavum septi pellucidi, *J. Neuropsychiatry Clin. Neurosci. 8*:147 (1996).

205. C. M. Shaw and E. C. Award, Cava septi pellucidi et vergae: their normal and pathological states, *Brain 92*:213 (1969).

206. S. W. Lewis and C. G. Mezey, Clinical correlates of septum pellucidum cavities: an unusual association with psychosis, *Psychol. Med. 15*:43 (1985).

207. R. J. Mathew, C. L. Partain, M. V. Prakash, M. V. Kulkarni, T. P. Logan, and W. H. Wilson, A study of the septum pellucidum and corpus callosum in schizophrenia with MR imaging, *Acta Psychiatr. Scand. 72*:414 (1985).

208. G. Degreef, G. Lantos, B. Bogerts, M. Ashtari, and J. Lieberman, Abnormalities of the septum pellucidum on MR scans in first-episode schizophrenic patients, *Am. J. Neuroradiol. 13*:835 (1992).

209. G. Degreef, B. Bogerts, P. Falkai, B. Greve, G. Lantos, M. Ashtari, and J. Lieberman, Increased prevalence of the cavum septum pellucidum in magnetic resonance scans and post-mortem brains of schizophrenic patients, *Psych. Res. Neuroimaging 45*:1 (1992).

210. L. E. DeLisi, A. L. Hoff, M. Kushner, and G. Degreef, Increased prevalence of cavum septum pellucidum in schizophrenia, *Psychiatry Res. Neuroimaging 50*:193 (1993).

211. T. F. Scott, T. P. Price, M. S. George, J. Brillman, and W. Rothfus, Cerebral malformations and schizophrenia, *J. Neuropsychiatry Clin. Neurosci. 5*:287 (1993).

212. G. J. Jurjus, H. A. Nasrallah, S. C. Olson, and S. B. Schwarzkopf, Cavum septum pellucidum in schizophrenia, affective disorder, and healthy controls: a magnetic resonance imaging study, *Psychol. Med. 23*:319 (1993).

213. M. E. Shenton, Temporal lobe structural abnormalities in schizophrenia: a selective review and presentation of new MR findings, *Psychopathology: The Evolving Science of Mental Disorders* (S. Matthysse, D. Levy, J. Kagan, and F. M. Benes, eds.), Cambridge University Press, New York, 1996, p. 51.

214. R. W. McCarley, M. E. Shenton, B. F. O'Donnell, and P. G. Nestor, Uniting Kraepelin and Bleuler: the psychology of schizophrenia and the biology of temporal lobe abnormalities, *Harvard Rev. Psychiatry 1*:36 (1993).

215. R. E. Gur and G. D. Pearlson, Neuroimaging in schizophrenia research, *Schizophr. Bull. 19*:337 (1993).

13

Magnetic Resonance Spectroscopy in Schizophrenia and Psychotic Disorders

Matcheri S. Keshavan and Jay W. Pettegrew
University of Pittsburgh, Western Psychiatric Institute and Clinic, Pittsburgh, Pennsylvania

I. INTRODUCTION

The advent of in vivo structural and functional imaging techniques over the last two decades has led to a substantial surge in our knowledge about the biological basis of schizophrenia and other major psychotic disorders. Over the past few years, magnetic resonance spectroscopy (MRS), a novel noninvasive approach to examination of brain chemistry, has been applied in the study of these disorders. While still not ready for clinical use, MRS has the potential to characterize the pathophysiological substrate of disorders hitherto considered as "functional" psychoses for lack of evidence of a neuroanatomical basis. Two pivotal questions pose themselves in this regard:

1. What neuroanatomical systems, e.g., frontostriatopallidothalamic, and frontotemporal, are involved in the generation of the positive and negative symptoms characteristic of these disorders?
2. What pathophysiological mechanisms, i.e., neurodevelopmental or neurodegenerative, are likely to mediate these abnormalities?

Being noninvasive, MRS can address these questions in a longitudinal framework; a good deal of literature has already accumulated in this area and is worthy of a review and reappraisal. Among the various approaches available, phosphorus MRS and proton MRS have been most frequently applied. In this chapter, we focus on MRS studies in schizophrenia, with special emphasis on proton and phosphorus MRS. We will also review MRS literature on other major psychotic disorders, but only to place the schizophrenia findings in perspective. Details of the basic physics, instrumentation, and principles underlying MRS are beyond the scope of this chapter and are covered elsewhere in this volume; the reader is also referred to more detailed works for this purpose [1,2].

II. ^{31}P MRS STUDIES

The phosphorus nucleus has been used extensively in both in vivo and in vitro MRS studies. The advantage of ^{31}P is its 100% natural abundance and the fairly wide range of chemical shift (about 30 parts per million, or ppm) for biologically relevant ^{31}P-containing compounds. However, since the concentration of ^{31}P nuclei is much less (about 10 mM) than that of ^{1}H (about 50 M), it has a substantially smaller signal-to-noise ratio (SNR). The SNR of ^{31}P is also diminished because of its relatively shorter T_2 and longer T_1 relaxation times. Because of SNR constraints, the resolution of ^{31}P MRS is rather poor, i.e., about 10 cm^3, while that of ^{1}H MRI is 1 cm^3.

A. What ^{31}P MRS Reveals

Phosphorus MRS provides important information about both energy and membrane metabolism. The ^{31}P MRS resonance of α (esterified ends), β (middles), and γ phosphate moieties (ionized ends) of adenosine triphosphate (ATP), phosphocreatine (PCr), ADP, and inorganic phosphate (Pi) provide information about energy metabolism. α- and γ-Phosphate resonances contain a mixture of ATP and other phosphates. β-ATP, on the other hand, is generally thought to most reliably reflect tissue ATP levels. ATP serves as the high-energy reservoir in the metabolism of carbohydrates, lipids, and proteins via the Krebs cycle; any excess is saved as PCr. PCr, catalyzed by creative kinase (PCr + ADP $\rightarrow$ ATP + creatine), serves as an "energy shuttle," which helps brain ATP levels to be constant. Pathological states associated with hypoxia, ischemia, anaerobic metabolism, and impaired energy utilization perturb the levels of ATP, PCr, and Pi. When oxygen is lacking, a shift occurs to anaerobic metabolism; lactate is generated from pyruvate, and pH is reduced.

^{31}P MRS also reveals important insights into the metabolism of cell membranes, which are integral for the maintenance of structure, ion conduction, and signal transduction as well as maintenance of concentration gradients; cell membranes are comprised of a phospholipid bilayer. Phosphomonoesters (PME) are the precursors, and phosphodiesters (PDE) are the breakdown products of membrane phospholipids [e.g., phosphatidyl choline (PtdC), phosphatidyl ethanolamine (PtdE), and phosphatidyl serine (PtdS)]. PMEs include phosphorylcholine, phosphorylserine, phosphorylethanolamine, and α-glycerophosphate; PDEs include glycerophosphorylcholine and glycerophosphorylethanolamine. PME and PDE resonances reflect membrane turnover and may differ between healthy and disease states. Phospholipids themselves constitute a large part of the broad resonance underlying the PDE and PME peaks. The intracellular pH can be calculated indirectly from the separation between the ionized and esterified ends [3] intracellular magnesium (Mg^{2+}) also can be similarly estimated [4].

B. Studies in Schizophrenia

Reduced activity of the prefrontal cortex ("hypofrontality") is seen in schizophrenia as evidenced by decreased glucose utilization and regional blood flow in positron emission tomography (PET) and single photon emission computed tomography (SPECT) studies [5]. These observations, and evidence that schizophrenia is associated with membrane phospholipid alterations in peripheral cells (for review see Ref. 6), stimulated our studies of brain energy and membrane phospholipid metabolism using ^{31}P MRS. We predicted that (a) schizophrenia would be associated with abnormal utilization of high-energy phosphates such as ATP and PCr in the prefrontal cortex and (b) schizophrenia would be associated with neurochemical abnormalities in membrane phospholipid metabolism, as evidenced by a reduction in PME and an increase in PDEs. To test these hypotheses, we examined brain high-energy phosphate and membrane phospholipid metabolism in the dorsal prefrontal cortex of neuroleptic-naive, first-episode schizophrenic patients and matched healthy controls; analysis of the ^{31}P MRS spectra demonstrated decreased levels of PME and P_i compared to control subjects. The schizophrenic group also showed increased levels of PDE and ATP [7,8].

Several other in vivo ^{31}P MRS studies of schizophrenic patients [9–14] have now appeared in the literature (Table 1). The phospholipid findings of Pettegrew et al.'s 1991 study [8] have been replicated in part by three independent groups examining the frontal lobe [12–14]. Stanley et al. [14] examined a 2- to 3-cm slice of the prefrontal cortex by ^{31}P MRS using a fast-rotating gradient spectroscopy pulse sequence to localize a 15- to 20-cm^3 region. They compared 11 drug-naive, 8 newly diagnosed medicated, and 10 chronic medicated schizophrenia patients with matched controls and found significantly lower PME levels in all of the schizophrenia groups and significantly higher PDE levels in the drug-naive group compared to controls.

In contrast to the findings concerning membrane phospholipid metabolism, the results with respect to alterations in frontal lobe high-energy phosphate metabolism in schizophrenia have been variable across studies. The most recent study of Stanley et al. [14] found no significant differences in the high-energy phosphate metabolite levels in schizophrenic patients versus controls. The differences across these studies may lie in the MRS methodology or may relate to variability in the clinical status of the schizophrenic patients, e.g., medicated or unmedicated, acute or chronic.

Studies of the temporal lobe using ^{31}P MRS have also been relatively less consistent. O'Callaghan et al. [9] found no evidence for alterations in membrane phospholipid or energy metabolism in a series of chronic schizophrenic patients. However, their control subjects were somewhat older, and spectral contamination by superficial tissues next to the coil could not be ruled out. Fukuzako et al. [11] found evidence of increased PDE in both the medial temporal lobes in schizophrenia. They also found reduced β-ATP in the left medial temporal lobe in schizophrenia, suggesting a lateralized abnormality in high-energy phosphate metabolism. Deicken [12] observed that PCr:Pi and PCr:β-ATP ratios were higher in the right temporal lobes of schizophrenia patients, suggesting a right/left asymmetry in the patients but not in the controls. They suggested two possible explanations for these findings: a right temporal hypometabolism or a left temporal hypermetabolism. A similar metabolic asymmetry in the temporal lobes has been observed in previous PET studies of schizophrenia.

Table 1 Phosphorus MRS Studies in Schizophrenia

Study	Population studied	MRS technique	Brain region of interest	Main findings	Ref
Pettegrew et al., 1991	11 first-episode neuroleptic-naive SCZ; 10 HCN	Surface coil	Dorsal prefrontal cortex	Decreased PME, Pi; increased PDE, and ATP	8
O'Callaghan et al., 1991	18 medicated SCZ and 10 HCN	Surface coil	Left temporal lobe	Mean pH higher in patients; no other differences	9
Deicken et al., 1994	20 chronic SCZ and 16 HCN	Head coil; ISIS pulse sequence	Frontal lobes	Increased PDE, and decreased PCr	12
Fukuzako et al., 1994	16 medicated chronic SCZ; 16 HCN	Three-dimensional chemical shift imaging	Medial temporal lobes	Increased PDE bilaterally; decreased ATP on left side	11
Kato et al., 1995	27 medicated chronic SCZ; 26 HCN	One-dimensional chemical shift imaging	Frontal lobes	Bilaterally decreased PME; increased ATP, and Pcr on the left side	13
Stanley et al., 1995	11 first-episode drug-naive, 8 newly diagnosed medicated, and 10 chronic medicated SCZ	Fast-rotating gradient spectroscopy (FROGS)	Frontal lobes	Decreased PME, increased PDE, increased Mg	14

SCZ = Schizophrenia; HCN = healthy controls; ISIS = image selected in vivo spectroscopy.

C. Specificity Issues

Membrane phospholipid alterations, as observed by ^{31}P MRS, may not be confined to schizophrenic illness. Few studies to date have reported ^{31}P MRS data in patients with nonschizophrenic psychotic illness, such as delusional disorders. Decreases in PME and PDE have been noted in cocaine-dependent polysubstance abusers [15]. In vivo ^{31}P MRS studies of affective disorder have also been carried out. Kato et al. [16] compared ^{31}P MRS parameters between manic subjects on lithium to their euthymic state as well as with normal controls. A significant elevation of PME was seen and was attributed to the possible accumulation of inositol-1-phosphate in brain induced by lithium. ^{31}P MRS investigations have also reported increases in PME in the frontal lobes in depressive patients [17]. By contrast, bipolar patients have decreased PME during the euthymic state [18]. Patients with Alzheimer's disease have ^{31}P MRS findings of increased PME and PDE [19]; autism is associated with decreased PCr suggesting increased energy utilization, consistent with a hypermetabolic picture [20]. No alterations were observed in PME or PDE in this disorder.

Thus, the ^{31}P MRS findings of schizophrenia may have some measure of specificity as compared to other major neuropsychiatric disorders. Interestingly, however, observations similar to schizophrenia are seen with normal aging. This supports one model of schizophrenia being viewed as a form of premature aging of select brain structures [8].

D. State-Trait Issues

Alterations in phospholipid metabolites similar to those observed in schizophrenia (decreased PME, increased PDE) were seen in a presumed "healthy" control subject who was studied 2 years before her first psychotic episode [21]. This suggests that the phospholipid alterations seen in schizophrenia may represent "trait" markers and underscores the importance of longitudinal MRS studies in schizophrenia. In a cross-sectional comparison of patients at different stages of schizophrenic illness, Stanley et al. [14] showed that PMEs were reduced in both newly diagnosed and chronic patients, but the PDE elevations were seen only in the first-episode cases. This suggests that the PME reductions may be trait markers, while the PDE changes may reflect state-related phenomena. These findings need to be confirmed in prospective longitudinal follow-up studies. In an ongoing study using this design, we found that the PME reductions appear to persist with neuroleptic treatment (J. W. Pettegrew et al., unpublished findings). Longitudinal studies of subjects at risk for schizophrenia (e.g., first-degree relatives of schizophrenic probands) are also valuable in our efforts to clarify state-trait issues.

E. Clinical Correlates

An association has been observed between reduced PME levels in the prefrontal cortex and negative symptoms in one study [22]. These authors also observed that patients with prominent negative symptoms had higher β-ATP levels. Thus, MRS measures of decreased frontal lobe metabolism correlate with negative symptoms, consistent with observations of hypofrontality as measured by PET studies correlating with negative symptoms [6]. Deicken et al. [23] observed an association between reduced left frontal PME and poorer performance on the Wisconsin card sort test (fewer categories achieved, lower percent conceptual level, and greater total errors). An association has also been reported between reduced PME levels and abnormalities in saccadic eye movements, considered to reflect frontal lobe integrity [24]. Thus, PME reductions appear to correlate with trait-related abnormalities in schizophrenia.

Calabrese et al. [25] initially observed a significant negative correlation between total BPRS scores and PCr-β-ATP ratios in both right and left temporal lobes. This correlation appeared to be largely accounted for by thinking disturbance. This group subsequently reported that the degree of metabolic asymmetry of PCr in the temporal lobes (right minus left/right plus left) was positively correlated with the BPRS thinking disturbance subscale score [23]. Thus, temporal lobe metabolic activity may parallel positive symptomatology, in contrast to frontal metabolic activity, which may correlate with negative symptoms and deficits in cognitive functioning.

Observations, reviewed above, suggesting that PME reductions may be trait phenomena raise the question as to whether this is a familially transmitted marker. In a preliminary analysis of subgroups divided by family history, Keshavan et al. [26] observed the PME levels were more reduced in the patients with a family history of schizophrenia.

Few studies have systematically examined the neuroanatomical correlates of ^{31}P MRS findings in schizophrenia. In a preliminary study, it was observed that the PDE levels correlate significantly with corpus callosal size, particularly the anterior quartile [27]. The pathophysiological significance of this finding remains to be clarified.

F. Possible Pathophysiological Mechanisms

Decreased PME and increased PDE levels could suggest decreased synthesis and increased breakdown of membrane phospholipids in schizophrenia. Demisch et al. [28] have reported a significantly decreased incorporation of ^{14}C-labeled arachidonic acid in membrane phospholipids in patients with schizoaffective and schizophreniform disorders, which could suggest decreased membrane phospholipid synthesis. Decreased levels of membrane PtdC have been observed in erythrocytes in some schizophrenics [29], and decreased PtdE has been reported as well [6]. Gattaz et al. [30] has reported increased activity of phospholipase A_2 in plasma from schizophrenic patients. It is possible, therefore, that the PME and PDE alterations represent membrane alterations that antedate the onset of anatomical changes.

The ^{31}P MRS findings observed in schizophrenia are similar to what happens during normative postnatal development. Preliminary data from our group on normal neurodevelopmental changes show an exponential decrease in PME levels and oxidative metabolic rate during the period of normal synaptic pruning, which occurs during late childhood and early adolescence [31]. These findings are consistent with Buchli et al.'s [32] observation that human brain levels of PME decrease from the neonatal to the adult period. Adolescence is also characterized by reductions in gray matter volumes, regional brain metabolism, and delta sleep. Taken together, it has been proposed [8,33–35] that the abnormality in membrane and energy metabolism in schizophrenia may be related to an exaggeration of normative peri-adolescent synaptic pruning that occurs in nonhuman primates [36] and humans [37]. Such synaptic loss is also consistent with observations of predominant reductions in gray but not white matter [38–41]. It is unlikely that normal neuronal cell death is exaggerated (which should decrease numbers of neurons and their axons and, thus, reduce the volume of both gray and white matter). Recent neuropathological work by Selemon et al. [42] showing neurophil reductions in the dorsolateral prefrontal cortex of schizophrenic patients supports the possibility of exaggerated synaptic pruning in this disorder. Nonsynaptic components (such as glial cell bodies and processes, neuronal cell bodies and processes without synapses) may, on the other hand, increase proportionately. O_2 consumption is higher for neurons compared to neuroglia Sokoloff [43,44]; a preferential reduction in synapses is therefore consistent with observations of reduced cortical energy utilization in schizophrenia [8].

The view that schizophrenia results from an abnormality in postnatal (or "late") synaptic elimination processes is consistent with its typical onset in adolescence. However, alternative models must be considered as well. Abnormal neurodevelopment in schizophrenia may also result from faulty myelination processes in critical brain regions [45]. "Early" neurodevelopmental models postulate a disruption in intrauterine or perinatal brain development resulting from infections, malnutrition, or obstetric complications [46–48]. Observations of premorbid abnormalities in socialization and neuromotor function in some schizophrenic patients are in support of this model. However, not all patients have such premorbid abnormalities, and not all subjects with these abnormalities go on to develop schizophrenia. It is therefore more likely that schizophrenic illness results from an interaction between early disruption in brain development and postnatal brain maturation processes, i.e., a "two-hit" model.

The synaptic loss associated with normal pruning is predominantly of presumably glutamatergic asymmetrical junctions on dendritic spines [49]. The prefrontal-limbic glutamatergic neurons are therefore likely to be involved in the pathophysiology of schizophrenia. Stanley et al.'s [14] observation of increased Mg^+ in schizophrenic patients is of interest in this regard. Intracellular Mg^+ voltage dependently blocks NMDA receptor channels; thus, abnormal Mg levels could lead to reduction of glutamatergic neuronal function, consistent with the hypoglutamatergic hypothesis of schizophrenia [50].

G. Psychopharmacological Studies

The noninvasive nature of ^{31}P MRS studies allows them to be repeated before and after administration of pharmacological agents. Renshaw et al. [51] showed accumulation of PMEs following lithium administration to cats in therapeutically meaningful doses. It is possible that such effects could parallel lithium's therapeutic effects; using ^{31}P MRS one can noninvasively monitor second messenger–mediated events, which may mediate lithium's effects. ^{31}P MRS has been used to detect the muscarinic agonist–induced accumulation of phosphomonoesters (possibly related to changes in inositol phosphates) in cats [51]. It is thus possible to carry out longitudinal and drug-related monitoring of changes in phospholipid metabolism in neuropsychiatric disorders. We recently examined ^{31}P MRS data in schizophrenic and schizoaffective patients before and after 1 and 2 weeks of treatment with lithium: reduced pretreatment PME and increases in nucleotide phosphates at 1 week predicted therapeutic response [52]. Few studies have examined the question of whether ^{31}P MRS data before treatment predict therapeutic response to antipsychotic drugs.

III. PROTON MRS STUDIES

A. What ^{1}H MRS Reveals

The main advantage of ^{1}H MRS is its relatively better sensitivity and, hence, SNR. Localized ^{1}H MRS can therefore be carried out using voxels of interest as small as 1 cm^3. Since water protons in living tissue dominate signals from protons bound to other chemical species, techniques of water supression are needed to obtain ^{1}H MR spectra. One limitation of ^{1}H MRS is that the range of visible chemical shifts is much narrower (10 ppm) than that of ^{31}P MRS. Thus, the detection of individual resonances is more difficult. ^{1}H MRS can be used to measure resonances from (a) amino acids, neurotransmitters, and their derivatives, (b) metabolites related to energy metabolism such as glucose, phosphocreatine, creatine, lactate, and acetate and N-acetyl aspartate (NAA), (c) metabolites related to phospholipid metabolism such as phosphorylcholine, phosphorylethanolamine, glycerophosphorylcholine, and glycerophosphorylethanolamine, and (d) metabolites related to nucleotide metabolism such as adenine, guanine, uracil, and cytosine. NAA is considered to be primarily intraneuronal, although some glial cells may also contain

NAA [53] and provide an index of neuronal mass and integrity. The role of brain NAA remains unclear. Its neuronal co-localization with N-acetylaspartylglutamate (NAAG) suggests a possible relation to excitatory amino acids. NAAG, when cleaved by a dipeptidase, yields NAA and glutamate. ^{1}H MRS also provides information about (a) choline-containing metabolites, which may represent putative neuronal and extraneuronal markers, (b) creatine, which is a biproduct of high-energy and protein metabolism, (c) inositol, an intermediary in the phosphoinositide cycle, a second messenger system, (d) γ-amino butyric acid, an inhibitory neurotransmitter, and (e) glutamate, an excitatory neurotransmitter.

B. ^{1}H MRS Studies in Schizophrenia

^{1}H MRS studies have revealed a fairly consistent body of evidence, suggesting metabolic abnormalities in the temporal cortex of schizophrenic patients (Table 2). Nasrallah et al. [54] reported a significant reduction in NAA in the right hippocampus/amygdala complex of schizophrenic patients. Renshaw et al. [55] observed a reduction in NAA:Cr ratio in both the right and left temporal lobes of schizophrenic patients. Fukuzako et al. [56] recently reported a 23% reduction in the NAA:Ch + Cr ratios in the medial temporal lobe of schizophrenic patients. Meier et al. [57] observed a 22% of NAA in left hippocampus, as well as a biateral reduction in choline and creatine. These findings are consistent with observations of reductions in the volume of temporal cortex in schizophrenic patients [58,59].

These studies used somewhat variable approaches to MRS. All of them assumed that the relaxation times for the ^{1}H MRS metabolites do not differ between schizophrenic and control subjects and that these relaxation times remain constant during brain development. However, preliminary evidence suggests that T_1 and T_2 relaxation times are relatively unaffected in pathological conditions [60] and during neurodevelopment [61]. All of these studies, except that of Maier et al. [57], have chosen to present NAA data as ratios to other metabolites such as creatine; observations that creatine might change as well in the illness suggest that this approach is problematic. Another source of variance is that most of these studies have examined chronic schizophrenic patients, and the potential confounds of treatment and illness chronicity can not be excluded. Interestingly, Hendren et al. [62] reported a trend for a reduction in NAA:Cr ratios in a series of children with early schizotypal personality disorder or schizophrenia as compared to a group of young healthy controls. No data were provided about prior treatment or illness duration. If confirmed, this preliminary observation points to the possibility that NAA alterations occur in children at risk for schizophrenia illness.

Table 2   Proton MRS Studies in Schizophrenia

Study	Population studied	MRS technique	Brain region	Main findings	Ref
Nasrallah et al., 1994	11 chronic medicated SCZ; 11 HCN	STEAM (TE = 50 ms)	Medial temporal lobes	Reduced NAA in right limbic temporal lobe	54
Hendren et al., 1994	9 children (ages 8–12) with SCZ and SCZTY and age/sex-matched HCN	Localized spin echo proton MRS (TE = 136 ms)	Left frontal cortex	Trend for reduction in NAA/Cr in SCZ	
Renshaw et al., 1995	13 first-episode psychoses patients and 15 HCN	STEAM (TE = 30 ms)	Temporal lobes	NAA/PCr reduced and choline/creatine ratios increased on the left side	55
Buckley and Waddington, 1994	28 SCZ; 20 HCN	STEAM (TE = 68 ms)	Frontal, temporal	Reduction in frontal but not temporal NAA	77
Stanley et al., 1995	6 first-episode SCZ; 9 male controls	STEAM (TE = 20 ms)	Left dorsolateral prefrontal cortex	Glutamate reduced and glutamine increased; no changes in NAA choline or creatine	63
Maier et al., 1995	25 chronic SCZ; 32 HCN	STEAM (TE = 135 ms); water in tissue as internal standard	Hippocampus	22% reduction in NAA in left, choline and creatine reduced bilaterally	57
Fukuzako et al., 1995	15 chronic SCZ; 5 HCN	STEAM (TE = 15 ms)	Frontal and medial temporal lobes	Reduction in NAA in left medial temporal lobe.	56

SCZ = Schizophrenia; SCZTY = schizotypal personality disorder; HCN = health controls; NAA = N-acetyl aspatate; STEAM = stimulated echo acquisition mode; TE = echo-time.

To date, only one study has appeared in the literature describing ^{1}H MRS findings in first-episode, treatment-naive schizophrenic patients. Stanley et al. [63] reported reductions in the glutamate and aspartate signals and an increase in the glutamine signal in six schizophrenic patients; no alterations were seen in the levels of NAA, creatine, or choline resonances. They interpreted these findings to reflect decreased glutamatergic neurotransmission. However, they urge caution in the interpretation of these findings because of the small sample size and the difficulties in quantification of small resonances such as glutamate. In particular, studies that acquire MR spectra with a short echotime (e.g., 20 ms) result in complex spectra because of overlap between multiple proton-containing metabolites. Such overlap makes it difficult to assign the spectral metabolites; in vitro experiments are needed to address this issue.

C. Specificity Issues

Preliminary reports of ^{1}H MRS in major depression also have appeared in the literature [64,65], showing increases in choline resonances. Sharma et al. [66] obtained ^{1}H spectra from the frontal and occipital regions of nine psychiatric patients and nine healthy controls. The patients, notably lithium-treated bipolar disorders, showed an increased NAA:PCr ratio compared to controls. Charles et al. [67] recently observed a trend for increased choline among elderly depressives; these levels subsided following treatment. ^{1}H MRS studies have been carried out recently in lithium-treated patients with bipolar disorder and lithium-free controls [68]. Contrary to erythrocyte data showing accumulations of choline with lithium treatment, no changes were seen in the brain content of choline or related compounds. Thus, in contrast to studies in schizophrenia, none of the ^{1}H MRS studies of affective disorder have shown alterations in NAA. Thus NAA reductions in the temporal lobe may have some measure of specificity for schizophrenic illness.

D. Pathophysiological Significance

Reductions in brain NAA levels have been reported to parallel the progressive brain volume loss in neurodegenerative disorders [69]. NAA decreases after selective neuronal loss both in animal models as well as in a variety of neurological disorders characterized by neuronal loss [70]. It is therefore conceivable that NAA reductions in the temporal lobe may reflect volume loss in this brain region, reported in neuropathological as well as imaging studies of schizophrenia [58,59]. Thus, the question may arise as to whether the reductions in NAA are simply due to inclusion of more CSF in the voxel of interest. However, a recent study [57], in which care was taken to address these issues, also showed substantial reductions in NAA in the temporal lobes. This metabolic abnormality could be related to reductions in the number, density, or neuronal volume in this brain region. The NAA reductions could also result from loss of neuropil, comprised largely by synapses (also containing NAA) due to an exaggerated synaptic pruning process discussed above. However, such NAA reductions could be offset to some extent by the fact that neuropil reductions also lead to increased neuronal packing, which in effect would elevate NAA levels in the voxel of interest. A combination of reduced neuronal number and synaptic density, however, could lead to an overall decrement in NAA. Reductions in the choline signal observed in some studies [57] is also consistent with this; a reduction in choline signal in MRS could result from an overall reduction in synthesis of phospholipids observed in vitro [7] and in vivo, as reviewed earlier. Such metabolic alterations in the temporal and frontal cortex would be consistent with the neurodevelopmental models proposed to underlie schizophrenic illness. The preliminary observations of reductions in glutamate and increases in glutamine in the frontal lobes in schizophrenia [63] would also be of great interest in the context of this model and need to be replicated.

IV. FLUORINE MRS STUDIES

A number of studies have dealt with ^{19}F MRS. This nucleus is 100% naturally abundant and has high NMR sensitivity and a fairly large chemical shift range. However, negligible fluorine concentrations in the human body rule out its use for studying endogenous metabolites. Since a number of fluorinated psychopharmacological drugs are currently in clinical use, this approach offers a powerful technique to monitor their pharmacokinetics. ^{19}F MRS has been used to follow the kinetics of fluorinated drugs in animals [71,72]. Fluorinated antipsychotic drugs amenable to ^{19}F MRS studies include trifluperazine, triflupromazine, fluphenazine, trifluperidol, Pimozide, and haloperidol. Recently, ^{19}F MRS studies have been conducted in patients being treated with Fluphenazine and Fluoxetine [73,74]. ^{19}F MRS therefore offers a safe way to measure psychoactive drugs directly in brain tissue. This is particularly valuable because of the unreliable relationship between serum concentration of neuroleptics and their clinical effects. The ability to spectroscopically detect fluorine containing metabolies is related to the equivalent weight; thus, trifluperazine is more "MRS visible" than haloperidol [75]. A major limitation of in vivo ^{19}F MRS is the difficulty to satisfactorily resolve metabolites of the fluorinated psychoactive drugs. Improvements in NMR technique are needed before attempting to correlate serum concentrations with brain levels of these fluorinated drugs. Other potential uses of ^{19}F MRS include monitoring therapeutic response and side effects and eventually even studies of receptor populations using fluorinated medications as biological "traces" [76].

V. CONCLUSIONS AND FUTURE DIRECTIONS

In summary, the "first-generation" MRS studies of schizophrenic illness have been promising in illuminating important aspects of the pathophysiology of this disorder. Noteworthy findings include reduction in NAA in temporal lobes, evidence of membrane alterations in the prefrontal and temporal cortex, and possible asymmetrical alteration in energy metabolism in schizophrenia. However, several substantial methodological hurdles still need to be overcome in this nascent field [77]. The following are among the central problems that need to be, and are being, addressed:

1. Precise localization of the voxels of interest (VOI) for MRS continues to be a problem; morphometric measurements of the regions of interest deploying MR images acquired in the same setting, as well as the use of MRI-compatible brain atlases, are likely to improve accurate localization (78).

2. Heterogeneity of tissue in the voxel of interest (e.g., gray vs. white matter or CSF) is likely to lead to conflicting findings; approaches to address this include quantification of tissue types within VOI (by developing an interface between MRI segmentation software and MRS) as well as use of the smallest VOI permissible for the experiment.

3. The MRS technique has poor sensitivity, leading to difficulties in quantifying MR spectral resonances; an example of this difficulty is the problem in separating the glutamate from the glutamine signal in efforts to examine the glutamate hypothesis of schizophrenia [16]. Studies using high field magnets (e.g., 3 or 4 Tesla magnets) can improve spectral resolution, since SNR increases linearly with static magnetic field strength; however, the highest usable field strengths are limited by the extent of patient radio frequency power absorption.

4. Nonreplication of findings often results from too much subjective interpretation of MRS data; fully automated spectral processing routines are likely to help minimize such operator bias.

5. Different compounds and different tissues have varying relaxation times (longitudinal relaxation or T_1 and transverse relaxation or T_2). The observed ^{31}P MRS signal, which consists of long T_1 species, does not fully recover its magnetization when the repetition time is short. Thus, changes in T_1 will lead to different peak areas for the techniques such as proton decoupling. It is, therefore, possible that patient control differences in MRS metabolites may be confounded by potential group differences in relaxation times (T_1 and T_2) of these metabolites; further research is needed to examine these possible sources of systematic error.

6. The careful choice of patient populations with a view to minimize potential confounds of illness chronicity and medication is critical; the first-episode strategy is valuable in this regard [79].

One of the central advantages of MRS is its noninvasiveness and the fact that it reveals insights about aspects of neurochemistry, unavailable with other techniques, such as membrane metabolism, cytosolic metabolites, and intracellular pH. The noninvasiveness of MRS lends itself to repeated application over the course of the illness. This aspect of MRS is especially attractive to research in schizophrenia, a chronic illness with a variable course. MRS studies are likely to shed light on the critical task of separating state from trait markers and of distinguishing progressive versus static aspects of the pathobiology of schizophrenia. An exciting new direction would be to use MRS in prospective longitudinal follow-up studies of offspring at high risk for schizophrenia with a view to identify early predictors of vulnerability to this illness; such insights will potentially aid in both early diagnosis and prevention of this devastating disorder.

REFERENCES

1. M. S. Keshavan, S. Kapur, and J. W. Pettegrew, Magnetic resonance spectroscopy in psychiatry: potential, pitfalls, and promise, *Am. J. Psychiatry 148*(8): 976 (1991).
2. S. R. Dager and R. G. Steen, Applications of magnetic resonance spectroscopy to the investigation of neuropsychiatric disorders, *Neuropsychopharmacology 62*:249 (1992).
3. J. W. Pettegrew, G. Withers, K. Panchalingam, et al. Considerations for brain pH assessment by ^{31}P NMR. *Magn. Resonance Imaging 6*:135 (1988).
4. R. K. Gupta, P. Gupta, and R. P. Moore, NMR studies of intracellular metal ions in intact cells and tissues, *Ann. Rev. Biophys. Bioeng. 13*:221 (1984).
5. N. C. Andreasen, K. Rezzi, R. Alliger, I. I. Swayze, M. Falum, P. Kirchenr, G. Cohen, and D. S. O'Leary, Hypofrontality in neuroleptic-naive patients and in patients with chronic schizophrenia, *Arch. Gen. Psychiatry 49*:943 (1992).
6. J. Rotrosen and A. Wolkin, Phospholipid and prostaglandin hypothesis in schizophrenia, *Psychopharmacology: The Third Generation of Progress* (H. Y. Meltzer, ed.), Raven Press, New York, 1987, p. 759.
7. M. S. Keshavan, J. W. Pettegrew, K. Panchalingam, D. Kaplan, J. Brar, and K. Campbell, In vivo 31P Nuclear magnetic resonance (NMR) spectroscopy of the frontal Lobe metabolism in neuroleptic naive first episode psychoses: preliminary studies, schizophrenia research (1989).
8. J. W. Pettegrew, M. S. Keshavan, K. Panchalingam, S. Strychor, D. B. Kaplan, M. G. Tretta, and M. Allen, Alterations in brain high-energy phosphate and phospholipid metabolism in first episode, drug-naive schizophrenia. A pilot study of the dorsal prefrontal cortex by in vivo ^{31}P NMR spectroscopy, *Arch. Gen. Psychiatry 48*:563 (1991).
9. E. O. O'Callaghan, O. Redmond, R. Ennis, J. Stack, A. Kinsella, J. T. Ennis, L. Conall, and J. L. Waddington, Initial investigation of the left temporoparietal

region in schizophrenia by ^{31}P magnetic resonance spectroscopy, *Biol. Psychiatry* 29:1149 (1991).

10. P. Williamson, D. Drost, J. Stanley, T. Carr, S. Morrison, and H. Merskey, Localized phosphorus 31 magnetic resonance spectroscopy in chronic schizophrenic patients and normal controls [letter], *Arch. Gen. Psychiatry* 48:578 (1991).

11. H. Fukuzako, K. Takeuchi, K. Ueyama, T. Fukuzako, Y. Hokazono, K. Hirakawa, K. Yamada, T. Hashiguchi, M. Takigawa, and T. Fujimoto, ^{31}P magnetic resonance spectroscopy of the medial temporal lobe of schizophrenic patients with neuroleptic-resistant marked positive symptoms, *Eur. Arch. Psych. Clin. Neurosci.* 244:236 (1994).

12. R. F. Deicken, G. Calabrese, E. L. Merrin, D. J. Meyerhoff, W. P. Dillon, M. W. Weiner, and G. Fein, [31]Phosphorus magnetic resonance spectroscopy of the frontal and parietal lobes in chronic schizophrenia *Biol. Psychiatry* 36:503 (1994).

13. T. Kato, T. Shioiri, J. Murashita, H. Hamakawa, T. Inubushi, and S. Takahashi, Lateralized abnormality of high-energy phosphate and bilateral reduction of phosphomonoester measured by phosphorus-31 magnetic resonance spectroscopy of the frontal lobes in schizophrenia, *Psychiatry Res.* 61:151 (1995).

14. J. A. Stanley, P. C. Williamson, D. J. Drost, T. J. Carr, J. Rylett, A. Malla, and R. T. Thompson, An in vivo study of the prefrontal cortex of schizophrenic patients at different stages of illness via phosphorus magnetic resonance spectroscopy, *Arch. Gen. Psychiatry* 52:399 (1995).

15. S. MacKay, D. J. Meyerhoff, W. P. Dillon, M. W. Weiner, and G. Fein, Alteration of brain phospholipid metabolites in cocaine-dependent polysubstance abusers, *Biol. Psychiatry* 34:261 (1993).

16. T. Kato, T. Shiori, S. Takahashi, and I. Inubushi, Measurement of brain phosphoinositide metabolism in bipolar patients using in vivo 31P-MRS, *J. Affect. Disord.* 22:185 (1991).

17. T. Kato, S. Takahashi, T. Shiori, and T. Inubushi, Alterations in brain phosphorous metabolism in bipolar disorder detected by in vivo 31P and [7]Li magnetic resonance spectroscopy, *J. Affect. Disord.* 27:53 (1993).

18. R. F. Deiken, M. W. Weiner, and G. Fein, Decreased temporal lobe phosphomonoesters in bipolar disorder, *J. Affect. Disord.* 33:195 (1995).

19. J. W. Pettegrew, K. Panchalngam, J. Moossy, J. Martinez, G. Rao, and F. Boller, Correlation of phosphorus-31 magnetic resonance spectroscopy and morphologic findings in Alzheimer's disease, *Arch. Neurol.* 45:235 (1988).

20. N. J. Minshew, G. Goldstein, S. M. Dombrowski, K. Panchalingam, and J. W. Pettegrew, A preliminary ^{31}P MRS study of autism: evidence for undersynthesis and increased degradation of brain membranes, *Biol. Psychiatry* 33:762 (1993).

21. M. S. Keshavan, J. W. Pettegrew, K. Panchalingam, D. Kaplan, and E. Bozik, Phosphorus 31 magnetic resonance spectroscopy detects altered brain metabolism before onset of schizophrenia, *Arch. Gen. Psychiatry* 48:1112 (1991).

22. T. Shioiri, T. Kato, T. Inubushi, J. Murashita, and S. Takahashi, Correlations of phosphomonoesters measured by phosphorus-31 magnetic resonance spec-

troscopy in the frontal lobes and negative symptoms in schizophrenia, *Psych. Res. 55*:223 (1994).

23. R. F. Deicken, E. L. Merrin, T. C. Floyd, and M. W. Weiner, Correlation between left frontal phospholipids and Wisconsin Card Sort Test performance in schizophrenia, *Schizophr. Res. 14*:177 (1995).

24. J. A. Sweeney, M. S. Keshavan, J. R. Carl, G. L. Haas, and J. W. Pettegrew, ^{31}P MRS studies in schizophrenia: relation to eye movement abnormalities, *Biol. Psychiatry 33*:21A (1993).

25. G. Calabrese, R. F. Deiken, G. Fein, E. L. Merrin, F. Schoenfeld, and M. W. Weiner, [31]Phosphorous magnetic resonance spectroscopy of the temporal lobes in schizophrenia, *Biol. Psychiatry 32*:26 (1992).

26. M. S. Keshavan, J. W. Pettegrew, and R. Ward, Are membrane changes in schizophrenia familial?, *Biol. Psychiatry 33*:45A (1993).

27. M. S. Keshavan, R. D. Sanders, J. W. Pettegrew, S. M. Dombrowsky, and C. S. Panchalingam, Frontal lobe metabolism and cerebral morphology in schizophrenia: ^{31}P MRS and MRI studies, *Schizophr. Res. 10*:241 (1993).

28. L. Demisch, H. Gebaldo, K. Heinz, and R. Kirsten, Transmembranal signalling in schizophrenic and affective disorders: studies on arachidonic acid and phospholipids, *Schizophr. Res. 22*:275 (1987).

29. J. D. Stevens, The distribution of phospholipid fractions in the red cell membrane of schizophrenics, *Schizophr. Bull. 6*:60 (1972).

30. W. F. Gattaz, M. Kolisch, T. Thuren, J. A. Virtanen, and P. K. J. Kinnunen, Increased plasma phospholipase A2 activity in schizophrenic patients: reduction after neuroleptic therapy, *Biol. Psychiatry 22*:421 (1987).

31. K. Panchalingam, J. W. Pettegrew, S. Strychor, and M. Trette, Effect of normal aging on membrane phospholipid metabolism by 31 P in vivo MR spectroscopy (abstr). *Soc Neurosci 349*:20 (1990).

32. R. Buchli, E. Martin, P. Boesiger, and H. Rumpel, Developmental changes of phosphorus metabolite concentrations in the human brain: a ^{31}P magnetic resonance spectroscopy study in vivo, *Pediatr. Res. 35*:431 (1994).

33. I. Feinberg, Schizophrenia: Caused by a fault in programmed synaptic elimination during adolescence?, *J. Psychiatr. Res. 17*(suppl. 4):319 (1982).

34. R. E. Hoffman and T. H. McGlashan, Parallel distributed processing and the emergence of schizophrenic symptoms, *Schizophr. Bull. 19*:119 (1993).

35. M. S. Keshavan, S. Anderson, and J. W. Pettegrew, Is schizophrenia due to excessive synaptic pruning in the prefrontal cortex? *J. Psychiatr. Res. 28*:239 (1994).

36. P. Rakic, J.-P. Bourgeois, M. F. Eckenhoff, N. Zecevic, and P. S. Goldman-Rakic, Concurrent overproduction of synapses in diverse regions of the primate cerebral cortex, *Science 232*:232 (1986).

37. P. R. Huttenlocher, Synaptic density in human frontal cortex. Developmental changes and effects of aging, *Brain Res. 163*:195 (1979).

38. B. Pakkenberg, Post-mortem study of chronic schizophrenic brains, *Br. J. Psychiatry 151*:744 (1987).

39. R. B. Zipursky, K. O. Lim, E. V. Sullivan, B. W. Brown, and A. Pfefferbaum,

Widespread cerebral gray matter volume deficits in schizophrenia, *Arch. Gen. Psychiatry 49*:195 (1992).

40. I. Harvey, M. A. Ron, G. DuBoulay, D. Wicks, S. W. Lewis, and R. M. Murray, Reduction of cortical volume in schizophrenia on magnetic resonance imaging, *Psychol. Med. 23*:591 (1993).
41. T. E. Schlaepfer, Decreased regional cortical gray matter volume in schizophrenia, *Am. J. Psychiatry 151*:842 (1994).
42. L. D. Selemon, G. Rajkowska, and P. S. Goldman-Rakic, Abnormally high neuronal density in the schizophrenic cortex. A morphometric analysis of prefrontal area 9 and occipital area 17, *Arch. Gen. Psychiatry 52*:805 (1995).
43. L. Sokoloff, Measurement of local cerebral glucose utilization and its relation to local functional activity in the brain, *Adv. Exp. Med. Biol. 291*:21 (1991).
44. L. Sokoloff, Function-related changes in energy metabolism in the nervous system: localization and mechanisms, *Keio J. Med. 42*:95 (1993).
45. F. M. Benes, M. Turtle, Y. Khan, and P. Farol, Myelination of a key relay zone in the hippocampal formation occurs in the human brain during childhood, adolescence and adulthood, *Arch. Gen. Psychiatry 51*:477 (1994).
46. R. M. Murray and S. W. Lewis, Is schizophrenia a neurodevelopmental disorder?, *Br. Med. J. 295*:681 (1987).
47. D. R. Weinberger, Implications of normal brain development for the pathogenesis of schizophrenia, *Arch. Gen. Psychiatry 44*:464 (1987).
48. J. L. Waddington, Schizophrenia: developmental neuroscience and pathobiology, *Lancet 341*:531 (1993).
49. J. Storm-Matisen and O. P. Otterson, Immunocytochemistry of glutamate at the synaptic level, *J. Histochem. Cytochem. 38*:1733 (1990).
50. J. S. Kim, H. H. Kornhuber, W. Schid-Burgk, et al., Low cerebrospinal fluid glutamate in schizophrenic patients and a new hypothesis on schizophrenia, *Neurosci. Lett. 20*:379 (1980).
51. P. F. Renshaw, M. D. Schnall, and J. S. Leigh, Jr., In vivo 31P NMR spectroscopy of agonist-stimulated phosphatidylinositol metabolism in cat brain, *Magn. Resonance Med. 4*:221 (1987).
52. M. S. Keshavan, J. W. Pettegrew, and K. Panchalingam, MRS in the study of psychoses: psychopharmacological studies, *NMR Spectroscopy in Psychiatric Brain Disorders* (H. A. Nasrallah and J. W. Pettegrew, eds.), American Psychiatric Press, Washington, DC, 1995, p. 131.
53. J. Urenjak, S. R. Williams, D. G. Gadian, and M. Noble, Proton nuclear magnetic resonance spectroscopy unambiguously identifies different neural cell types, *J. Neurosci. 13*:981 (1993).
54. H. Nasrallah, T. E. Skinner, P. Schmalbrock, and P. M. Robitaille, Proton magnetic resonance spectroscopy (^{1}H MRS) of the hippocampal formation in schizophrenia: a pilot study, *Br. J. Psychiatry 165*:481 (1994).
55. P. F. Renshaw, D. A. Yurgelun-Todd, M. Tohen, S. Gruber, and B. M. Cohen, Temporal lobe proton magnetic resonance spectroscopy of patients with first-episode psychosis, *Am. J. Psychiatry 152*:444 (1995).
56. H. Fukuzako, K. Takeuchi, Y. Kokazono, T. Fukuzako, K. Yamada, T. Hashi-

guchi, Y. Obo, K. Ueyama, M. Takigawa, and T. Fujimoto, Proton magnetic resonance spectroscopy of the left medial temporal and frontal lobes in chronic schizophrenia: preliminary report, *Psych. Res. 61*:193 (1995).

57. M. Maier, M. A. Ron, G. J. Barker, and P. S. Tofts, Proton magnetic resonance spectroscopy: an in vivo method of estimating hippocampal neuronal depletion in schizophrenia, *Psych. Med. 25*:1201 (1995).

58. P. Falkai, B. Bogerts, and M. Rosumek, Cell loss and volume reduction in the entorhinal cortex of schizophrenics, *Eur. Arch. Psychiatry Neurol. Sci. 24*:515 (1988).

59. R. L. Suddath, M. F. Casanova, T. E. Goldberg, D. G. Daniel, J. R. Kelsoe, and D. R. Weinberger, Temporal lobe pathology in chizophrenia: a quantitative magnetic resonance imaging study, *Am. J. Psychiatry 146*:464 (1989).

60. B. A. Inglis, R. E. Brenner, P. M. G. Munro, S. C. R. Williams, W. I. McDonald, and K. D. Sales, Measurement to proton NMR relaxation times for NAA Cr, and Cho in acute EAE, *Soc. Magn. Resonance Med. 2*:2162 (1992).

61. P. B. Toft, P. Christiansen, O. Pryds, H. C. Lou, and O. Henriksen, T_1, T_2, and concentrations of brain metabolites in neonates and adolescents estimated with H-1 MR spectroscopy, *J. Magn. Resonance Imaging 4*:1 (1994).

62. R. L. Hendren, J. Hodde-Vargas, R. A. Yeo, L. A. Vargas, W. M. Brooks, and C. Ford, Neuropsychophysiological study of children at risk for schizophrenia: a preliminary report, *J. Am. Acad. Child. Adolesc. Psychiatry 34*:1284 (1995).

63. J. F. Stanley, D. J. Drost, P. C. Williamson, and T. J. Carr, In vivo proton MRS study of glutamate and schizophrenia, *NMR Spectroscopy in Psychiatric Brain Disorders* (H. A. Nasrallah and J. W. Pettegrew, eds.), American Psychiatric Press, Washington, DC, 1995, p. 21.

64. H. C. Charles, F. Lazeyras, K. R. R. Krishnan, O. B. Boyko, M. Payne, and D. Moore, Brain choline in depression: in vivo detection of potential pharmaco-dynamic effects of antidepressant therapy using hydrogen localized spectroscopy, *Prog. Neuropsychopharmacol. Biol. Psychiatry 18*:1121 (1994).

65. P. F. Renshaw, A. L. Stoll, A. Rothschild, M. Fava, and B. M. Cohen, Multiple brain ^{1}H MRS abnormalities in depressed patients suggest impaired second messenger cycling, *Biol. Psychiatry 33*:441 (1993).

66. R. Sharma, P. N. Venkatasubramanian, M. Barany, and J. M. Davis, Proton magnetic resonance spectroscopy of the brain in schizophrenic and affective patients, *Schiz. Res. 8*:43 (1992).

67. H. C. Charles, F. Lazeyras, O. Boyko, A. Allen, and K. R. R. Krishnan, Elevated choline concentrations in basal ganglia of depressed patients, *Biol. Psychiatry 31*:99A (1993).

68. A. L. Stoll, P. F. Renshaw, G. S. Sachs, A. R. Guimaraes, C. Miller, B. M. Cohen, B. Lafer, and R. G. Gonzalez, The human brain resonance of choline-containing compounds is similar in patients receiving lithium treatment and controls: an in vivo proton magnetic resonance spectroscopy study, *Biol. Psychiatry 32*:944 (1992).

69. F. A. Howe, R. J. Maxwell, D. E. Saunder, M. M. Brown, and J. R. Griffiths, Proton spectroscopy in vivo, *Magn. Resonance O. 9*:33 (1993).

70. D. L. Birken and W. H. Oldendorf, N-Acetyl-l-aspartic acid: a literature review of a compound promonent in 1 H NMR spectroscopic studies of the brain, *Neurosci. Biobehav. Rev. 13*:23 (1989).

71. M. Bartels, K. Albert, G. Kruppa, K. Mann, G. Schroth, S. Tabarelli, and M. Zabel, Fluorinated psychopharmacological agents: noninvasive observation by fluorinated psychopharmacological agents: noninvasive observation by fluorine-19 nuclear magnetic resonance, *Psychiatry Res. 18*:197 (1986).

72. D. C. Arndt, A. V. Ratner, K. F. Faull, J. D. Barchas, and S. W. Young, ^{19}F magnetic resonance imaging and spectroscopy of a fluorinated neuroleptic ligand: in vivo and in vitro studies, *Psychiatry Res. 25*:73 (1988).

73. M. Bartels, U. Gunther, K. Albert, K. Mann, N. Schuff, and H. Stuckstedte, ^{19}F nuclear magnetic resonance spectroscopy of neuroleptics: the first in vivo pharmacokinetics of trifluoperazine in the rat brain and the first in vivo spectrum of fluphenazine in the human brain, *Biol. Psychiatry 30*:656 (1991).

74. R. A. Komoroski, J. E. Newton, C. Karson, D. Cardwell, and J. Sprigg, Detection of psychoactive drugs in vivo in humans using ^{19}F NMR spectroscopy, *Biol. Psychiatry 29*:711 (1991).

75. C. N. Karson, J. Newton, R. Komoroski, P. Mohanakrishnan, et al., Fluoxetine and trifluoperazine in human brain: a ^{19}F-nuclear magnetic resonance spectroscopy study, *Psych. Res. 45*:95 (1992).

76. C. Heimberg, R. A. Komoroski, J. E. O. Newton, and C. Carson, ^{19}F MRS: a new tool for psychopharmacology, *NMR Spectroscopy in Psychiatric Brain Disorders* (H. A. Nasarallah and J. W. Pettegrew, eds.), American Psychiatric Press, Inc., Washington, DC, 1995, p. 213.

77. P. F. Buckley and J. L. Waddington, Magnetic resonance spectroscopy in schizophrenia: a nascent technology for a neurodevelopmental disorder?, *Biol. Psychiatry 36*:789 (1994).

78. J. Rademacher, A. M. Galaburda, D. N. Kennedy, P. A. Filipek, and V. S. Caviness, Human cerebral cortex: localization, parcellation, and morphometry with magnetic resonance imaging, *J. Cog. Neurosci. 4*:352 (1992).

79. M. S. Keshavan and N. R. Schooler, First episode studies in schizophrenia: criteria and characterization, *Schizo. Bull. 18*:491 (1992).

14

Positron Emission Tomography Studies of Cerebral Metabolism and Blood Flow in Schizophrenia

Charlie L. Swanson, Jr., Lyn M. Harper Mozley, and Raquel E. Gur
Mental Health Clinical Research Center, University of Pennsylvania, Philadelphia, Pennsylvania

I. INTRODUCTION

Most positron emission tomography (PET) investigations have examined cerebral metabolism (CMR) or blood flow (rCBF) in the resting condition along anterior-posterior dimensions in patients with schizophrenia, while some studies have analyzed subcortical-cortical or laterality dimensions. A subset of these investigations has related physiology to medication status or clinical phenomenology. More recent studies have employed activation techniques to characterize task-related cerebral activity. In this chapter, we summarize the PET literature across isotopes,, imaging conditions, and image analysis techniques. The interpretation of this growing literature as a whole is complicated by many factors, including differences in subject selection or characterization, sample sizes, parameters of data acquisition and scanner properties, imaging conditions, and image analysis techniques (see Ref. 1 for review). Nonetheless, we attempt to highlight previous findings and to suggest directions for future PET research in schizophrenia. In Table 1 we provide information about sample size and demographics, isotopes, scanning conditions, data analysis, and major findings. We then summarize the findings of the relevant studies in the categories of (a) resting conditions, anterior-posterior, laterality or subcortical-cortical dimensions (including baseline measures in medication studies); (b) medication effects; (c) relationship to clinical symptomatology; and (d) activation conditions, and follow with our conclusions.

II. ANTERIOR-POSTERIOR

The majority of PET studies in schizophrenia have examined cerebral metabolism or blood flow along the anterior-posterior dimension, following the pioneering [133]Xenon study of Ingvar and Franzen [2]. These authors found that patients who were chronically ill with schizophrenia had relatively low frontal lobe blood flow and high temporal-occipital flow compared to both patients who were more acutely ill and alcoholic, neurologically intact comparison subjects. Relative "hypofrontality" in schizophrenia was reported in one of the first studies to use PET [3]. Using resting uptake conditions and FDG, these authors observed decreased glucose use in the frontal lobes of patients, relative to hyperfrontality in control subjects. Thirteen years and approximately 20 studies later, the answer to the "hypofrontality" question is somewhat unclear when one looks across studies, although consistent findings are often reported within laboratories. Most of these investigations of frontal lobe physiology have employed FDG and resting uptake conditions. However, approximately half of these studies have reported "hypofrontality" or decreased anterior-posterior gradients in schizophrenia, while the other half have found either increased anterior/posterior ratios or no hypofrontality. With some exceptions, it appears that the most recent studies [4–6] have not supported findings of hypofrontality.

III. LATERALITY

As with the anterior-posterior dimension, authors have reported many different findings in laterality differences between patients with schizophrenia and

Table 1 Positron Emission Tomography Studies of Cerebral Metabolism and Blood Flow in Schizophrenia

Study	Patients	Controls	Isotope	Condition	Analysis	Major findings
Buchsbaum et al., 1982 [3]	n = 8 6M, 2F age = 22 yo 7RH, 1LH no rx 2 wk ip	n = 6 4M, 2F age = 26 yo all RH	FDG	Resting eyes closed, darkened, quiet room	Arteriolized venous blood 7-8 scans a) cortical peel (4 regions/ ea. hemisphere) on 3 slices based on anatomic landmarks (supraventr, midventr, infventr) b) central gray matter—squares with 1 corner in center in ea. quadrant of midventr slice rel ROI CMR/total slice CMR	Dec fro glucose use and lower fro cortex ratios; dec uptake in L vs R hemis; dec central gray matter CMR on left; hyperfro in ctls, no L-R diffs
Sheppard et al., 1983 [8]	n = 12 8M, 4F age = 30 all RH ip 1st psych adm (n = 10) no previous rx (n = 6)	n = 12 8M, 4F age = 31 all RH	15O	Eyes closed, minimal external sensory stim; 3 conditions ea. subject: 1) contin inhal of 15-O2, 2) contin inhal of 15-CO2; 3) external positron-emitting ring source	Femoral A-line, samples condition 1, 2; 2 axial slices selected rel to c-m and o-m lines for analysis, ea. with 1 image for cond 1 and 2; 4 methods of analysis: 1) central block, 2) outer cerebral segment, 3) inner cerebral segment, 4) central squares	No dec in fro rCBF or CMR in pts; no ant/post ratio diffs; dec BG in pts using 2 methods; overall, R > L asymmetry in ctls, not pts
Brodie et al., 1984 [16]	n = 6 chronic ip no rx 2 wk	n = 5 age-matched	FDG	Resting eyes open, ears plugged darkened room scanned before and after thiothixene tx	Abs ROI CT anatomical landmarks also, pattern analysis using fast Fourier transformation of 422 images, incl 12 ctls and 13 pts with schiz	L hypofro pre-tx; hypofro not affected by rx; whole slice CMR at level of BG inc by 25% after rx

(continued)

Table 1 (*continued*)

Study	Patients	Controls	Isotope	Condition	Analysis	Major findings
Buchsbaum et al., 1984 [12]	n = 16 11M, 5F age = 28 yo 15RH, 1LH n = 11 (aff. pts.) 7M, 4F age = 42 no rx 2 wk ip + op	n = 13 7M, 6F age = 31 yo 11RH, 2LH	FDG	Eyes closed, darkened quiet room, electrical stim R forearm	Arteriolized venous blood 7–8 slices abs ROI CMR a) chose scans showing top of somatosensory strip b) cortical peel (4 regions/ ea. hemisphere) on 3 slices (supraventr, midventr, infventr)	Higher abs CMR in posterior regions in pts, c/w relative hypofro in pts; significant anteroposterior gradient in ctls, diminished in pts, esp. superiorly; higher CMR in L hemis, esp. ant and midant in ctls
Clark et al., 1984 [42]	n = 7 all M age = 18–29 yo all RH off rx at least 2 wk	n = 9 all M age = 18–30 yo all RH	FDG	Eyes closed; darkened quiet room; somatosensory stim to R forearm	Arteriolized venous blood 4 slices selected based on 'standard referent' c–m line rel ROI CMR/ whole slice CMR; ROI's n = 30; outlined rectangular regions of varying dimensions and constant area; examined PPMC coeff of regions w/in a plane; areas judged to be coupled if corr coeff sig	Patterns of metabolic coupling existed for each group and were signif diff on 2 slices; med ant/post coupling and fro coupling in pts; fro coupling, some L-sided, some R-sided in ctls; corr maps consistent with sensory input in ctls
Farkas et al., 1984 [24]	n = 13 (w/ scans) all M med age = 26 yo 6 on rx	n = 11 (w/ scans) med age = 24 yo	FDG	No eating or caffeinated beverages for 2 hr. before; eyes closed white noise	A-line 2 slices (BG and semioval center); superimposed CT scans ROI-ant-entire fro; post-rest of brain	No whole slice diffs btn pts and ctls; dec fro, relative to posterior in pts; no diffs btn. rx and no rx
DeLisi et al., 1985 [10]	n = 9 6M, 3F age = 26 yo dur 7 yr 3 op, 5 ip both scans; 1 ip then op	Matched on age and gender	FDG	Sound tx, darkened room; scan 1 off rx; scan 2 on rx, mean 11.2 mo later, on rx 7.4 mo	Arteriolized venous blood 7–8 scan slices; abs; cortical peel for ant/post grad; boundary-fitting algorithm for BG	Higher abs activity in pts; inc total cortical, temp (esp L), BG uptake on rx with no change in ant/post grad

Reference	Patients	Controls	Tracer	Conditions	Methods/ROI	Results
DeLisi et al., 1985 [7]	n = 21, 15M, 6F, age = 28 yo, 20 RH, ip and op, no rx 2 wk	n = 21, 15 M, 6 F, age = 32, 21 RH	FDG	Darkened, quiet room, somatosensory stim of R arm	7–8 slices, used lowest slice above lat ventr that showed centrum semiovale to calculate ant/post ratios; abs	Dec ant/post ratios in pts; no L/R diffs in pts or ctls; CT measured atrophy and clinical status not assoc with metabolic abnormalities; no WB diffs btn M, F
Jernigan et al., 1985 [43]	n = 6, all M, no rx 2 wk, chronic ip	n = 6, all M, age-match	FDG	Blindfolded; no coffee or rx on day of scan; no food 3 hrs before inject; auditory vigilance task	Arteriolized venous blood; rel ROI CMR/all ROI in hemis; facial markers for PET and CT positioning; 3–4 nonoverlapping images; 1 level in all subjects; 8 ROI's a) semi-automated (computer-defined cortical zones) b) 2 manual: "manual regions", "manual quadrants"	No effects when adjustments were made for multiple comparison
Wolkin et al., 1985 [21]	n = 10, all M, RH, age = 38 yo, ip, no rx 2 wk, 3 pts with movement disorders	n = 8, age = 27, 7 RH, 1 LH, CT 'nml' slight sulcal prominence in several pts + ctls	FDG	Eyes open, ears plugged; dimly lit room; pts scanned pre/post tx, incl ECT (1pt)	3 slices - infraventr, midventr, supraventr abs; rel ROI CMR/slice CMR; 40 ROI's - anatomically-defined, some estab by "geometric criteria"; 17 final ROI's	Pre-tx: dec abs L fro and temp; post-tx: hypofro with abs values, not ant/post grad general inc in CMR, sig for R ten pre-tx, withdrawal-motor retardation negatively corr with R lenticular CMR
Volkow et al., 1986 [17]	n = 4, all M, RH, age = 28 yo, dur 8 yr off rx	n = 12, all M, RH, age = 29 yo	CDG	Scanned off rx and after injection of thiothixene	Arteriolized venous blood atlas-based ROI's (n = 6) superimposed on subject's CT, outlined with light pen	No hypofro; higher CMR than ctls, not statis signif; rx had no sig effect on metabolic pattern; inc BG metab after inject in neuroleptic-naive pts

(continued)

Table 1 (*continued*)

Study	Patients	Controls	Isotope	Condition	Analysis	Major findings
Buchsbaum et al., 1987 [14]	n = 8 6 M, 2 F age = 27 yo (8 of 21 pts in Buchsbaum et al 1984)	n = 24 age- and sex-matched;	FDG	Scanned pre/post rx, 11.2 mo apart, on rx for 8.6 mo before 2nd scan; electrical stim of R forearm during uptake	7–8 slices; 3 selected for analysis (supraventr, midventr, infventr); 1) ROI cortical peel; 2) ROI using neuroanatomical atlas-box placed in each structure; 7 ROI's; abs; rel ROI/slice CMR	Dec BG CMR in pts. vs. ctls; ant CMR than post in pts, not affected by rx; rx assoc with inc BG CMR, L > R, put > caudate
Cohen et al., 1987 [34]	n = 16 12M, 4F age = 27 yo no rx 2 wk 1 NN 7 ip	n = 27 15M, 12F age = 33 yo	FDG	Eyes patched auditory CPT	Arterialized venous blood 7–8 slices global CMR = estimate of avg value for sampled grey matter rich areas ROI CMR: ROI/global CMR ROI's: 2.9 cm² boxes over 5 planes w/ atlas; 55 ROI's	No diff pt & ctls in global CMR mid prefro CMR assoc w/ task accuracy in ctrl but not pts med par, L ant temp, 5 midfro diff in pts than ctrls
Gur et al., 1987 [11]	n = 12 11 M, 1 F all RH off rx or never rx age = 30 yo educ = 13 yr	n = 12 11 M, 1 F age = 25 yo educ = 15.5 10 with NL neuropsy, 2 mild imp	FDG	Resting, eyes open, ears unoccluded; dimly lit room, minimal noise	A-line; scans examined for adequacy of counts, etc., then superimposed on standard anatomic atlas; semi-automated procedure for ROI placement; abs; rel ROI CMR/WB CMR; 8 ROI	Dec WB CMR in pts; in pts and ctls, abs and rel subcort CMR > cort CMR, and L > R; no hypofro in pts; pts had dec abs CMR cort and subcort and steeper rel subcort/cort grad; higher BPRS score assoc with > abs CMR and > L CMR
Gur et al., 1987 [44]	n = 15 all RH age = 28 yo educ = 13 yr off rx, 1st study	n = 8 all RH age = 27 yo educ = 15 yr	FDG	Resting, eyes open, ears unoccluded; dimly lit room, minimal noise pts: 2 scans, 11.6 wk apart; ctls: 2 scans, 12 wk apart	A-line; scans examined for adequacy of counts, etc., then superimposed on standard anatomic atlas; semi-automated procedure for ROI placement; abs; rel ROI CMR/WB CMR; 8 ROI	No changes in ave WB CMR, laterality, regional cort CMR, or subcort/cort CMR; steeper subcort/cort grad in pts in study I persisted; changes in subcort/cort grad not assoc with changes in clinical status; changes toward higher R CMR, rel to L, assoc. with clinical improvement

Kishimoto et al., 1987 [45]	n = 20; 18 M, 2 F; age = 38; 19 RH; 19 op, 1 ip ill for 12 yr; 17 on rx	CDG	Eyes closed, darkened room	6 slices based on o-m line; used human brain map for computed tomography; sorted photos of PET images into 3 piles (hypofro, hypopar, NL)	No total brain count diffs btn pts and ctls, but ctls had > frontal counts; no ctls were hypofro or hypopar; 6 pts (all M) were hypofro w/ 38% dec fro counts; 8 pts (all M) were hypopar w/ 26% dec par counts; 6 pts (4M, 2F) were NL; concluded 3 subtypes of chronic schizophrenia identified by PET
Volkow et al., 1987 [38]	n = 18; age = 32 yo; all RH M on meds: antipsy & antichol 10 def, 8 nondef all ip	CDG	Two conditions: rest-eyes open, ears plugged eye tracking task-3 hrs later, shape recognition	14 slices WB CMR = 10 slices (exc 2 top & 2 bottom) avg value ROI CMR = weighted avg across slices R&L fro, par, temp, occ, caud, GP, put, thal id on CT & coreg with PET rel ROI/WB CMR	Dec L&R abs and rel fro metab in baseline and task; def scz: dec global CMR dur baseline and task, dec fro during task, no task related inc in CMR; sig cor btn occ CMR and pos sx more sig corr btn ROI CMR's & sxs during task than rest
Wiesel et al., 1987 [46]	n = 20; 15 M, 5 F; age = 27 yo off rx at least 3 wk. illness dur. 10 yr. max. 8—1st episode, 4—subchronic, 8 chronic	CDG	Dimly lit room, minimal noise, eyes covered; EEG to ensure wakefulness	A-line (15 pts, 9 ctls) or arteriolized venous blood abs (A-line subj only); rel ROI CMR/ WB CMR (all subj) 7 slices; 35 ROI's, drawn on indiv's CT, transferred to corresponding PET slices	No abs. WB diffs; dec abs and rel sup temp, bilat med fro in pts; dec rel inf par; L/R asymmetries: dec temp, L baseline fro in pts, pts w/ L < R abs lent CMR ctls with L > R lenticular CMR, R > L rel sup temp in pts, R < L sup temp in ctls; lower mear CMR assoc w/ subchronic/chronic course; lower CMR assoc with new sx; CMR not assoc with atrophy
Resnick et al., 1988 [15]	n = 18; 17 M, 1 F; age = 26 yo; educ = 15 yr; all RH; no rx 1st scan: 2 NN, 14 < 6 mo, 4 > 6 mo	FDG	Resting, eyes/ears open; 12 pts, on rx, had 2nd scan 8.7 wk later; 11 ctls had 2nd scan 12.9 wk later	A-line; scans examined for count adequacy, etc, computerized anatomic atlas used; abs and rel ROI CMR/ WB CMR and abs	Inc subcort/cort grad. in pts (both dec cort. CMR and inc subcort); rel hypermetab of thal and lentic nuc; lower cort and bilat caud abs CMR in unmed pts; higher L than R subcort metab in pts; no consistent rx effects for pts who were re-scanned after tx

(continued)

Table 1 (*continued*)

Study	Patients	Controls	Isotope	Condition	Analysis	Major findings
Szechtman et al., 1988 [47]	2 groups 1) n = 5, 4 M, 1 F, age = 21 yo, educ = 14 yr, rx 1 yr; 2) n = 12, all M, age = 29, educ = 11.8, rx 7.4 yr	n = 10, all M, 9 RH, 1 LH, age = 28 yo, educ = 18 yr	FDG	Eyes closed, quiet lighted room	16 slices, 3 selected for analysis (midthalamic-midstriatal, midcallosal, supracallosal); rel ROI CMR/whole cortical rim CMR	Dec L CMR in sup temp. gyrus in pts and ctls; 1 yr rx inc corpus striatal CMR, but did not change overall pattern of fro hyperactiv, post hypoactiv; 7.4 yr rx pts had fro hyperactivity and post hypoactiv, but pattern was more similar to ctls
Volkow et al., 1988 [39]	n = 18, age = 32 yo, all RH M on meds: antipsy & antichol	n = 12, age = 29 yo, all RH M	CDG	Two conditions: baseline—eyes open, ears plugged; eye tracking task—3 hrs later, shape recognition	14 slices WB CMR = 10 slices (exc 2 top & 2 bottom) avg value ROI CMR = weighted avg across slices R&L fro, par, temp, occ, caud, GP, put, thal id on CT & coreg with PET	Scz: inc ROI CMR variability; dec corr between ROI CMR's; dec corr btn: ant and post, thal and ct pts less change baseline to task
Wolkin et al., 1988 [48]	n = 13, all M, all RH, age = 34 yo, chronic 9 ip, 4 op off rx 10 d	n = 8, age = 33	FDG	Not given	abs indiv's CT scan superimposed on matched PET images	Dec ant/post ratios in pts dec abs fro and post CMR in pts, not explained by atrophy on CT
Clark et al., 1989 [49]	3 twin sets, nml/scz, prodr/scz, sczaff/sczaff	6 twin sets, age = 28 yo, educ = 14 yr	FDG	Eyes covered, ears not occluded	arteriolized venous blood; 14 slices, 5 selected; fixed area 1.7 cm²; elliptical ROI's; 26 total ROI's; (see [54])	Scz: dec orb prefro CMR
Cleghorn et al., 1989 [50]	n = 8, 6M, 2F, age = 23 yo, educ = 13 yr	n = 10, age = 28 yo, educ = 18 yr, 8RH, 2LH	FDG	Eyes closed	Arteriolized venous blood 16 slices, 3 selected for analysis 1) with thal and striatum 2) above	No diffs in WB CMR; inc rel fro (prefro, not orb fro) CMR in pts, no laterality effect; dec rel inf par CMR; fro/par ratios > in pts than ctls

Study	Subjects		Tracer	Condition	Method	Results
(continued)	6RH, 2LH never rx 7 ill < 2 yr IQ = 97 1 pt with truncal tic	IQ = 123			BG through cc 3) above cc vortex through cing; computer algorithm used to divide cortical rim of each slice into 36 ROI's; rel ROI/whole slice CMR	
Cohen et al., 1989 [35]	n = 33 dx = 16 scz, 17 aff d/o *h/o SA in 13 pts		FDG	Eyes closed aud discrim (CPT)	Arteriolized venous blood; atlas based ROI's; 2.9 cm² boxes over ROI's; 7–8 slices, parallel to CML; 13 areas of interest	No diff btn scz, aff and n/c in global CMR; aff pts: dec temp and L BG than scz aff and scz dec mid prefro during task (not rel to perf)
DeLisi et al., 1989 [13]	n = 21 15M, 6F age = 28 yo 20 RH off rx at least 15 d ip, op		FDG	Darkened, quiet room; forearm shocks	7–8 slices based on c-m line; 3 sets of slices and image analysis methods: 1) temporal lobe - standard atlas to select best slice showing region, computer boundary-fitting program; 2) peel analysis based on atlas slice; 3) ROI analysis based on atlas slice; abs and rel ROI CMR/ whole slice CMR	(Varied with analysis method) > CMR in pts than ctls; > CMR in L ant temp vs R ant temp in pts, proportional to severity of psychopathology; > bilat CMR (mean and max) in pts relative to ctls; > L CMR in pts, more marked for temp than fro areas; no temp asymmetry in ctls; ant CMR > post CMR in pts; ant L/R ratios > in pts
Guich et al., 1989 [36]	n = 15 14M, 1F age = 27 yo 13RH, 2LH no rx 1 mo educ = 13 yr		FDG	CPT coincident EEG	9 planes at 10mm increment chose supravent slice, outlined boundary, 2 cm ring of ctx identified fro/occ ratio calculated	Scz: inc delta in fro; corr inc fro delta w/ rel dec fro CMR

(continued)

Table 1 (*continued*)

Study	Patients	Controls	Isotope	Condition	Analysis	Major findings
Gur et al., 1989 [51]	n = 20, 19M, 1 F, age = 29 yo, educ = 15, all RH, no rx (same as Resnick et al., 1988)	none	FDG	Resting, fasting, eyes/ears open	A-line; scans examined for count adequacy, etc., computerized anatomic atlas used; 7 cortical ROI's only; derived laterality (L-R hemis) and frontality (fro-post) values	Laterality disturbances, not fro abnormalities, are related to sx specific to schiz
Levy et al., 1989 [9]	n = 42, all M, 21-50 yo, all RH, 20 rx, 20 off rx at least 2 wk	n = 40, all M, 20-50 yo, all RH	CDG	Resting	Arteriolized venous blood; metabolic centroid (MC) method of analysis	Mean MC in ctls is superior to mean geometric centroid; mean MC of pts is lower and more post to the mean geometric centroid, particularly for pts w/ rx consistent w/ hypofro; no signific hemis laterality in pts or ctls. ave metab activity in pts < ctls
Luchins et al., 1989 [52]	n = 1, 22 yo AA F	none	FDG	Visual monitor task scan while catatonic repeated 17 d later - not catatonic	5 slices; 14 ROI's, z normalized to avg of all ROI's	Catatonic: avg WB CMR 'nml' L BG CMR > R BG CMR; after catatonia: 10% inc WB CMR, L BG = R BG CMR
Wik et al., 1989 [22]	Sulpiride n = 11, 7M, 4F, age = 28 yo; CPZ n = 6, 5M, 1F, age = 23 yo	n = 7, all M, age = 29 yo	CDG	Eyes covered baseline scan & then 5-6 wks rx w/ CPZ 400 mg/d or sulpiride 800 mg/d, then rescan	Arteriolized venous blood; some with A-lines; absolute CMR only if A-line, o/w rel ROI to WB CMR; ROI drawn on CT & then coreg w/ PET slice; 7 slices	Sulpiride: lower global CMR than & CPZ pts; sulpiride: inc R abs & rel R lent nml no changes with CPZ group
Buchsbaum et al., 1990 [37]	n = 13, 11M, 2F, age = 28 yo, 11 RH, 2LH, educ = 13 yr	n = 18, 14M, 4F, age = 26 yo, all RH, educ = 15 yr	FDG	CPT	Arteriolized venous blood; 9 planes at 10 mm increment; chose supra, mid, & inf vent slices; outlined boundary, 2 cm ring of ctx identified; 8 ROI's for each slice	Scz: dec rel and abs fro, temp-par CMR; ctl: inc rel R fro and R temp-par CMR with task; scz: worse CPT perf assoc w/ inc R temp-par CMR

Study	Patients	Controls	Tracer	Conditions	Method	Results
Bartlett et al., 1991 [53]	n = 8 all M age = 32 yo all RH chronic off rx	n = 11 all M age = 21 all RH	CDG or FDG	Resting, eyes open; ctls scanned 2x with CDG in 1 d; 6 pts scanned 2x in 1 d with CDG; 2 pts rescanned after 24 and 120h with FDG	Arteriolized venous blood; 14 interleaved images; 7 ROI's (4 cort, 2 subcort, 1 WB) located on 9 slices; abs and rel ROI CMR/WB CMR	No diff in % change scan 1 to scan 2 in any ROI in pts or ctls, but rel regional CMR showed fro changes, esp for pts; no diffs btn pts with diff clinical status scan 1 to scan 2
Bartlett et al., 1991 [23]	Thiothixine n = 8 age = 36 yo dur = 15 yr HPL n = 12 age = 35 yo dur = 10 yr	none	FDG	Scanned pre tx and then 4–11 wks post tx thiothixine & 5–6 wks post tx HPL	Arteriolized venous blood 14 slices whole brain = 10 slices (exc 2 top & 2 bottom) BG = id on CT and coreg with PET on single slice DLPFC = id on CT and coreg with PET on single slice	Thiothix: inc WB, BG, DLPFC C (had lower WB CMR pre tx); HPL: dec WB, BG, DLPFC CMR
Clark et al., 1991 [54]	nml olf n = 8 M age = 25 yo on meds olf agnosia n = 8 M age = 27 yo on meds	n = 8 8 M age = 24 yo educ = 14 yr	FDG	Eyes covered light breakfast	Arteriolized venous blood; 14 slices, 5 selected; fixed area 1.7 cm² elliptical ROI's; 26 total ROI's: cortical mantle, paired lat vent, caud, put, orb fro, lat temp, cer	Scz: dec fro; olf agnosia: dec R BG & thal (comp to scz w/ nml olf)
Cleghorn et al., 1991 [25]	n = 11 8M, 3F age = 26 yo educ = 12 yr 9RH, 2LH never tx'd	n = 8 8M age = 27 yo educ = 18 yr 7RH, 1LH	FDG	Eyes closed scans with saline vs. apomorphine infusion	Arteriolized venous blood; relative CMR; 16 slices, 3 selected for analysis; cortical peel, striatum, thal, ant & post cing	Dec rel striatal CMR in scz after apomorphine but not in controls
Levy et al., 1991 [55]	n = 12 12M all RH	n = 11 11M all RH	CDG	Eyes opened, ears plugged; rescan with visual eye-tracking task	14 slices FOI's not previously defined functional image analysis	Scz: cort-subcort grad sig in A-P L ant-R post; BG & thal best distinction btn scz ctls

(continued)

Table 1 (*continued*)

Study	Patients	Controls	Isotope	Condition	Analysis	Major findings
Buchsbaum et al., 1992 [19]	n = 12 11M, 1F age = 29 yo 7 clozapine 5 thiothix	none	FDG	CPT scan after 14 d med free, then repeated after 28–49 d of tx	Arteriolized venous blood 9 slices cortical peel: abs ROI CMR/WB CMR stereotaxic subcortical: abs ROI CMR/slice CMR	Cloz: inc BG (R > L); thiothixine: dec BG (sup inf grad) R inf caud differentiates responder
Buchsbaum et al., 1992 [18]	n = 25 21M, 4F age = 35 yo 11ip, 14op	none	FDG	CPT 10 wk double-blind, crossover HPL v plac scan @ 5 & 10 weeks	Arteriolized venous blood 9 slices cortical peel: abs ROI CMR/WB CMR stereotaxic subcortical: abs ROI CMR/slice CMR	Response correlated with: dec striatum on placebo & inc striatum on HPL; placebo R inf put & L caud is best predictor of HPL resp: stri rel CMR assoc w/ resp
Buchsbaum et al., 1992 [56]	n = 18 18M 17RH, 1LH never rx'd	n = 20 all RH	FDG	CPT	Arteriolized venous blood abs ROI CMR/WB CMR 9 slices at 10 mm increment automated edge, cortical peel subcortical stereotaxic ROI's: 32 ctx, 126 subctx	Dec inf & med fro/occ ratio; dec caud & put
Cleghorn et al., 1992 [27]	With AH n = 12 8M, 4F age = 24 yo educ = 11 yr	Without AH n = 10 8M, 2F age = 29 yo educ = 13 yr	FDG	Eyes closed	Arteriolized venous blood absolute CMR 16 slices, 3 for analysis (mid thal-mid striatal, mid callosal, Broca) cortical peel	AH: dec aud ctx & L Wernicke, inc striatum & ant cing, trend inc R Broca's
Friston et al., 1992 [57]	n = 30 25M, 5F age = 36 yo 27 RH ip chronic ill for 15 yr onset age = 22 yr rx 3 groups of clinical sx	none	^{15}O	Eyes closed, darkened quiet room	15 original slices interpolated to 43 planes and cubic voxels; intercommisural line identified and images transfixed into standard stereotactic space; canonical analysis - 10 rCBF regions and sum of all subsyndrome scores; SPM	Global rCBF was not assoc. with any subsyndrome; > severity of psychopathology assoc with inc rCBF in L med temp, mesencephalic, thalamic, and L striatal areas, esp. L phpc

Study	Subjects	Controls	Tracer	Conditions	Method	Results
Gunther, 1992 [41]	n = 13 all M age = 32 yo	n = 14	FDG	Three conditions: rest-eyes closed; simple motor—ext/flex R hand; complex motor—R thumb touches other fingers	ROI CMR normalized to WB 16 ROI's: R&L SM & PM, R&L pre fro, R&L thal, R&L BG, med fro, inf fro, R&L par, R&L temp	Simple motor: no changes; complex motor: nmls inc med fro L SM, scz no activation
Liddle et al., 1992 [30]	n = 30 25M, 5F age = 36 yo 27RH, 3LH on meds	None	$^{15}O_2$	Eyes closed	A-line SPM	Correlations with sx groups: deficit: pos R&L caud, neg L DL neg L sup par assn ctx; disorganization: pos R ant cing, pos R dors thal, neg R VLPFC neg R&L ang g; reality distortion: pos L phpc g, pos L vent striatum neg R post cing
Tamminga et al., 1992 [4]	n = 12 off rx at least 1 mo 4 def, 7 nondef, 1 ? 8 with TD	n = 12 matched	FDG	Fasting, eyes patched, ears plugged	Arteriolized venous blood; 5 axial slices; abs from animal model; rel ROI CMR/cereb CMR; 9 neocortical, 3 limbic, 3 BG, 1 thal areas	No dec fro CMR in pts; no L/R diffs btn pts and ctls; dec CMR in hippoc in pts; dec cing CMR in ctls; dec hippoc and ant cing CMR in def and nondef pts; also dec thal, fro, and par CMR in def pts, but NL in nondef pts
Volkow et al., 1992 [58]	n = 18 age = 27 yo on rx for 7 yr ip	n = 12 23–47 yo	CDG		R and L cerebellum marked on indiv's CT; regions then projected onto corresp. PET planes; abs and rel cereb CMR/WB CMR (WB = ave activ in 10 central slices)	Dec abs and rel cereb CMR in pts, no L/R diffs; no corr btn cereb and fro rel metab
Wolkin et al., 1992 [31]	n = 20 20M 16RH, 4LH no rx 2 wk 13AA, 6W, 1H	None	FDG	Eyes open ears unoccluded	Arteriolized venous blood abs ROI CMR/WB CMR CT based ROI's 7 ROI's per hemisphere: DLPFC, orb mrf PFC, temp, stri, thal, mes temp, cer	Inc neg sxs assox with dec R DLPF

(continued)

Table 1 (*continued*)

Study	Patients	Controls	Isotope	Condition	Analysis	Major findings
Clark et al., 1993 [59]	n = 17 8M, 9F age = 29 yo on meds	n = 16 8M, 8F age = 26 yo	FDG	Eyes covered light breakfast	Arteriolized venous blood 14 slices, 5 selected fixed area 1.7 cm² elliptical ROI's 26 total ROI's	Factor analysis of ROI's CMR rev 3 factors: scz I-dec gen CMR; scz II-dec fro, par; ctls
Dolan et al., 1993 [5]	n = 30 25M, 5F age = 36 yo on meds	Depressed n = 40 25M, 15F age = 57 yo	¹⁵O₂	Eyes closed	A-line SPM	Sx effect but no dx effect or dx - sx interaction; no hypofrontality
Siegel et al., 1993 [60]	n = 70 70M age = 30 yo 61RH, 9LH no rx 1 mo	n = 30 30M age = 30 yo all RH	FDG	Degraded stimulus CPT	Arteriolized venous blood abs ROI CMR/WB CMR 9 slices at 10 mm increment automated edge, cortical peel subcortical stereotaxic ROI's: 32 ctx, 126 subctx	Scz: dec med fro, cing, med temp cc, vent caud CMR; inc L lat temp & occ; "hypofrontality" due to inc occ; dec R > L asymmetry temp/fro in scz dec BG and med fro CMR
Potkin et al., 1994 [20]	n = 18 16M, 2F op	None	FDG	CPT 10 wk double blind, cross over cloz v plac scan @ 5 & 10 weeks	Arteriolized venous blood 9 slices cortical peel: abs ROI CMR/WB CMR stereotaxic subcortical: abs ROI CMR/slice CMR	Clozapine: inc rel striatum CMR (R > L) dec rel fro CMR (L > R) inc rel occ CMR
Schroeder et al., 1994 [61]	n = 83 76M, 7F age = 30 yo 76RH, 7LH no rx 1 mo	n = 47 30M, 17F age = 30 yo all RH	FDG	Degraded stimulus CPT	Arteriolized venous blood abs ROI CMR/WB CMR 10 slices cortical peel 16 ROI in ea hemisphere	Scz: L > R temp CMR; canonical analysis: hypofrontality parietal ctx/motor strip distinguish scz from ctl
Wolkin et al.,	n = 23 23M	None	FDG	Eyes open baseline scan & then	Arteriolized venous blood abs CMR and rel to	Amph: dec abs CMR all ROI x/ ce dec rel CMR L temp

Study	Subjects	Controls	Tracer	Condition	Method	Results
1994 [26]	age = 35 yo 18RH, 5LH			repeat: 16 with amphetamine, 7 without	WB CMR ROI's CT based and mapped ROI's:DLPFC, orb med PFC, temp, striatum, thal, mes temp, cer	
Frith et al., 1995 [40]	n = 18 14M, 4F 6 NL VF, 4 'odd' VF, 7 poor VF ip age = 31 yo	n = 6 5M, 1F age = 57 yo	$^{15}O_2$	Verbal fluency (VF)	A-line SPM	N/c: dec L sup temp during VF scz: no chng L sup temp during VF
Gur et al., 1995 [6]	n = 42 29M, 13F age = 28 yo educ 12 yr 20W, 22AA off meds	n = 42 29M, 13F age = 28 yo educ = 15 yr 24W, 18AA	FDG	Resting fasting eyes open ears unoccluded	A-line absolute CMR coregistered to MRI 42 ROI's per hemisphere: template fitted to MRI slices	Scz: rel inc L midtemp (esp neg and Schneider sxs, not paranoid sxs); general higher metabolism and lo relative L hemisphere assoc with better premorbid and outcome; inc subcort-cort gradient in FE pts no hypofrontality
Silbersweig et al., 1995 [28]	n = 6 6M age = 32 yo 5 chronic AH 1 AH + VH	None	$H_2^{15}O$	Eyes closed, push button during scan when having AH	SPM	Statistical maxima: in pts with AH - R and L thal, R put, P and L phcp g, R caud, L cer, R ant cing, L subcal g; in pt with AH and VH - vis assn ctx, aud and ling assn ctx

<, > = greater, less; abs = absolute; ant = anterior; assoc = associated; BG = basal ganglia; bilat = bilateral; btn = between; c-m = canthomeatal; c/w = consistent with; caud = caudate; cing = cingulate; CMR = metabolic rate; coeff = coefficient; cond = condition; contin = continuous; ctl = control; d/o = disorder; dec = decrease; dur = duration; ea = each; esp = especially; estab = established; fro = frontal; grad = gradient; hemis = hemisphere; imp = improvement; inc = increase; incl = include; indiv = individual; infraventr = infraventricular; inhal = inhaled; inj = injection; ip = injection; op = inpatient, outpatient; L, R = left, right; lat = lateral; M, F = male, female; max = maximum; med = medication; midventr = midventricular; neg = negative; NL = normal; o-m = orbitomeatal; olf = olfactory; orb = orbital; par = parietal; post = posterior; prodr = prodromal; pt = patient; put = putamen; rCBF = blood flow; rel = relative; RH, LH = right-, left-handed; rx = medication treatment; scz = schizophrenia; sczaff = schizoaffective; sig = significant; signif = significant; stim = stimulation; subj = subject; supraventr = supraventricular; thal = thalamus; tx = general treatment; w/ = with; w/in = within; WB = whole brain; yo = years old; yr = year(s).

controls. With regard to laterality in patients, most studies find either no hemispheric asymmetries [7–9] or increased metabolism or blood flow in the left hemisphere, particularly in temporal areas [6,10,11]. One study [3] noted decreased FDG uptake in the left hemisphere relative to the right in patients. In the case of control subjects, most studies have reported no left-right differences [3,7]. However, both Buchsbaum et al. [12] and Gur et al. [11] found higher left than right metabolism in controls. In contrast, Sheppard et al. [8] reported greater blood flow in the right hemisphere than in the left in their comparison sample. Most of the studies examining laterality have used FDG in resting conditions; the three studies employing somatosensory stimulation during uptake [7,12,13] have dissimilar findings with regard to laterality in patients and controls.

IV. SUBCORTICAL-CORTICAL

Relative to examinations of anterior-posterior or left-right differences, few investigators have addressed subcortical-cortical gradients. Although decreased resting basal ganglia metabolism and blood flow have been noted by Buchsbaum et al. [14] and Sheppard et al. [8], respectively, only metabolic studies from the University of Pennsylvania have reported ratios of subcortical/cortical metabolism. Both of these studies [11,15] reported a higher subcortical/cortical metabolic gradient in patients with schizophrenia using FDG and resting uptake conditions. An additional finding in the Gur et al. [11] paper was higher subcortical than cortical metabolism in both patients and healthy controls.

V. MEDICATION

Investigators have also described the relationship of brain blood flow and metabolism with neuroleptic treatment in schizophrenia. A common, but not universal, finding is an association between treatment and increased striatal/basal ganglia metabolic rate. Brodie et al. [16], Volkow et al. [17], and Buchsbaum et al. [14,18] showed an increase in basal ganglia CMR with typical neuroleptic treatment. Although clozapine is an "atypical" neuroleptic, Buchsbaum et al. [19] and Potkin et al. [20] both demonstrated increases in metabolic rate in striatum or basal ganglia with clozapine treatment.

In addition to striatal and regional effects, neuroleptics can be associated with more global brain metabolism effects. Wolkin et al. [21] demonstrated a general increase in CMR and a decrease in relative hypofrontality with neuroleptic treatment. DeLisi et al. [10] also showed global increases in CMR (especially left temporal and basal ganglia) with neuroleptics.

Not all studies demonstrated an increase in basal ganglia metabolism with neuroleptic treatment. In 1989, Wik et al. [22] examined the effects of sulpiride and chlorpromazine in patients over 5–6 weeks of treatment. They showed that at the end of treatment, sulpiride alone caused changes. Sulpiride treatment was associated with an increase in the glucose metabolic rate in the right lentiform nucleus. However, the sulpiride patients were more chronic and had lower global absolute and relative CMR than the controls or chlorpromazine patients at baseline and posttreatment. Bartlett et al. [23] compared the effects of thiothixine versus haloperidol on glucose metabolism. They demonstrated an association of increased CMR in whole brain, basal ganglia, and DLPFC with thiothixine treatment, while haloperidol was associated with decreases in the same areas. It is important to note that the patients were not randomly assigned to treatment groups and that the thiothixine patients were more chronic with lower whole brain CMR pretreatment.

Some investigators showed no neuroleptic effect on brain metabolic rate. Farkas et al. [24] found no difference between six patients treated with neuroleptics and seven untreated patients. Resnick et al. [15] showed no consistent treatment effects in 12 patients on uncontrolled neuroleptic treatment for an average of 9 weeks.

Another method to understand medication effects on brain metabolism is to use dopaminergic agents acutely. Cleghorn et al. [25] demonstrated a decrease in relative striatal CMR after apomorphine administration in patients but not controls. Wolkin et al. [26] found that acute amphetamine administration in patients with schizophrenia was associated with decreases in absolute CMR in all ROIs except the cerebellum and a decrease in the left temporal lobe relative to whole brain CMR.

In summary, most, but not all, studies have shown an association between neuroleptic treatment and increase in basal ganglia glucose metabolism. This association holds for the atypical neuroleptic clozapine as well. These results are not surprising in light of the high D2 receptor density in the basal ganglia. Further work is necessary to describe how central this phenomenon is to the pathophysiology of schizophrenia and its treatment.

VI. PHENOMENOLOGY

Investigators have also examined the association between symptomatology and brain blood flow and metabolism. In 1992, Cleghorn et al. [27] compared 12 schizophrenic patients with auditory hallucinations (AH) to 10 schizophrenic patients without AH. The patients with AH were distinguished on the basis of the following ROI CMR: decreased auditory cortex and left Wernicke's region and increased striatum and anterior cingulate. In an oxygen-15 study, Silbersweig et al. [28] examined five patients with chronic AH. Using statistical parametric mapping (SPM) for analysis, they found these statistical maxima: right and left thalamus, right putamen, right and left para-hippocampal gyrus, right caudate, left cerebellum, right anterior cingulate, and left subcallosal gyrus.

Deficit symptoms are an important area of investigation in schizophrenia. They are associated with prognostic and neurobiological variables [29]. Accordingly, there has been ample interest in examining deficit symptoms and their relationship to brain blood flow and metabolism, especially in light of the hypofrontality hypothesis. Tamminga et al. [4] demonstrated correlations with decreases in the thalamus, frontal and parietal CMR in the deficit subtype. Liddle et al. [30], in an oxygen-15 study, investigated 30 patients and then correlated ROIs with three main symptom groups. Deficit symptoms were correlated with the right and left caudate positively and the left DLPFC and left superior parietal association cortex negatively (for ROI correlations with the other two symptom groups, see Table 1). In 1992, Wolkin et al. [31] demonstrated an association between deficit symptoms and decreased right DLPFC CMR. Gur et al. [6] showed an increase in relative left midtemporal CMR associated with deficit symptoms.

An important consideration with all symptom-neurobiology associations is disease specificity. Is the neurobiology simply associated with the symptom complex and not specific to the disease process? Dolan et al. [5] examined this issue in a study of 30 patients with schizophrenia and 40 depressed patients with oxygen-15 and SPM analysis. They compared the two patient groups on psychomotor poverty. In their analysis they found a symptom effect but no diagnosis effect or diagnosis by symptom interaction. Interpretation of symptom-PET ROI relationships should be conservative and question the degree of disease specificity.

VII. COGNITIVE ACTIVATION

A number of cognitive deficits have been shown in patients with schizophrenia [32]. A tool to understand the pathophysiology of schizophrenia is the use of cognitive tasks to "activate" the brain during a PET scan. In addition, there is concern that scans of patients at rest have increased variability compared to controls. Activation studies may limit this variability and increase effect size allowing for more meaningful comparisons between patients and controls [1,33]. Yet a lack of a standard resting baseline across activation procedures, within and across laboratories, poses a limitation on data interpretation.

Three investigators have examined forms of the continuous performance test (CPT) as an activation task in schizophrenia. Cohen et al. [34] showed differences in schizophrenia versus controls in the medial parietal, left anterior temporal, and five midfrontal regions during an auditory form of the CPT.

In controls but not patients, task accuracy was associated with midprefrontal CMR. Subsequently, Cohen et al. [35] found no difference in the patient groups (schizophrenia vs. affective disorder) on global CMR, but a decrease in the middle prefrontal CMR during an auditory discrimination CPT for both patient groups. Affective disorder patients had decreased temporal and left basal ganglia CMR that was different from patients with schizophrenia. It is important to note that 13 of the 33 patients had a history of substance abuse. Guich et al. [36] studied patient CPT performance with FDG scans and coincident EEG. The 15 schizophrenic patients had an increase in frontal delta activity, which correlated with a decrease in relative frontal CMR. Buchsbaum et al. [37] showed a decrease in relative and absolute frontal CMR by patients during the CPT. These patients also exhibited a decreased relative and absolute temporal-parietal CMR during the task. Even with this task-related variability in the CPT, it is now often used as a "baseline" task in the study of brain physiology in schizophrenia.

Three investigators have also shown changes in metabolism or flow during cognitive activation with controls but not patients, suggesting inefficiencies in the pathways underlying task performance in schizophrenia. Volkow et al. examined an eye-tracking task as an activation paradigm in two published studies [38,39]. They found less change from baseline to task for patients as compared to controls. The patients also had increased variability in ROI CMRs with decreased correlations between ROIs as compared to controls. They also examined the relationship of performance on the task to schizophrenic symptomatology. They found that patients with deficit symptomatology had decreased frontal CMR during the task. There was a significant correlation between positive symptoms and occipital CMR during the task. In general, there were more correlations between symptomatology and ROI CMRs during the task than at rest. In an oxygen-15 study, Frith et al. [40] demonstrated that controls decrease left superior temporal flow during a verbal fluency task while schizophrenics exhibited no change. Gunther [41] showed increases in medial frontal and left sensorimotor cortex CMR by controls during a complex motor task, while patients with schizophrenia showed no change.

VIII. CONCLUSION

Most of the results of PET studies involving anterior-posterior and laterality dimensions, phenomenology, and cognitive activation are equivocal. Somewhat consistent findings are found with subcortical-cortical and medication effects. Patients with schizophrenia appear to have steeper subcortical-cortical gradients than controls. Neuroleptic treatment seems to be associated with an increase in basal ganglia metabolism.

There are a number of potential sources for variability in these findings. There are important methodological considerations related to selection and characterization of patients and controls, acquisition parameters, scanner characteristics, and image and data analysis. For example, many early studies had limited numbers of patients, many of whom had other comorbid diagnoses such as substance abuse. There are hints that there are symptom-related differences; therefore, it is of utmost importance that patients be well characterized clinically. In addition, there are sometimes differences between the controls and patients, such as education and IQ, that might produce findings that are not representative of the pathophysiological process of schizophrenia itself.

Another potential confound is the use of cognitive paradigms as a baseline. With the hopes that cognitive activation will decrease subject variability and increase effect sizes, investigators are increasingly relying on paradigms involving cognitive tasks without a true resting state. However, the variability of and within activation conditions also limits interpretation across studies.

Perhaps the largest variability across studies relates to data acquisition and image analysis. Standard atlas or individualized anatomical CT- or MRI-based techniques are most often employed, followed by the cortical peel method. Most investigators currently use MRI-based cross-registration. More recently, researchers have used statistical parametric mapping. Other techniques include, but are not limited to, pattern analysis, metabolic coupling, mean centroid analysis, factor or canonical analysis, and other boundary-fitting algorithms. While it is beyond the scope of this chapter to critique specific methods, cross-registration of PET images with corresponding MRI images appears to be the most rigorous method currently available for resolving these sources of variability and characterizing brain physiology in schizophrenia.

REFERENCES

1. M. S. Buchsbaum, The frontal lobes, basal ganglia, and temporal lobes as sites for schizophrenia, *Schizophr. Bull. 16*(3):379 (1990).
2. D. H. Ingvar and G. Franzen, Distribution of cerebral activity in chronic schizophrenia, *Lancet 2*(7895):1484 (1974).
3. M. S. Buchsbaum, D. H. Ingvar, R. Kessler, et al., Cerebral glucography with positron tomography. Use in normal subjects and in patients with schizophrenia, *Arch. Gen. Psychiatry 39*(3):251 (1982).
4. C. A. Tamminga, G. K. Thaker, R. Buchanan, B. Kirkpatrick, L. D. Alphs, T. N. Chase, and W. T. Carpenter, Limbic system abnormalities identified in schizophrenia using positron emission tomography with fluorodeoxyglucose and

neocortical alterations with deficit syndrome, *Arch. Gen. Psychiatry 49*(7):522 (1992).

5. R. J. Dolan, C. J. Bench, P. F. Liddle, K. J. Friston, C. D. Frith, P. M. Grasby, and R. S. Frackowiak, Dorsolateral prefrontal cortex dysfunction in the major psychoses; symptom or disease specificity? *J. Neurol. Neurosurg. Psychiatry 56*(12):1290 (1993).

6. R. E. Gur, P. D. Mozley, S. M. Resnick, et al., Resting cerebral glucose metabolism in first-episode and previously treated patients with schizophrenia relates to clinical features, *Arch. Gen. Psychiatry 52*(8):657 (1995).

7. L. E. DeLisi, M. S. Buchsbaum, H. H. Holcomb, et al., Clinical correlates of decreased anteroposterior metabolic gradients in positron emission tomography (PET) of schizophrenic patients, *Am. J. Psychiatry 142*(1):78 (1985).

8. G. Sheppard, J. Gruzelier, R. Manchanda, S. R. Hirsch, R. Wise, R. Frackowiak, and T. Jones, 15O positron emission tomographic scanning in predominantly never-treated acute schizophrenic patients, *Lancet 2*(8365–66):1448 (1983).

9. A. V. Levy, J. D. Brodie, A. G. Russell, N. D. Volkow, E. Laska, and A. P. Wolf, The metabolic centroid method for PET brain image analysis, *J. Cereb. Blood Flow Metab. 9*(3):388 (1989).

10. L. E. DeLisi, H. H. Holcomb, R. M. Cohen, D. Pickar, W. Carpenter, J. M. Morihisa, A. C. King, R. Kessler, and M. S. Buchsbaum, Positron emission tomography in schizophrenic patients with and without neuroleptic medication, *J. Cereb. Blood Flow Metab. 5*(2):201 (1985).

11. R. E. Gur, S. M. Resnick, A. Alavi, et al., Regional brain function in schizophrenia. I. A positron emission tomography study, *Arch. Gen. Psychiatry 44*(2):119 (1987).

12. M. S. Buchsbaum, L. E. DeLisi, H. H. Holcomb, et al., Anteroposterior gradients in cerebral glucose use in schizophrenia and affective disorders, *Arch. Gen. Psychiatry 41*(12):1159 (1984).

13. L. E. DeLisi, M. S. Buchsbaum, H. H. Holcomb, et al., Increased temporal lobe glucose use in chronic schizophrenic patients, *Biol. Psychiatry 25*(7):835 (1989).

14. M. S. Buchsbaum, J. C. Wu, L. E. DeLisi, H. H. Holcomb, E. Hazlett, K. Cooper-Langston, and R. Kessler, Positron emission tomography studies of basal ganglia and somatosensory cortex neuroleptic drug effects: differences between normal controls and schizophrenic patients, *Biol. Psychiatry 22*(4):479 (1987).

15. S. M. Resnick, R. E. Gur, A. Alavi, R. C. Gur, and M. Reivich, Positron emission tomography and subcortical glucose metabolism in schizophrenia, *Psychiatry Res. 24*(1):1 (1988).

16. J. D. Brodie, D. R. Christman, J. F. Corona, et al., Patterns of metabolic activity in the treatment of schizophrenia, *Ann. Neurol. 15*(suppl):S166 (1984).

17. N. D. Volkow, J. D. Brodie, A. P. Wolf, B. Angrist, J. Russell, and R. Cancro, Brain metabolism in patients with schizophrenia before and after acute neuroleptic administration, *J. Neurol. Neurosurg. Psychiatry 49*(10):1199 (1986).

18. M. S. Buchsbaum, S. G. Potkin, B. V. Siegel, Jr., et al., Striatal metabolic rate and clinical response to neuroleptics in schizophrenia, *Arch. Gen. Psychiatry* *49*(12):966 (1992).

19. M. S. Buchsbaum, S. G. Potkin, J. F. Marshall, et al., Effects of clozapine and thiothixene on glucose metabolic rate in schizophrenia, *Neuropsychopharmacology* *6*(3):155 (1992).

20. S. G. Potkin, M. S. Buchsbaum, Y. Jin, et al., Clozapine effects on glucose metabolic rate in striatum and frontal cortex, *J. Clin. Psychiatry* *55*(suppl B): 63 (1994).

21. A. Wolkin, J. Jaeger, J. D. Brodie, A. P. Wolf, J. Fowler, J. Rotrosen, F. Gomez-Mont, and R. Cancro, Persistence of cerebral metabolic abnormalities in chronic schizophrenia as determined by positron emission tomography, *Am. J. Psychiatry* *142*(5):564 (1985).

22. G. Wik, F. A. Wiesel, I. Sjogren, G. Blomqvist, T. Greitz, and S. Stone-Elander, Effects of sulpiride and chlorpromazine on regional cerebral glucose metabolism in schizophrenic patients as determined by positron emission tomography, *Psychopharmacology* *97*(3):309 (1989).

23. E. J. Bartlett, A. Wolkin, J. D. Brodie, E. M. Laska, A. P. Wolf, and M. Sanfilipo, Importance of pharmacologic control in PET studies: effects of thiothixene and haloperidol on cerebral glucose utilization in chronic schizophrenia, *Psychiatry Res.* *40*(2):115 (1991).

24. T. Farkas, A. P. Wolf, J. Jaeger, J. D. Brodie, D. R. Christman, and J. S. Fowler, Regional brain glucose metabolism in chronic schizophrenia. A positron emission transaxial tomographic study, *Arch. Gen. Psychiatry* *41*(3):293 (1984).

25. J. M. Cleghorn, H. Szechtman, E. S. Garnett, C. Nahmias, G. M. Brown, R. D. Kaplan, B. Szechtman, and S. Franco, Apomorphine effects on brain metabolism in neuroleptic-naive schizophrenic patients, *Psychiatry Res.* *40*(2): 135 (1991).

26. A. Wolkin, M. Sanfilipo, B. Angrist, E. Duncan, S. Wieland, A. P. Wolf, J. D. Brodie, T. B. Cooper, E. Laska, and J. P. Rotrosen, Acute d-amphetamine challenge in schizophrenia: effects on cerebral glucose utilization and clinical symptomatology, *Biol. Psychiatry* *36*(5):317 (1994).

27. J. M. Cleghorn, S. Franco, B. Szechtman, R. D. Kaplan, H. Szechtman, G. M. Brown, C. Nahmias, and E. S. Garnett, Toward a brain map of auditory hallucinations [see comments], *Am. J. Psychiatry* *149*(8):1062 (1992).

28. D. A. Silbersweig, E. Stern, C. Frith, et al., A functional neuroanatomy of hallucinations in schizophrenia, *Nature* *378*:176 (1995).

29. T. H. McGlashan and W. S. Fenton, The positive-negative symptom distinction in schizophrenia: review of natural history validators, *Arch. Gen. Psychiatry* *49*:63 (1992).

30. P. F. Liddle, K. J. Friston, C. D. Frith, S. R. Hirsch, T. Jones, and R. S. Frackowiak, Patterns of cerebral blood flow in schizophrenia, *Br. J. Psychiatry* *160*:179 (1992).

31. A. Wolkin, M. Sanfilipo, A. P. Wolf, B. Angrist, J. D. Brodie, and J. Rotrosen, Negative symptoms and hypofrontality in chronic schizophrenia, *Arch. Gen. Psychiatry* *49*(12):959 (1992).

32. A. J. Saykin, D. L. Shtasel, R. E. Gur, D. B. Kester, L. H. Mozley, P. Stafiniak, and R. C. Gur, Neuropsychological deficits in neuroleptic naive patients with first episode schizophrenia, *Arch. Gen. Psychiatry 51*:124 (1994).
33. J. M. Cleghorn, R. B. Zipursky, and S. J. List, Structural and functional brain imaging in schizophrenia, *J. Psychiatry Neurosci. 16*(2):53 (1991).
34. R. M. Cohen, W. E. Semple, M. Gross, T. E. Nordahl, L. E. DeLisi, H. H. Holcomb, A. C. King, J. M. Morihisa, and D. Pickar, Dysfunction in a prefrontal substrate of sustained attention in schizophrenia, *Life Sci. 40*(20):2031 (1987).
35. R. M. Cohen, W. E. Semple, M. Gross, T. E. Nordahl, A. C. King, D. Pickar, and R. M. Post, Evidence for common alterations in cerebral glucose metabolism in major affective disorders and schizophrenia, *Neuropsychopharmacology 2*(4):241 (1989).
36. S. M. Guich, M. S. Buchsbaum, L. Burgwald, J. Wu, R. Haier, R. Asarnow, K. Nuechterlein, and S. Potkin, Effect of attention on frontal distribution of delta activity and cerebral metabolic rate in schizophrenia, *Schizophr. Res. 2*(6):439 (1989).
37. M. S. Buchsbaum, K. H. Nuechterlein, R. J. Haier, J. Wu, N. Sicotte, E. Hazlett, R. Asarnow, S. Potkin, and S. Guich, Glucose metabolic rate in normals and schizophrenics during the Continuous Performance Test assessed by positron emission tomography, *Br. J. Psychiatry 156*:216 (1990).
38. N. D. Volkow, A. P. Wolf, P. Van Gelder, J. D. Brodie, J. E. Overall, R. Cancro, and F. Gomez-Mont, Phenomenological correlates of metabolic activity in 18 patients with chronic schizophrenia, *Am. J. Psychiatry 144*(2):151 (1987).
39. N. D. Volkow, A. P. Wolf, J. D. Brodie, R. Cancro, J. E. Overall, H. Rhoades, and P. Van Gelder, Brain interactions in chronic schizophrenics under resting and activation conditions, *Schizophr. Res. 1*(1):47 (1988).
40. C. D. Frith, K. J. Friston, S. Herold, D. Silbersweig, P. Fletcher, C. Cahill, R. J. Dolan, R. S. J. Frackowiak, and P. F. Liddle, Regional brain activity in chronic schizophrenic patients during the performance of a verbal fluency task, *Br. J. Psychiatry 167*:343 (1995).
41. W. Gunther, MRI-SPECT and PET-EEG findings on brain dysfunction in schizophrenia, *Prog. Neuropsychopharmacol. Biol. Psychiatry 16*(4):445 (1992).
42. C. M. Clark, R. Kessler, M. S. Buchsbaum, R. A. Margolin, and H. H. Holcomb, Correlational methods for determining regional coupling of cerebral glucose metabolism: a pilot study, *Biol. Psychiatry 19*(5):663 (1984).
43. T. L. Jernigan, T. D. Sargent, A. Pfefferbaum, N. Kusubov, and S. M. Stahl, 18-Fluorodeoxyglucose PET in schizophrenia, *Psychiatry Res. 16*(4):317 (1985).
44. R. E. Gur, S. M. Resnick, R. C. Gur, A. Alavi, S. Caroff, M. Kushner, and M. Reivich, Regional brain function in schizophrenia. II. Repeated evaluation with positron emission tomography, *Arch. Gen. Psychiatry 44*(2):126 (1987).
45. H. Kishimoto, H. Kuwahara, S. Ohno, et al., Three subtypes of chronic schizophrenia identified using 11C-glucose positron emission tomography [published erratum *Psychiatry Res 23*(3):353 (1988)], *Psychiatry Res. 21*(4):285 (1987).
46. F. A. Wiesel, G. Wik, I. Sjogren, G. Blomqvist, T. Greitz, and S. Stone-Elander, Regional brain glucose metabolism in drug free schizophrenic patients and clinical correlates, *Acta Psychiatr. Scand. 76*(6):628 (1987).

47. H. Szechtman, C. Nahmias, E. S. Garnett, G. Firnau, G. M. Brown, R. D. Kaplan, and J. M. Cleghorn, Effect of neuroleptics on altered cerebral glucose metabolism in schizophrenia, *Arch. Gen. Psychiatry 45*(6):523 (1988).
48. A. Wolkin, B. Angrist, A. Wolf, J. D. Brodie, B. Wolkin, J. Jaeger, R. Cancro, and J. Rotrosen, Low frontal glucose utilization in chronic schizophrenia: a replication study, *Am. J. Psychiatry 145*(2):251 (1988).
49. C. Clark, H. Klonoff, J. S. Tyhurst, D. Li, W. Martin, and B. D. Pate, Regional cerebral glucose metabolism in three sets of identical twins with psychotic symptoms, *Can. J. Psychiatry 34*(4):263 (1989).
50. J. M. Cleghorn, E. S. Garnett, C. Nahmias, G. Firnau, G. M. Brown, R. Kaplan, H. Szechtman, and B. Szechtman, Increased frontal and reduced parietal glucose metabolism in acute untreated schizophrenia, *Psychiatry Res. 28*(2):119 (1989).
51. R. E. Gur, S. M. Resnick, and R. C. Gur, Laterality and frontality of cerebral blood flow and metabolism in schizophrenia: relationship to symptom specificity, *Psychiatry Res. 27*(3):325 (1989).
52. D. J. Luchins, J. T. Metz, R. C. Marks, and M. D. Cooper, Basal ganglia regional glucose metabolism asymmetry during a catatonic episode, *Biol. Psychiatry 26*:725 (1989).
53. E. J. Bartlett, F. Barouche, J. D. Brodie, A. Wolkin, B. Angrist, J. Rotrosen, and A. P. Wolf, Stability of resting deoxyglucose metabolic values in PET studies of schizophrenia, *Psychiatry Res. 40*(1):11 (1991).
54. C. Clark, L. Kopala, T. Hurwitz, and D. Li, Regional metabolism in microsmic patients with schizophrenia, *Can. J. Psychiatry 36*(9):645 (1991).
55. A. V. Levy, F. Gomez-Mont, N. D. Volkow, J. F. Corona, J. D. Brodie, and R. Cancro, Spatial low frequency pattern analysis in positron emission tomography: a study between normals and schizophrenics, *J. Nuclear Med. 33*(2):287 (1991).
56. M. S. Buchsbaum, R. J. Haier, S. G. Potkin, et al., Frontostriatal disorder of cerebral metabolism in never-medicated schizophrenics, *Arch. Gen. Psychiatry. 49*(12):935 (1992).
57. K. J. Friston, P. F. Liddle, C. D. Frith, S. R. Hirsch, and R. S. Frackowiak, The left medial temporal region and schizophrenia. A PET study, *Brain 115*(Pt 2):367 (1992).
58. N. D. Volkow, A. Levy, J. D. Brodie, A. P. Wolf, R. Cancro, P. Van Gelder, and F. Henn, Low cerebellar metabolism in medicated patients with chronic schizophrenia, *Am. J. Psychiatry 149*(5):686 (1992).
59. C. M. Clark, L. Kopala, G. James, T. Hurwitz, and D. Li, Metabolic subtypes in patients with schizophrenia, *Biol. Psychiatry 33*(2):86 (1993).
60. B. V. Siegel, Jr., M. S. Buchsbaum, W. E. Bunney, Jr., et al., Cortical-striatal-thalamic circuits and brain glucose metabolic activity in 70 unmedicated male schizophrenic patients, *Am. J. Psychiatry 150*(9):1325 (1993).
61. J. Schroeder, M. S. Buchsbaum, B. V. Siegel, F. J. Geider, R. J. Haier, J. Lohr, J. Wu, and S. G. Potkin, Patterns of cortical activity in schizophrenia, *Psychol. Med. 24*(4):947 (1994).

15

Neuroimaging in Late-Life Psychosis

Laura L. Symonds
University of California—San Diego, San Diego, California

Dilip V. Jeste
University of California—San Diego, and
VA Medical Center, San Diego, California

425

I. INTRODUCTION

The relatively sudden appearance of psychosis in a previously normally functioning individual is a puzzling phenomenon, and may well be, as Kraepelin
and Bleuler [1] said, ". . . the darkest area of psychiatry." The application
of modern neuroimaging techniques in the 1980s launched a search for structural abnormalities in the brains of individuals with late onset of psychiatric
symptoms. Most of these initial investigations began by selecting patients
solely on the basis of any psychiatric diagnosis with onset of symptoms in
later life. Thus, patients such as those with tumors or metabolic encephalopathies were included [2–5]. The results of these investigations made clear that
a majority of such patients had abnormal brain scans. The most common
abnormalities were large, confluent white matter lesions, and multiple or
scattered lacunae in the basal ganglia or cortex. Tumors, hydrocephalus,
and evidence of traumatic brain injury were also observed. In one study [3],
the authors observed that it appeared that the patients "with the most dramatic and radical changes in personality in late life were more likely to have
detectable lesions." The question remained: Can psychoses not associated
with the progressive dementias, tumors, and traumatic insults also be linked
to brain abnormalities visible on CT or MR scans?

    This chapter reviews neuroimaging studies that have addressed the issue
of brain abnormalities related to psychosis in later life. In contrast to the
relative explosion of structural and functional neuroimaging studies of schizophrenia and other psychoses in younger individuals, neuroimaging studies
of late-life psychosis have been relatively few (see Table 1). Furthermore,
such reports have been primarily limited to qualitative ratings of white matter
changes and ventricle size or to two-dimensional quantitative measurements
of ventricles. All but two studies [6,7] used structural neuroimaging techniques (CT or MRI). Most of the studies reviewed here sought to come to
a better understanding of the biological basis of the psychotic disorders. One
of the purposes of this chapter is to determine to what extent some late-
onset psychoses (e.g., schizophrenia), and not others, are associated with
specific brain abnormalities. We have chosen, therefore, to organize this
review by diagnosis and to be as rigorous as possible in determining the
similarities of diagnostic criteria among the various studies. The following
sections of this chapter discuss studies pertinent to (a) late-life "paraphrenia", (b) early-onset schizophrenia in older patients, (c) late-onset schizo-

Table 1 Neuroimaging Studies in Late-Life Psychosis

Study and Ref.	Subjects (N & diagnosis)	Imaging method	Imaging measurements	Results
Miller et al., 1986 [2]	5 late paraphrenia	CT	Clinical inspection of white matter lucencies, infarcts, etc.	4/5 patients had clinical abnormalities, including white matter lucencies, infarcts, hydrocephalus
Naguib and Levy, 1987 [20]	43 late paraphrenia 40 age-matched NC	CT	VBR (planimeter)	VBR: patients (13.09 ± 4.34) > NC (9.75 ± 4.35), $p < 0.001$
Rabins et al., 1987 [37]	29 LOS 23 AD 23 NC	CT	VBR (planimeter)	VBR: AD (17.5 ± 5.0) > LOS (13.3 ± 3.4), $p < 0.001$; LOS > NC (8.6 ± 5.2), $p < 0.001$
Pearlson et al., 1987 [24]	8 late paraphrenia 14 NC	CT	VBR (planimeter) Sulcal width	VBR: patients (12.3 ± 2.4) > NC (10.8 ± 3.0), trend VBR, age correlation: patients $r = -0.13$, $p < 0.05$, NC $r = 45$, n.s.
Weinberger et al., 1987 [32]	17 EOS, elderly 16 NC	CT	VBR (planimeter) Sulcal width	VBR: patients > NC, $p < 0.005$ Sucli: patients > NC, trend
Miller and Lesser, 1988 [3]	25 late-onset psychosis, various diagnoses	CT/MRI	Clinical readings of scans	40% had normal scans; 60% had evidence for silent stroke, dementia, tumors
Miller et al., 1989 [4]	5 late-onset psychosis (1 LOS, 3 delusional disorder, 1 mania) 60 NC	CT/MRI	Qualitative descriptions of white matter abnormalities	5/5 patients had large, subfrontal lesions 0/60 NC had similar lesions
Hymas et al., 1989 [21]	42 late paraphrenia 23 NC (subjects same as in (20))	CT	VBR (planimeter)	45% patients had decline in memory/orientation which was not correlated with VBR.
Burns et al., 1989 [22]	42 late paraphrenia 39 NC (subjects same as in (20))	CT	Qualitative ratings of sulci (overall cortical atrophy)	Cortical atrophy: no difference between patients & NC.
Broadhead and Jacoby, 1990 [54]	14 "early-onset mania" (<52 yrs) 21 "late-onset mania" (>55 yrs) 20 age-comparable NC	CT	Qualitative ratings of cortical atrophy VBR (planimeter)	Cortical atrophy: manic patients > NC, $p < .01$; No difference between early- & late-onset mania VBR: no difference between patients & NC (% not reported)
Breitner et al., 1990 [38]	8 late-onset psychosis 8 NC	MRI	Qualitative ratings of atrophy, vascular lesions, signal hyper-intensities	8/8 patients, but 0/8 NC had at least 1 white matter lesion > 10 mm diameter in temporo-parietal or occipital area 7/8 patients, but 0/8 NC had lesions in pons or basal ganglia
Flint et al., 1991 [31]	12 LOS 4 late-onset delusional disorder	CT	Clinical description of cerebral infarcts	4/4 delusional disorder, and 1/12 LOS patients had cerebral infarcts

(continued)

Table 1   *(continued)*

Study and Ref.	Subjects (N & diagnosis)	Imaging method	Imaging measurements	Results
Krull et al., 1991 [39]	11 LOS 9 AD 9 NC	MRI	Qualitative ratings of ventricular enlargement and white matter hyperintensities.	*Ventricular enlargement*: AD > NC, $p < 0.005$; LOS > NC, n.s. $p < 0.1$ *White matter abnormalities*: no significant differences among groups
Miller et al., 1991 [5]	24 late-onset psychosis, various diagnoses 72 NC	MRI/CT	VBR Clinical description of brain abnormalities, including tumor, stroke, etc.	*VBR*: patients (10.6 ± 3.2) > NC (8.8 ± 3.6), n.s. $p < 0.1$ *Clinical abnormalities*: 42% of patients, 8% of NC, $p < 0.001$
Pearlson et al., 1991 [41]	11 LOS 12 AD 18 NC	MRI	Quantitative volume measurements of whole brain and grey matter structures	Both LOS and AD patients: decreased volumes of several medial temporal grey matter structures, but decreased volume in anterior superior temporal gyrus only for LOS
Lesser et al., 1992 [57]	12 late-onset psychosis, NOS	MRI/CT	Clinical description of brain abnormalities White matter lesion measurements	8/12 patients had clinical abnormalities, including white matter lesions, infarcts, cyst, cortical atrophy
Howard et al., 1992 [23]	41 late paraphrenia, 16 with FRS, 25 without FRS 40 NC (subjects same as in (20))	CT	Qualitative ratings of ventricular enlargement, cortical atrophy	*Ventricular enlargement*: no differences among groups *Cortical atrophy*: patients without FRS > patients with FRS or NC, $p < 0.01$
Lesser et al., 1993 [26]	22 late-onset psychosis, including LOS, delusional disorder & NOS NC, N not specified	MRI	Quantitative measurements of white matter hyperintensities	Approximately 50% of both patients & NC had white matter hyperintensities but more patients (18%) than NC (2%) had hyperintensities > 10 cm
Pearlson et al., 1993 [7]	11 LOS 12 AD 18 NC	MRI	Quantitative measurements of third ventricle and VBR Volume measurements of CSF and whole brain	*3rd ventricle*: LOS > NC; AD > NC, $p < 0.01$ *VBR*: LOS (9.0 ± 2.8) > NC (7.1 ± 4.7), trend; AD > NC, $p < 0.05$ *%CSF*: LOS > NC, trend: AD > NC, $p < 0.05$
Pearlson et al., 1993 [7]	11 LOS (6 from above study) 11 EOS	MRI	Qualitative ratings of atrophy (sulci and ventricle)	No difference between EOS and LOS
Howard et al., 1994 [28]	47 late paraphrenia 31 paranoid schizophrenia 16 delusional disorder 33 NC	MRI	Quantitative measurements of CSF, brain, and ventricular volumes	*Volume of lateral and 3rd ventricles*: delusional disorder > NC, $p < 0.03$ paranoid schizophrenia > NC, n.s.

Table 1 (*continued*)

Study and Ref.	Subjects (N & diagnosis)	Imaging method	Imaging measurements	Results
Foerstl et al., 1994 [25]	14 late-onset paranoid psychosis AD & NC, Ns not specified	CT, EEG	VBR (planimeter) Qualitative ratings of clinical abnormalities, including infarcts	*VBR*: AD (16.9 ± 5.08) > NC (7.83 ± 3.50); psychosis patients (12.22 ± 4.14) > NC Non FRS (14.7 ± 3.8) > FRS (10.6 ± 4.3), $p < 0.05$
Dupont et al., 1994 [6]	4 LOS 7 EOS 11 NC	SPECT, IMP	Global and regional uptake	*Global uptake*: NC > patients, $p < 0.05$ *Regional uptake corrected for mean cortical uptake*: NC > patients for left posterior frontal ($p < 0.001$) and bilateral anterior inferior temporal ($p < 0.005$ left & $p < 0.01$ right)
Corey-Bloom et al., 1995 [8]	16 LOS 14 EOS 28 NC	MRI	Quantitative volume measurements of CSF, ventricles, white matter abnormalities, and grey matter structures	*Ventricles*: LOS > NC, $p < 0.05$ *Thalamus*: LOS > EOS, $p < 0.05$
Howard et al., 1995 [27]	38 late paraphrenia 31 NC	MRI	Qualitative ratings of white matter hyperintensities and changes in grey matter nuclei	*White matter hyperintensities*: no differences between patients and NC; positive correlation with age and with blood pressure
Fujikawa et al., 1995 [55]	20 late-onset mania 20 early-onset affective disorder 20 late-onset major depression	MRI	Type and diameter of cerebral infarcts measured on T_1- and T_2-weighted images	Both late-onset patient groups had more infarcts than NC Late-onset mania had more "mixed" type of infarcts than late-onset major depression patients or NC
Symonds et al., 1996 [40]	24 LOS 30 EOS 15 other late-life psychosis patients 41 NC	MRI	Qualitative ratings of MRI report narrative of white matter hyperintensities, ventricular enlargement, atrophy, and infarcts	No differences among any of the groups

AD = Alzheimer's disease; CSF = cerebrospinal fluid; CT = computed tomography; EOS = early-onset schizophrenia; FRS = first-rank symptoms (Schneiderian); LOS = late-onset schizophrenia; MRI = magnetic resonance imaging; NC = normal comparison subjects; NOS = not otherwise specified; n.s. = not significant (statistically); VBR = ventricle/brain ratio.

phrenia, (d) late-onset delusional disorder, and (e) late-onset mania. Many studies cited here used patient groups from more than one of the above diagnostic categories and are therefore reviewed in more than one section of this chapter. For example, Corey-Bloom et al. [8] compared late-onset schizophrenia patients, early-onset schizophrenia patients, and normal comparison subjects. Therefore, the reader will find their study cited in both the early-onset schizophrenia and the late-onset schizophrenia sections of this chapter. Before we describe imaging characteristics of these various psychotic disorders that occur in late life, however, we need to clarify the diagnoses themselves.

II. DIAGNOSIS OF LATE-ONSET PSYCHOSIS

Several different terms have been used to describe patients with an onset of psychosis in late life in whom there is no known organic or affective disorder. Included among these terms are "late-onset schizophrenia," "paraphrenia," and "late paraphrenia." Even more confusing, different investigators have sometimes used the same term in different ways. Reviews of the historical development and diagnostic confusion of the terms can be found in Harris and Jeste [9] and Reicher-Roessler et al. [10].

Kraepelin [11,12] first distinguished dementia praecox (i.e., schizophrenia) from paraphrenia. The latter, while sharing a number of the features of dementia praecox, did not involve severe disturbances of emotion or volition, and the majority of Kraepelin's paraphrenia patients had onset of illness in later life, after age 40. Follow-up of these same paraphrenia patients suggested that many of them (at least 38%) had, in fact, a course similar to that of dementia praecox [13]. Bleuler [1] was the first to describe late-onset schizophrenia per se and to make explicit that the symptoms of late-onset schizophrenia were similar to those of early-onset schizophrenia.

In the 1950s and 1960s, Roth and collaborators evolved a concept of "paraphrenia" and "late paraphrenia," which described patients similar to Kraepelin's paraphrenia patients, but with onset after age 60 [14,15]. These late paraphrenia patients had a complex of paranoid symptoms in the absence of organic disorder, confusion, or primary affective disorder. The patients all had some type of delusions either with or without hallucinations.

The ICD-9 [16] included a category for paraphrenia separate from schizophrenia. The primary distinction was that in the diagnosis of paraphrenia, as opposed to schizophrenia, personality had to be well preserved, and if affective symptoms or disordered thinking were present, they could not dominate the clinical picture.

The DSM-III [17] did not include a category for paraphrenia, but did include a separate category of paranoid disorder, which, unlike the diagnosis of schizophrenia, did not restrict age of onset. The DSM-III-R [18] allowed for the diagnosis of schizophrenia after age 45; such patients were given the diagnosis of late-onset schizophrenia. The DSM-IV [19] removed the distinction between early-onset and late-onset schizophrenia and allowed diagnosis of schizophrenia without regard to age of onset of illness.

In view of the different diagnostic criteria applied to psychosis patients who develop the disorder in later life, we have separated our review of relevant neuroimaging studies into different sections. The following section on paraphrenia undoubtedly includes some patients with schizophrenia, but it is nearly impossible to separate such patients from other "paraphrenia" patients. The results, therefore, may or may not apply to late-onset schizophrenia.

III. LATE "PARAPHRENIA"

This section reviews the neuroimaging results of eight studies that used paraphrenia as a diagnostic category. We chose to separate these studies from those of schizophrenia and delusional disorder for two reasons. First, as discussed above, there is considerable evidence that paraphrenia is a heterogeneous diagnostic category which often includes organic and delusional disorders as well as schizophrenia. Second, some of the neuroimaging literature on so-called paraphrenia indicates that rather severe brain abnormalities are often associated with this diagnosis.

"Paraphrenia" has been variously defined, but in general the studies summarized below used ICD-9 criteria or those of Roth [14] and Kay and Roth [15]: patients experienced a late onset of psychotic symptoms, which included delusions and sometimes hallucinations; they had preserved intellect, personality, and affective responses; and there was no history of cerebrovascular accidents or neurological disorders. Thus, the patient groups in the following studies on paraphrenia most likely included some bona fide schizophrenia patients, but it is unclear how many, or what other diagnoses may have been represented. Furthermore, because most investigators relied upon Kay and Roth [15] diagnostic criteria for paraphrenia, the patient groups were generally restricted to those with onset of illness after age 60, which is considerably older than the DSM-III-R categorization of late-onset schizophrenia. (Other details of subjects in the separate studies are provided below.)

Four of the eight studies on late paraphrenia summarized below used the same subject group. All eight studies looked for evidence of either cortical atrophy, usually by calculating the ventricular: brain ratio (VBR), or clinical abnormalities such as white matter changes or infarcts. In general, differences in VBR between patient groups and normal comparison groups were rather robust, and there was some indication that the result might be due primarily to inclusion of patients without Schneider's first rank symptoms. Conversely, there was little support in the studies (from three separate groups) that white matter changes or other clinical abnormalities characterized the brains of late paraphrenia patients.

A. Ventricular Size

Naguib and Levy [20] calculated the VBR from CT scans of 43 late paraphrenia patients, all with onset of symptoms after the age of 60 (mean ~ 72 years), and 40 normal comparison subjects. As in all the studies of late paraphrenia patients reported here, approximately 85% of the patients were women. The mean age of the patients was 75.8 years. The mean VBR of the patients was significantly larger than that of the comparison subjects ($p < 0.001$). The same group of investigators determined that the VBR was not related in these patients to clinical symptoms, cognitive symptoms, or course of disease [21]. The scans of these same patients were then rated qualitatively on a 3- to 4-point scale to determine if cortical sulci were also larger in patients than in normal comparison subjects [22]. No differences between the two groups were found, suggesting to the authors that brain abnormalities in late paraphrenia patients were not cortical, but ventricular (or subcortical). The fourth study to make use of the same CT scans provided one possible explanation as to why VBR was observed to be larger in patients. Howard et al. [23] rated the CT scans qualitatively for ventricular enlargement, cortical atrophy (width of sulci and fissures), and temporal lobe atrophy, using a 4-point scale. These authors divided the paraphrenia patients into two groups based upon whether they had Schneider's first rank symptoms (16 patients) or did not have such symptoms (25 patients). Whereas there were no differences among the two patient groups and the normal comparison group in the ratings of ventricular enlargement or temporal lobe atrophy, there was a statistically significant difference between those patients with first rank symptoms and those without. The patients without first rank symptoms had significantly greater widths of cortical sulci, indicating that only a subgroup of the paraphrenia patients demonstrated signs of cortical atrophy.

Pearlson et al. [24] also investigated the VBR in a smaller group of eight late paraphrenia patients, all diagnosed according to the criteria of Kay and Roth [15]. The average age of the patients was 71.6 years, and mean age of onset of symptoms was approximately 68 years; comparison subjects were 14 nonpsychiatric patients (mean age 72.9 years) referred for CT evaluation of headaches or dizziness, whose CT scans were normal. Although the VBR was larger in paraphrenia patients than that in the comparison subjects, the difference did not reach statistical significance, perhaps because of the relatively small sample size. Another possibility, however, is that the paraphrenia patients consisted of subgroups of patients with different structural brain abnormalities. A recent study by Foerstl et al. [25] supports this idea. These authors compared the VBRs of 14 paraphrenia patients diagnosed according to ICD-9 criteria to 14 normal control subjects and found that the patients had significantly larger VBRs ($p < 0.001$). When these authors divided the group of 14 paraphrenia patients into those with first rank symptoms and those without (the Ns for the two groups were not specified), they found that those without first rank symptoms had significantly larger VBRs. This parallels Howard et al.'s result for cortical atrophy in a similar group of patients, and lends some weight to the idea that paraphrenia patients with first rank symptoms may be different from the paraphrenia patients who have the most obvious or severe cerebral atrophy.

B. Gray or White Matter Lesions

Three studies investigated the degree to which paraphrenia patients had a greater degree of white matter abnormalities and other brain lesions than normal healthy subjects [25–27]. The Lesser et al. [26] study, however, did not specifically use the term "paraphrenia," but instead their group of patients had a mixture of DSM-III diagnoses, including "late-onset schizophrenia," "late-onset delusional disorder," and "late-onset psychosis, not otherwise specified." Two of the studies found no significant differences between paraphrenia patients and normal comparison subjects [25,27], and the third study did find a difference, although not in overall incidence of white matter abnormality [26]. A fourth study examined white matter abnormalities in paraphrenia patients and compared their frequency of occurrence to that in another group of psychosis patients diagnosed with late-onset delusional disorder [28].

Foerstl et al. [25] qualitatively rated the CT scans of paraphrenia patients and normal comparison subjects for the presence and severity of clinical abnormalities including infarcts, white matter hyperintensities, and basal ganglia calcifications. The investigators found no significant differences between the two groups on any of the qualitative measures, even when they took into account whether patients had first rank symptoms or not.

Howard et al. [27] qualitatively rated the T_2-weighted MR scans of 38 paraphrenia patients diagnosed according to ICD-9 criteria and 31 normal comparison subjects. The patients all had an onset of symptoms after age 60, and the mean age of both patients and comparison subjects was approximately 80 years. The authors rated white matter hyperintensities and changes in gray matter nuclei using a standardized grading system modified from Fazekas et al. [29] by Coffey et al. [30]. There were no significant differences between patients and normal comparison subjects on any of the qualitative ratings, though the degree of white matter hyperintensities correlated significantly with both age and blood pressure.

Lesser et al. [26] compared the MR scans of 22 "late-onset psychosis" patients to those of an unspecified number of normal subjects. The patients included those with late-onset schizophrenia, delusional disorder, and psychosis not otherwise specified, all diagnosed using DSM-III-R [18] criteria. The area of each white matter hyperintensity on every 10-mm-thick slice was measured to 0.01 cm^2. Although the same percentage of patients and controls demonstrated white matter abnormalities (in keeping with the two studies cited above), the distribution was different, so that more patients than controls (18% vs. 2%) had areas of hyperintensity >10 cm^2, whereas, more controls than patients had smaller areas of hyperintensity (<1 cm^2 or 1–10 cm^2).

Flint et al. [31] examined the neuroradiologists' narrative reports of the CT scans of 16 psychosis patients with onset of psychosis after age 60. Twelve patients had both delusions and hallucinations and carried an ICD-9 diagnosis of paraphrenia. The remaining four patients met ICD-9 criteria for paranoia (some might have met DSM-IIIR criteria for delusional disorder). The scans of all four of the probable delusional disorder patients showed evidence of cerebral infarction, primarily in the basal ganglia or frontal lobe; only one of the 12 paraphrenia patients had similar lesions.

IV. EARLY-ONSET SCHIZOPHRENIA PATIENTS IN LATE LIFE

Two structural imaging studies compared the sizes of ventricles and other CSF-filled spaces in older schizophrenia patients to those of normal, healthy individuals of similar ages. One functional neuroimaging study used SPECT to assess cerebral blood flow in older schizophrenia patients. The results of these three studies are briefly described below.

Weinberger et al. [32] reported a significant increase in the VBR and a trend toward larger cortical and interhemispheric sulci in a group of 17 severely psychotic schizophrenia inpatients (mean age = 72 years) compared to controls. VBR and sulcal widths were measured with a planimeter in at least one CT slice. Not surprisingly, increased VBR and increased variability in VBR were also correlated with increasing age in both patients and controls.

A recent study by Corey-Bloom et al. [8], which included 14 early-onset schizophrenia patients in addition to 16 late-onset schizophrenia patients and 28 normal comparison subjects, all over the age of 45 years, used a quantitative semiautomated computerized method to determine the volumes on MR scans of several gray matter structures including the caudate nucleus, lenticular nucleus, and thalamus as well as frontal and temporal cortex. There were no significant differences between early-onset schizophrenia patients and normal comparison subjects in any of these specific brain regions, although relatively small numbers of subjects may have contributed to this negative result.

Finally, Dupont et al. examined global and regional blood flow in a SPECT study of a group of 11 middle-aged and elderly schizophrenia patients (mean age = 56.7), a majority with an early onset of the disease, i.e., onset before age 45 [6]. Global uptake of the tracer, iodoamphetamine, was significantly lower in patients than in comparison subjects. Sixteen regional areas of interest were also examined in this study, and, after correcting for average cortical uptake, three areas demonstrated significantly lower cerebral blood flow in the patients: the left posterior frontal region and both left and right anterior inferior temporal regions. These brain regions have been found in several studies of younger schizophrenia patients to have both perfusion defects as well as smaller volumes [33–36].

V. LATE-ONSET SCHIZOPHRENIA

We found 10 neuroimaging studies that had examined brain abnormalities in late-onset schizophrenia patients, although in one of these [28], late-onset patients were given the ICD-10 diagnosis of "paranoid schizophrenia," which the authors referred to as "late paraphrenia with paranoid schizophrenia" [2,4,7,8,28,37–41] (see Table 1). Five main findings emerge from these studies related to size of ventricular spaces, presence of white or gray matter lesions, volume of medial and lateral temporal cortex, volume of thalamus, and density of dopamine D_2 receptors.

A. Ventricular Size

The most widely reported and consistent neuroimaging result in late-onset schizophrenia patients was that, as in early-onset schizophrenia patients, there was an increase in size of the ventricles compared to age-comparable normal subjects. Three studies indicated a statistically significant increase in size of lateral or third ventricles in late-onset patients than in normal comparison subjects [7,8,37], one study indicated a trend toward an increase in ventricular size [39], and one study reported a nonsignificant ventricle size difference in the same direction [28]. To our knowledge, no studies reported a significant difference in the opposite direction.

Each of the studies that reported a statistically significant difference in ventricular size used quantitative methods for measuring two-dimensional or three-dimensional spaces. Rabins et al. [37] measured the VBR in 29 patients with late-onset schizophrenia diagnosed according to DSM-III [17] criteria (except that age of onset of symptoms was greater than 44 years, which in the DSM-III precluded a diagnosis of schizophrenia) and 23 controls. They chose the single 8-mm-thick CT slice in each subject's scan that contained the widest portion of the bodies of the lateral ventricles. The slice was enlarged to approximately life-size on a radiographic projector. Areas of lateral ventricles and of the region inside the inner skull margin were determined using a digitizing planimeter, and the VBR was computed. Measured in this way, the VBR was significantly larger in the late-onset schizo-phrenia patients than in the normal comparison subjects.

Pearlson et al. [7] used a similar method to determine the VBR in the MR scans of 11 late-onset patients (all of whom met the DSM-III-R criteria for late-onset schizophrenia and experienced their first positive symptoms of illness after age 55) and 18 normal comparison subjects. For each subject they chose the single 5-mm-thick T_2 axial slice in which the lateral ventricles had their maximal area. These authors also determined volumes of the third ventricles in the same scans by summing the areas of the third ventricle from two consecutive 3-mm-thick coronal slices. The volume of the third ventricle was significantly larger in the schizophrenia patients than in normal compari-son subjects. The VBR also was larger in the patients, but the difference failed to reach statistical significance. The number of patients in this study was rather small and may explain the lack of statistical significance, though the same study also looked at the VBR in patients with Alzheimer's dementia and found that the Alzheimer's patients had significantly larger VBRs than normal comparison subjects. This result serves to underscore the point that brain abnormalities in schizophrenia patients tend to be of a much more subtle nature than in other neurologically based diseases such as Alzheimer's disease.

Krull et al. [39] applied qualitative rating methods to the MR films of late-onset schizophrenia patients (DSM-III-R) and normal comparison sub-jects. The investigators rated the degree of ventricular enlargement and of white matter abnormality (reviewed below). The late-onset schizophrenia patients had a nonsignificantly greater degree of ventricular enlargement than normal controls. It is possible, however, that subjective rating methods may not be sensitive enough to pick up subtle differences in brain abnormalities. For example, in a study of late paraphrenia using a subjective rating method of ventricular enlargement, Howard et al. [23] were unable to find differences between patients and normal comparison subjects, even though two previous studies using the same set of patients found significant increases in lateral ventricular volume when the investigators measured the VBR quantitatively [20,22].

Corey-Bloom et al. [8] measured the total volume of all ventricles in 5-mm-thick axial MR slices from MR scans of 16 patients who had a DSM-III-R diagnosis of late-onset schizophrenia and 28 normal comparison sub-jects. The mean age of the patients in this study was just over 59 years, and all patients experienced their first prodromal symptoms after the age of 45. Volume of ventricles was determined by summing the areas of ventricular spaces in all slices throughout the brain. The ventricular volume of the late-onset schizophrenia patient group was significantly larger than in the compar-ison group.

The only quantitative study that has failed to show statistically significant or trend differences in ventricle size between late-onset schizophrenia patients and normal comparison subjects is that by Howard et al. [28]. These authors computed the volumes of the third and lateral ventricles by summing pixel areas of all 27 5-mm-thick MR slices of the scans of 47 late paraphrenia patients, 31 of whom met ICD-10 criteria for paranoid schizophrenia. The other 16 met ICD-10 criteria for delusional disorder. Although late-onset schizophrenia patients had larger ventricular volumes than normal comparison subjects, they were at best marginally larger. One possible explanation for the difference between the findings of this study and the others cited above may be that Howard et al.'s patients included only the paranoid schizophrenia subtype, whereas the other four studies most likely included other schizophrenia subtypes in their patient groups. In addition, Howard et al.'s patients were both significantly older (mean age = 78.1 years) and had a later age of disease onset (mean = 72.4 years). It can be more difficult to reveal differences between patient groups and comparison groups as they age because the variability of the measured areas and volumes tends to increase with age. An interesting finding emerged from the Howard et al. study: whereas the schizophrenia patients did not have significantly larger ventricles than normal comparison subjects, the delusional disorder patients *did* have markedly larger ventricular volumes. This suggests that late-onset delusional disorder and late-onset schizophrenia may be associated with different brain pathology, a subject discussed later.

B. Gray or White Matter Lesions

The second finding that emerged from the neuroimaging literature on late-onset schizophrenia related to the presence of brain lesions. In two separate case report studies, Miller et al. [2,4] described a total of 10 patients, all of whom were brought to the psychiatric hospital with prominent delusions or symptoms similar to those of schizophrenia. Possibly some of these patients might have been diagnosed with late-onset schizophrenia by DSM-III-R [18] criteria. In 9 of the 10 patients, CT scans revealed significant structural brain pathology, primarily white matter lucencies. Based upon the first 5 patients [2], the authors offered the etiological interpretation that the "organic disorders altered previously functioning monitoring systems, allowing development of a fixed delusion." The second series of 5 patients [4] were specifically selected from a group of 27 patients because their CT scans had particularly large white matter lesions. All lesions were large, confluent, and in subfrontal white matter regions.

A separate study by Breitner et al. [38] examined the MR scans of eight patients diagnosed with late-onset schizophrenia according to DSM-III-R

[18] criteria (although on follow-up, one of the patients appeared to have a dementing disease) and compared them to eight normal subjects of similar age. The average age of the patients was 76.9 years and that of controls was 71.1 years; the age of onset of symptoms in the patients ranged from approximately 60 to 80 years. Scans were qualitatively rated using the method of Fazekas et al. [29] for describing cerebral atrophy, based on the appearance of ventricles and sulci, white matter lesions not including lacunes, hemorrhages, and infarcts, which were rated separately. All of the patients and none of the controls had at least one white matter lesion larger than 10 mm in diameter in temporoparietal or occipital regions. In addition, seven of the eight patients, but none of the controls, had small lesions in the gray matter of pons or basal ganglia. These three papers suggest that large white matter lesions may be associated with the development of psychotic symptoms.

We have taken a somewhat different approach to the study of brain lesions in psychosis. We compared groups of patients to normal comparison subjects and selected their study groups on the basis of psychiatric diagnosis rather than the presence of white matter lesions [39,40].

In the initial study, Krull et al. [39] used subjective qualitative ratings of MR scans of nine late-onset schizophrenia patients and nine normal comparison subjects. There were no significant differences between schizophrenia patients and normal subjects in scores for the degree of abnormal white matter hyperintensities, though the late-onset group did show a nonsignificant trend for large ventricles (reviewed above). Recently, Symonds et al. [40] reviewed the MRI reports of 24 late-onset schizophrenia patients as well as 30 early-onset schizophrenia and 15 other psychosis patients (including nine from the earlier study by Krull et al. [39]), all diagnosed using DSM-III-R criteria, and 41 normal comparison subjects (including nine from the study by Krull et al. [39]). A qualitative rating scheme was employed to determine the frequency, type, and severity of several measures of abnormality, including infarcts, lacunae, and white matter hyperintensities. The vast majority of the MRIs were reported to be within normal limits, and there were no significant differences either between psychosis patients and normal comparison subjects or between early-onset and late-onset schizophrenia patients in terms of frequency, type, or severity of the structural abnormalities. The authors concluded that late-onset schizophrenia could exist without clinically significant structural abnormalities in the brain and that, in this respect, it was similar to early-onset schizophrenia.

C. Temporal Lobe Volume

The literature on young, early-onset schizophrenia patients contains studies reporting that early-onset schizophrenia is associated with smaller volumes of medial and/or lateral areas of the temporal lobe than in normal healthy individuals [35,42–44]. Barta et al. [41] sought to investigate whether the same differences would also be found in schizophrenia patients with a later age of onset. These investigators identified temporal lobe regions of interest on MRI films of 11 late-onset schizophrenia patients, 12 Alzheimer's disease patients, and 18 healthy age-comparable subjects. Superior temporal gyrus, amygdala, entorhinal cortex, and hippocampus as well as whole temporal lobes were interactively outlined on a graphics workstation, and the areas were summed across contiguous images to arrive at volume estimates for the various regions. Four of the six regions were significantly smaller in late-onset schizophrenia patients than in normal comparison subjects: entorhinal cortex, amygdala, hippocampus, and superior temporal gyrus. Interestingly, all of these regions were also smaller in Alzheimer's disease patients except for the superior temporal gyrus, thus showing some possible specificity of brain abnormality in schizophrenia.

D. Thalamic Volume

The thalamus has only recently entered the arena of interest in neuroimaging studies in schizophrenia, and there are now a few reports that the thalamus is smaller in schizophrenia patients with an early onset of the disease [45,46]. Corey-Bloom et al. [8] investigated whether the thalamus is similarly affected in late-onset schizophrenia patients. These authors used quantitative volume estimates of several brain regions in 16 late-onset and 14 early-onset schizophrenia patients in addition to 28 age-comparable healthy controls. The investigators discovered that the thalamus in late-onset patients was significantly larger than that in early-onset schizophrenia patients and that the volumes in the normal comparison subjects were intermediate between the early- and late-onset patient groups. It will be interesting to see if the difference in the volume of the thalamus between normal comparison subjects and late-onset schizophrenia patients is indeed statistically significant in studies with larger sample sizes. The possibility that long-term neuroleptic treatment contributes to structural brain changes also needs to be ruled out. The pathophysiological significance of larger brain nuclei is not clear. There are, however, a few other reports in the psychiatric neuroimaging literature of younger patients with larger, rather than smaller, brain regions. For example, Jernigan et al. [47] found that the lenticular nuclei were significantly larger in early-onset schizophrenia patients compared to normal subjects. Dupont et al. [48] reported that the thalamus was significantly larger in bipolar patients compared to unipolar patients and that the volumes of the normal comparison subjects were intermediate and significantly different from both patient groups.

E. Dopamine D$_2$ Receptor Density

A hotly debated issue in the current literature is whether the brains of schizophrenia patients differ from healthy individuals in the densities of dopamine receptors that bind typical neuroleptics such as haloperidol. Several groups, using PET techniques, found differences between groups of younger schizophrenia patients and age-comparable controls; schizophrenia patients displayed greater density of dopamine D$_2$ receptor, especially in the caudate nucleus [49,50]. Other groups, however, observed no such differences [51].

Pearlson et al. [7] investigated D$_2$ receptor density in a group of 13 late-onset schizophrenia patients (mean age = 74 years), all neuroleptic-naive, and 17 healthy controls (mean age = 39 years). After a CT localization scan, two PET scans were obtained, the second scan 4 hours after administration of unlabeled oral haloperidol, to reveal binding under conditions of virtually completely blocked dopamine D$_2$ receptors. After attempting to account for age and gender differences in dopamine receptor densities by using a two-variable regression equation to yield standardized residual values, the investigators found a modest but statistically significant (using a one-tailed t-test) increase in the density of D$_2$ receptor density in the caudate nucleus. The authors cautiously concluded that late-onset schizophrenia patients had elevated dopamine receptor density in their caudate nuclei and that they were similar to early-onset patients in this regard.

Taken together, the results from the neuroimaging studies of late-onset schizophrenia indicate that the late-onset patients have several of the same brain abnormalities reported in early-onset schizophrenia. Neuroimaging similarities between early-onset and late-onset schizophrenia include a tendency to have larger ventricles than healthy normal individuals and smaller regions of temporal lobe, as well as increased density of dopamine D$_2$ receptors in the caudate nucleus. There are also indications of possible differences (e.g., larger thalamus in late-onset schizophrenia) between those patients who are afflicted earlier in life compared to those who do not show obvious signs of the disease until middle age of later. Many other regions that have been reported to be abnormal in volume or activity (i.e., blood flow or glucose utilization) in younger schizophrenia patients have not yet been investigated in late-onset patients. Neuroimaging studies of normal aging have indicated that almost all measures of regional brain volume and activity show markedly increased variability among older compared to younger individuals [52]. This increased variability in sizes of structures renders it more difficult to demonstrate a significant difference, if one exists, between late-onset schizophrenia patients and similarly aged normal comparison subjects. Studies that include both large sample sizes and more refined measurement techniques should help sort out the relative contributions of aging and psychosis in the brains of late-onset psychosis patients.

The extent to which early-onset and late-onset schizophrenia are separate clinical entities is relevant to the current controversy regarding the role of brain lesions in the etiology of schizophrenia. Several groups have suggested that gray and white matter lesions seen on CT or MR scans of late-onset psychosis patients are the cause of the psychosis symptoms. For example, Miller and colleagues have documented many cases where this appears to be the case [2,4], indicating that late-onset psychosis can occur as a result of insults to the brain, which are typically more common later in life. It appears, however, that late-onset schizophrenia can occur in the absence of such brain insults [40]. The role that brain lesions, particularly white matter abnormalities, play in the pathophysiology of various neurological disorders is at present not clear, and it will be important to learn how brain lesions contribute to the development of late-onset schizophrenia.

VI. LATE-ONSET DELUSIONAL DISORDER

Three separate studies used neuroimaging techniques to investigate structural abnormalities in the brains of patents diagnosed with late-onset delusional disorder [4,28,31]. The two major findings to emerge from these CT and MRI studies were related to size of ventricles and white matter lesions. Two studies that compared the abnormalities in delusional disorder patients to those in patients with either paraphrenia [31] or late-onset schizophrenia [28] found these abnormalities to be more pronounced in delusional disorder patients.

A. Ventricular Size

A study by Howard et al. [28], which was described in the earlier section on late-onset schizophrenia, compared quantitative volume measurements of whole brain, extracerebral CSF spaces, and third and lateral ventricles in 31 late-onset schizophrenia patients, 16 late-onset delusional disorder patients, and 33 normal comparison subjects. When the two patient subgroups were compared to the normal comparison group, only delusional disorder patients had significantly larger ventricle sizes. The extent to which these results are due to diagnosis, however, is not clear; the delusional patients were significantly older than either late-onset schizophrenia patients or normal comparison subjects (83 vs. 78 and 79 years, respectively, $p = 0.047$) and had nonsignificantly later age of onset of illness (76 vs. 72 years, $p = 0.114$) and lower Mini-Mental State Examination [53] scores than schizophrenia patients (27.5 vs. 28.6, $p = 0.071$), all of which would be expected to be associated with cortical atrophy and enlarged ventricles.

B. Gray or White Matter Lesions

In a case study of five late-onset psychosis patents selected because of large white matter lesions visible on CT scans, Miller et al. [4] noted that three of the patients were diagnosed with late-onset delusional disorder (range of onset about 60–80 years). All three of these patients, as well as the remaining two (one late-onset schizophrenia, one late-onset mania) had large subfrontal lesions of deep white matter, and two patients, both with delusional disorder, also had infarcts in the basal ganglia.

Flint et al. [31] set out to examine how the diagnosis of delusional disorder with onset after age 60 might differ from that of paraphrenia. Within the context of a larger study, they were able to obtain CT brain scans on a subset of their patients diagnosed using ICD-9 or ICD-10 criteria. Twelve of the 16 patients had a diagnosis of paraphrenia (i.e., they had delusions without hallucinations), and four patients had a diagnosis of paranoia (delusional disorder). The narratives of the neuroradiologists' CT reports were examined for mention of "silent (clinically unsuspected) cerebral infarction." Five of the 16 patients had such infarcts, primarily located in the basal ganglia or frontal lobe. Of these five patients, four were delusional disorder patients. In other words, all of the delusional disorder patients compared to only one of the paraphrenia patients had evidence of silent infarction.

The available neuroimaging evidence in late-onset delusional disorder, then, suggests that patients who carry this diagnosis may have enlarged ventricles, a structural abnormality they share with late-onset schizophrenia. In addition, there is some evidence that late-onset delusional patients tend to have gray and white matter lesions in deep white matter and basal ganglia.

VII. LATE-ONSET MANIA

There were at least two neuroimaging investigations of brain abnormalities associated with the psychiatric diagnosis of late-onset mania. Mania tends to appear later in life than the other psychoses already discussed, and early-onset mania is often considered to have an onset before the age of 50 (or even 60; see Broadhead and Jacoby [54], while late-onset mania denotes onset after the age of 50 or 60. Three separate papers reported structural abnormalities associated with late-onset mania; one of the papers specifically compared late-onset to early-onset mania [54]. A second paper compared late-onset mania to both late-onset major depression and early-onset major depression [55]. The third paper consisted of a single case report and has been discussed previously [4]. The abnormalities focused on in these papers were, as in other investigations, ventricular size, cortical atrophy, and gray/white matter lesions.

A. Size of Ventricles and Cortical Atrophy

Broadhead and Jacoby [54] obtained CT scans on a group of 35 manic patients over the age of 60 and 20 age-comparable normal subjects. They rated on a four-point scale the degree of cortical atrophy of the four individual lobes of the brain and also determined the VBR of lateral ventricles as well as areas of the Sylvian and interhemispheric fissures. The patients had a range of onset of illness, both early (before age 60) and late (after age 60). Mania was diagnosed according to Feighner's diagnostic criteria (56) except that Broadhead and Jacoby did not exclude patients who had evidence of contributing organic factors, because they were interested in determining the relationship of organic factors to the development of mania later in life. VBR was not different between the mania group and the control group. On ratings of cortical atrophy, however, the elderly mania group (including both late-onset and early-onset patients) had significantly more cortical atrophy than did the normal comparison subjects. Early-onset and late-onset patents did not differ from each other in either VBR or cortical atrophy.

B. Gray or White Matter Lesions

A recent study by Fujikawa et al. [55] compared three similarly aged groups of patients: late-onset mania (onset after 50, mean = 58.0), early-onset affective disorder (onset before age 50, mean = 38.1; half of them bipolar, and the other half major depression), and late-onset major depression (onset after 50, mean = 58.1). These authors were particularly interested to know if silent infarctions of gray or white matter could have contributed to the etiology of the psychosis or affective disorder. There were two major findings of this study. First, the late-onset mania patient group had significantly more silent infarctions (65%) than the early-onset affective disorder patient group (25%), but not statistically more than the late-onset major depression group (55%). The two late-onset groups were significantly different from each other, however, in the type of infarction; one-half of the late-onset mania group had more severe "mixed" types of infarcts, i.e., both perforating gray and white matter lesions. The authors suggested, therefore, that approximately half of the cases of late-onset mania and late-onset major depression might be secondary to silent cerebral infarctions and, furthermore, that the specific types of infarctions characteristic of late-onset mania were more widespread and severe. Neuroimaging results suggested to these authors, then, that late-onset mania was a more serious form of affective illness than major depression.

VIII. SUMMARY

Beginning in the 1980s when modern neuroimaging techniques became readily available, the initial studies sought to determine if there were brain abnormalities associated with late-life psychosis, and particularly with a later onset of illness. Such studies made clear that it was possible for patients to develop psychosis in association with structural brain abnormalities such as multiple infarctions or large, confluent white matter lesions. This finding was in contrast to what was known about the majority of early-onset psychosis patients who developed their psychotic symptoms in the absence of obvious structural abnormalities. In the past several years investigators have attempted to discover if such lesions are necessary to cause psychosis. To answer this question, investigators have made attempts to carefully define diagnosis of subjects, to make explicit the inclusion and exclusion criteria, and, more recently, to make use of more refined quantitative analysis techniques.

So far, most of these studies have dealt with either the size of CSF-filled spaces, particularly the lateral ventricles, as an indicator of cerebral atrophy or with the presence of gray or white matter lesions in CT or MR scans. There is evidence that some, but not all, types of late-onset psychoses are associated with increased size in ventricles and changes in white matter. Lesions of gray matter structures or of deep white matter have also been reported in patients with late-onset psychoses. Finally, there are a few reports of other abnormalities associated with late-onset schizophrenia, including smaller anterior superior temporal gyrus, increased D_2 receptor density in the caudate, and increased size of thalamus. The first two findings parallel those of younger early-onset schizophrenia patents, whereas an increased size in thalamus is in contrast to what has been found so far for younger schizophrenia patients.

The published literature in this area is limited by small sample sizes. Larger and well-controlled studies including longitudinal investigations are warranted. Further studies will be very helpful in determining which of the many structural and functional abnormalities found in neuroimaging experiments with younger schizophrenia patients are also found in late-onset patients and if the areas in which the results diverge can be related to the clinical differences between them.

This work is supported in part by the National Institute of Mental Health grants #5 P30 MH49671, #5 R37 MH43693, #5 P30 MH49671-01S1, and by the Department of Veterans Affairs.

REFERENCES

1. M. Bleuler, Late schizophrenic clinical pictures, *Fortschr. Neurol. Psychiatry* 15:259 (1943).
2. B. L. Miller, F. D. Benson, J. L. Cummings, and R. Neshkes, Late-life paraphrenia: an organic delusional system, *J. Clin. Psychiatry* 47:204 (1986).

3. B. L. Miller and I. M. Lesser, Late-life psychosis and modern neuroimaging, *Psychiatr. Clin. North Am. 11*:33 (1988).

4. B. L. Miller, I. M. Lesser, K. Boone, M. Goldberg, E. Hill, M. H. Miller, D. F. Benson, and M. Mehringer, Brain white-matter lesions and psychosis, *Br. J. Psychiatry 155*:73 (1989).

5. B. L. Miller, I. M. Lesser, K. B. Boone, E. Hill, C. M. Mehringer, and K. Wong, Brain lesions and cognitive function in late-life psychosis. *Br. J. Psychiatry 158*: 76 (1991).

6. R. M. Dupont, P. Lehr, G. Lamoureaux, S. Halpern, M. J. Harris, and D. V. Jeste, Preliminary report: cerebral blood flow abnormalities in older schizophrenic patients, *Psychiatry Res. 55*:121 (1994).

7. G. D. Pearlson, L. E. Tune, D. F. Wong, E. H. Aylward, P. E. Barta, R. E. Powers, G. A. Chase, G. J. Harris, and P. V. Rabins, Quantitative D2 dopamine receptor PET and structural MRI changes in late onset schizophrenia, *Schizophr. Bull. 19*:783 (1993).

8. J. Corey-Bloom, T. Jernigan, S. Archibald, M. J. Harris, and D. V. Jeste, Quantitative magnetic resonance imaging in late-life schizophrenia, *Am. J. Psychiatry 152*:447 (1995).

9. M. J. Harris and D. V. Jeste, Late-onset schizophrenia: an overview. *Schizophr. Bull. 14*:39 (1988).

10. A. Riecher-Rossler, W. Rossler, H. Foerstl, and U. Meise, Late-onset schizophrenia and late paraphrenia, *Schizophr. Bull. 21*:345 (1995).

11. E. Kraepelin, On paranoid diseases (in German), *Z. Gesamte Neurol. Psychiatr. 11*:617 (1919).

12. E. Kraepelin, *Dementia Praecox and Paraphrenia* (R. M. Barclay, trans.), Krieger, Huntington, NY, 1971.

13. W. Mayer, On paraphrenic psychoses (in German), *Z. Gesamte Neurol. Psychiatr. 71*:187 (1921).

14. M. Roth, The natural history of mental disorder in old age, *J. Mental Sci. 101*: 281 (1955).

15. D. W. K. Kay and M. Roth, Environmental and hereditary factors in the schizophrenias of old age ("late paraphrenia") and their bearing on the general problem of causation in schizophrenia, *J. Mental Sci. 107*:649 (1961).

16. World Health Organization, *Mental Disorders: Glossary and Guide to Their Classification in Accordance with the Ninth Revision of the International Classification of Diseases*, World Health Organization, Geneva, 1978.

17. American Psychiatric Association, *Diagnostic and Statistical Manual of Mental Disorders*, American Psychiatric Press, Washington, DC, 1980.

18. American Psychiatric Association, *Diagnostic and Statistical Manual of Mental Disorders*, 3rd ed. rev., American Psychiatric Press, Washington, DC, 1987.

19. American Psychiatric Association, *Diagnostic and Statistical Manual of Mental Disorders*, 4th ed., American Psychiatric Association, Washington, DC, 1994.

20. M. Naguib and R. Levy, Late paraphrenia: neuropsychological impairment and structural brain abnormalities on computed tomography, *Int. J. Geriatr. Psychiatry 2*:83 (1987).

21. N. Hymas, M. Naguib, and R. Levy, Late paraphrenia—a follow-up study, *Int. J. Geriatr. Psychiatry 4*:23 (1989).

22. A. Burns, J. Carrick, D. Ames, M. Naguib, and R. Levy, The cerebral cortical appearance in late paraphrenia, *Int. J. Geriatr. Psychiatry 4*:31 (1989).

23. R. J. Howard, H. Forstl, O. Almeida, A. Burns, and R. Levy, Computer-assisted CT measurements in late paraphrenics with and without Schneiderian first-rank symptoms: a preliminary report, *Int. J. Geriatr. Psychiatry 7*:35 (1992).

24. G. D. Pearlson, D. Garbacz, H. O. Ahn, and P. V. Rabins, Lateral cerebral ventricular size in late onset schizophrenia, *Schizophrenia and Aging* (N. E. Miller, et al., eds.), Guilford Press, New York, 1987, pp. 246–248.

25. H. Foerstl, P. Dalgalarrondo, A. Reicher-Roessler, M. Lotz, C. Geiger-Kabisch, and F. Hentschel, Organic factors and the clinical features of late paranoid psychosis: a comparison with Alzheimer's disease and normal aging, *Acta Psychiatr. Scand. 89*:335 (1994).

26. I. M. Lesser, B. L. Miller, J. R. Swartz, K. B. Boone, C. M. Mehringer, and I. Mena, Brain imaging in late-life schizophrenia and related psychoses, *Schizophr. Bull. 19*:773 (1993).

27. R. Howard, T. Cox, O. Almeida, R. Mullen, P. Graves, A. Reveley, and R. Levy, White matter signal hyperintensities in the brains of patients with late paraphrenia and the normal community-living elderly, *Biol. Psychiatry 38*:86 (1995).

28. R. J. Howard, O. Almeida, R. Levy, P. Graves, and M. Graves, Quantitative magnetic resonance imaging volumetry distinguishes delusional disorder from late-onset schizophrenia, *Br. J. Psychiatry 165*:474 (1994).

29. F. Fazekas, J. B. Chawluck, A. Alavi, H. I. Hurtig, and R. Zimmerman, MR signal abnormalities at 1.5T in Alzheimer's dementia and normal aging, *AJNR 8*:421 (1987).

30. C. E. Coffey, G. S. Figiel, W. T. Djang, and R. D. Weiner, Subcortical hyperintensity on magnetic resonance imaging: a comparison of normal and depressed elderly subjects, *Am. J. Psychiatry 47*:187 (1990).

31. A. J. Flint, S. I. Rifat, and M. R. Eastwood, Late-onset paranoia: distinct from paraphrenia?, *Int. J. Geriatr. Psychiatry 6*:103 (1991).

32. D. R. Weinberger, D. V. Jeste, R. J. Wyatt, and P. F. Teychenne, Cerebral atrophy in elderly schizophrenic patients: effects of aging and of long-term institutionalization and neuroleptic therapy, *Schizophrenia and Aging: Schizophrenia, Paranoid and Schizophreniform Disorders in Later Life* (N. E. Miller et al., eds.), Guilford Press, New York, 1987, pp. 109–118.

33. K. F. Berman, E. F. Torrey, D. G. Daniel, and D. R. Weinberger, Regional cerebral blood flow in monozygotic twins discordant and concordant for schizophrenia, *Arch. Gen. Psychiatry 49*:927 (1992).

34. E. Gordon, R. J. Barry, J. Anderson, R. Fawdry, C. Yong, S. Grunewald, and R. A. Meares, Single photon emission computed tomography (SPECT) measures of brain function in schizophrenia, *Aust. NZ J. Psychiatry 28*:446 (1994).

35. T. E. Schlaepfer, G. J. Harris, A. Y. Tien, L. W. Peng, S. Lee, E. B. Federman,

G. A. Chase, P. E. Barta, and G. D. Pearlson, Decreased regional cortical gray matter volume in schizophrenia, *Am. J. Psychiatry 151*:842 (1994).

36. J. Schroeder, M. S. Buchsbaum, B. V. Siegel, F. J. Geider, R. J. Haier, J. Lohr, J. Wu, and S. G. Potkin, Patterns of cortical activity in schizophrenia, *Psychol. Med. 24*:947 (1994).

37. P. Rabins, G. Pearlson, G. Jayaram, C. Steele, and L. Tune, Increased ventricle-to-brain ratio in late-onset schizophrenia, *Am. J. Psychiatry 144*:1216 (1987).

38. J. Breitner, M. Husain, G. Figiel, K. Krishnan, and O. Boyko, Cerebral white matter disease in late-onset psychosis, *Biol. Psychiatry 28*:266 (1990).

39. A. J. Krull, G. Press, R. Dupont, M. J. Harris, and D. V. Jeste, Brain imaging in late-onset schizophrenia and related psychoses, *Int. J. Geriatr. Psychiatry 6*:651 (1991).

40. L. L. Symonds, J. M. Olichney, T. L. Jernigan, J. Corey-Bloom, J. F. Healy, and D. V. Jeste, Lack of clinically significant gross structural abnormalities in MRIs of older patients with schizophrenia and related psychoses (in press).

41. G. D. Pearlson, R. Powers, P. E. Barta, E. H. Aylward, P. V. Rabins, L. D. Raimundo, G. A. Chase, and L. E. Tune, MRI volume in late-life onset schizophrenia, New Research Program and Abstracts, *Amer. Psychiatr. Assoc.* p. 164 (1991).

42. M. E. Shenton, R. Kikinis, F. A. Jolesz, S. D. Pollak, M. LeMay, C. Wible, H. Hokama, J. Martin, D. Metcalf, M. Coleman, and R. W. McCarley, Abnormalities of the left temporal lobe and thought disorder in schizophrenia: a quantitative magnetic resonance imaging study, *N. Engl. J. Med. 327*:604 (1992).

43. B. Bogerts, J. A. Lieberman, M. Ashtari, R. M. Bilder, G. Degreef, G. Lerner, C. Johns, and S. Masiar, Hippocampus-amygdala volumes and psychopathology in chronic schizophrenia, *Biol. Psychiatry 33*:236 (1993).

44. M. Flaum, V. W. Swayze, D. S. O'Leary, W. T. C. Yuh, J. C. Ehrhardt, S. V. Arndt, and N. C. Andreasen, Effects of diagnosis, laterality, and gender on brain morphology in schizophrenia, *Am. J. Psychiatry 152*:704 (1995).

45. N. C. Andreasen, J. C. Ehrhardt, V. W. Swayze, R. J. Alliger, W. T. C. Yuh, G. Cohen, and S. Ziebell, Magnetic resonance imaging of the brain in schizophrenia, *Arch. Gen. Psychiatry 47*:35 (1990).

46. N. C. Andreasen, L. Flashman, M. Flaum, S. Arndt, V. W. Swayze, D. S. O'Leary, J. C. Ehrhardt, and W. T. C. Yuh, Regional brain abnormalities in schizophrenia measured with magnetic resonance imaging, *JAMA 272*:1763 (1994).

47. T. L. Jernigan, S. Zisook, R. K. Heaton, J. T. Moranville, J. R. Hesselink, and D. L. Braff, Magnetic resonance imaging abnormalities in lenticular nuclei and cerebral cortex in schizophrenia, *Arch. Gen. Psychiatry 48*:881 (1991).

48. R. M. Dupont, T. L. Jernigan, W. Heindel, N. Butters, K. Shafer, T. Wilson, J. Hesselink, and J. C. Gillin, Magnetic resonance imaging and mood disorders. Localization of white matter and other subcortical abnormalities, *Arch. Gen. Psychiatry 52*:747 (1995).

49. D. Wong, H. Wagner, and L. Tune, Positron emission tomography reveals elevated D2 dopamine receptors in drug-naive schizophrenic patients, *Science 234*:1558 (1986).

50. L. E. Tune, D. F. Wong, G. Pearlson, M. Strauss, T. Young, E. K. Shaya, R. F. Dannals, A. A. Wilson, H. T. Ravert, J. Sapp, T. Cooper, G. A. Chase, and H. N. Wagner, Dopamine D2 receptor density estimates in schizophrenia: a positron emission tomography study with 11C-N-methylspiperone, *Psychiatry Res. 49*:219 (1993).

51. L. Farde, F. Wiesel, and S. Stone-Elander, D2 dopamine receptors in neuroleptic-naive schizophrenic patients: a positron emission tomography study with [11C] raclopride, *Arch. Gen. Psychiatry 47*:213 (1990).

52. T. L. Jernigan, G. A. Press, and J. R. Hesselink, Methods for measuring brain morphologic features on magnetic resonance images: validation and normal aging, *Arch. Neurol. 47*:27 (1990).

53. M. F. Folstein, S. E. Folstein, and P. R. McHugh, Mini-Mental State: a practical method for grading the cognitive state of patients for the clinician. *J. Psychiatr. Res. 12*:189 (1975).

54. J. Broadhead and R. Jacoby, Mania in old age: a first prospective study, *Int. J. Geriatr. Psychiatry 5*:215 (1990).

55. T. Fujikawa, S. Yamawaki, and Y. Touhouda, Silent cerebral infarctions in patients with late-onset mania, *Stroke 26*:946 (1995).

56. J. P. Feighner, E. Robins, S. B. Guze, R. A. Woodruff, G. Winokur, and R. Munoz, Diagnostic criteria for use in psychiatric research, *Arch. Gen. Psychiatry 26*:57 (1972).

57. I. M. Lesser, D. V. Jeste, K. B. Boone, M. J. Harris, B. L. Miller, R. K. Heaton, and E. Hill-Gutierrez, Late-onset psychotic disorder, not otherwise specified: clinical and neuroimaging findings, *Biol. Psychiatry 31*:419 (1992).

16

Brain Imaging in Phobic Disorders

**Nicholas L. S. Potts, John Travers, and
Jonathan R. T. Davidson**
Duke University Medical Center, Durham, North Carolina

I. INTRODUCTION

The introduction of DSM-III in 1980 along with the advent of modern imaging techniques stimulated researchers to begin to directly examine in vivo how individuals with specific anxiety disorders might be neurobiologically different from the general population. This led to a number of studies examining patients using a variety of brain imaging techniques, from computerized axial tomography (CT), magnetic resonance imaging (MRI), and magnetic resonance spectroscopy (MRS) to positron emission tomography (PET) and single photon emission tomography (SPECT). These studies have been performed in both asymptomatic states and in response to certain visual or chemical challenges. This work in general, although relatively new and limited in quantity, appears to support the concept that these disorders are separate and biologically distinct from each other as well as the general population.

Anxiety disorders make up the largest percentage of psychiatric disorders seen in the United States. In the recent National Comorbidity Study (NCS), almost 25% of respondents met criteria for at least one anxiety disorder during their lifetime, with 17% of the population meeting criteria for such a disorder within the previous 12 months [1]. Long-term studies have revealed that these disorders are associated with marked social and occupational impairment. Anxiety disorders have a number of consequences that highlight their devastating impact. They are often chronic disorders and cause progressive restriction and impairment in functioning. One study [2] found that patients with panic disorder or social phobia have lifetime suicide attempt rates of 18% and 12%, respectively. Davidson et al. [3] found that depression was 10 times more likely to occur in subjects with posttraumatic stress disorder (PTSD) compared to non-PTSD subjects and that subjects with PTSD were more than 8 times more likely to attempt suicide, even after controlling for comorbid depression. Anxiety disorders are associated with high comorbidity of other psychiatric disorders, mainly substance abuse, depression, and other anxiety disorders [1]. Because of their high prevalence, chronicity, and impairment, it has become clear that we need to better understand the cause of these disorders and how to treat them. This chapter will discuss the findings of brain imaging studies in anxiety disorders [except for obsessive-compulsive disorder (OCD), reviewed in a previous chapter by Book et al.]. Each sections reviewing a separate disorder, is divided into structural studies (CT and MRI) followed by functional imaging studies (MRS, PET, and SPECT).

II. PANIC DISORDER

Based on neuroimaging studies, panic disorder (except for OCD) is the most widely investigated anxiety disorder. Numerous studies have been conducted over the last two decades demonstrating physiological abnormalities in people suffering from panic disorder with or without the presence of agoraphobia. However, these abnormalities do not point to one specific neurotransmitter system in the brain; rather they have implicated all the major systems, i.e., noradrenaline, serotonin, dopamine, gamma-aminobutyric acid (GABA), and more recently cholecystokinin [4].

The initial neuroimaging study in panic disorder was performed by Uhde and Kellner [5]. This study compared the mean ventricular-brain ratio (VBR) of 25 patients with panic disorder to those of previously published normal controls. Patients over 50 and those with histories of alcohol or drug abuse, significant weight loss or gain, and suspected neurological disorders were excluded. Patients with a prior history of benzodiazepine use were, however, included. No difference in mean VBR was found between panic disorder patients and controls. There was a significant association between VBR and duration of prior benzodiazepine use and percentage treated with benzodiazepines, although the mean VBR of panic patients who had received prior benzodiazepine treatment was not significantly different from patients with no previous benzodiazepine exposure. This finding is consistent with a previous study, which demonstrated increased ventricular enlargement in high-dose benzodiazepine users compared to normal controls or low-dose benzodiazepine users [6]. A second CT study was performed by Lepola et al [7], which had a slightly larger sample size but did not study VBR compared to normal controls. In this study CT scans were not compared to normal controls. The aim of this study was to determine the prevalence of neuroimaging abnormalities in patients with panic disorder. Of the 30 patients scanned, 20% (6/30) had some type of detectable abnormality. Three patients had mild cerebral atrophy, two had small lacunar infarctions, and one had enlarged lateral ventricles. This study was very limited in its focus of analysis, and consequently few conclusions can be drawn. It does replicate the previous finding by Uhde and Kellner [5].

Another group of studies used MRI to detect neurological abnormalities. The first, by Ontiveros et al [8], compared brain MRI images in 30 right-handed patients with proven lactate-sensitive panic disorder to those in 30 right-handed age- and sex-matched normal controls. Scans were rated on a scale from 0 to 4, with 0 being normal and 4 being severely abnormal. All scans were rated by three separate radiologists blind to the diagnosis. The MRI scans of 43% panic disorder patients were rated abnormal compared to 10% of normal controls. The most common feature seen in this panic disorder group was right-sided temporal lobe abnormalities. The most common of these findings was an abnormal signal intensity in the temporal lobe region, mainly signal intensity abnormalities. These abnormal temporal lobe scans were associated with patients who had earlier age of onset of symptoms, current symptom severity, and greater duration of illness. Another study, by Fontaine et al. [9], replicated these results. This study compared MRI scans on 31 patients with panic disorder to 20 age- and sex-matched controls. All patients and subjects were right-handed. As in the Ontiveros study, Fontaine found right temporal lobe abnormalities in 40% of panic patients compared to 10% of normal controls. The main abnormalities seen were abnormal signal activity and asymmetrical atrophy of the temporal lobes, mostly involving the right side.

There have been more functional than structural studies of panic disorder. These include MRS, PET, and SPECT studies. Besides the two MRI studies, there has been one MRS study in panic disorder. The purpose of this study was to evaluate the effects of hyperventilation on brain lactate levels in patients with panic disorder compared to normal controls [10]. Seven panic patients and seven matched controls had baseline brain lactate levels measured using MRS, followed by 20 minutes of sustained hyperventilation. Repeat measurements of brain lactate using MRS revealed a greater increase in brain lactate levels in the panic disorder patients compared to the normal controls, despite similar serum lactate levels in both groups. This increase in brain lactate levels in the panic disorder group may reflect a greater decrease in cerebral blood flow (CBF) due to hypocapnia. This greater decrease in CBF may be secondary to increased sensitivity and reactivity to hypocapnia in people with panic disorder.

The next group of neuroimaging studies of panic disorder are those using PET. Four of the five studies of panic disorder using PET were performed by Reiman et al. [11–14]. The first of these compared resting CBF in panic patients with lactate-sensitive panic disorder, panic patients with lactate-nonsensitive panic disorder, and normal controls. The first study found that patients with lactate-sensitive panic disorder had significant asymmetry of CBF (left < right) located in the region of the parahippocampal gyrus [11]. The next three studies by Reiman et al. [12–14] confirmed the initial findings. It was also found [12–14] that lactate-sensitive panic patients had significant asymmetry of the parahippocampal blood flow (left < right), blood volume (left < right), and oxygenation (left < right) compared with lactate-nonsensitive patients and normal controls. Overall, lactate-sensitive panic patients also demonstrated higher whole brain metabolic activity and an abnormal susceptibility to hyperventilation, as indicated by their mild respiratory alkalosis during the resting scans. This latter finding is consistent with the findings of Dager et al. [10] that lactate-sensitive panic disorder patients may have a resting decrease in cerebral blood flow due to hypocapnia and that people with panic disorder may have an increased sensitivity to this regulatory mechanism. In 1990, Nordahl et al. [15] attempted to replicate the studies of Reiman et al. [12–14]. While confirming asymmetrical hippocampal activity (left < right) in panic patients compared to normal controls, they did not discover global differences between panic patients and normal controls. This inability to replicate the Reiman et al.'s findings may be explained by Nordahl's subject population. In this study, patients did not have to have proven lactate-sensitive panic disorder, thus the panic patient population may not be comparable.

The last group of studies used SPECT imaging in panic disorder patients. The first SPECT study, performed by Stewart et al. [16], compared 10 patients with panic disorder with or without agoraphobia to 5 normal controls. Using inhaled xenon-133 as the isotope, regional CBF was determined in both panic patients and normal controls after a saline infusion and after a lactate infusion. No resting measure was obtained after it was determined in the first three patients that baseline SPECT results were not different from saline infusion results. This method was implemented after the third patient to minimize patient exposure to radiation. Six of the 10 panic patients experienced lactate-induced panic attacks. Lactate infusion was associated with a marked increase in hemispheric blood flow levels in both panic patients and normal controls. Panic patients with lactate-induced panic attacks did not demonstrate a significant change in CBF compared with lactate-nonsensitive patients and normal controls. A second SPECT study using 99m-Tc labeled hexamethypropyleneamine oxime (HMPAO) compared CBF alterations in six panic patients and six controls after the administration of yohimbine [17]. Yohimbine caused a significant and consistent decrease in frontal cortical blood flow in panic patients, but not in controls. Another study [18] used xenon-133 to measure changes in CBF in panic and generalized anxiety disorder (GAD) patients and controls before and after intravenous caffeine infusion. The anxiety disorder patients showed no increase in anxiety symptoms after the administration of caffeine. Both groups of patients and normal controls showed similar patterns of reduced CBF following the caffeine infusion, but no change was seen after saline administration in normal controls. It appears that the CBF changes found in this study following the administration of caffeine were probably secondary to the caffeine directly rather than any underlying defective pathophysiological disturbance. The latest SPECT study [19] compared regional CBF in seven lactate-sensitive panic disorder patients compared to five normal controls. This study used HMPAO to measure CBF in both groups. Significant differences found in panic patients compared to controls included right-left asymmetry in the inferior frontal cortex, greater CBF in the inferior occipital cortex, and decreased CBF to the hippocampal regions bilaterally. These results further support the previous study, which indicated hippocampal abnormalities in panic disorder patients, more specifically lactate-sensitive panic disorder.

III. POSTTRAUMATIC STRESS DISORDER

In a recent NCS epidemiological survey, Kessler et al. [20] found a national lifetime prevalence of 7.8%, with females having a higher lifetime prevalence of PTSD than males (10.4% vs. 5%). A neurobiological basis for PTSD is suggested by studies that have demonstrated dysregulation of certain neurotransmitter pathways, hypothalamic-pituitary-adrenal (HPA) axis disturbances [21], and abnormal psychophysiological responses [22] in subjects with PTSD. These reports suggest that chronic PTSD may lead to brain architecture changes in areas related to memory and intellect, i.e., the hippocampus.

The first neuroimaging study of patients with PTSD used CT images in 10 former prisoners of war [23]. All 10 subjects were American World War II veterans, with a mean age of 68.5 years old (range 62–72 years). These 10 patients were divided into two groups based on the presence or absence of EEG-measured stage 4 sleep. This study found that 60% of patients had no stage 4 sleep. When this group of patients was compared to the group with stage 4 sleep present on EEG, they had increased VBRs and global sulcal widening (GSW). There are two major problems with the interpretation of this study's results. The first is that no normal controls were used; instead, the increased VBRs and GSW are based on a comparison of the VBRs and GSW of these six subjects with the four patients in the study. The separation of these two groups was based on the presence or absence of EEG-measured stage 4 sleep. The other problem is that the generalized findings of ventricular enlargement and GSW are also associated with aging of late life and dementia of an Alzheimer's type. Bremner et al. [24] compared standard MRI brain images in 26 Vietnam veterans and 22 matched controls. Right hippocampal volumes were significantly reduced (8% smaller) in combat-PTSD subjects compared to control subjects. Measurements of caudate volumes and temporal lobe regions revealed no difference in volumes between patients and controls. Deficits in short-term verbal memory were associated with smaller right hippocampal volumes.

Two functional brain studies have been conducted in combat-related PTSD patients: one using PET and the other SPECT. The PET study by Semple et al. [25] compared six subjects with PTSD and concurrent diagnosis of substance abuse with seven normal controls who had no history of substance abuse. There was a trend for patients with PTSD and concurrent substance abuse to have increased orbital frontal cortex regions and reduced hippocampal left/right ratio, but neither reached statistical significance. Liberzon et al. [26] studied the effects of exposure to combat sound activation compared to background white noise in the same subject population using SPECT. CBF was measured using 99m-Tc-HMPAO. Preliminary results found increased regional blood flow in both parahippocampal regions and left striatum after exposure to combat sound activation compared to background white noise in the same subject population using SPECT. These results suggested hippocampal and parahippocampal abnormalities in patients with chronic PTSD.

One limitation of these PTSD studies is that all patient subjects were males with combat-related trauma. Studies in noncombat and female trauma victims are currently underway.

IV. SOCIAL PHOBIA

Like panic disorder, social phobia is a common, severe, anxiety disorder that can cause significant social and occupational impairment. While there is high comorbidity between social phobia and panic disorder, many differences separate them. These differences include age at onset, specificity of associated physiological symptoms, gender distribution, sleep patterns, and sensitivity to caffeine and lactate [27]. Both dopaminergic and serotonergic theories have been proposed for social phobia, and each is supported by certain investigational studies and pharmacotherapy trials [28].

Neuroimaging has recently been applied as a method of investigation into the neurobiology of social phobia. Potts et al. [29] measured total cerebral volumes and basal ganglia volumes in 22 patients with social phobia compared to 22 age- and sex-matched normal controls using MRI. No statistically significant difference was demonstrated between social phobia patients and normal control subjects with respect to total cerebral, caudate, putamen, and thalamic volumes. Although this study failed to demonstrate any specific cerebral structural abnormalities in patients with social phobia, it did reveal an age-related reduction in putamen volumes in patients with social phobia that was greater than that seen in controls. This age-related reduction in putamen values in patients with social phobia was not correlated with the severity of their illness.

This led to a follow-up MRS study by Davidson et al. [30], which found significant differences on proton-localized MRS findings in 20 social phobics compared to 20 age- and sex-matched normal controls. The social phobia group demonstrated significantly lower choline and creatinine in cortical and subcortical regions compared to controls. Choline, creatinine, and NAA SNRs in the thalamic area were all inversely proportional to the severity of social phobia and/or the fear subscale of the Duke Brief Social Phobia Scale. Thus, it appears that the most severely symptomatic social phobia group demonstrated the lowest metabolic activity. These findings may also suggest that social phobia is associated with altered energy activity, membrane function, and neuronal activity in the cortical, basal ganglia, and thalamic regions, with some of the changes being related to symptom severity. Our group has replicated the finding of lowered NAA/choline ratios in a second study of

MRS in social phobics compared to normal controls. In another study of social phobia, MRS was used to measure cerebral concentrations of fluoxetine concentrations in patients being treated with fluoxetine. In this study, Miner et al. [31] measured brain fluoxetine levels in patients with social phobia using fluorine magnetic resonance spectroscopy. This study found that the five responders all had larger cerebral fluoxetine concentrations than the three nonresponders, suggesting a possible threshold level of fluoxetine being necessary before a response is seen.

V. GENERALIZED ANXIETY DISORDER

There have been few neuroimaging studies involving patients with GAD. To date there have been two PET studies and one SPECT study. The first study [32] involved 18 patients with GAD who had PET studies before and after being randomized in a placebo-controlled double-blind study of clorazepate for 21 days. Clorazepate was given at a daily dose of 22.5 mg/day. 18F-Deoxyglucose was used to assess glucose metabolism pre- and posttreatment. An asymmetrical decrease (left < right) in glucose metabolism was seen in the visual cortex, and relative increases in glucose metabolism were found in the basal ganglia and thalamus after the 21 days of treatment with clorazepate. The PET scans taken at day 21 were then compared to human autopsy atlas images that contained benzodiazepine receptor-binding site concentrations. When this analysis was performed, the degree of altered glucose metabolism was directly related to the concentration of benzodiazepine receptors in that region. This is consistent with the inhibitory role of the GABA system, i.e., activation of the system by benzodiazepines should lead to greater neuronal inhibition and thus decreased neuronal activity.

A second PET study [33] was performed by the same research group. The aim of this second study was to directly compare possible differences in regional cerebral metabolism between normal controls and patients with GAD. Eighteen right-handed patients who met criteria for GAD and were medication-free for at least 3 weeks were compared to 15 normal controls who did not have any medical or psychiatric diagnoses and were medication-free. The GAD patients entered a 21-day double-blind placebo-controlled trial with 22.5 mg/day of clorazepate versus placebo. The results showed that in a medication-free, resting no-task state, patients with GAD had greater occipital lobe, temporal lobe, and frontal lobe metabolism relative to normal controls. After 21 days of clordiazepate, GAD patients had a significant decrease in glucose metabolism in cortical lobes, the limbic system, and basal ganglia compared to the GAD group that received placebo. The relative occipital cortex activity at baseline in this study is consistent with the previous findings by Buchsbaum et al. [31] in GAD patients compared to controls.

The one published SPECT study in GAD was performed by Mathew and Wilson [18]. This study used xenon-133 to measure changes in CBF in panic disorder and GAD patients and controls before and after an intravenous caffeine infusion. Both groups of anxiety disorder patients showed no increase in anxiety symptoms after the administration of caffeine. Both groups of patients and normal controls showed similar patterns of reduced CBF following the caffeine infusion, but no change was seen after saline administration in normal controls. The CBF changes found in this study following the administration of caffeine were probably secondary to the caffeine directly rather than any underlying defective pathophysiological disturbance.

VI. SIMPLE PHOBIA

While simple phobia is the most common phobic disorder, very little is known about its biological roots. To date five studies have been published in patients with simple phobia: four PET and one SPECT. The first of these studies investigated the effects of confrontation with a phobic object on CBF in patients with simple phobia [34]. Seven patients with simple phobia related to small animals and eight matched controls underwent a series of five PET scans in a rest-fear-rest-fear-rest paradigm. In each of the patients exposure to the phobic object produced marked physiological arousal and anxiety. Baseline and repeated resting scans did not differ at any time between patients with simple phobia and controls. Absolute global and some regional CBF was significantly lower during object exposure in the patient group. However, when the measurements were corrected to account for the effects of hypocapnia secondary to hyperventilation, no detectable differences between populations were seen.

Wik et al. [35] used a series of three 4-minute videos played twice to measure the effects of phobic confrontation on CBF in six patients with snake phobia. After an initial 30- to 60-minute rest period, patients were shown the three videos in varying order. The videotapes consisted of one neutral scene of people walking in a park, a scene of snakes in the wild or in captivity, and one aversive scene of war and torture. 15-0-Butanol, which has a very short half-life, was the radioactive isotope used to measure CBF. This study found that phobic confrontation led to CBF increases in the secondary visual cortex and a CBF reduction in the hippocampus, orbitofrontal, prefrontal, temporopolar and posterior cingulate cortex compared to CBF during the neutral stimulus. The effects of the aversive video lay almost directly between the effects of the neutral and phobic confrontation. When Frederickson et al. [36] examined another set of six patients with snake phobia, repeating the same study protocol employed by Wik et al. [34], they also noted increased CBF to the secondary visual cortex, which was not seen in scans taken during aversive or neutral videos. Of note was the fact that the thalamus showed increased CBF in response to the phobic video. This latter result was also seen in a PET study done by Rauch et al. [37]. Rather than using three different videos, this group used a simpler paradigm of two control neutral stimuli, each followed by an individually tailored phobic object confrontation.

O'Carroll et al. [38] performed a SPECT imaging study. Ten patients with simple phobia had SPECT studies performed while listening to a 4-minute relaxation tape and again after an appropriate interval listening to a 4-minute tape describing exposure to the feared stimulus. Exposure to the feared stimulus led to reduced tracer uptake in the right occipital and right posterior temporal regions. These results, while occuring in roughly the same region as the PET studies in patients with simple phobia, show the opposite effect on blood flow, i.e., it decreased rather than increased.

VII. SUMMARY

Neuroimaging studies of phobic disorders have helped provide evidence that biological factors are involved in these disorders. In panic disorder, initial CT studies [5,7] provided nonspecific findings but imply that prolonged high-dose benzodiazepines may be associated with increased VBR. It is important to mention that the patients given high-dose benzodiazepine did not have prebenzodiazepine baseline MRI studies, and these MRI findings may pre-date treatment. The MRI studies suggest temporal lobe involvement panic disorder, particularly in the presence of comorbid agoraphobia. PET studies [11–15] have consistently showed asymmetrical CBF in the hippocampal and parahippocampal regions, while SPECT [16–19] studies have found varying and inconsistent results. This may be due to different radioisotopes being used, different patient selection criteria, and varying provocation methods, i.e., lactate vs. yohimbine.

The PTSD studies have yielded mixed results. The initial CT study [23] had a number of problems that made interpretation of the studies data difficult. The more recent MRI [24] and SPECT [26] studies suggest hippocampal and parahippocampal involvement. However, one problem common to all of the PTSD studies is that their patient populations reflect only one subgroup of the overall PTSD population. Further studies in other trauma populations are now underway.

The one MRI study of social phobia [29] revealed an age-related reduction in putamen volumes in patients. This finding is consistent with biological theories of social phobia, which have implicated the basal ganglia as having some role in its etiology [28]. MRS studies have shown that more severe symptomotology is proportional to reduced metabolic activity. A study by Miner et al. [31] found that a minimum level of fluoxetine in the brain may be necessary before a clinical response is seen.

The first GAD PET study [32] found an increase in glucose metabolism in the thalamus and a relative decrease in glucose metabolism in the visual cortex (left < right) after treatment with clorazapate. The follow-up GAD PET study [33] confirmed the decrease in occipital lobe activity after treatment with a benzodiazepine. The SPECT study [18] failed to find any abnormality specific to GAD or panic disorder, but rather was able to attribute all changes in CBF to a direct effect of the caffeine. Finally, simple phobia studies [34–38] showed mixed results. The first study [34] was unable to detect any difference between baseline and phobic confrontation scans once they were corrected for the effects of hyperventilation. The results of the next study [35] appear to correlate with the degree of physiological arousal precipitated by aversive and phobic confrontation videos. This may mean that the changes seen in CBF are on a spectrum of severity that correlates with the degree of physiological arousal or anxiety and are not specific to simple phobia. The SPECT study in simple phobia, while localizing changes to the same brain region as the PET studies, showed the opposite effect on CBF, i.e., SPECT demonstrated a decease in CBF rather than the increase in CBF seen in the PET simple phobia studies.

While these studies have helped to elucidate possible biological factors in phobic disorders, most have yet to be thoroughly replicated. An important factor in these replication studies will be consistency in patient selection. It may be that the panic disorder studies were not consistently similar because patient selection varied in the presence or absence of agoraphobia and whether the panic disorder was lactate-sensitive. Three areas of research that will help to shed light on the etiology and treatment of these disorders are (a) neuroimaging pre- and posttreatment intervention, (b) the use of MRS to determine the site of action of psychotropic compounds like the fluoxetine in social phobia study, and (c) the emergence of functional MRI. Functional MRI is a new area of research with great potential as a research tool in psychiatry. The advantages of functional MRI include that it is noninvasive, does not involve exposure to radiation, is able to capture images as they are occurring, and with the development of more powerful magnets for clinical use will have greater spatial resolution than either PET or SPECT. With this combination of research tools, it may not be much longer before we are able to develop a greater understanding of phobic disorders and how best to treat them.

REFERENCES

1. R. Kessler, K. McGonagle, S. Zhao, C. Nelson, M. Hughes, S. Eshleman, H. Wittchen, and K. Kendler, Lifetime and 12 month prevalence of DSM-III-R psychiatric disorders in the United States, *Arch. Gen. Psychiatry 51*:8 (1994).
2. P. Cox, D. Direnfeld, R. Swinson, and G. Norton, Suicidal ideation and suicide attempts in panic disorder and social phobia, *Am. J. Psychiatry, 151*(6):882 (1994).
3. J. Davidson, D. Hughes, D. Blazer, and L. George, Posttraumatic stress disorder in the community: an epidemiological study, *Psychol. Med. 22*:713 (1991).
4. M. Johnson, R. Lydiard, and J. Ballenger, Panic disorder: pathophysiology and drug treatment, *Drugs 49*(3):328 (1995).
5. T. Uhde and C. Kellner, Cerebral ventricular size in panic disorder, *J. Affective Disord. 12*:175 (1987).
6. M. Lader, M. Ron, and H. Petursson, Computed axial brain tomography in long term benzodiazepine users, *Psychol. Med. 14*:203 (1984).
7. U. Lepola, U. Nousiainen, M. Puranen, P. Riekkinen, and R. Rimon, EEG and CT findings in panic disorder, *Biol. Psychiatry 28*:721 (1990).
8. A. Ontiveros, R. Fontaine, G. Breton, R. Elie, S. Fontaine, and R. Dery, Correlation of severity of panic disorder and neuroanatomical changes on magnetic resonance imaging, *J. Neuropsychiatry 1*(4):404 (1989).
9. R. Fontaine, G. Breton, R. Dery, S. Fontaine, and R. Elie, Temporal lobe abnormalities in panic disorder: an MRI study, *Biol. Psychiatry 27*:304 (1990).
10. S. Dager, W. Strauss, K. Marro, T. Richards, G. Metzger, and A. Artru, Proton magnetic resonance spectroscopy investigation of hyperventilation in subjects with panic disorder and comparison subjects, *Am. J. Psychiatry 152*(5):666 (1995).
11. E. Reiman, M. Raichle, F. Butler, P. Herscovitch, and E. Robins, A focal brain abnormality in panic disorder, a severe form of anxiety, *Nature 310*:683 (1984).
12. E. Reiman, M. Raichle, E. Robins, K. Butler, P. Herscovitch, P. Fox, and J. Perlmutter, The application of positron emission tomography to the study of panic disorder, *Am. J. Psychiatry 143*(4):469 (1986).
13. E. Reiman, The study of panic disorder using positron emission tomography, *Psychiatr. Dev. 1*:63 (1987).
14. E. Reiman, M. Raichle, E. Robins, M. Mintun, Fusselman, P. Fox, J. Price, and K. Hackman, Neuroanatomical correlates of a lactate induced anxiety attack, *Arch. Gen. Psychiatry 46*:493 (1989).
15. T. Nordahl, W. Semple, M. Gross, T. Mellman, P. Stein, P. Goyer, A. King, T. Uhde, and R. Cohen, Cerebral glucose metabolic differences in patients with panic disorder, *Neuropsychopharmacology 3*(4):261 (1990).
16. R. Stewart, M. Devous, J. Rush, L. Lane, and F. Bonte, Cerebral blood flow changes during sodium-lactate-induced panic attacks, *Am. J. Psychiatry 145*(4):442 (1988).
17. S. Woods, K. Koster, J. Krystal, E. Smith, I. Zubral, P. Hoffer, and D. Charney, Yohimbine alters regional cerebral blood flow in panic disorder, *Lancet 11*:678 (1988).

18. R. Mathew and W. Wilson, Behavioral and cerebrovascular effects of caffeine in patients with anxiety disorders, *Acta Psychiatr. Scand. 82*(1):17 (1990).
19. M. Cristofaro, A. Sessarego, A. Pupi, F. Biondi, and C. Faravelli, Brain perfusion abnormalities in drug naive, lactate-sensitive panic patients: a SPECT study, *Biol. Psychiatry 33*:505 (1993).
20. R. Kessler, A. Sonnega, E. Bromet, M. Hughes, and C. Nelson, Posttraumatic stress disorder in the National Comorbidity Survey, *Arch. Gen. Psychiatry 52*: 1048 (1995).
21. D. Charney, A. Deutch, J. Krystal, S. Southwick, and M. Davies, Psychobiologic mechanisms in posttraumatic stress disorder, *Arch. Gen. Psychiatry 50*: 294 (1993).
22. Pitman, S. Orr, D. Forgue, J. deJong, and J. Claiborn, Psychophysiologic assessment of posttraumatic stress disorder imagery in Vietnam combat veterans, *Arch. Gen. Psychiatry 44*:970 (1987).
23. J. Peters, D. van Kammen, W. van Kammen, and T. Neylan, Sleep disturbance and computerized axial tomographic scan findings in former prisoners of war, *Comp. Psychiatry 31*(6):535 (1990).
24. J. Bremner, P. Randall, T. Scott, R. Bronen, J. Seibyl, S. Southwick, G. Laney, G. McCarthy D., Charney, and R. Innis, MRI-based measurements of hippocampal volume in patients with combat-related posttraumatic stress disorder, *Am. J. Psychiatry 152*(7):973 (1995).
25. W. Semple, P. Goyer, R. McCormack, E. Morris, B. Compton, G. Muswick, D. Nelson, B. Donovan, G. Leisure, M. Berridge, F. Miraldi, and C. Schultz, Preliminary report: brain blood flow using PET in patients with posttraumatic stress disorder and substance abuse histories, *Biol. Psychiatry 34*:115 (1993).
26. L. Liberzon, L. Fig, and T. Jung, Brain blood flow in posttraumatic stress disorder: SPECT Activation, *Biol. Psychiatry 37*:622 (1995).
27. T. Uhde, M. Tancer, B. Black, and T. Brown, Phenomenology and neurobiology of social phobia: comparison with panic disorder, *J. Clin. Psychiatry 52*: 31 (1991).
28. N. Potts and J. Davidson, Social phobia: biological aspects and pharmacotherapy, *Prog. Neuro-Psychopharmacol. Biol. Psychiatry 16*(5):635 (1992).
29. N. Potts, J. Davidson, K. Krishnan, and P. Doraiswamy, Magnetic resonance imaging in patients with social phobia, *Psychiatry Res. 52*:35 (1994).
30. J. Davidson, K. Krishnan, H. Charles, O. Boyko, N. Potts, S. Ford, and L. Patterson, Magnetic resonance spectroscopy in social phobia: preliminary findings, *J. Clin. Psychiatry 54*:19 (1993).
31. C. Miner, J. Davidson, N. Potts, L. Tupler, H. Charles, and K. Krishnan, Brain fluoxetine measurements using fluorine magnetic resonance spectroscopy in patients with social phobia, *Biol. Psychiatry 38*:696 (1995).
32. M. Buchsbaum, J. Wu, R. Haier, E. Hazlett, R. Ball, M. Katz, K. Sokolski, M. Lagunas-Solar, and D. Langer, Positron emission tomography assessments of effects of benzodiazepines on regional glucose metabolic rates in patients with anxiety disorder, *Life Sci. 40*:2393 (1987).
33. J. Wu, M. Buchsbaum, T. Hershey, E. Hazlett, N. Sicotte, and J. Johnson, PET in generalized anxiety disorder, *Biol. Psychiatry 29*:1181 (1991).

34. J. Mountz, J. Modell, M. Wilson, G. Curtis, M. Lee, S. Schmaltz, and D. Kuhl, Positron emission tomography evaluation of cerebral blood flow during state anxiety in simple phobia, *Arch. Gen. Psychiatry 46*:501 (1989).
35. G. Wik, M. Fredrikson, K. Ericson, L. Eriksson, S. Stone-Elander, and T. Greitz, A functional cerebral response to frightening visual stimulation, *Psychiatry Res. Neuroimaging 50*:15 (1993).
36. M. Fredrikson, G. Wik, T. Greitz, L. Eriksson, S. Stone-Elander, S. Stone-Elander, and G. Sedvall, Regional cerebral blood flow during experimental phobic fear, *Psychophysiology 30*:126 (1993).
37. S. Rauch, C. Savage, N. Alpert, E. Miguel, L. Baer, H. Breiter, A. Fischman, P. Manzo, C. Moretti, and M. Jenike, A positron emission tomographic study of simple phobic symptom provocation, *Arch. Gen. Psychiatry 52*:20 (1995).
38. R. Carroll, A. Moffoot, M. Van Beck, N. Dougall, C. Murray, K. Ebmeier, and G. Goodwin, The effect of anxiety induction on the regional uptake of 99m-Tc-Exametazime in simple phobia as shown by single photon emission tomography, *J. Affective Disord. 28*:203 (1993).

17

Neuroimaging in Obsessive-Compulsive Disorder

Sarah W. Book, Gerardo Villarreal,* Olga Brawman-Mintzer, Mark S. George, and R. Bruce Lydiard
Medical University of South Carolina, Charleston, South Carolina

I. INTRODUCTION

Obsessive-compulsive disorder (OCD) is a disabling anxiety disorder characterized by obsessions or compulsions. Obsessions are recurrent and persistent thoughts, impulses, and images which are experienced, at some time of the disturbance, as intrusive and inappropriate, causing marked anxiety. Compulsions are repetitive behaviors or mental acts which may be aimed at reducing distress. Once widely regarded as a rare, predominantly psychological illness refractory to therapeutic intervention, OCD is now recognized as a common (lifetime prevalence 1.9–3%) [1], often treatable neurobiological condition.

---

* *Current affiliation*: Appalachian Regional Healthcare, Harlan, Kentucky

The etiology of the illness is still not understood. However, OCD is phenomenologically and biologically distinct from other anxiety disorders such as panic disorder. For example, the selective therapeutic response of OCD patients to serotonin uptake inhibitors [clomipramine and the selective serotonin reuptake inhibitors SSRIs] but not to other antidepressants or anxiolytic agents, which are effective in the treatment of other anxiety disorders, has led to research in the direction of potential specific abnormalities in the serotonin neurotransmitter system. Additionally, researchers observed that treatment with the antiobsessional agent clomipramine decreased obsessional symptoms, which in turn correlated with decreases in the concentration of the serotonin metabolite 5-hydroxyindoleacetic acid (5-HIAA) in the cerebrospinal fluid (CSF) and in blood platelets [2]. Perturbation of serotonin function via challenge with serotonin agonists or antagonists can increase or decrease (respectively) obsessions and anxiety in patients with OCD [2]. Further, treatment with antiobsessionals appears to attenuate these effects [3].

In OCD there may be a disturbance in a theoretic loop of neurobiological action, the cortical-striatal-thalamic-cortical loop [4]. This loop includes the orbital frontal cortex, which, when activated, theoretically activates the caudate nucleus, which in turn deactivates the globus pallidus, which deactivates the thalamus, which in turn activates the orbitofrontal cortex (Fig. 1). In

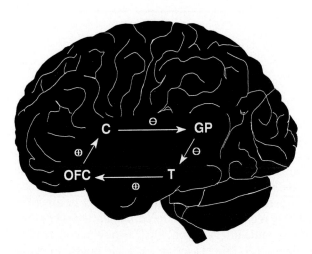

Fig. 1 Theoretical cortical-striatal-thalamic-cortical loop. OFC: Orbitalfrontal cortex; C: caudate; GP: globus pallidus; T: thalamus; ⊖: inhibitory pathway; ⊕: excitatory pathway.

OCD, there is perhaps a deregulation of this particular orbitofrontal loop. Neuroimaging studies support this theory, showing increased activity of orbitofrontal cortex and caudate nucleus in OCD patients when compared to control subjects (Fig. 2).

Computer-assisted imaging technologies are conventionally divided into those examining brain structure (i.e., structural imaging) and those measuring metabolic or biochemical function, (i.e., functional imaging). Structural imaging techniques include computed tomography (CT) and magnetic resonance imaging (MRI). Functional imaging techniques include single photon emission tomography (SPECT), positron emission tomography (PET), and fast or functional MRI (fMRI). All of these methods have been used to study OCD.

This chapter will highlight the major findings in brain imaging research of patients with OCD.

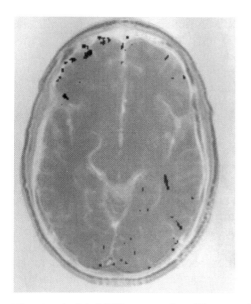

Fig. 2 Axial MRI scan of a 37-year-old man with severe OCD. Serial echoplanar bold images were taken during a resting period (thinking, but not obsessing) and then when the patient was actively obsessing. The regional activity was compared across these two conditions using paired t-tests. The grey image represents brain structure (T_1-weighted MRI), and the dark areas are regions that were significantly more active during obsessing than during the control state ($p < 0.05$). (MUSC Picker 1.5 Tesla MRI scanner.)

II. STRUCTURAL BRAIN IMAGING IN OCD

MRI and CT imaging techniques have been employed to examine brain structures in patients with OCD. Specifically, there have been four targeted areas: (a) the ratio of ventricle volumes to whole brain volumes, or ventricular brain ratio (VBR), (b) lateral ventricle volumes, (c) caudate size, and (d) the volume of the retrocallosal parieto-occipital white matter.

Two groups have looked at VBR in subjects with OCD, and their findings are not consistent. Behar and colleagues [5] compared CT scans of 16 adolescents with OCD and 16 age-, sex-, race-, handedness-, and IQ-matched normal controls and found that the OCD patients had significantly higher VBR than controls. In fact, four OCD patients had VBRs that were more than two standard deviations above the control mean. However, other studies failed to confirm these findings. Insel et al. [6] compared CT scans of 10 OCD patients and 10 age- and gender-matched nonpsychiatric controls and found no differences, not only in VBR but also in left to right hemisphere asymmetry and sulcal prominence.

Other researchers have examined ventricular volumes, especially the lateral ventricles, in patients with OCD and controls, and these studies, too, have yielded conflicting findings. Stein et al. [7] utilized CT to evaluate lateral ventricular volumes in OCD patients ($n = 16$) and in nonpsychiatric patients complaining of headaches ($n = 8$). The OCD group was divided into those with evidence of significant neurological soft sign abnormalities ($n = 8$) vs. those with minimal abnormalities ($n = 8$) in fine motor function, involuntary and mirror movements, and visuospatial function. The authors found that a subgroup of OCD patients with high soft sign scores had significantly larger lateral ventricular volumes than did both the "low soft sign" OCD patients and comparison subjects.

Although this subgroup of "soft sign" OCD patients has not again been investigated, Luxenberg and colleagues [8] compared CT scans of OCD patients ($n = 10$) with those of normal comparison subjects ($n = 10$). They found no differences in the size of the lateral and the third ventricle between these two groups. They did find a difference in the size of the caudate nucleus. Their sample of patients with OCD had significantly smaller caudates than did the control subjects.

Luxenberg's finding of reduced caudate volume was replicated in an MRI study by Robinson et al. [9], who evaluated MRI scans of 26 subjects with OCD and 26 normal controls. In addition to caudate size, they also compared volumes of prefrontal cortex, lateral and third ventricles, and whole brain. The authors found a significant reduction in bilateral caudate nuclei volumes in OCD patients compared to normal controls. However, there were no significant differences in prefrontal cortex, lateral and third ventricular volumes, or whole brain volumes. Scarone and colleagues [10] obtained MRI scans from 20 OCD patients and 16 normal comparison subjects. Interestingly, they found that in the right hemispheres of OCD patients, the head of the caudate was larger compared to normal comparison subjects, but found no significant differences between the left caudate volume of OCD patients and normal controls. In contrast, Kellner et al. [11] compared MRI scans of 12 patients with OCD with those of 12 normal controls by measuring areas of the head of the caudate, cingulate gyrus thickness, corpus callosum, and intracaudate/frontal horn ration. The authors found no significant differences in these measures between OCD patients and normal comparison subjects.

Consistent with the negative findings by Kellner, Breiter et al. [12] failed to discern differences between female OCD patients (n = 6) and normal female controls (n = 8). They analyzed volumes of the retrocallosal white and gray matter, which includes the parieto-occipital area, as well as the retrocallosal lateral ventricles. They also measured the anterior-posterior length and the total area of the midsagittal corpus callosum to ensure that any differences in retrocallosal volume could not be attributed to a change of the landmark that defines its perimeter. The authors found significantly smaller right-sided retrocallosal volumes, but no significant differences in the sizes of the corpus callosum in OCD patients compared to controls.

Finally, Garber and colleagues [13] examined the brain structure of OCD patients and normal controls using T_1 images of MRIs of 32 subjects with OCD and 14 normal controls. Regional T_1 mapping measures the amount of water in membrane and fluids, roughly representing extracellular fluid and intracellular tissue volumes. Garber et al. hypothesized that if the brains of OCD patients differed from those of controls on a cellular level, the T_1 should also be different. Results demonstrated that patients with OCD had greater asymmetry between their right and left frontal regions than did the normal controls. Further, OCD patients with one or more first-degree relative with OCD had more T_1 abnormalities in the anterior cingulate gyrus than did other patients and normal controls. In addition, right to left T_1 differences for the orbital cortex had significant correlation with symptom severity in unmedicated OCD patients and OCD patients with a family history positive for OCD.

In summary, the results of structural studies of the brains of subjects with OCD have been varied. These variations can be explained by many factors including technical differences between studies, sample size, and lack of a homogeneous population (e.g., sex, age, medication status, presence of neurological soft signs, duration and severity of illness). Nevertheless, several findings emerge. Specifically, there are data indicating that OCD patients may have abnormal caudate volumes, abnormal ventricular volumes, and frontal abnormalities. These findings could be consistent with the theory that the pathophysiology of OCD includes dysfunction of the cortical-striatal-thalamic-cortical loop.

III. FUNCTIONAL BRAIN IMAGING IN OCD

Important advances have been made in the past several years in functional neuroimaging research in OCD. To date, researchers have used primarily PET and SPECT, high-resolution imaging techniques using tracer amounts of biochemicals labeled with radiation emitters, which are subsequently localized in different brain areas. SPECT technique is used to measure regional cerebral blood flow (rCBF), which is highly correlated with cerebral metabolism, and PET is used to measure rCBF as well as more direct measurements of basal cerebral glucose or oxygen metabolic rates. The most popular SPECT radionucleotides used in studies of OCD is technetium 99m hexamethylpropylenamine oxime (HMPAO), which is given intravenously, and xenon 133 (^{133}Xe), an inert lipophilic gas given by inhalation. SPECT can measure the relative ratios of the uptake of HMPAO in different regions of the brain, which directly correlates to the rate of four events: (a) HMPAO crossing the blood-brain barrier, (b) cerebral blood flow, (c) uptake of HMPAO by cells, and (d) intracellular conversion of HMPAO to a hydrophilic form. The clearance of ^{133}Xe, which freely diffuses throughout the extracellular area of the brain, is used to determine absolute blood flow values. PET studies in OCD have used as their tracer F-fluorodeoxyglucose (FDG) or ^{11}C-glucose.

Using PET and SPECT, researchers have found abnormalities in the frontal lobe, in particular the orbital frontal cortex, and the basal ganglia, specifically the caudate nuclei, which normalize with treatment. In addition, there are also data indicating possible abnormalities in other brain areas in OCD patients, such as the thalamus, the cingulate, the temporal lobe, as well as the whole cerebral hemispheres. This section will review the recent advances in the functional neuroimaging studies in OCD.

A. SPECT Studies in OCD

Machlin et al. [14] used high-resolution HMPAO SPECT in 10 OCD patients and 8 age- and sex-matched controls. They calculated uptake in specific brain regions relative to whole cortex uptake. In patients with OCD, medial frontal but not orbital frontal ratios were increased compared to controls. Medial frontal ratios correlated negatively with Hamilton Anxiety rating scale scores but not with OCD-specific (Yale-Brown Obsessive Compulsive Scale) ratings. Rubin and colleagues [15] performed ^{133}Xe and HMPAO

SPECT in 10 adult unmedicated OCD patients and 10 age-matched adult male normal controls. They found no differences between the two groups using the ^{133}Xe SPECT. However, they found significantly higher uptake using HMPAO SPECT in OCD patients in the bilateral orbital frontal and dorsal parietal cerebral cortex, the left area of the posterofrontal cortex, and decreased uptake in the head of the caudate bilaterally when compared to controls. There were no differences in the putamen or the thalamus bilaterally. The authors postulated that the HMPAO findings may be due to a difference in blood-brain barrier permeability between patients and normals not detected with ^{133}Xe. Differences in resolution between HMPAO (2–9 nm) and ^{133}Xe (13–20 nm) may also explain the differences in study results using both techniques. Because of this resolution difference, xenon SPECT can accurately yield information about cortex, not subcortical structures. Edmonstone et al. [16] used SPECT to evaluate 12 OCD patients, 12 patients with major depression, and 12 normal controls. Compared with controls, OCD patients showed decreased uptake in the right caudate and the putamen bilaterally. In addition, the bilateral caudate and left putamen uptake correlated positively with anxiety scores in the OCD group. Adams et al. [17] used HMPAO SPECT to find left basal ganglia hypoperfusion in 6 of 11 OCD patients. Recently, Lucey and colleagues [18] compared 30 OCD patients and 30 healthy controls. Using HMPAO SPECT, they found decreased rCBF in OCD patients in the superior frontal cortex bilaterally, the right inferior frontal cortex, the left temporal cortex, the left parietal cortex, the right caudate, and the right thalamus.

Functional neuroimaging has also been utilized to evaluate brain changes in OCD patients following pharmacological treatment of OCD. Hoehn-Saric et al. [19] examined six OCD patients after 3–4 months of treatment with fluoxetine at doses ranging from 80 to 100 mg/day. The authors reported decreased medial frontal to whole cortex HMPAO uptake following effective treatment with fluoxetine. In a case report, Hoehn-Saric et al. [20] also reported decreased frontal metabolism on HMPAO SPECT in one OCD patient who developed a frontal lobe syndrome (i.e., apathy and indifference) while taking up to 100 mg of fluoxetine per day for 4 months. The symptoms disappeared 4 months after discontinuing fluoxetine. The authors concluded that high doses of fluoxetine may significantly decrease frontal metabolism in OCD patients.

Finally, researchers also utilized SPECT techniques to investigate differences in regional cerebral blood flow during symptom provocation in OCD patients. For example, Zohar et al. [21] used ^{133}Xe SPECT to evaluate 10 OCD patients with contamination obsessions and washing compulsions during relaxation state, imaginal flooding, and in vivo exposure to phobic stimuli, which induces contamination obsessions and washing rituals. Surprisingly, the authors found that when compared to the state of relaxation, the imaginal flooding caused an increase in rCBF in the temporal areas whereas the in vivo exposure caused a decrease in rCBF in all cortical regions studied (including the cerebrum, prefrontal, precentral, parietal, temporal, and posterior regions). The authors speculated that during a highly anxiety-provoking in vivo exposure, blood may be shunted away from the cortical areas of the brain to other areas such as the caudate, which is not visualized with ^{133}Xe.

In summary, although SPECT studies in OCD have been limited and often yielded conflicting results, the available data suggest that OCD patients may have abnormalities in the frontal lobe, in particular the orbital frontal cortex, and the basal ganglia, specifically the caudate nuclei, which normalize with pharmacological treatment. Abnormalities in the caudate and the orbital frontal cortex are consistent with the theory of a cortical-striatal-thalamic-cortical loop disturbance in OCD. The differing results could be due to a lack of consistency between studies in terms of subject demographics, illness severity and duration, as well as the small number of subjects in some studies. Also, further research utilizing specific tracers, which can image specific neurotransmitter systems such as the serotonergic system, are clearly needed.

B.   PET Studies in OCD

There are several advantages to the use of PET technology for assessing functional abnormalities in OCD and other psychiatric disorders. First, PET often provides images with higher resolution than SPECT, and localization of different brain areas is probably more accurate. Further, PET technology can incorporate pharmaceuticals and organic compounds as vehicles, whereas SPECT technology is more limited by the type of vehicle that can be coupled to a radionucleotide.

To date 11 studies have used PET to examine functional brain abnormalities in patients with OCD. In the first study, Baxter et al. [22] evaluated 14 OCD patients, 14 patients with unipolar depression, and 14 normal controls. They found that compared with controls and depressed patients, OCD patients had significantly increased metabolic rates in the whole cerebral hemispheres, caudate nuclei, and orbital gyri. Metabolic rates in the left orbital gyrus divided by those of the ipsilateral hemisphere (''normalized'' rates) were significantly higher than controls with a trend toward significance in the right hemisphere. Normalized caudate metabolic rates in OCD did not differ from controls. Further, 10 OCD patients were rescanned after treatment with trazadone with or without a monoamine oxidase inhibitor for an unspecified period of time. Patients who responded to treatment with considerable symptom reduction had a significant increase in both left and right normalized caudate metabolic rates compared to nonresponders. There were no changes in the orbital-hemisphere ratios. Baxter et al. [23] replicated these findings in a study of 10 medication-free, nondepressed OCD patients and 10 age-, sex-, and handedness-matched controls. In this study they observed increased metabolic rates in the whole cerebral hemispheres, the orbital gyri, the heads of the caudate nuclei, and an increased orbital/hemisphere ratio ("normalized" ratio) bilaterally compared to controls. The differences in the orbital/hemisphere ratios between the two studies may be explained by the unbalanced ratio of female to male subjects in the first study. Similarly, Nordahl et al. [24] compared PET scans of 8 nondepressed OCD patients and 30 normal controls during an auditory continuous performance task, which evaluates functional localization of sustained attention. They also found increased normalized metabolic rates in both orbital gyri, but not in the caudate, in OCD patients compared to controls.

Swedo et al. [25] used PET to compare 18 adults with childhood onset OCD and 18 controls. Study results demonstrated an increase in metabolic rates in the left orbital frontal region, the right sensorimotor region, and bilaterally in the prefrontal and anterior cingulate regions. In addition, OCD severity correlated positively with metabolism in the right orbital region. Recently, Perani et al. [26] also found an increase in metabolic rates in PET study of 11 patients with OCD and 15 controls. The authors demonstrated a significantly increased metabolism in the cingulate gyrus, the pallidum/putamen, and the thalamus as well as a trend toward increased metabolism in the caudate.

In contrast, Martinot et al. [27] found decreased, rather than increased, metabolic rates on PET scans of OCD patients. The authors examined PET scans of 16 nondepressed patients with OCD and 8 normal controls and found lower absolute metabolic rates in the whole cortex. The normalized metabolic rates were also significantly lower in the prefrontal lateral cortex in OCD patents compared to controls. In addition, they could not confirm orbital gyrus differences between OCD patients and their controls. Further, OCD patients had a negative correlation between prefrontal lateral cortex metabolism and attention test scores, which assess frontal lobe function. The authors suggested that the differences in study results may be due to differences in sample selection. For example, OCD patients in their study had a longer duration of illness and were more anxious than OCD patients in other PET studies. In addition, control subjects in this study had higher overall metabolic rates than normal controls in other studies.

PET technology has also been used to evaluate changes in metabolic rates following pharmacological treatment of OCD. To date, three studies have looked at the effect of treatment on metabolic rates in patients with

OCD. Benkelfat et al. [28] examined PET scans of eight OCD patients following treatment with clomipramine at doses ranging from 125 to 300 mg per
day for a minimum of 12 weeks. They found that successful treatment correlated with a decrease in metabolic rates in the left caudate and in the bilateral
orbital frontal gyrus. A similar study by Swedo and colleagues [29] repro-
duced these findings. They reexamined 13 OCD adult patients with childhood
onset OCD after at least one year of treatment (mean of 20 months) with
clomipramine and fluoxetine. Eight patients received clomipramine, two fluoxetine, and three were drug-free. Seven patients were rated as treatment
responders, and six patients were rated nonresponders. The authors found
that clinical improvement correlated with a decrease in the normalized metabolic rates in the orbitofrontal region bilaterally. In a third study, Baxter et
al. [30] examined the effects of 10-week treatment with either fluoxetine
or behavioral therapy on metabolic rates in 18 patients with OCD. In both
treatment groups, clinical responders showed decreased normalized metabolism in the head of the right caudate. Thus, increased caudate and orbitofrontal activity is state related and resolves with symptom resolution irrespective
of the treatment method.

Finally, researchers have also utilized PET to examine changes in brain
metabolism during symptom provocation in OCD patients. For example,
Rauch et al. [31] looked at the PET scans of eight patients with OCD during
rest and during symptom provocation. When compared to the resting state,
they found that symptom provocation caused an increase in rCBF in the
right caudate, left anterior cingulate cortex, and bilateral orbitofrontal cortex. These findings were replicated and extended in a study by McGuire and
colleagues [32]. They looked at 12 PET scans each of four patients in a
hierarchy of symptom producing stimuli. The researchers customized an
anxiety-producing protocol for each patient in which they exposed them to 12
different stimuli while in the scanner, which produced 12 levels of increasing
anxiety. They found that symptom severity correlated positively to rCBF
on the right side in the inferior frontal gyrus, caudate, putamen, globus pallidus, and thalamus and on the left side in the hippocampus and posterior
cingulate gyrus. The authors hypothesized that increases in rCBF may be
caused by urges to perform compulsive movements in the orbitofrontal cortex, thalamus, neostriatum, and globus pallidus and by anxiety in the hippocampus and posterior cingulate cortex.

In summary, despite some conflicting results, the available PET data
further suggest that OCD patients may have abnormalities in the orbitofron-
tal-caudate system, which may mediate the expression of some of the symptoms of OCD. These findings complement the findings of SPECT studies
and further support a cortical-striatal-thalamic-cortical loop theory in the
pathology of OCD.

IV. THE NEUROANATOMY OF OCD

Recent brain imaging studies provide important clues as to which brain areas may be involved in the mediation of cognitions and behaviors associated with OCD. Current data support the potential involvement of the orbitofrontal white matter, the cingulate gyrus, the caudate, and the globus pallidus, which in part make up the cortical-striatal-thalamic-cortical loop, in the pathophysiology of OCD. As we have discussed, there are numerous interconnections between these brain structures. For example, excitatory projections flow out of the orbitofrontal and cingulate cortex to the caudate nucleus and the nucleus accumbens. Inhibitory projections in turn flow from the caudate to the globus pallidus, which sends inhibitory fibers to the thalamus, which projects back to the cortex. Several researchers hypothesized that in OCD there may be an increase in the activity of the caudate nucleus [2,4]. This could occur when either the orbitofrontal cortex or the caudate itself becomes hyperactive. An increase in caudate activity would cause increased inhibition of the globus pallidus, leading to the disinhibition of the thalamus and subsequently the deregulation of this cortical-striatal-thalamic-cortical loop. Baxter has suggested [33] that the main dysfunction in OCD is in the striatum, which causes the cortex, particularly the orbitofrontal and cingulate cortex, to overfunction in order to compensate. According to this theory, the striatum, which normally screens out sensations, thoughts, and impulses related to aggression, danger, hygiene, and sex during everyday routine activities, is not doing its job. The cortex would then compensate with conscious efforts towards distraction (e.g., rituals and avoidance). Neuroimaging studies have supported this model. Structural studies show abnormalities in the striatum, particularly the caudate, and functional studies have shown that both the orbitofrontal cortex and the caudate of subjects with OCD have distinct metabolic patterns. Thus, the cortical-striatal-thalamic-cortical loop may begin to explain the unregulated disinhibition of actions and thoughts in patients with obsessive-compulsive disorder.

REFERENCES

1. Karno, J. M. Golding, S. B. Sorenson, and M. A. Burnam, The epidemiology of obsessive-compulsive disorder in five US communities, *Arch. Gen. Psychiatry* 45(12):1094 (1988).
2. T. R. Insel and J. T. Winslow, Neurobiology of obsessive compulsive disorder, *Psychiatr. Clin. North Am.* 15(4):813 (1992).
3. J. Zohar, T. R. Insel, R. C. Zohar-Kadouch, J. L. Hill, and D. L. Murphy, Serotonergic resposivity in obsessive-compulsive disorder. Effects of chronic clomipramine treatment, *Arch. Gen. Psychiatry* 45:167 (1988).

4. G. E. Alexander, M. R. DeLong, and P. L. Strick, Parallel organization of functionally segregated circuits linking basal ganglia and cortex, *Ann. Rev Neurosci. 9*:357 (1986).
5. Behar, D., Rapoport, J. L., Berg, C. J., Denckla, M. B., Mann, L., Cox, C., Fedio, P., Zahn, T., and Wolfman, M. G., Computerized tomography and neuropsychological test measures in adolescents with obsessive-compulsive disorder. *Am. J. Psychiatry 141*(3):363 (1984).
6. T. R. Insel, E. F. Donnelly, M. L. Lalakea, I. S. Alterman, and D. L. Murphy, Neurological and neuropsychological studies of patients with obsessive-compulsive disorder, *Biol Psychiatry 18*(7):741 (1983).
7. D. J. Stein, E. Hollander, S. Chan, C. M. De Caria, S. Hilal, M. R. Liebowitz, and D. F. Klein, Computed tomography and neurological soft signs in obsessive-compulsive disorder, *Psychiatry Res. 50*(3):143 (1993).
8. J. S. Luxenberg, S. E. Swedo, M. F. Flament, R. P. Friedland, J. Rapoport, and S. I. Rapoport, Neuroanatomical abnormalities in obsessive-compulsive disorder detected with quantitative X-ray computed tomography, *Am. J. Psychiatry 145*(9):1089 (1988).
9. D. Robinson, H. Wu, R. Munne, M. Ashtari, J. M. J. Alvir, G. Lerner, A. Koreen, K. Cole, and B. Bogerts, Reduced caudate nucleus volume in obsessive-compulsive disorder, *Arch. Gen. Psychiatry 52*(5):393 (1995).
10. S. Scarone, S. Colombo, S. Livian, M. Abbruzzese, P. Ronchi, M. Locatelli, G. Scotti, and E. Smeraldi, Increased right caudate nucleus size in obsessive-compulsive disorder: detection with magnetic resonance imaging, *Psychiatr. Res. 45*:115 (1992).
11. C. H. Kellner, R. R. Jolley, R. C. Holgate, L. Austin, R. B. Lydiard, M. Laraia, and J. C. Ballenger, Brain MRI in obsessive-compulsive disorder, *Psychiatry Res. 36*(1):45 (1991).
12. H. C. Breiter, P. A. Filipek, D. N. Kennedy, L. Baer, D. A. Pitcher, M. J. Olivares, P. F. Renshaw, V. S. Caviness, and M. A. Jenike, Retrocallosal white matter abnormalities in patients with obsessive-compulsive disorder, *Arch. Gen. Psychiatry 51*:663 (1994).
13. H. J. Garber, J. V. Ananth, L. C. Chiu, V. J. Griswold, and W. H. Oldendorf, Nuclear magnetic resonance study of obsessive-compulsive disorder, *Am. J. Psychiatry 146*(8):1001 (1989).
14. S. R. Machlin, G. J. Harris, G. D. Pearlson, R. Hoehn-Saric, P. Jeffery, and E. E. Camargo, Elevated medial-frontal cerebral blood flow in obsessive-compulsive patients: a SPECT study, *Am. J. Psychiatry 148*(9):1240 (1991).
15. R. T. Rubin, J. Villanueva-Meyer, J. Ananth, P. G. Trajmar, and I. Mena, Regional xenon 133 cerebral blood flow and cerebral technetium 99m HMPAO uptake in unmedicated patients with obsessive-compulsive disorder and matched normal control subjects. Determination by high-resolution single-photon emission computed tomography, *Arch. Gen. Psychiatry 49*(9):695 (1992).
16. Y. Edmonstone, M. P. Austin, N. Prentice, N. Dougall, C. L. P. Freeman, K. P. Ebmeier, and G. M. Goodwin, Uptake of 99mTc-exametazine shown by single photon emission computerized tomography in obsessive-compulsive dis-

order compared with major depression and normal controls, *Acta Psychiatr. Scand. 90*:298 (1994).

17. B. L. Adams, L. B. Warneke, A. J. McEwan, and B. A. Fraser, Single photon emission computerized tomography in obsessive compulsive disorder: a preliminary study, *J. Psychiatry Neurosci. 18*(3):109 (1993).

18. J. V. Lucey, D. C. Costa, T. Blanes, G. F. Busatto, L. S. Pilowsky, N. Takei, I. M. Marks, P. J. Ell, and R. W. Kerwin, Regional cerebral blood flow in obsessive compulsive disorder patients at rest, *Br. J. Psych. 167*:629 (1995).

19. R. Hoehn-Saric, G. D. Pearlson, G. J. Harris, S. R. Machlin, and E. E. Camargo, Effects of fluoxetine on regional cerebral blood flow in obsessive-compulsive patients, *Am. J. Psychiatry 148*(9):1243 (1991).

20. R. Hoehn-Saric, G. J. Harris, G. D. Pearlson, C. S. Cox, S. R. Machlin, and E. E. Camargo, A fluoxetine-induced frontal lobe syndrome in an obsessive compulsive patient, *J. Clin. Psychiatry 52*:3 (1991).

21. J. Zohar, T. R. Insel, K. F. Berman, E. B. Foa, J. L. Hill, and D. R. Weinberger, Anxiety and cerebral blood flow during behavioral challenge. Dissociation of central from peripheral and subjective measures, *Arch. Gen. Psychiatry 46*(6): 505 (1989).

22. L. J. Baxter, M. E. Phelps, J. C. Mazziotta, B. H. Guze, J. M. Schwartz, and C. E. Selin, Local cerebral glucose metabolic rates in obsessive-compulsive disorder. A comparison with rates in unipolar depression and in normal controls [published erratum appears in *Arch. Gen. Psychiatry 44*(9):800 (1987)], *Arch. Gen. Psychiatry 44*(3):211 (1987).

23. L. J. Baxter, J. M. Schwartz, J. C. Mazziotta, M. E. Phelps, J. J. Pahl, B. H. Guze, and L. Fairbanks, Cerebral glucose metabolic rates in nondepressed patients with obsessive-compulsive disorder, *Am. J. Psychiatry 145*(12):1560 (1988).

24. T. E. Nordahl, C. Benkelfat, W. E. Semple, M. Gross, A. C. King, and R. M. Cohen, Cerebral glucose metabolic rates in obsessive compulsive disorder, *Neuropsychopharmacology 2*(1):23 (1989).

25. S. E. Swedo, M. B. Schapiro, C. L. Grady, D. L. Cheslow, H. L. Leonard, A. Kumar, R. Friedland, S. I. Rapoport, and J. L. Rapoport, Cerebral glucose metabolism in childhood-onset obsessive-compulsive disorder, *Arch. Gen. Psychiatry 46*(6):518 (1989).

26. D. Perani, C. Colombo, S. Bressi, A. Bonfanti, F. Grassi, S. Scarone, L. Bellodi, E. Smeraldi, and F. Fazio, FDG PET study of obsessive-compulsive disorder: A clinical/metabolic correlation study after treatment, *Br. J. Psychiatry 166*:244 (1995).

27. J. L. Martinot, J. F. Allilaire, B. M. Mazoyer, E. Hantouche, J. D. Huret, F. Legaut-Demare, A. G. Deslauriers, P. Hardy, S. Pappata, J. C. Baron, et al., Obsessive-compulsive disorder: a clinical, neuropsychological and positron emission tomography study, *Acta Psychiatr. Scand. 82*(3):233 (1990).

28. C. Benkelfat, T. G. Nordahl, W. E. Semple, A. C. King, D. L. Murphy, and R. M. Cohen, Local cerebral glucose metabolic rates in obsessive-compulsive disorder. Patients treated with clomipramine, *Arch. Gen. Psychiatry 47*(9):840 (1990).

29. S. E. Swedo, P. Pietrini, H. L. Leonard, M. B. Schapiro, D. C. Rettew, E. L. Goldberger, S. I. Rapoport, J. L. Rapoport, and C. L. Grady, Cerebral glucose metabolism in childhood-onset obsessive-compulsive disorder. Revisualization during pharmacotherapy, *Arch. Gen. Psychiatry 49*(9):690 (1992).
30. L. J. Baxter, J. M. Schwartz, K. S. Bergman, M. P. Szuba, B. H. Guze, J. C. Mazziotta, A. Alazraki, C. P. Selin, H. K. Ferng, P. Munford, et al., Caudate glucose metabolic rate changes with both drug and behavior therapy for obsessive-compulsive disorder, *Arch. Gen. Psychiatry 49*(9):681 (1992).
31. S. L. Rauch, M. A. Jenike, N. M. Alpert, L. Baer, H. C. Breiter, C. R. Savage, and A. J. Fischman, Regional cerebral blood flow measured during symptom provocation in obsessive-compulsive disorder using oxygen 15-labeled carbon dioxide and positron emission tomography, *Arch. Gen. Psychiatry 51*(1):62 (1994).
32. P. K. McGuire, C. D. Bench, C. D. Frith, I. M. Marks, R. S. J. Frackowiak, and R. J. Dolan, Functional anatomy of obsessive-compulsive phenomena, *Br. J. Psychiatry 164*:459 (1994).
33. L. R. Baxter, J. M. Schwartz, B. H. Guze, K. Bergman, and M. P. Szuba, Neuroimaging in obsessive compulsive disorder: seeking the mediating neuroanatomy, *Obsessive Compulsive Disorders: Theory and Management*, 2nd ed. (M. E. Jenike, L. Baer, W. E. Minichiello, eds.), Year Book Medical Publishers, Inc., Chicago, 1990, p. 166.

18

Brain Imaging and Personality Disorders

Ingrid Kemperman, David Silbersweig, and Emily Stern
The New York Hospital—Cornell Medical Center,
New York, New York

Mark J. Russ
Hillside Hospital, Long Island Jewish Medical Center,
Glen Oaks, New York

I. INTRODUCTION

The tendency until recently has been to emphasize the role of developmental and psychosocial factors to describe the source of personality and personality disorders. The biological plausibility of brain dysfunction in personality disorders is provided by the known behavioral effects of traumatic brain injury, epilepsy (especially with temporal lobe foci), developmental disturbances, and other organic mental syndromes. Further, there is substantial evidence for a genetic basis for many personality traits in normals [1]. Neurobiological approaches to understanding personality and personality disorders are beginning to receive increasing attention.

Neurological findings in borderline personality disorder (BPD) include reports of a higher incidence of electroencephalographic abnormalities [2,3], event-related potential abnormalities [4], abnormalities on neuropsychological tests [5], and an increase of neurological soft signs [6]. Genetic, biochemical, and electrophysiological correlates of psychopathy and antisocial personality disorder are reviewed by Dolan [7]. Neurobiological studies of schizotypal personality disorder suggest a strong relationship to schizophrenia [8]. Recent studies have shown promise in elucidating the biology of particular behaviors and traits frequently exhibited in certain personality disorders. For example, low measures of serotonin activity have been associated with aggression, impulsivity, and high rates of suicide [9,10]. Recently, a specific genetic locus for the D4-dopamine receptor gene has been identified that appears to contribute to the genetic variation in the trait of novelty seeking [11,12].

Relatively little work, however, has been done to localize brain abnormalities in patients with a personality disorder diagnosis. New imaging techniques provide direct in vivo measurements of brain structure and function. In this chapter, we will provide a critical review of studies that utilize structural [computed tomography (CT) and magnetic resonance imaging (MRI)] and functional [single photon emission tomography (SPECT) and positron emission tomography (PET)] brain-imaging techniques that are relevant to the study of personality disorders. There is a growing consensus that personality disorders are not discrete categories but, instead, are aggregates of dimensional traits. These traits may lie on a spectrum of severity between normal and disordered personality. Therefore, we will review both structural and functional imaging studies of subjects with categorical diagnoses of personality disorder as well as studies that address dimensions of personality.

II. STRUCTURAL IMAGING IN PERSONALITY DISORDERS

Five structural imaging studies are reviewed (see Table 1). These provide preliminary findings on the use of MRI to look at nonspecific abnormalities in personality disorders in general, CT to find evidence of gross structural abnormalities in borderline personality disorder, and both MRI and CT along with the Wisconsin Card Sorting Test (WCST) to study schizotypal personality disorder. These studies demonstrate both the shortcomings and great potential of the use of structural imaging in personality research.

A. Personality Disorders (General)

A number of studies have found that, compared to age-matched controls, there is a greater incidence of certain brain-imaging abnormalities (e.g., ventricular enlargement, cortical atrophy, or white matter abnormalities) in a variety of psychiatric populations, including depression [13], bipolar disorder [14], and schizophrenia [15]. Depending on the their location and nature, such lesions may have specific effects on behavior and cognition and thus be variably associated with different psychiatric populations. For example, in a study of psychiatric patients (diagnoses not given) by Becker et al. [16], bifrontal white matter lesions were found to be associated with thought incoherence and right frontal-temporal white matter lesions with affective symptoms.

Woods et al. [17] performed the only published study looking at nonspecific structural imaging abnormalities, which includes patients with a diagnosis of personality disorder. The study utilizes MRI scan reports from 536 psychiatric inpatients in 10 DSM-III-R diagnostic categories (which included a general category of "personality disorder") and 51 normal control subjects. Scans were reviewed for incidence and severity of four types of abnormality: deep white matter hyperintensities, periventricular hyperintensities, ventricular enlargement, and cortical atrophy. The diagnostic categories were assigned based on the clinical diagnoses made during the hospital stay and charted in the hospital files. The personality disorder group, comprised of 60 subjects, included the 10 DSM-III-R personality disorders, personality disorder not otherwise specified, as well as multiple other diagnostic categories including the eating disorders, impulse control disorders, and posttraumatic stress disorder.

Ventricular enlargement was found to be significantly greater for the personality disorder group than for the control subjects. This was also true for the schizoaffective, substance abuse, and dementia/delirium, depressed nonpsychotic, and bipolar psychotic groups. Also, compared to controls, a significant excess of periventricular hyperintensities was present for the personality disorder group as well as the schizoaffective and dementia/delirium groups. Thus, imaging abnormalities were present in increased numbers of inpatients in multiple major psychiatric diagnostic groups, including but not specific to those with a diagnosis of personality disorder.

Table 1 Structural Imaging in Personality Disorders

N	Type; setting	Method; measures	Findings	Ref.
536/60	General psychiatric patients/ subgroup of these patients categorized as having a personality disorder	Magnetic resonance imaging (MRI) scans analyzed for deep white matter hyperintensities, periventricular hyperintensities (PVH), ventricular enlargement (VE), and cortical atrophy	Excessive ventricular enlargement and periventricular hyperintensities compared to normals in patients with the primary diagnosis of personality disorder ↑ VE in other disorders- schizoaffective disorder, substance abuse, dementia ↑ PVH in schizoaffective disorder and dementia	17
51	normal controls			
26	Patients with borderline personality disorder	CT scans qualitatively read	All scans were normal.	21
8	Patients with borderline personality disorder	CT scans-Ventricular brain rations (VBR) were calculated	The ventricular brain ratio of the borderline patients and normal controls did not differ. The teenage schizophrenic/ schizophreniform group had significantly enlarged ventricles (and VBRs) compared to the borderline patients and normal controls.	22
15	Schizophrenic/ schizophreniform pts			
18	Normal controls			
31	Patients with borderline personality disorder	Computed Tomography (CT)-analyzed for ventricle-brain ratios, third ventricular size, frontal lobe atrophy	A narrower third ventricle in borderlines was the only difference between borderline patients and normal controls.	23
28	Normal controls			
17	Normal volunteers	MRI scans; Wisconsin Card Sorting Test (WCST); Non-frontal cognitive measures; 3 scales to assess for traits of schizotypy	Higher scores on schizotypal personality measures were associated with both reduced prefrontal area and more perseveration and percentage of perseveration errors on the WCST.	26
36	Patients with schizotypal personality disorder (SPD)	CT scans; WCST; plasma HVA; MRI scans of a subset of these patients	SPD pts had larger lateral ventricles than OPD patients, no difference from schizophrenic patients. Correlations of increased lateral ventricles and frontal horn volumes with perseverative errors on the WCST in the SPD but not OPD group. Reduced plasma HVA also tended to correlate with enlarged frontal horns and impaired WCST performance in the SPD group. An MRI study of a subset of these patients demonstrated a	27
23	Patients with nonodd other personality disorders (OPD)			
133	Patients with schizophrenia			

Table 1 (*continued*)

N	Type; setting	Method; measures	Findings	Ref.
			tendency for schizophrenic patients to have less frontal region gray matter than healthy controls and SPD patients, who tended to have greater than normal grey matter. In SPD group, reduced frontal region gray matter correlated with increased perseverative errors and tended to correlate with DSM-III criteria for deficit-like symptoms.	

However, the study has significant limitations. One potential limitation is the use of multiple neuroradiologist readers and nonquantitative assessment of the MRI abnormalities; the interrater reliability cannot be reliably assessed. The diagnoses were entirely clinical, and furthermore, the "personality disorder" group included patients with other diagnoses (see above). Neuroanatomical changes such as white matter hyperintensities are known to be associated with age (probably as a result of vascular changes associated with concurrent medical illness) and abnormal neurological examinations [18,19]. This is important as Woods and colleagues note a significant interaction among age and diagnosis for the four types of abnormalities as well as significant differences in age of the various diagnostic groups. Furthermore, there is a probable selection bias: the decisions to refer for scans were made by clinicians who suspected some neurological abnormality. Therefore, although this study is of interest, a prospective study involving age-matched control subjects and a more quantitative analysis of these interactions might yield more insights into the pathophysiology of personality disorders.

B. Borderline Personality Disorder

As previously mentioned, studies of patients with borderline personality disorder (BPD) have found evidence of neurological dysfunction. An excellent discussion of the strength of the association between BPD and brain dysfunction is provided by van Reekum [20]. Evidence of structural brain abnormalities in patients with BPD have been sought in three CT scan studies [21–23].

Snyder et al. [21] obtained CT scans of 26 patients fulfilling DSM-III criteria for BPD. All scans were qualitatively read by the same neuroradiologist, who found no evidence of abnormalities. It was noted that, in particular, there was no evidence of ventricular enlargement. Schultz [22] compared the CT scans of a group of BPD patients with those of a schizophrenic and a normal population. The schizophrenic group had significantly larger ventricular-brain ratios than either of the other two groups. The borderline patients and the normal controls did not differ. Lucas et al. [23] conducted a blind study comparing 31 patients who met DSM-III and Diagnostic Interview for Borderlines (DIB) criteria for borderline personality and 28 normal controls with no concurrent neurological or medical illnesses. They used quantitative measures of ventricular-brain ratios, third ventricular size, and evidence of frontal lobe atrophy. There were no significant differences between the two groups on any of these measures except for a narrower third ventricle in borderline patients, which could be accounted for by the narrower third ventricle observed in female subjects overall. A trend toward more CT scan abnormalities was found in a small group of patients with BPD studied by van Reekum et al. (unpublished). Given the lack of significant findings from these studies and the relatively low spatial resolution of CT compared to MRI, further studies of CT scans of patients with BPD are not likely to yield significantly new information.

C. Schizotypal Personality Disorder

Schizotypal personality disorder (SPD) has long been thought to be linked to schizophrenia. Recent research has further supported this hypothesis on the basis of evidence of shared phenomenology, genetics, biology, and treatment response [8]. Structural and functional studies in schizophrenia have found evidence of ventricular enlargement, reduced frontal lobe area [24], reduced cerebral metabolism in the frontal cortex using PET, and increased perseveration errors on the WCST [25]. Two studies test the hypothesis that the structural and performance abnormalities frequently found in schizophrenia underlie schizotypal personality disorder as well as schizotypal traits in the normal population.

Raine et al. [26] tested the hypothesis that prefrontal deficits underlie schizotypal personality traits in the normal population. As part of a larger study on schizophrenia, 17 hospital workers functioning as the normal control group completed three scales used to measure schizotypal personality disorder as well as two "control" questionnaires which did not tap into the defining features of schizotypal personality disorder. These subjects underwent MRI and were tested with neuropsychological measures of prefrontal functioning—the WCST as well as two nonfrontal cognitive measures. High schizotypal scores were significantly associated with reduced prefrontal area and more WCST perseveration errors; conversely no relationships were observed between prefrontal area and measures unrelated to SPD traits. This study does not preclude the possibility that other deficits may underlie schizotypal personality disorder, as other areas of the brain were not studied.

Siegel et al. [27] performed a computed tomographic study of 36 patients with SPD, 23 patients with nonodd other personality disorder (OPD), and 133 schizophrenic patients. SPD patients were found to have larger lateral ventricles than OPD patients and no significant differences from schizophrenic patients. Increased lateral and frontal horn volumes were correlated with increased perseveration errors on the WCST, a putative frontal dopaminergic task, in the SPD group, but not in the OPD group. Reduced plasma HVA also tended to correlate with enlarged frontal horns and with impaired WCST performance in the SPD group. An MRI study of a subset of these patients demonstrated a tendency for schizophrenic patients to have less frontal region gray matter than healthy controls and SPD patients, who tended to have more than normal gray matter. In the SPD group, reduced frontal region gray matter correlated with perseverative errors on the WCST and tended to correlate with DSM-III criteria for deficitlike symptoms. Siegel and colleagues conclude that these findings suggest a relationship between deficitlike symptoms, prefrontal neuropsychological symptoms, prefrontal neuropsychological deficits, prefrontal hypodopaminergia, and reduced prefrontal cortical volume in schizotypal personality disorder.

III. FUNCTIONAL IMAGING IN PERSONALITY DISORDERS AND PERSONALITY DIMENSIONS

Ten functional imaging studies will be reviewed here (Table 2). These provide preliminary findings on the use of SPECT and PET with frontal challenge tests to study schizotypal personality disorder, PET to look for functional abnormalities in borderline and antisocial personality disorder as well as in patients with a history of violence, SPECT during a lexical decision task to study psychopathy, and PET to study normal personality traits. These methods have great promise for increasing our understanding of the physiology and structural substrates of disordered personality.

A. Schizotypal Personality Disorder

As in the above structural imaging studies, yet unpublished functional imaging studies have found evidence that schizotypy is a disorder in the spectrum of schizophrenia. Trestman et al. [28] utilized SPECT imaging to compare prefrontal functioning in males with schizotypal personality disorder with normal controls. Trestman and colleagues compared regional cerebral blood flow (rCBF) during an automated version of the WCST with that during a symbol matching test (SMT). These preliminary data suggest that, compared to normal controls, SPD patients may increase blood flow in regions of the

Table 2 Functional Imaging in Personality Disorders and Personality Dimensions

N	Type; setting	Method; measures	Findings	Ref.
10 9	Patients with schizotypal PD Normal controls	SPECT; Wisconsin Card Sorting task (WCST); Symbol Matching Test (SMT-a control task)	Patients with schizotypal PD had greater increase in blood flow to dorsolateral prefrontal cortex (DLPFC) in response to the WCST, particularly the left DLPFC. Blood flow in the medial temporal lobe decreased on the left and increased on the right during WCST vs. SMT in schizotypal PD, while the opposite occurs in normals.	28
12 10 22	Patients with schizotypal pd Patients with schizophrenia Normal controls	FDG-PET of subcortical regions; California Verbal Learning Test	In the caudate nucleus, both patient groups showed left greater than right glucose metabolism asymmetry, while controls had right greater than left asymmetry. Controls and schizophrenic patients showed a small right greater than left asymmetry of metabolism in the putamen, schizotypal patients showed a significantly more prominent asymmetry in the same direction.	29
12 19 21	Patients with schizotypal pd Patients with schizophrenia Normal controls	FDG-PET of region of interest from anterior cingulate cortex to the posterior cingulate cortex; California Verbal Learning Test	Glucose metabolic rates in the anterior cingulate cortex was lowest in the SPD group and highest in the control group, with that of schizophrenics falling between. Glucose metabolic rate in the posterior cingulate cortex was lowest in the control group and highest in the SPD group, with that of schizophrenics falling between.	30
10 15	Patients with borderline pd Normal controls	FDG-PET	Trend towards higher right than left FDG uptake in borderline patients compared to normal controls.	31
17 43	Patients with Pds: 6 antisocial PD 6 borderline PD 2 dependent PD 3 narcisistic PD Normal controls	FDG-PET; Life history of aggression scale	Borderline PD: Higher glucose metabolism in the prefrontal cortex, Lower metabolism in inferior portions of the frontal cortex, the posterior cingulate, and the left parietal area. Antisocial PD: No significant difference compared to normals. History of aggressive impulse behavior inversely correlated with glucose metabolism in the orbital and prefrontal cortex and the right temporal cortex.	35
NA	Substance abusers: Psychopaths Nonpsychopaths	SPECT imaging: lexical decision task	Psychopaths had near normal increase in right basal ganglia blood flow when they recognized neutral words. They had no expected, normal, further increase in blood flow if the word had affective content. Psychopaths also had more ventral occipital and less left temporoparietal cortical activation than normals with the affective task.	42

Table 2 (*continued*)

N	Type; setting	Method; measures	Findings	Ref.
22 22	Murderers Normal controls	FDG-PET; Continuous performance task	Murderers had lower glucose metabolism in lateral and medial frontal cortex relative to controls.	48
4 4	Psychiatric patients with history of arrests for violent behavior Normal controls	PET (FDG and H₂¹⁵O) CT; EEG	All violent patients had lower blood flow and glucose metabolism on the left temporal cortex than the right. The two patients with marked cortical atrophy on CT scans had relatively minimal dysfunction in the temporal cortex. The two violent patients with normal CT scans (one of which had a normal EEG) had a larger defect in blood flow and metabolism in the frontal and temporal cortex. Three violent patients had spiking activity in the left temporal cortex.	52
NA	Normal controls; medical school	FDG-PET; Eysenck Personality Questionnaire	Lower frontal glucose metabolism was associated with psychoticism. Higher frontal glucose metabolism was associated with neuroticism.	56
10	Normal volunteers	FDG-PET; Symptom Checklist 90 (SCL-90)	Correlations between the SCL-90 obsessive-compulsive subscale and regional orbital frontal cortical metabolism were significant for the left orbital frontal gyrus but not for the right orbital frontal gyrus. No significant correlations were found for basal ganglia metabolism and obsessive compulsive symptoms.	57
13	Healthy volunteers	H₂ ¹⁵O1PET; Cloninger's Tridimensional Personality Questionnaire	Blood flow in the brainstem and cerebellum positively correlated with higher scores on the harm-avoidance subscale. There was a trend for scores on the novelty seeking subscale to correlate positively with blood flow in the brainstem and left caudate.	58
9	Patients with bilateral Parkinson's disease	(¹⁸F)-dopa-PET; Cloninger's Tridimensional Personality Questionnaire	Dopamine uptake in the left caudate positively correlated with scores on novelty seeking.	62

NA = Number of subjects not available from meeting abstract.

dorsolateral prefrontal cortex (DLPFC) during the WCST. Schizotypal patients appear to have a dissociation of performance from rCBF in the left DLPFC, while in normals left DLPFC rCBF is inversely related to rate of perseverative errors. In addition, unlike normals, SPD patients significantly increase the DLPFC/occipital lobe ratio of rCBF during the WCST compared to the SMT. This evidence of frontal blood flow increase during the WCST is the opposite of that seen in schizophrenia, implicating a possible compensatory mechanism functioning in schizotypal personality disorder. On the other hand, Trestman and colleagues found that the rCBF of SPD patients parallels the abnormalities seen in schizophrenia in the medial temporal lobes (including the hippocampus and adjacent structures): blood flow decreases on the left and increases on the right during WCST versus SMT, while the opposite pattern occurs in normal controls.

In another study, Siegel et al. [29] utilized PET to examine the subcortical regions of 22 healthy controls, 10 schizophrenic patients, and 12 SPD patients. The subjects performed a modified version of the California Verbal Learning Test during the 18-fluoro-2-deoxyglucose uptake period preceding PET scan acquisition. The three groups showed different patterns of striatal metabolism. While controls and schizophrenic patients showed a right greater than left asymmetry of metabolism in the putamen, SPD patients showed significantly more prominent asymmetry in the same direction. In the caudate nucleus, both patient groups demonstrated left greater than right metabolic asymmetry, while controls had a right greater than left asymmetry in that region. These findings suggest abnormal striatal function in SPD, which may reflect a particular form of dopaminergic system dysfunction in schizophrenia spectrum illness.

Haznedar et al. [30] examine the role of cingulate pathology and the concept of hypofrontality in schizophrenia spectrum illness. The authors point out that the anterior cingulate cortex is of particular interest in schizophrenia, as it has been implicated in both attentional and affective behaviors, and postmortem studies have shown cytoarchitectural changes of the cingulate in schizophrenic subjects. In this study, glucose metabolism was measured during the California Verbal Learning Test using PET in 12 SPD patients, 19 schizophrenic patients, and 21 normal controls. Patients were off all psychoactive medication for at least 2 weeks and had negative urine screens for drug abuse. Cingulate glucose metabolic rate (GMR) was measured in 12 regions of interest from the anterior cingulate cortex to the posterior cingulate cortex. Measurements of GMR in the medial frontal regions anterior to the anterior cingulate cortex was done for comparison. Glucose metabolic rate in the anterior cingulate cortex was lowest in the SPD group and highest in the control group, with that of the schizophrenics falling between. In contrast, glucose metabolism in the posterior cingulate cortex was highest in the SPD group, with that of the schizophrenics falling between.

B. Borderline Personality Disorder

De la Fuente et al. [31] conducted a PET study with 18-F-fluorodeoxyglucose (FDG) of the temporal lobes of 10 patients with borderline personality disorder and 15 controls. This study tests the hypothesis that temporal epileptic phenomena are involved in the etiology of BPD. This hypothesis has been put forth for a number of reasons. It has been noted that certain clinical features in BPD such as the paroxysmal and brief changes in affect and behavior, the lack of control of anger, impulsivity, and the high incidence of dissociative experiences are examples of symptoms also shared by patients with temporal lobe foci and complex partial seizures (CPS). A pilot study indicated that carbamazepine, the most effective treatment for CPS, might be effective in BPD [32]. For the detection of temporal lobe foci in CPS, the sensitivity and specificity of surface EEG recordings are relatively low [33], while PET has been found to be useful [34].

De la Fuente and colleagues found no significant differences between the patient and control groups. Although this finding does not support the involvement of temporal lobe epilepsy in the etiology of BPD, it does not specifically exclude a role for overactivity of the limbic system. De la Fuente and colleagues did report a trend towards higher right than left FDG uptake in the posterior part of the temporal lobe in BPD patients compared with control subjects.

Goyer et al. [35] used PET to examine regional cerebral metabolic rates of glucose (rCMRG) in patients with personality disorders, with a particular focus on the frontal lobes. An auditory cortical activation procedure with a continuous performance task (CPT) was used during the scan. Goyer studied 43 normal controls and 17 personality disorder patients. The diagnostic groups included antisocial ($n = 6$), borderline ($n = 6$), dependent ($n = 2$), and narcissistic ($n = 3$) personality disorder. The dependent and narcissistic personality disorder group were not separately analyzed due to the small number of patients in each group. Both the patients and the normal controls were without significant medical or neurological illnesses, medication-free for at least 2 weeks, and not abusing alcohol or substances during the study period. All subjects were screened for psychiatric illness with a semistructured clinical interview. Thirteen of the personality disorder patients had a past history of either major depression or adjustment disorder; the axis I disorder had resolved in 10 of them at the time of the PET scan.

Goyer and colleagues found a number of differences between normals and patients with borderline personality disorder. Within the frontal lobes, patients with BPD demonstrated two significant differences between normalized rCMRG compared to the controls: an increase in the prefrontal cortex (superior frontal and inferior frontal gyrus) and a decrease in more inferior portions of the frontal lobes (middle frontal/inferior frontal/precentral gyri). With regard to the frontal lobe findings, this group of borderline patients shares some findings with other diagnostic groups but appears to exhibit a unique combination of area of increases and decreases in cerebral metabolic rates of glucose.

For example, frontal lobe increases in rCMRG for other nonpsychotic and nonsubstance abuse diagnostic groups (i.e., panic disorder [36], obsessive-compulsive disorder [37]) have been documented; these findings, however, have been localized predominant in the orbital frontal cortex or a combination of orbital frontal and prefrontal cortex. In a PET study of adults with hyperactivity of childhood onset, Zametkin et al. [38] reported significant bilateral decreases in absolute rCMRG in the same frontal lobe regions on which Goyer found decreases, but normalized rCMRG in Zametkin's study was significantly decreased only on the left.

When nonfrontal regions of interest of the borderline patients were explored in Goyer's study, it was found that mean normalized rCMRG was lower in the posterior cingulate and left parietal area. These areas are involved in sensory integration. No differences were found for subcortical regions in the basal ganglia and thalamus. The finding of decreased normalized rCMRG in the left posterior parietal region in borderline patients has been reported by Nordahl et al. [36] for panic disorder and Goyer et al. [39] for summer seasonal affective disorder. In a study by Nordahl et al. [40], a trend for a decrease in normalized rCMRG ($p = 0.06$) was also reported in a study of patients with obsessive-compulsive disorder. Goyer hypothesizes that a biological correlate for anxiety may exist in the posterior parietal area. However, in a study of patients with major depression examined categorically and dimensionally [41], decreased regional cerebral blood flow (rCBF) in the left inferior parietal lobule correlated with psychomotor retardation and depressed mood, while measures of anxiety were related to *increased* blood flow in the inferior parietal lobules bilaterally (along with posterior cingulate cortex). In the future, correlational analyses with dimensional measures of depression and anxiety could be utilized in functional imaging studies of BPD to test such hypotheses.

More PET studies are needed to explore the significance of Goyer's preliminary findings. Goyer and colleagues note that the borderline subjects scored relatively low on the Diagnostic Interview for Borderlines (DIB), suggesting that this group may not be as severely ill as other groups of patients with BPD. This is further supported by the absence of any axis I diagnosis in five of the six BPD patients at the time of the scan. Consequently, glucose metabolic findings that tend to distinguish this group of BPD patients may differ in a more severely ill group.

C. Antisocial Personality Disorder

In the study by Goyer and colleagues [35], no differences were found in normalized rCMRG metabolism between normals and patients with antisocial personality disorder. Activation studies that target suspected defects in the disorder being studied can reveal useful information (as seen with the use of the WCST in the studies of schizotypal personality disorder previously described). This is illustrated in a study described below [42], which utilized an activation procedure related to findings from previous studies of psychopathy.

Antisocial personality disorder is characterized by a number of features including a tendency to not conform to social norms. It is well known that sociopaths fail to demonstrate appropriate levels of anxiety in situations involving punishment or threat of punishment. This failure is evident in observable behavior and is indexed by measures such as skin conductance response (SCR). Sociopaths show poor SCR conditioning with aversive unconditioned stimuli such as shock and defective SCRs on anticipation of aversive stimuli [43,44]. Utilizing SCRs, Damasio [45] found that patients with acquired sociopathy due to bifrontal lesions had abnormal autonomic responses to socially meaningful stimuli such as pictures depicting social disaster, mutilation, and nudity. These findings have been interpreted as indicating that the sociopath's inability to avoid punishment is related to a failure to respond emotionally to perceived consequences of behavior [45,46].

Utilizing SPECT, Intrator et al. [42] studied psychopaths' response to negative affective verbal stimuli by comparing cerebral blood flow in psychopath and nonpsychopath substance abusers in a veterans hospital during a lexical decision task. She found that psychopaths had a near normal increase in right basal ganglia blood flow when they recognized neutral words but no expected, normal, further increase in blood flow when the words had a negative affective content. It was also found that the psychopaths had more ventral occipital and less temporoparietal cortical activation than normals with the affective task. Although this study is preliminary, it provides support for the hypothesis that psychopaths respond abnormally to stimuli with aversive emotional significance.

D. Aggression and Violence

Goyer et al. [35] also explored the relationship between frontal lobe rCMRG and aggressive impulse difficulties in a group of 17 patients with personality disorders. A modified version of the life history of aggression rating scale [47] was administered to the patients, which includes rating of history of aggression directed towards people, property, or self (i.e., suicide attempts). Goyer and colleagues found an inverse correlation of rCMRG in the orbital and prefrontal cortex as well as the right temporal cortex and history of aggressive behavior impulse difficulties. These findings in a group of subjects with various personality disorders attest to the importance of looking at dimensions of personality, which often cut across diagnostic groups.

Consistent with Goyer's finding in relation to aggression, Raine et al. [48] found decreased rCMRG in the prefrontal cortex of murderers. In this study, 20 subjects charged with murder, 2 charged with attempted murder (labeled below as "murderers" for ease of reference), and 22 age-matched and gender-matched controls were studied with PET to measure local cerebral uptake of glucose during the continuous performance task (CPT). A degraded stimulus version of the CPT was employed as a frontal challenge task because it has been shown to produce increases in relative glucose metabolic rate in the frontal lobes of normal controls in addition to increases in the right temporal and parietal lobes. The subjects had been referred for imaging to obtain evidence relating to an insanity defense or to determine capability of understanding the judicial process (incompetent to stand trial), although some who had been found guilty were referred to obtain information for diminished capacity as an ameliorating circumstance in the sentencing phase of the trial. The particular reasons for referral were diverse and included a history of schizophrenia, organic brain damage, substance abuse, affective disorder, hyperactivity and learning disability, and paranoid and passive-aggressive personality disorder. The control groups were age and sex matched and, like the patient group, included three schizophrenics. It is important to recognize that the findings of Raine's study relate specifically to subjects accused of murder in whom questions regarding mental illness or organic brain injury have been raised.

Raine and colleagues [48] found widespread reduced prefrontal glucose metabolism in the murderer group compared to controls. More detailed analyses of specific subareas indicated the effect was the strongest for anterior medial and for the higher supraventricular superior frontal cortex (relative to lower ventricular levels). Murderers had lower lateral prefrontal activity for the left but not the right hemisphere relative to controls. There was also a trend towards reduced activity in the orbital frontal cortex. The prefrontal deficit found in their sample of murderers appears to be specific and does not appear to reflect generalized brain dysfunction. Groups did not differ on posterior frontal, temporal, or parietal lobe measures. Glucose levels for a particular area were expressed as a ratio of all other brain areas in that slice and therefore reflect relative glucose metabolic deficits. When prefrontal/occipital ratios were compared, reduced prefrontal activation relative to occipital cortex was found in the murderers. There were no group differences in behavioral performance on the CPT, indicating that the prefrontal deficits cannot be attributed to a motivational deficit. Raine et al. postulated that other cortical or subcortical regions not normally utilized on this task compensated for the prefrontal dysfunction in murderers, thus allowing them to perform as well as controls on the CPT.

Although it is likely that a diagnosis of personality disorder (especially antisocial personality disorder) may be overrepresented in a study of murderers, psychiatric diagnoses were not made in the subjects of Raine's study [48]. The systematic finding of the prefrontal deficit in a heterogeneous group of violent offenders points to the likely importance of this finding in relation to violence. Using data from several sources, individual differences in violence committed within the murderer group were assessed (i.e., planned vs. impulsive, sexual involvement vs. nonsexual, etc.). There were no significant differences in the two global prefrontal measures when the murderer subgroups were compared. However, the sample size was reduced and a substantial effect size was observed in the direction of impulsive murderers having lower prefrontal glucose metabolism than murderers who planned their act. Future studies of larger samples of violent offenders may tell us the significance of the type of violence in relation to deficits in the prefrontal area.

Although frontal deficits have been observed in various axis I disorders, the pattern of findings for murderers differs from these groups. Schizophrenics, in addition to showing frontal deficits, also show right temporal and right parietal deficits to the CPT [49], whereas no such deficits were observed in murderers. Major depression has most often been associated with a deficit in the left dorsolateral prefrontal cortex [50], but has also been associated with bilateral changes [51]. Murderers show largely a bilateral deficit that extends beyond dorsolateral prefrontal cortex.

Volkow and Tancredi [52] evaluated four males from an in-patient psychiatric unit with a history of at least three legal arrests because of violent behavior, using EEG, CT, and PET with both 15-oxygen–labeled water for determination of cerebral blood flow and FDG for determination of glucose metabolism. The patients carried multiple and diverse psychiatric diagnoses, which included bipolar disorder, posttraumatic stress disorder, and substance abuse. One of the four patient subjects carried the clinical diagnosis of borderline personality disorder. This patient had a history of outbursts of violent behavior since the age of 15, for which he had no recall. Two of the four patients exhibited violent behavior while intoxicated. The left temporal/right temporal (LT/RT) and frontal/occipital (F/O) ratios of the four violent patients for FDG and CBF were compared to the LT/RT and F/O for CBF of four normal controls.

The PET scans for all four patients in Volkow and Tancredi's study [52] showed temporal cortex asymmetry, with left showing lower blood flow and metabolism than the right. The CT scans of two patients (one of which carried the diagnosis of BPD) revealed marked cortical atrophy, and their PET scans showed relatively minimal dysfunction—a relatively mild decrease in blood flow in the left temporal cortex. The other two patients showed comparatively larger areas of defect (decreased metabolism and blood flow) in the frontal and temporal cortex, yet their CT scans were normal. This illustrates that new functional imaging techniques such as PET allow us to detect cerebral pathology, which was henceforth unrecognized by the CT scan. It is interesting to note that the two patients who experienced no remorse for their actions also demonstrated hypofrontality on their PET scans.

Volkow and Tancredi point out that the analysis of the violent act is of importance in understanding possible neural system implications in its occurrence. Particular areas of cerebral dysfunction may facilitate violent outbursts through various mechanisms. Defects in the prefrontal area, which is implicated in higher cognitive functions such as abstraction [53], could facilitate the occurrence of violent behavior because of the inability to understand concepts such as right or wrong or to appraise the consequences of, or inhibit, the violent act. Abnormalities in the limbic areas (including the medial temporal cortex), which appear to be involved in generation of affects and emotions, could elicit feelings that arise in vacuo [54]. This type of patient will tend to show random outbursts of rage and violence with very poor impulse control [55]. This subtype of violent individual appears to have a higher incidence of EEG abnormalities [7]. Abnormalities in the association areas of the brain that lead to derangements in perception may evoke assaultive behavior when a stimulus is perceived as threatening.

E. Personality Traits in the Normal Population

A few recent, yet unpublished, studies correlate specific personality factors with measures of brain function. Semple [56] reported a PET study of normal medical students who completed the Eysenck personality questionnaire. This study found that lower frontal glucose metabolism was associated with psychoticism. Higher frontal glucose metabolism was associated with neuroticism. Kraft et al. [57] looked at the relationship of obsessionality in normals with orbital frontal and basal ganglia metabolism. In Kraft's study 10 normal volunteers underwent FDG-PET scans and were administered the Symptom Checklist 90, which includes an assessment of obsessive-compulsive symptoms. Correlation between the obsessive-compulsive subscale and regional orbital frontal cortical metabolism was significant for the left orbital frontal gyrus, but not for the right orbital frontal gyrus or basal ganglia.

In a $H_2^{15}O$-PET study of 13 normal volunteers, George et al. [58] correlated regional brain activity and three personality dimensions from the Cloninger's Tridimensional Questionnaire (TPQ): novelty seeking, harm avoidance, and reward dependence, putatively related to distributed brain networks regulated by dopamine, norepinephrine, and serotonin, respectively. rCBF in the brainstem and cerebellum positively correlated with higher scores on the harm-avoidance subscale. There was a trend for scores on the novelty-seeking subscale to correlate positively with rCBF in the brainstem and left caudate, an area rich in dopamine.

The relationship between dopamine and novelty seeking is supported by evidence that dopamine mediates exploratory and self-stimulation behavior in experimental animals [59,60] and that the rewarding effects of amphetamines and cocaine in both humans and animals are related to dopamine release [61]. Other recent studies have also related dopamine to the novelty-seeking trait. Clinicians have long observed an association between Parkinson's disease and certain personality traits (such as seriousness), both premorbidly and after the onset of the motor symptoms. Menza et al. [62] examined the relationship between dopaminergic function, as reflected by (^{18}F) dopa uptake on PET scanning, and Cloninger's TPQ personality measures in nine patients with bilateral Parkinson's disease. Antiparkinsonian medication was stopped 12 hours prior to the scan. Correlational analysis between scores on the TPQ and the (^{18}F) dopa uptake values for the left, right, and mean caudate and putamen were performed. Scores on novelty seeking were significantly correlated with uptake in left caudate. No significant correlation was found between novelty seeking, harm avoidance, or reward dependence and uptake in other striatal sites. Other relevant areas, such as the mesolimbic dopamine system (which can impact on caudate function), were not studied. Two groups, Ebstein et al. [11] and Benjamin et al. [12], have now identified a specific genetic locus for the D4 dopamine receptor gene that contributes to the genetic variation in the novelty-seeking trait.

IV. CONCLUSION

Many of the studies presented in this chapter are recent and the findings preliminary. The most consistent findings were in the studies of SPD, which utilized performance tasks to target suspected deficits, and in the studies looking at the dimension of violence and aggression. The findings in both these areas demonstrate the utility of a dimensional view of psychopathology when conducting research.

The structural imaging studies support an association of impairment of the WCST with reduced prefrontal area in SPD patients. These changes were also correlated with deficitlike symptoms of SPD in the normal population. In Siegel's study [27], impaired WCST also tended to correlate with reduced plasma HVA, reflecting hypodopaminergia. The reduced frontal region gray matter, impaired frontal lobe function, and associated hypodopaminergia parallels the abnormalities found in schizophrenics. In contrast, SPECT imaging utilizing the WCST revealed that blood flow is increased in the prefrontal cortex in SPD patients compared to normals (even in the face of normal to slightly subnormal performance on the WCST), rather than decreased as usually seen in schizophrenia [63]. However, Frith et al. [64] showed increased activation of the frontal lobes with word-generation task in schizophrenics, demonstrating that failure to activate the frontal lobes is not always present in schizophrenics. Other areas of abnormality demonstrated in the functional imaging studies of schizotypal personality disorder include the cingulate, striatum, and temporal lobe. Again, although these areas are also known to be affected in schizophrenia, the findings in these regions do not consistently parallel those of schizophrenics. It has been suggested that some of the differences between SPD and schizophrenia reflect a compensatory strategy in SPD patients for inefficient cortical processing. In any case, the differences go against the view that SPD is simply a mild form of schizophrenia. Nevertheless, the study of Cluster A personality disorders such as schizotypal personality disorder suggests a close relationship with schizophrenia and affords an unusual opportunity to disentangle the neurophysiological dimensions underlying the schizophrenia spectrum disorders.

Another finding emerging from functional imaging of personality dimensions is the association of decreased frontal activity and history of aggression. This association was found in patients with a variety of personality disorders [35] as well as studies that included an even more heterogeneous group of subjects [48,52]. The systematic finding of frontal lobe deficits in relation to a history of violence and aggression in a heterogeneous group of patients points to the importance of this finding in relation to violence. Abnormalities in the temporal lobe may also facilitate violence as demonstrated in Volkow and Tancredi's study [52]. This may be related to emotional dysregulation leading to sudden outbursts of rage. As violence can be facilitated by a number of factors, it is important that the nature of the violent acts be analyzed. Raine's study [48] found a tendency for impulsive murderers to have lower prefrontal glucose metabolism than murderers who planned their act.

Future studies of larger samples of subjects with a history of aggressive and violent behaviors can tell us the significance of the type of violence in relation to particular localized brain deficits. In previous biological studies of violent offenders, low CSF concentrations of 5-hydroxyindoleatic acid (5-HIAA) were found in impulsive violent offenders and not in those whose violence was planned [65]. The bridge between such peripheral chemical studies and functional anatomical studies could be made with chemically specific SPECT or PET ligands, which provide central, localized measures of specific neurochemical function. Alternatively, pharmacological challenges can be performed in which a patient's blood flow or metabolism is assessed before and after a specific pharmacological agent is administered.

Other brain-imaging studies of categorical personality disorders were done on patients with borderline and antisocial personality disorder. CT studies found no evidence of gross brain abnormalities in patients with borderline personality disorder compared to normals. Future structural imaging may employ MRI-based computerized morphometric analyses, which have recently been developed [66]. These quantitative measures provide high resolution of specific brain structures and show promise as a more rigorous approach that could be applied to the study of personality disorders. Voxel-by-voxel analyses of magnetic resonance images are also being explored [67]. In any event, an absence of findings in structural imaging studies does not rule out functional brain dysfunction, as illustrated by Volkow and Tancredi's study [52] in which PET detected abnormalities unrecognized in the CT scans on the same patients.

A number of differences in brain glucose metabolism were found in borderline patients compared to normals [35]. Although a number of these regional differences can be found in other diagnostic groups, the combination of increases and decreases in cerebral metabolism appears to be unique to BPD. This highlights the point that functional imaging studies in psychiatry may need to focus more on observing specific patterns of deficits in order to obtain neuroanatomical specificity for the condition under scrutiny. Although Goyer and colleagues found no difference in brain function between normals and patients with antisocial personality disorder, differences were found by Intrator [42] utilizing an activation paradigm. This points to the power of activation studies that target suspected areas of dysfunction of the disorder under study. Correlational analyses with dimensional measures may also help with the interpretation of the findings.

Findings from recent preliminary PET studies suggest that there may be links between stable personality traits in the normal population and regional brain function. This is exemplified by preliminary evidence for brain correlates of such traits as harm avoidance, novelty seeking, and obsessionality. As with the finding that prefrontal deficits underlie schizotypal personality traits in the normal population [26], some of these normal personality traits may reflect an attenuated version of a spectrum disorder.

The study of axis II pathology is complex due to the heterogeneity of patients with the same personality disorder diagnosis. The multiple criteria in DSM allow many ways to reach the same diagnosis, and patients with one axis II diagnosis often have other personality disorder diagnoses as well [68]. Furthermore, patients with personality disorders have high frequencies of concurrent or lifetime axis I disorders [69]. The issue of comorbidity in patients with a personality disorder diagnosis has led to much controversy, as exemplified in the debate about borderline personality disorder. On the one hand, it has been pointed out that BPD has unique symptomatology which can be reliably discriminated from other axis II disorders [70] and that the comorbidity between BPD and axis I disorders is nonspecific [69]. Yet it has also been suggested that BPD could be alternatively classified as a variant of an affective disorder, schizophrenia, posttraumatic stress disorder, and the impulse control disorders [71–74]. The overlap between the phenomenology of borderline personality disorder and the axis I disorders raises questions about their relationship. Are they separate but comorbid disorders? Does one contribute to the development of the other? Do they share common etiological backgrounds to the point that they are a variant of the same disorder? In general, the literature supports the growing recognition of differences among subtypes as well as etiologies of personality disorders [7,20,75]. The central, in vivo neurobiological correlates that functional neuroimaging provides can help to clarify these issues.

Conversely, these issues are important when considering neurobiological studies of personality disorders, as they point to the necessity of a careful characterization of the subjects being studied. This includes an assessment of axis I and axis II disorders, with attention to dimensional features, as well as a thorough developmental and neurological history. This process of assessment will help avoid the confound of comorbidity and aid the development of more homogeneous study populations or a more sophisticated assessment of clinical variance. By knowing precisely what factors are being studied, the probability of achieving positive research results will be increased.

New, high-sensitivity, 3-D $H_2^{15}O$-PET activation techniques [76] allow the study of individual subjects, and hence their neurobiological variability, as well as groups. Although PET is the current gold standard for high-sensitivity imaging of neural systems throughout the entire brain, functional MRI (fMRI) is another technique that is extremely promising and is advancing rapidly [77]. The higher resolution and lack of radiation are attractive attributes of fMRI, although areas of signal void at the ventral aspect of the brain (which are of particular interest in psychiatric disease) may be problematic and will require continued technical advances to overcome. There have also been advances in image processing and analysis that will aid in the study of personality disorders. These include image realignment (to correct for slight interscan head movement), image co-registration across modalities (such as PET and MRI), image transformation to standardized coordinate spaces (for group comparisons), and the complementary use of categorical and correlational study designs and statistical analyses.

Clinically, structural imaging should be used when a neurological disorder is suspected or with patients presenting with a change in personality. Functional neuroimaging of personality disorders is not clinically indicated at this time. Neuroimaging studies are, however, increasing our understanding of the basic mechanisms underlying personality disorders. This is a prerequisite for developing biologically specific diagnostic and therapeutic clinical strategies for the axis II disorders. As such, neuroimaging studies, if well designed, hold the promise of shedding light on many of the controversies within the personality literature and aiding in the development of strategies for the treatment of personality disorders.

REFERENCES

1. W. J. Lively, K. L. Jang, D. N. Jackson, and P. A. Vernon, Genetic and environmental contributions to dimensions of personality disorder, *Am. J. Psychiatry 150*:1826 (1993).
2. R. W. Cowdry, D. Pickar, and R. Davies, Symptoms and EEG findings in the borderline syndrome, *Int. J. Psychiatry Med. 15*:201 (1985).
3. S. Snyder and W. M. 'Pitts Jr, Electroencephalography of DSM-III borderline personality disorder, *Acta Psychiatr. Scand. 69*:129 (1984).
4. S. P. Kutcher, H. R. Blackwood, D. St Clair, D. F. Gaskell, and W. J. Muir, Auditory P300 in borderline personality disorder and schizophrenia, *Arch. Gen. Psychiatry 44*:645 (1987).
5. K. M. O'Leary, P. Brouwers, D. L. Gardner, et al., Neuropsychological testing of patients with borderline personality disorder, *Am. J. Psychiatry 148*:106 (1991).
6. D. Gardner, P. B. Lucas, R. W. Cowdry, Soft sign neurologic abnormalities in borderline personality disorder and normal control subjects, *J. Nerv. Ment. Dis. 175*:117 (1987).
7. M. Dolan, Psychopathy—a neurobiological perspective, *Br. J. Psychiatry 165*:151 (1994).
8. L. J. Siever, Biologic factors in schizotypal personal disorders, *Acta Pschiatr. Scand. 90*:45 (1994).
9. A. Roy, J. DeJong, and M. Linnoila, Cerebrospinal fluid monamine oxidase metabolites and suicidal behavior in depressed patients: a five year follow-up study, *Arch. Gen. Psychiatry 46*:609 (1989).
10. E. F. Coccaro, L. J. Siever, H. M. Klar, et al., Serotonergic studies in patients with affective and personality disorder: correlates with suicidal and impulsive aggressive behavior, *Arch. Gen. Psychiatry 49*:587 (1989).
11. R. P. Ebstein, O. Novick, R. Umansky, et al., Dopamine D4 receptor (D4DR) exon III polymorphism associated with the human personality trait of novelty seeking, *Nature Genetics 12*:78 (1996).
12. J. Benjamin, L. Li, C. Patterson, et al., Population and familial association between the D4 dopamine receptor gene and measures of novelty seeking, *Nature Genetics 12*:81 (1996).
13. K. Krishnan, V. Goli, E. H. Ellinwood, et al., Leukoencephalopathy in patients diagnosed as major depressive, *Biol. Psychiatry 23*:519 (1988).
14. G. S. Figiel, K. R. R. Krishnan, V. P. Rao, M. Doraiswamy, et al., Subcortical hyperintensities on brain magnetic resonance imaging: a comparison of normal and bipolar subjects, *J. Neuropsychiatry Clin. Neurosci. 3*:18 (1991).
15. J. C. Breitner, M. M. Husain, G. S. Figiel, et al., Cerebral white matter disease in late-onset paranoid psychosis, *Biol. Psychiatry 28*:266 (1990).
16. T. Becker, A. Schmidtke, G. Stober, et al., Hyperintense Marklagerlasionen bei psychiatrischen Patienten, *Nervenaerzt 65*:191 (1994).

17. B. T. Woods, S. Brennan, D. Yurgelun-Todd, et al., MRI abnormalities in major psychiatric disorders: an exploratory comparative study, *J. Neuropsychiatry Clin. Neurosci. 7*:49 (1995).

18. R. F. Deicken, V. I. Reus, L. Manfredi, and O. M. Wolkowitz, MRI deep white matter hyperintensities in a psychiatric population, *Biol. Psychiatry 29*:918 (1991).

19. F. W. Brown, R. J. Lewine, P. A. Hudgins, and S. C. Risch, White matter hyperintensity signals in psychiatric and nonpsychiatric subjects, *Am. J. Psychiatry 149*:620 (1992).

20. R. van Reekum, Acquired and developmental brain dysfunction in borderline personality disorder, *Can. J. Psychiatry 38*:S4 (1993).

21. S. Snyder, W. M. Pitts Jr., and Q. Gustin, CT scans of patients with borderline personality disorder, *Am. J. Psychiatry 140*:272 (1983).

22. S. C. Schultz, M. K. Miriam, P. R. Kishore, et al., Ventricular enlargement in teenage patients with schizophrenia spectrum disorder, *Am. J. Psychiatry 140*: 1592 (1983).

23. P. B. Lucas, D. L. Gardner, R. W. Cowdry, and D. Pickar, Cerebral structure in borderline personality disorder, *Psychiatry Res. 27*:111 (1989).

24. N. Andreasen, H. A. Nasarallah, V. Dunn, et al., Structural abnormalities in the frontal system in schizophrenia, *Arch. Gen. Psychiatry 43*:136 (1986).

25. D. R. Weinberger, K. F. Berman, and R. F. Zec, Physiologic dysfunction of dorsolateral prefrontal cortex in schizophrenia, *Arch. Gen. Psychiatry 43*:114 (1986).

26. A. Raine, C. Sheard, G. P. Reynolds, and T. Lencz, Pre-frontal structural and functional deficits associated with individual differences in schizotypal personality, *Schizophr. Res. 7*:237 (1992).

27. B. V. Siegel, M. S. Buchsbaum, L. J. Siever, and R. L. Trestman, Dopamine function and MRI measures in schizotypy, Annual Psychiatric Association Annual Meeting '95, Miami, Syllabus & Proceedings Summary (Symposium), p. 76.

28. R. L. Trestman, M. S. Buchsbaum, B. V. Siegel, et al., SPECT imaging of cognition in schizotypals, American Psychiatric Association Annual Meeting '95, Miami, Syllabus & Proceedings Summary, p. 76.

29. B. V. Siegel, L. J. Siever, R. L. Trestman, and M. S. Buchsbaum, Regional brain glucose metabolism in schizotypal personality disorder, American College of Neuropsychopharmacology 33rd Annual Meeting '94, San Juan, Peurto Rico, Abstracts of panels and posters, p. 148.

30. M. M. Haznedar, M. S. Buchsbaum, B. V. Siegel, et al., Cingulate metabolism in schizophrenia spectrum, American Psychiatric Association Annual Meeting '95, Miami, New Research and Abstracts, p. 152.

31. J. M. De la Fuente, F. Lotstra, S. Goldman, et al., Temporal glucose metabolism in borderline personality disorder, *Psychiatr. Res. 55*:237 (1994).

32. R. W. Cowdry, and D. L. Gardner, Pharmacotherapy of borderline personality disorder, *Arch. Gen. Psychiatry 45*:111 (1988).

33. J. R. Stevens, Emotional activation of the electroencephalogram in patients with convulsive disorders, *J. Nerv. Ment. Dis. 128*:339 (1959).

34. W. H. Theodore, B. Jabbari, D. Leiderman, et al., Positron emission tomography in epilepsy: comparison of cerebral blood flow and glucose metabolism, *Ann. Neurol. 28*:262 (1990).
35. P. F. Goyer, P. J. Andreason, W. E. Semple, et al., Positron-emission tomography and personality disorders, *Neuropsychopharmacology 10*:21 (1994).
36. T. E. Nordahl, W. E. Semple, M. Gross, et al., Cerebral glucose metabolic differences in patients with panic disorder, *Neuropsychopharmacology 3*:261 (1990).
37. C. Benkelfat, D. L. Murphy, J. Zohar, et al., Clomipramine in obsessive-compulsive disorder. Further evidence of serotonergic mechanisms of action, *Arch. Gen. Psychiatry 46*:23 (1989).
38. A. J. Zametkin, T. E. Nordahl, M. Gross, et al., Cerebral glucose metabolism in adults with hyperactivity of childhood onset, *N. Engl. J. Med. 323*:1361 (1990).
39. P. F. Goyer, P. M. Schulz, W. E. Semple, et al., Cerebral glucose metabolism in patients with summer seasonal affective disorder, *Neuropsychopharmacology 7*:233 (1992).
40. T. E. Nordahl, C. Benkelfat, W. E. Semple, et al., Cerebral glucose metabolic rates in obsessive-compulsive disorder, *Neuropsychopharmacology 2*:23 (1989).
41. C. J. Bench, K. J. Friston, R. G. Brown, R. S. Frackowiak, and R. J. Dolan, Regional cerebral blood flow in depression measured by positron emission tomography: the relationship with clinical dimensions, *Psychol. Med. 23*:579 (1993).
42. J. Intrator, SPECT imaging in psychopaths during the lexical decision task, Third International Conference of the International Society for the Study of Personality Disorders '93, Cambridge, MA.
43. R. D. Hare, Electrodermal and cardiovascular correlates of psychopathy, *Psychopathic Behavior: Approaches to Research* (R. D. Hare and D. Schalling, eds.), Wiley, New York, 1970, p. 107.
44. D. T. Lykken, A study of anxiety in the sociopathic personality, *J. Abnormal Social Psychol. 55*:6 (1957).
45. A. R. Damasio, D. Tranel, and H. Damasio, Individuals with sociopathic behavior caused by frontal damage fail to respond autonomically to social stimuli, *Behav. Brain Res. 41*:81 (1990).
46. R. D. Hare and M. J. Quinn, Psychopathy and autonomic conditioning, *J. Abnormal Psychol. 7*:408 (1971).
47. G. L. Brown, F. K. Goodwin, J. C. Ballenger, et al., Aggression in humans correlates with cerebrospinal fluid amine metabolites, *Psychiatry Res. 1*:131 (1979).
48. A. Raine, M. S. Buchsbaum, J. Stanley, et al., Selective reductions in prefrontal glucose metabolism in murderers, *Biol. Psychiatry 36*:365 (1994).
49. M. S. Buchsbaum, K. H. Neuchterlein, R. J. Haier, et al., Glucose metabolic rate in normals and schizophrenics during the continuous performance test assessed by positron emission tomography, *Br. J. Psychiatry 156*:216 (1990).
50. L. R. Baxter, J. M. Schwartz, and M. E. Phelps, Reduction of prefrontal cortex

glucose metabolism common to three types of depression, *Arch. Gen. Psychiatry 46*:243 (1989).

51. H. S. Mayberg, Functional imaging studies in secondary depression, *Psychiatr. Ann. 24*:643 (1994).
52. N. D. Volkow and L. Tancredi, Neural substrates of violent behavior. A preliminary study with positron emission tomography, *Br. J. Psychiatry 151*:668 (1987).
53. A. R. Luria, *Higher Cortical Functions in Man*, Basic Books, New York, 1966.
54. D. P. Blumer, H. W. Williams, V. H. Mark, The study and treatment on a neurological ward of aggressive patients with focal brain disease, *Confinia Neurol. 36*:125 (1974).
55. D. Mungas, An empirical analysis of specific syndromes of violent behavior, *J. Nerv. Ment. Disorders 171*:609 (1983).
56. W. Semple, Eysenck personality traits and frontal glucose metabolism by PET, Third International Conference of the International Society for the Study of Personality Disorders '93, Cambridge, MA.
57. L. W. Kraft, R. Kusubov, R. Tang, et al., Orbital frontal cortex metabolism and obsessionality in normal volunteers, Biological Psychiatry Forty-Ninth Annual Convention and Scientific Program '94, Philadelphia, Program and Abstracts, p. 684.
58. M. S. George, T. A. Ketter, P. J. Parekh, et al., Personality traits correlate with resting rCBF, American Psychiatric Association Annual Meeting '94, Philadelphia, New Research, p. 173.
59. S. D. Iversen, Brain dopamine systems and behavior, *Handbook of Psychopharmacology*, (L. L. Iversen, S. D. Iversen and S. H. Snyder, eds.), Plenum Press, New York, 1977, p. 33.
60. T. J. Crow, A map of the rat mesencephalon for electrical self-stimulation, *Brain Res. 36*:265 (1972).
61. T. J. Crow, J. F. W. Deakin, Neurohumoral transmissions, behavior and mental disorder, *Handbook of Psychiatry*, (S. M. Cambridge, ed.), Cambridge University Press, Cambridge, UK, 1985, p. 137.
62. M. A. Menza, M. H. Mark, D. J. Burn, and D. J. Burn, D. J. Brooks, Personality correlates of (^{18}F) dopa striatial uptake: Results of positron-emission tomography in parkinson's disease, *J. Neuropsychiatry Clin. Neurosci. 7*:176 (1995).
63. D. R. Weinberger and K. F. Berman, Speculation on the meaning of cerebral metabolic hypofrontality in schizophrenia, *Schizophr. Bull. 14*:157 (1988).
64. C. D. Frith, J. Friston, S. Herold, D. Silbersweig, et al., Regional brain activity in chronic schizophrenic patients during the performance of a verbal fluency task, *Br. J. Psychiatry 167*:343 (1995).
65. M. Linnoila and M. Virkkunen, Aggression, suicidality, and serotonin, symposium: brain serotonin and its relation to psychiatric diseases, *J. Clin. Psychiatry 53*:46 (1992).
66. P. A. Filipek, C. Richelme, D. N. Kennedy, V. S. Caviness, Jr., The young adult brain: an MRI-based morphometric analysis, *Cereb. Cortex 4*:344 (1994).
67. I. C. Wright, P. K. McGuire, J. B. Poline, et al., A voxel-based method for the statistical analysis of gray and white matter density applied to schizophrenia. *Neuroimage 2*:244 (1995).

68. J. F. Clarkin, T. A. Widiger, A. Frances, S. W. Hurt and M. Gilmore, Prototypic typology and the borderline personality disorder, *J. Abnormal Psychology 92*: 263 (1983).

69. J. G. Gunderson and K. A. Phillips, A current view of their interface between borderline personality disorder and depression, *Am. J. Psychiatry 148*:967 (1991).

70. M. C. Zanarini, J. G. Gunderson, F. R. Frankenburg, and D. L. Chauncey, Discriminating borderline personality disorder from other axis II disorders, *Am. J. Psychiatry 147*:161 (1990).

71. H. S. Akiskal, Subaffective disorders: disthymic, cyclothymic and bipolar II disorders in the "borderline" realm, *Psychiatr. Clin. North Am. 4*:25 (1981).

72. R. L. Spitzer, J. Endicott, and M. Gibbon, Crossing the border into borderline personality and borderline schizophrenia: the development of criteria, *Arch. Gen. Psychiatry 36*:17 (1979).

73. J. G. Gunderson and A. N. Sabo, The phenomenological and conceptual interface between borderline personality disorder and PTSD, *Am. J. Psychiatry 150*: 19 (1993).

74. M. C. Zanarini, Borderline personality disorder as as impulse spectrum disorder, *Borderline Personality Disorder—Etiology and Treatment* (J. Paris, ed.), American Psychiatric Press, Washington, DC. 1993, p. 67.

75. P. A. Andrulonis, B. C. Glueck, C. F. Stroebel, and N. G. Vogel, Borderline personality subcategories, *J. Nerv. Ment. Dis. 170*:670 (1982).

76. D. A. Silbersweig, E. Stern, C. D. Frith, et al., Detection of thirty-second cognitive activations in single subjects with positron emission tomography: a new low-dose $H_2^{15}O$ regional cerebral blood flow three-dimensional imaging technique, *J. Cereb. Blood Flow Metab. 13*:617 (1993).

77. S. Ogawa, D. W. Tank, R. Menon, J. M. Ellermann, S. G. Kim, H. Merkle, and K. Ugurbil, Intrinsic signal changes accompanying sensory stimulation: functional brain mapping with magnetic resonance imaging, *Proc. Natl. Acad. Sci. 89*:5951 (1992).

19

MRI and MRS in Dementia

David C. Steffens
Duke University Medical Center, Durham, North Carolina

I. INTRODUCTION

Magnetic resonance imaging (MRI) has been applied extensively to the study
of Alzheimer's disease (AD), while magnetic resonance spectroscopy (MRS)
has just begun to be used as a research tool in AD. MRI studies have focused
on findings related to general cortical atrophy (cerebral atrophy, increased
cerebral spinal fluid, and ventricular enlargement), focal atrophy (within the
entire temporal lobe, hippocampus, amygdala, and corpus callosum) and
white matter pathological change (deep white matter hyperintensities and
periventricular white matter hyperintensities). MRS studies largely have examined phospholipid metabolism, myo-inositol, and the neuronal marker,
N-acetylaspartate. This chapter will focus on both general and specific findings as reported in the recent literature. In addition to reviewing specific
structural and spectroscopic findings, correlations between these findings
and both histopathological changes and neuropsychological test performance
will be discussed.

II. MAGNETIC RESONANCE IMAGING (MRI) STUDIES
IN ALZHEIMER'S DISEASE

In an attempt to standardize imaging and reporting of MR findings in AD
for use by neuroradiologists in multiple medical centers using a variety of MR
equipment, the Consortium to Establish a Registry for Alzheimer's Disease
(CERAD) tested a protocol with 14 participating neuroradiologists [1]. These
individuals evaluated 28 MR scans of elderly patients so that interrater agreement could be assessed. "Acceptable" intraclass correlations (>0.79) were
found for rating the size of lateral (0.82) and third (0.82) ventricles and of
the temporal horn (0.80). "Less than satisfactory" intraclass correlations
were found for ratings of other areas: global atrophy of the brain (0.70);
sylvian fissure enlargement (0.70); temporal lobe sulci dilatation (0.66); and
cerebral sulci dilatation (0.64). Ratings for presence and severity of white
matter lesions yielded an intraclass correlation of 0.77. The authors conclude
that multicenter MR data will require more objective techniques for evaluation of MR findings in subjects with AD.

Methodological issues such as interrater agreement on various MR measures must be kept in mind when reviewing the literature in this area. Articles
in this chapter have been included in part because of their methodological
rigor. In the following sections we will examine global and focal changes on
MRI in AD.

A. Global Changes

1. Global Cerebral Atrophy

Global cerebral atrophy is seen both in AD and in normal aging, but most studies have found significant increases in atrophy in AD patients compared to age-matched cognitively intact control subjects. The persistent overlap in the range of degree of atrophy between AD patients and controls prohibits the use of global atrophy as a diagnostic marker for AD. However, most studies agree that cortical gray matter is significantly decreased in AD.

Murphy et al. [2] compared MRI scans of 19 men with mild to severe dementia of AD and 18 age-matched healthy male controls. AD patients overall had significantly smaller mean cerebral brain matter volumes, and this finding held true for the 9 patients with mild dementia.

Jernigan et al. [3] examined 25 AD patients and 55 normal control subjects not matched for age and found widespread cortical volume reductions in 22 AD patients. Overall cortical gray matter volumes were significantly decreased in AD patients compared with control subjects when the effects of age were removed.

Rusinek et al. [4] measured distribution of cerebral gray matter, white matter, and CSF in 14 AD patients and 14 controls using two specifically designed MR inversion-recovery sequences to compensate for partial signal averaging. Percentage of gray matter in brains of AD patients was significantly lower than controls. While the most significant reduction was in temporal lobes and in a specifically defined central region, significant reductions were also seen in the frontal and occipital lobes.

Narkiewicz et al. [5] studied postmortem MRI brain changes in 7 AD patients and 5 controls followed by histopathological examination. They found that the size and shape of the brain in AD reflected the atrophy seen in the hippocampus and parahippocampal structures.

Seab et al. [6] examined overall brain size on MRI in 10 AD patients and 7 elderly controls. They found significant reductions in overall brain size in the AD group compared to the control group, but that individual values within the two groups had a significant amount of overlap. Additionally, there was a significant correlation between overall atrophy and dementia severity as measured by the Mini-Mental State Examination (MMSE) [7], a finding also reported by Murphy et al. [2].

2. Ventricular Size and CSF Volumes

Enlarging ventricles and sulci, as well as increased size of CSF spaces, indirectly reflect both global and regional cerebral atrophy. Several studies have therefore attempted to quantify and characterize changes in these areas in

AD. Generally, MRI studies have demonstrated global and regional sulcal and ventricular dilatation. However, there is often noted significant overlap between groups of AD patients and normal controls, a problem that reduces the discriminative utility of these measurements.

Murphy et al. [2] found significantly larger mean ventricular volumes in AD patients compared to controls. Rusinek et al. [4] found statistically significant increases in CSF volume in temporal, occipital, and frontal regions of 14 AD patients compared to 14 healthy control subjects.

Tanna et al. [8] employed a computerized segmentation technique to measure CSF on MR images of 16 AD patients and 16 healthy elderly control subjects. Patients with AD had significantly higher total CSF and higher extraventricular, total ventricular, and third ventricular CSF volumes (49, 37, 99, and 74%, respectively).

Meyerhoff et al. [9] studied 8 probable AD patients and 10 age-matched controls. They found significant ventricular enlargements on MRI in the AD patients.

Seab et al. [6] examined ventricular size and sulcal size in MRI scans of 10 AD patients and 7 elderly controls. They found significant increases in both measures in the AD group compared to controls.

Slansky et al. [10] examined neuropsychological performance and size of the third ventricle and of the left and right temporal horns on MRI in 26 patients with probable AD. Using the MMSE and other memory tests, the authors found strong correlations between severity of dementia as measured by these tests and enlargement of the third ventricle and of the temporal horns. In the same patients, they found MRI superior to positron emission tomography (PET) in reflecting changes in the brainstem and mesial temporal lobe of AD patients.

B. Focal Atrophy

1. Temporal Lobe Structures

Good memory function is dependent on the integration of the temporal lobe, hippocampus, and other structures in the limbic system. In AD, the hippocampal formation (HF) and the parahippocampal gyrus (PHG), especially the entorhinal cortex, are associated with early neuropathological changes, specifically neurofibrillary tangles and senile plaques [11–13]. Studies have focused on quantifying and characterizing changes within the temporal lobe, HF, and related structures to test the assumption that changes including atrophy within these areas will yield more specific information about AD than relatively nonspecific global changes.

Murphy et al. [2] found significantly decreased temporal lobe volumes and larger temporal lobe CSF volumes in 19 men with AD compared to 18 age-matched male volunteers. Jernigan et al. [3] found severe reductions in mesial cortical structures which were significant in AD patients compared to controls.

Seab et al. [6] examined MRI scans of 10 AD patients and 7 elderly controls to quantify the size of the hippocampus. They found a 40% reduction in mean normalized hippocampal area of the AD patients compared to controls. Severity of hippocampal atrophy did not correlate with severity of overall dementia as measured on MMSE in AD patients, nor did it correlate with severity of overall atrophy, age of onset of AD, or duration of AD.

Convit et al. [14] measured different regions of the temporal lobe on MRI of 15 AD patients, 18 elderly normal subjects, and 17 cognitively impaired individuals who did not meet criteria for AD. Volume reductions were found in AD relative to normals for both medial and lateral temporal lobe volumes. The minimally cognitively impaired group showed reductions only in hippocampal volume, and these reductions were similar to the AD group.

Ikeda et al. [15] examined HF, PHG, and the temporal lobe in 6 patients with possible AD, 8 patients with probable AD, and 8 age-matched controls. Coronal T_1-weighted images were used for area measurements. Both the normalized HF and PHG were significantly smaller in both AD groups than in the controls, but did not differ between the two AD groups. The normalized temporal lobe was significantly smaller in patients with probable AD than in those with possible AD and controls, but did not differ between patients with possible AD and controls. The authors conclude that hippocampal and parahippocampal atrophy occurs in early AD and is more useful than neocortical atrophy for early detection of the disease.

Kesslak et al. [16] examined the MRI scans of 8 patients with AD and 7 age-matched controls who were tested on a battery of cognitive and olfactory tests. Patients with AD showed a significant reduction of 48.8% in hippocampus, 37.7% in PHG, and a nonsignificant decrease of 11.1% in striatum volume compared to normal controls. The hippocampi of AD patients appeared to flatten, losing their oval shape, resulting in an enlarged ventricular space. Similar atrophy was observed in the PHG, with a marked reduction in the cortical mantle, suggesting a substantial loss of neurons in AD. Hippocampal and PHG atrophy correlated best with the MMSE and less well with olfactory and visual tests. The high correlation with scores on the MMSE (HF, 0.898; PHG, 0.913) suggests that both structures are involved in and reflect general cognitive processes.

Jack et al. [17] examined temporal lobe structures on MRI because of their known involvement in memory function and AD dementia. Regions examined included the anterior temporal lobe (ATL) and the HF. Volumetric measurements were normalized by total intracranial volume (TIV). Normalized ATL and HF volumetric measurements were significantly smaller ($p <$

0.001) in AD patients (N = 20) than in controls (N = 22), but the HF volumes provided much better separation between the two groups. Eighty-five percent of the DAT patients fell below the range of the HF/TIV measurement for the control subjects. This separation help up over the entire age range studied. According to the authors, these data support the contention that MR-based HF volumetric measurements are accurate in differentiating AD patients from cognitively normal elderly individuals.

Scheltens et al. [18] used a ranking procedure to assess the medial temporal lobe including the hippocampal formation and surrounding spaces occupied by CSF in 21 AD patients and in 21 age-matched controls. Patients with AD showed a significantly higher degree of subjectively assessed medial temporal lobe atrophy (MTA) than controls. Linear measurements correlated highly with subjective assessment of MTA and also showed significant differences between groups. In AD patients, the degree of MTA correlated significantly with scores on the MMSE and memory tests, but poorly with mental speed tests. The authors conclude that MTA may be assessed quickly and easily with plain MRI films.

O'Brien et al. [19] compared 43 AD patients with 32 depressed patients matched for age, sex, and level of education using temporal lobe MRI. They used a four-point atrophy scale to examine the hippocampus, amygdala, entorhinal cortex, parahippocampal gyrus, and cerebral cortex. Using a cutoff of 2 or more on the anterior hippocampal atrophy rating provided good discrimination between groups, with a sensitivity of 93%, specificity of 84%, and 89% of cases correctly grouped overall. Even among a subgroup of 9 mild AD subjects and 10 cognitively impaired depressed subjects (matched on MMSE scores), the same cutoff correctly grouped 84% (16/19) cases. Within the AD group there was a significant correlation between length of history and atrophy of the entorhinal cortex. The authors conclude that temporal lobe atrophy on MRI can discriminate between AD and depressed patients, including depressed individuals with cognitive impairment.

Lehericy et al. [20] examined the accuracy of hippocampal and amygdala volume measurements normalized for total intracranial volume (TIV) in 13 patients with early AD (MMSE scores ≥ 21) and 5 with moderate AD (MMSE scores between 10 and 21), and in 8 age-matched controls. For early AD patients, they found significant atrophy for the amygdala (amygdala/TIV decreased 36%) and hippocampal formation (HF/TIV decreased 25%), but not for the caudate nucleus. No significant ventricular enlargement was found. For individuals with moderate AD, significant atrophy was found in all structures studied (amygdala/TIV decreased 40%, HF/TIV decreased 45%, caudate nucleus/TIV decreased 21%), and there was significant (63%) ventricular enlargement. Hippocampal volumes correlated with MMSE scores in the

AD patients. The authors found no overlap between AD and control values for the amygdalohippocampal volume, even in the early AD patients. They conclude that volumetric measurements of the amygdala and the AHC appear more accurate than those of the hippocampal formation alone in distinguishing patients with AD.

Desmond et al. [21] examined MR images of 24 patients with AD and 15 age-matched controls to assess mesial temporal structures, including the amygdala, hippocampus, parahippocampal gyrus, and entorhinal cortex. Volumetric analysis demonstrated significant differences between the two groups (30% reduction in the hippocampus and 40% reduction in the amygdala), but showed overlap in individual cases. Discriminant function analysis, using the standardized volume measurements, correctly predicted group membership (AD vs. control) in 85% of cases. Visual assessment alone demonstrated a sensitivity of 92% and a specificity of 93% in distinguishing AD patients from controls. The authors conclude that both volumetric and visual techniques are useful in separating AD patients from age-matched controls.

Cuenod et al. [22] studied amygdala volumes on MRI of 11 patients with early probable AD and 6 age-matched controls. They found the AD group showed significant (33%) atrophy of the amygdala compared with the control group. The mean amygdala index (which normalized interindividual variation by taking midsagittal intracranial area into account) correlated with the MMSE scores, but the correlation was no longer significant when only the AD patients were analyzed. The authors conclude that measurement of the amygdala using this technique may be useful in the early diagnosis of AD.

Erkinjuntti et al. [23] examined MR images of 34 early AD patients and 39 age-matched controls using a four-point rating scale for atrophy of temporal structures as well as linear measurements of hippocampal area and maximal transverse width of the temporal horns. Receiver operating characteristics analysis for atrophy ratings revealed that ratings of the entorhinal cortex best discriminated patients from controls, followed by ratings of the temporal neocortex, temporal horns and hippocampal formation. Linear measurements of the temporal horns and of the hippocampal formation differentiated the two groups, although there was significant overlap. The authors suggest that the presence of rated atrophy in selected temporal structures makes the diagnosis of AD more likely, but that early AD cannot be ruled out by the absence of atrophy in these structures.

Pearlson et al. [24] examined MRI scans of 15 AD patients with dementia of moderate severity and 16 normal controls. For patients, the volumes of the left and right amygdalae, left hippocampus, and left and right entorhinal cortices were significantly smaller than control volumes. Volumes of the left amygdala and of the left entorhinal cortex, when combined, provided the best structural discrimination between patients and controls, identifying 67% of patients and 100% of controls. Additionally, when these measures were combined with a measure of left temporoparietal regional cerebral blood flow using SPECT, the overall discrimination of the two groups was 100%.

Killiany et al. [25] studied five brain regions on the MRI scans of 8 early probable AD patients and 7 age-matched controls. Three volumetric measures were significantly different between patients and controls: the hippocampus, the temporal horn of the lateral ventricles, and the temporal lobe. There were no volumetric differences between patients and controls for the amygdala or the basal forebrain. Using discriminant function analysis, the authors found that a linear combination of the volumes of the hippocampus and the temporal horn of the lateral ventricles differentiated 100% of the patients and controls, suggesting that these measurements may provide good antemortem diagnostic markers for AD.

Laasko et al. [26] studied 32 patients with early probable AD and 16 age-matched healthy controls. AD patients had significantly smaller volumes of the left and right hippocampus and the left frontal lobe, but not of the right frontal lobe, right amygdala or left amygdala. Using discriminant function analysis, inclusion of volumes of the left and right hippocampus, the left and right frontal lobe and the right amygdala into a model correctly identified 92% of subjects into AD and control groups. Using volumes of hippocampus, frontal lobes, or amygdala alone, the correct classification was achieved in 88, 65, and 58% of subjects, respectively. The authors conclude that hippocampal volume measurements may be useful in the diagnosis of early AD.

Matsuzawa et al. [27] examined the amygdala and hippocampus using MRI in 6 AD patients and 15 patients with multi-infarct dementia. By evaluating T_1 serial slices of 8 mm thickness taken parallel to the lateral posterior horn, the authors compared demented patients and 38 controls on a measure of the combined area of the amygdala and hippocampus/total cranial cavity area. Both the AD group and the MID group had significantly smaller combined amydala/hippocampal areas than did the controls. There was no difference between the two dementia groups.

Narkiewicz et al. [5] studied postmortem MRI changes in the transverse fissure in 7 AD patients and five controls followed by histopathological examination. Where the transverse fissure is a narrow cleft in normals, the enlarged size and shape of the lateral part of the transverse fissure in AD patients reflect the atrophy of the hippocampus and parahippocampal structures. In particular, the authors found that sector CA1, the subiculum, the entorhinal cortex, and parahippocampal isocortex were most affected, while the dentate gyrus and thalamic structures were much less affected with little contribution to transverse fissure changes.

2. Correlation of Temporal Lobe Structures with Neuropsychological Measures

Deweer et al. [28] examined volumetric measures on MRI of the HF, amygdala, caudate nucleus, normalized for TIV in relation to measures of cognitive function in 18 probable AD patients. Hippocampal volume (HF/TIV) was correlated with specific memory variables. No correlations were found between amygdala volume and memory variables (except for intrusions) or between caudate nuclei volume and any neuropsychological score. This study confirms previous findings associating the hippocampal formation with memory performance, here in a population of AD patients.

As part of the CERAD group, Davis et al. [29] compared MRI scans with neuropathological evidence of temporal lobe atrophy in 20 autopsy-confirmed AD cases. Ratings of temporal horn size on MRI correlated significantly with neuropathological evidence of hippocampal atrophy. The authors also found a significant correlation between overall cerebral atrophy on neuroimaging and the MMSE score obtained at the time closest to the scan.

3. Microanatomy of the Temporal Lobes

Magnetic resonance techniques have also been used to study microanatomy in AD. Huesgen et al. [30] used MR microscopy at 7 tesla to identify the anatomy of the degenerating hippocampus in AD, and then made histopathological correlations in the same specimens. Among 13 patients with confirmed AD, the mean cross-sectional area of the hippocampus was decreased by 31% compared with 9 age-matched controls. This atrophy was highly correlated with tangle counts within the hippocampus, but not with plaque counts. The width of the gray matter in hippocampal area CA1, as identified by MR, correlated with the total area of the hippocampus.

4. Interuncal Distance

One simple measure on MRI scans is the length between the unci of the temporal lobes, known as the interuncal distance (IUD). The IUD can be measured directly from the image section through the suprasellar cistern on transaxial images by measuring the distance between the unci using a dial caliper. IUD can also be measured on coronal sections be identifying the most anterior section showing the temporal horn and measuring the distance between the unci at that level. Some researchers will then adjust for brain size by dividing IUD by intracranial width or intracranial area. Dahlbeck et al. [3] first compared axial MR images of 10 AD patients and 10 control subjects and found significant differences between the two groups. Their preliminary results indicate that an IUD greater than 30 mm may indicate hippocampal atrophy of AD.

Howieson et al. [32] evaluated the utility of the interuncal distance (IUD) in AD. When IUD was corrected for head size, significant differences between 10 probable early AD cases and 10 normal controls were found on coronal measurement of IUD. There was overlap in IUD between disease and control groups. There were no differences on transaxial IUD. Significant positive correlations between MMSE score and CDR Scale stage were observed. Age was not significantly correlated with IUD. The authors conclude that IUD is not a useful screening measurement for AD.

Laasko et al. [33] examined IUD in 54 probable AD patients, 40 with age-associated memory impairment, 27 healthy older patients, and 20 control subjects younger than age 50. The AD group had significantly greater IUD/intracranial area and IUD/brain area compared with age-matched controls. A considerable overlap was found in the values of AD patients and controls. The cutoff point of 30 mm for IUD yielded 37% sensitivity and 72% specificity to distinguish between the two groups. There was a strong correlation between IUD and age in the whole study population and in nondemented subjects. The authors conclude that IUD is not a reliable diagnostic tool for patients with mild to moderate AD and that this measure has a strong age dependence.

To further explore the clinical utility of IUD, Early et al. [34] measured IUD on axial MR scans of 12 AD patients and 17 healthy controls. The authors compared IUD with volume of the amygdala-hippocampal complex and found no significant correlation. IUD measurement was not useful in distinguishing patients with mild to moderate from normal volunteers. They conclude that IUD appears to be a better measure of overall brain volume and that this measure is age-related.

5. *Corpus Callosum*

Several studies have noted callosal atrophy and attempted to describe more clearly the changes as well as to correlate them to changes in AD. Vermersch et al. [35] examined the thickness of the corpus callosum (CC) in 20 AD patients and 21 age-matched controls. AD patients had a significant reduction in CC thickness compared with age-matched controls ($p < 0.01$), particularly in senile dementia compared to presenile dementia. The authors found no association between CC changes and either age or ventricular volume. They conclude that CC volume may prove to be a very specific, although not very sensitive marker for AD, particularly late-onset AD.

Biegon et al. [36] examined the corpus callosum in 20 AD patients and 16 young and 13 old control subjects. Aging did not significantly affect the mean area of the CC, but a small significant reduction was seen in AD in comparison to the young control group. AD is accompanied by a large and statistically significant reduction in the genu area of the CC in comparison to young and old controls. The authors conclude that selective changes in the CC accompany both aging and AD pathology.

Yamauchi et al. [37] examined the corpus callosum in 10 male AD patients and 14 age- and sex-matched controls using both MRI and PET. The authors found significant reductions in the size of the corpus callosum on MRI in the AD group compared to controls. They also found regional variations in degree of callosal atrophy, with a posterior predominance in degree of atrophy. Using PET data, they found that in AD patients, callosal atrophy was significantly correlated with decreased cortical oxygen metabolism both generally and regionally (anterior and posterior halves). Finally, the degree of callosal atrophy was significantly correlated with neuropsychological decline as measured by the Wechsler Adult Intelligence Scale (WAIS) [38] total and verbal IQ scores, but not with the performance IQ.

6. Subcortical Structures

Murphy et al. [2] found no difference between 19 patients with AD and 18 control subjects in the volumes of the thalamus, lenticular nuclei and caudate nuclei. However, Jernigan et al. [3] found significant decreases in the volumes of caudate, lenticular, and diencephalic gray matter in AD patients compared to control subjects.

The nucleus basalis of Meynert in the substantia innominata contains large aggregates of cholinergic neurons and is thought to be an important and vulnerable site in Alzheimer's disease. While the nucleus basalis itself may be too small to reliably study using current techniques, the substantia innominata in which it exists may be more suitable. To that end, Sasaki et al. [39] examined 22 AD patients and 13 age-matched patients with other disorders, although patients with major neurological disorders were excluded. T_2-weighted images through the anterior commissure were used to evaluate the thickness of the substantia innominata. The average thickness of the narrowest portions on the right and left substantia innominatas ranged from 1.3 to 2.6 mm in AD and was 2.6–3.5 mm in the control group, a highly statistically significant difference. No statistically significant difference was found between the thickness of right and left substantia innominatas. The authors correctly point out that because the substantia innominata contains not only the nucleus basalis of Meynert, but also nerve tracts, atrophy of the substantia innominata does not necessarily indicate neuronal loss of the nucleus basalis. However, this atrophy clearly suggests that both the substantia innominata and the nucleus basalis play a role in AD. Clearly, more studies of the substantia innominata and of the nucleus basalis are required.

C. Discussion of Global Changes and Focal Atrophy on MRI

It is important to remember that global cerebral atrophy may be seen on MRI scans of both affected and unaffected individuals. Conversely, patients with AD may have brain MRIs with anywhere from no atrophy to marked atrophic changes. Most studies, however, have shown significant increases in cerebral atrophy on MRI in AD patients compared with age-matched normal controls. The same may be said for ventricular size and cerebrospinal fluid volumes.

In terms of specific, focal changes, atrophy is generally seen in the temporal lobe and in its component parts. The hippocampus, a brain structure long associated with memory function, is typically atrophied in AD. The degree of hippocampal atrophy does not necessarily correlate with overall severity of dementia, but it may correlate with specific tests of memory. Other temporal lobe structures that tend to show atrophy in AD include the parahippocampal gyrus, entorhinal cortex, and amygdala.

In other studies of specific brain structures on MRI, the length between the temporal lobes, termed the interuncal distance, does not reliably correlate with AD diagnosis. Likewise, size of the CC does not appear to predict presence of AD, although large reductions in callosal size seem to correlate with some neuropsychological testing parameters and measures of overall dementia severity. Findings also appear equivocal for subcortical structures such as the thalamus and basal ganglia.

The goal of many investigators is to find a radiographic marker for early AD that is both highly sensitive (i.e., detects all cases) and specific (i.e., is present only with AD). Thus far, this aim has proven elusive. As MRI technology improves, we may yet develop a "good" diagnostic imaging test. One area to target may be the nucleus basalis of Meynert. Other neuropathological correlations may allow us to scan very isolated brain areas specific to AD.

D. White Matter Changes on MRI in Alzheimer's Disease

Investigators have also examined changes in the white matter of AD patients. White matter abnormalities commonly appear in both normal and diseased elderly individuals [40,41]. Research has commonly focused on assessing the extent of white matter hyperintensities (WMH) and periventricular hyperintensities (PVH) as viewed on T_2-weighted images. Areas of confluent WMH or PVH have been termed "leukoaraiosis" [42]. In order to quantify hyperintensities on MRI, several researchers have sought to develop standardized criteria with high interrater reliability. For example, Fazekas et al. [44] developed a grading system, which provides a rough assessment of the extent of subcortical white and gray matter changes. Additionally, Scheltens et al. [44] designed a rating scale in which PVH and WMH as well as basal ganglia and infratentorial signal hyperintensities may be rated in a semi-quantitative way. Despite being more elaborate, the newer scale showed a better inter- and intraobserver agreement than Fazekas' scale for grading white matter abnormalities. The authors suggest that their scale is preferable in studies focusing specifically on deep white matter pathology.

The design of studies examining white matter changes has varied depending on the specific research question. Some authors have sought to quantify white matter changes in AD patients alone, while others have compared white matter changes in AD patients and controls, AD patients and patients with cerebrovascular disease, and AD patients and patients with other forms of dementia. The following sections review findings in each of these areas of research.

1. White Matter Changes in AD Patients

Bennett et al. [45] examined MRI scans of 106 patients with probable AD, excluding persons with treated vascular risk factors or symptomatic cerebrovascular or cardiovascular disease. Twenty-six (25%) had grade 2 periventricular high signal and 29 (18%) had scattered white matter changes. PVH were associated with advancing age and gait disturbance, and WML were associated with gait disturbance and incontinence. The authors conclude that the presence of PVH and WML should not preclude a diagnosis of AD; indeed, these lesions are common in AD patients.

Marder et al. [46] examined CT or MRI scans in 158 patients with probable AD to assess the relationship between small noncortical lesions or periventricular "caps" and two measures of disease severity, the MMSE and the Blessed Dementia Rating Scale (Part 1) [47]. They found no association between lesion number or periventricular caps and disease severity. The authors observe that AD patients with these well-defined radiographic abnormalities cannot be differentiated by severity from AD patients who do not have them.

Brilliant et al. [48] examined MRI scans of 94 probable AD patients and 45 possible AD patients to determine the prevalence and significance of rarefied cerebral white matter (leukoaraiosis) in patients with AD. Only 8.7% of probable AD patients and 11.1% of possible AD patients exhibited large confluent areas of subcortical leukoaraiosis. The magnitude of leukoaraiosis correlated with the patient's age but not with the Hachinski Ischemic Scale and MMSE scores. The authors conclude that large confluent areas of leukoaraiosis occur in a small minority of Alzheimer patients and are probably not caused by AD.

2. *White Matter Changes in AD Patients Versus Controls*

Rusinek et al. [4] found no significant differences in white matter content between AD patients and controls in several areas of the brain studied.

McDonald et al. [49] compared MR scans of 22 patients with early-onset AD with 16 normal age-matched controls. AD patients were significantly more likely to have evidence of PVH than controls, but there was no significant difference between the two groups in either the frequency of subcortical hyperintensities (SCH) or the size of the largest lesion. Patients with AD more frequently demonstrated ventriculomegaly and sulcal widening compared with controls. This study suggests that the SCH seen in early-onset AD patients on MRI are related more to the aging process than to the AD process and that the increased frequency of PVH may have a relationship to the disease process.

Erkinjuntti et al. [50] examined MR images of 34 early AD patients and 38 age-matched controls using a variety of rating scales including that by Fazekas et al. [43]. They found no difference in the ratings, frequency, or extent of the hyperintensities between patients with early AD and controls. In a logistic model, hyperintensities were associated with arterial hypertension, diabetes, cardiac disorder, and age in different combinations, but not with AD. The authors conclude that small hyperintensities on MRI are frequent in both AD patients and normals, and when age and vascular risk factors are taken into account, there is no difference between the two groups in hyperintensities on MRI.

Kumar et al. [51] examined 16 AD patients free of major vascular risk factors and 23 healthy age-matched control subjects for PVH and deep WMH on MRI. They found no difference between AD patients and controls on three measures of high signal intensities. Within the AD group, there were positive correlations between age and both PVH and deep WMH, and between high-intensity signals in the subcortical gray nuclei and MMSE scores.

Waldemar et al. [52] examined correlates of PVHs and DWMHs in 18 probable AD patients and in 10 age-matched controls, all without major cerebrovascular risk factors. Ratings for PVHs were significantly higher in AD and correlated significantly with ventricular volume and with systolic arterial blood pressure, but not with regional cerebral blood flow (rCBF) on SPECT. There were no differences between the two groups on ratings of deep WMH. In the AD group, the volume of DWMHs correlated well with rCBF in the hippocampal region but not in the frontal, temporal, parietal, or occipital regions.

Scheltens et al. [53] studied PVH, WMH, and basal ganglia hyperintensities (BGH) in 13 presenile-onset (less than 65 years) AD patients, 16 senile-onset AD patients, and 24 age-matched controls. Significantly greater PVH,

WMH, and BGH were found in senile-onset AD patients compared to age-matched controls. Cortical atrophy did not differ significantly between pre-senile- and senile-onset AD. Thus presenile-onset AD patients differed from senile-onset AD patients with respect to white matter involvement but not with respect to gray matter involvement on MRI. The authors suggest that AD may be heterogeneous, since cerebrovascular risk factors were excluded from analysis, with a "pure" early-onset form with few white matter changes, and a "mixed" later-onset form with more white matter MRI changes than normal for age.

Harrell et al. [54] studied cognition and psychiatric state in 18 patients with AD and depression, 45 AD patients without depression, 12 older depressed patients, and 25 older normal individuals. High-intensity signals in the cortex and subcortical regions were similar in number and proportions among all groups, even when hypertensive patients were excluded. The authors found no correlations to cognitive or psychiatric state. Patients with AD exhibited more severe periventricular changes than did normal subjects, and neuropsychological performance was significantly worse in patients with AD who had more severe periventricular changes. Harrell et al. conclude that periventricular changes may predict poor neuropsychological performance, but they also emphasize that neither deep white matter lesions nor periventricular changes are useful for diagnostic purposes.

Leys et al. [55] studied 17 AD patients and 10 controls who were normotensive, nondiabetic, and free of cardiac disorders and found no difference in severity of MRI WMH and PVH between patients and controls. No correlation was found between hyperintensities and either age or MMSE score. The authors conclude that PVH and WMH on MRI are frequent findings in the elderly, both in AD and in normals. They suggest that individuals with these abnormalities should followed with neuropsychological and imaging evaluation to determine if they are at risk to develop clinically significant cognitive disturbance.

Scheltens et al. [56] used postmortem MRI to examine white matter changes in 6 AD patients and 9 controls. AD patients displayed more white matter hyperintensities on MRI. MRI abnormalities correlated with the loss of myelinated axons in the deep white matter in AD brains and with denudation of the ventricular lining. They conclude that white matter abnormalities in AD patients and controls consist of loss of myelinated axons, probably caused by arterial changes and breakdown of the ventricular lining.

3. White Matter Changes in AD and Cerebrovascular Disease

Bennett et al. [57] reported the results of several studies of neurobehavioral manifestations of patients with Binswanger's disease and the clinical correlates of white matter changes in autopsy-proven AD patients. Compared to AD patients, those with Binswanger's disease had less impairment in episodic memory, more depressive symptoms, and a more variable rate of cognitive decline. The authors also note that in the AD group, some white matter lesions were associated with incontinence and gait disturbance, but did not appear to contribute to dementia severity.

Wahlund et al. [58] compared the occurrence and degree of WMH in 23 probable AD patients, 25 with possible AD, and 31 with vascular dementia. Patients with vascular dementia had significantly more changes in the posterior part of the brain and in the right hemisphere than did AD patients. The total volume of the WMH as well as the regional distribution of these changes differed significantly between vascular dementia and AD. No significant correlation was found between cognitive impairment and degree of WMH in any of the groups. WMH seem not to be related to the degree of global cognitive decline in dementia.

Reed et al. [59] used MRI to distinguish between 25 AD patients and 25 patients with multi-infarct dementia (MID). Patients were examined using the following six MRI criteria: ventricular-brain ratio, presence of subcortical infarcts, bifrontal ventricular ratio, bicaudate ventricular ratio, third ventricular ratio, and presence of diffuse periventricular high-intensity white matter lucencies. When all six criteria were used, comparison of classification by discriminant function analysis with clinical classification provided 84% agreement for MID patients, 92% for AD patients, and 88% agreement overall.

Schmidt [60] evaluated MRI scans of 27 patients with probable AD, 31 patients with vascular dementia, and 18 normal controls. A number of findings were significantly more common in vascular dementia than in the other subsets: (a) basal ganglionic/thalamic hyperintense foci (Fazekas criteria, [39]), (b) thromboembolic infarctions, (c) confluent white matter, and (d) irregular PVH. Signal abnormalities on intermediate T_2-weighted scans in the uncal-hippocampal or insular cortex were frequently and almost exclusively noted in AD. Selective atrophy measurements failed to separate dementia syndromes. The authors suggest that MRI has the potential to increase the accuracy of clinical diagnosis of AD and vascular dementia.

Charletta et al. [61] compared MRI findings in African American subjects. Forty-three had AD, 22 had vascular dementia, and 22 had stroke without dementia. Between the AD and vascular dementia groups, patients with AD had significantly more atrophy of the temporal horns, less atrophy of the third ventricle, fewer lacunar infarcts, and fewer left and right hemisphere and left cortical infarcts than did patients with vascular dementia. Multivariable analysis showed that atrophy of the temporal sulci (OR =

0.09, CI = 0.01–0.83) and atrophy of the temporal horns (OR = 0.12, CI = 0.02–0.87) were predictors of AD, and atrophy of the third ventricle (OR = 90.37, CI = 4.09–999.0) and right hemisphere infarcts (OR = 6.41, CI = 1.36–30.3) were predictors of vascular dementia. The authors point out that their findings in these African American patients were similar to those reported in other dementia studies.

In an attempt to develop a better method for differential diagnosis of AD and vascular dementia based on neuroimaging studies, Hanyu et al. [62] used both MRI and SPECT technology in 55 patients and 36 patients with vascular dementia. Severity of deep white matter lesions and medial temporal atrophy were assessed using MRI, while hypoperfusion in the frontal and temporoparietal areas was determined by SPECT. For each patient, a combination of scores using the two modalities was used to calculate a single value indicating the probability of AD or vascular dementia. This system correctly identified AD in 91% (50/55) of AD cases and vascular dementia in 89% (32/36) of these patients, for an overall discrimination of 90%.

4. White Matter Changes in AD and Other Dementias

Julin et al. [63] compared MRI brain scans of 28 AD patients and 8 frontal lobe dementia patients and found no significant difference between the two groups on ventricular size, total cortical atrophy, regional distribution of atrophy, or amount of white matter lesions. The frequency of white matter lesions was low, with 18 of 28 AD patients being rated as being without amy pathological white matter lesions. The authors also found that SPECT imaging was a better method than MRI to clinically differentiate AD from frontal lobe dementia.

E. Discussion of White Matter Changes

The meaning of white matter changes on MRI remains unclear. Present in AD patients, in normal controls, and in individuals with cerebrovascular disease and other neurological disorders, these changes initially may serve to confuse the differential diagnosis of demented patients. The two most frequently reported findings of white matter change are white matter hyperintensities (WMHs) and periventricular hyperintensities (PVHs) viewed on T_2-weighted images. Some investigators have hypothesized that such white matter changes may be part of the normal aging process of the human brain. Thought to be vascular in origin, these changes are also found in subjects without known cerebrovascular disease or even without vascular risk factors. Therefore, the presence of WMH or PVH in a demented individual should neither preclude a diagnosis of AD or establish a diagnosis of ischemic vascular dementia.

F. Other MRI Studies in AD

Kirsch et al. [64] examined T_2 MR relaxation time in the hippocampal formation (HF) in 13 patients with probable AD, 11 elderly normals, 23 young normals, and 9 subjects with multi-infarct dementia. T_2 relaxation times were significantly greater in AD patients compared to each of the other three groups. Degree of T_2 prolongation was also directly correlated to cognitive and functional deterioration in the AD patients. The authors suggest that hippocampal T_2 prolongation may provide a specific marker by which pathology in patients with suspected AD can be detected, quantified, and followed in vivo.

Bartzokis et al. [65] used the measure of Field-Dependent R2 Increase (FDRI) to quantify tissue iron. They based this new method on the fact that ferritin, the primary tissue iron-storage protein, affects R2 in a field-dependent manner. FDRI values were significantly higher among 5 AD patients in the caudate and globus pallidus compared to 8 age-matched controls. The authors suggest that AD may involve disturbances in brain iron metabolism, and this process can be investigated in vivo using MRI.

Howanitz et al. [66] studied 20 patients with probable AD with psychosis and 12 patients with probable AD without psychosis. Psychosis was defined as presence of delusions or hallucinations. Correlations were found between the presence of hallucinations and three MRI variables: overall degree of atrophy, right lateral ventricular size, and left lateral ventricular size. Each analysis was corrected for duration of illness. These were no significant correlations between the presence of white matter lesions, size of right or left temporal horns, third ventricle size, and the presence of delusions or hallucinations. These data suggest that AD patients with hallucinations may have more generalized or advanced brain disease than AD patients without hallucinations.

Lehtovirta et al. [67] examined volumes of the hippocampus, amygdala and frontal lobes in AD patients based on number of $\epsilon4$ alleles of *APOE*, the polymorphic genetic locus for apolipoprotein E [68–70]. The risk for AD is enhanced, and the mean age of symptom onset reduced, as the number of $\epsilon4$ alleles (0, 1, or 2) increases [71]. Lehtovirta et al. [67] found that demented individuals with the $\epsilon4/\epsilon4$ genotype ($n = 5$) had smaller hippocampal and amygdala volumes than those with $\epsilon3/\epsilon4$ ($n = 9$) and those with $\epsilon3/\epsilon3$ or $\epsilon2\epsilon3$ ($n = 12$). The difference was significant for the right hippocampus and the right amygdala. The volumes of the frontal lobes were similar across the Alzheimer subgroups.

III. MAGNETIC RESONANCE SPECTROSCOPY (MRS) STUDIES IN ALZHEIMER'S DISEASE

A. N-Acetylaspartate, Myo-Inositol, Creatine, and Choline

Several authors have used N-acetylaspartate (NAA), a neuronal marker, to investigate changes in the brains of AD patients in vivo. Often, these changes are reported as ratios of NAA to another measurable marker, such as choline, creatine or myo-inositol (MI). Longo et al. (72-1993) demonstrated using 1H MRS in 2 patients with severe AD that there is a marked decrease of NAA signal with respect to choline.

Meyerhoff et al. [9] used MRS to study a large section of the centrum semiovale in 8 probable AD patients and 10 age-matched controls and found that in the white matter of AD patients there was a decreased NAA:choline ratio and NAA:creatine ratio but no changes in the choline:creatine ratio. The NAA:choline ratio was lower and choline:creatine ratio higher in the mesial gray matter of AD patients relative to elderly controls. The authors found that AD patients showed increased choline:creatine and choline:NAA ratios and an unchanged NAA:creatine ratio in posterior portions of the centrum semiovale. These findings suggest diffuse axonal injury and membrane alterations in gray and white matter of the centrum semiovale in AD patients.

Shonk et al. [73] used proton MRS to examine 65 AD patients, 39 with other dementias, 10 with frontal lobe dementias, 98 patients without dementia, and 32 healthy controls. AD patients had decreased NAA and increased MI. Patients with other dementias had decreased NAA but normal, (MI) (p vs. AD < 0.0005). Using MI/NAA, AD patients were distinguished from normal controls with 83% sensitivity and 95% specificity, with a positive predictive value of 98%. Because reduced NAA was observed in virtually all dementia, the authors urge that further attention be made to the neurophysiological role of MI in AD and other dementias.

Miller et al. [74] used HI-MRS to examine 11 AD patients and 10 age-matched controls. Patients showed a significant (22%) increase in MI and a significant (11%) decrease in N-acetyl (NA). NA, which comprises mainly NAA, a neuronal marker, has been found to be reduced in brains of AD patients at autopsy. The authors suggest that the combination of high MI and low NA with H1 MRS shows promise as an early diagnostic test for AD.

Shiino et al. [75] compared 9 AD patients, 3 patients with normal pressure hydrocephalus (NPH), and 26 volunteers using localized proton MRS. The MR spectra showed three major peaks corresponding to NAA, creatine and phosphocreatine (Cr), and choline-containing compounds. They found a significantly reduced NAA:Cr ratio in AD patients, even in those patients with no significant brain atrophy. There were no changes in normals or in patients with NPH. The authors postulate that the NAA:Cr ratio might reflect the number and/or activity of neuronal cells in the brain. They conclude that proton MRS may prove to be a useful tool for early detection and further pathophysiological study of AD.

Klunk et al. [76] used proton MRS to examine the extracts of 12 AD subjects and 5 control brain samples to measure a variety of amino acid levels. No changes in taurine, aspartate, or glutamine were observed. NAA was lower in AD compared with controls, and this decrease correlated with the number of plaques and neurofibrillary tangles. GABA were also lower in AD brain. Glutamate levels were greater in AD patients and showed an inverse correlation with NAA levels. The authors suggest that the decrease in NAA reflects neuronal loss and that remaining neurons could be exposed to a relative excess of glutamate and a relative lack of GABA. This imbalance could result in neurotoxic damage.

Kwo-On-Yuen et al. [77] used MRS to study changes in NAA in the postmortem brain tissue of 7 AD patients and 7 controls. In AD patients, reductions in NAA were present in the gray matter of the neocortex but not in the white matter. Reductions were seen in both white and gray matter in the parahippocampal gyrus. Only cortical levels correlated with dementia severity clinically. The authors noted a pattern of increasing correlation of MMSE score and postmortem NAA levels in AD patients.

Christiansen et al. [78] examined NAA concentration in the brain of 12 probable AD patients and 8 healthy volunteers using proton MRS. They found a significant reduction in the calculated NAA concentration in the brain of the AD patients compared to the healthy controls. The NAA:choline ratio was significantly higher in the control group compared to the probable AD patients. No significant differences were found between the creatine or choline concentrations obtained in the two groups. Additionally, there was no correlation between the calculated NAA concentration and the MMSE score in the probable AD patients.

Block et al. [79] used proton MRS to examine NAA, choline, and creatine compounds in the hippocampal region of 16 AD patients and 17 healthy controls. They found that AD patients had increased ratios of choline to NAA and of creatine to NAA due to increased choline compounds and decreased NAA. These changes were observed in 11 of 12 cases in the hippocampal region and in 7 of 12 cases in the temporo-occipital region. Hippocampal choline to NAA ratios were significantly elevated compared with controls.

Constans et al. [80] combined MRI and proton MRS to investigate the association of WMH and H1 metabolites in 11 AD patients with WMHs, 8 MID patients with WMHs, 8 elderly controls with substantial WMHs, and 21 elderly controls without or with minimal WMHs. In AD patients, extensive WMHs showed lower NAA and higher choline-containing metabolites compared to contralateral normal-appearing white matter (NAWM). For MID patients, WMHs were associated with higher choline-containing and lower creatine-containing metabolites compared with contralateral NAWM. The authors assert that because regional metabolite concentrations may covary with the presence of white matter hyperintensities, the extent of WMH present must be accounted for in analysis of MR spectroscopic data.

B. Phosphorus and Its Metabolites

Bottomley et al. [81] examined brain phosphate metabolite concentrations and ratios in 11 probable AD patients with mild to moderate dementia and in 14 normal controls. They found no significant differences in phosphocreatine, nucleoside triphosphate, inorganic phosphate, PM, and PE. There was no correlation between P-31 NMR indexes and the severity of dementia. The authors conclude that high-energy phosphate and membrane metabolism do not appear to play a major role in the disease process, except as a direct consequence of atrophy quantified with H1 MR imaging.

Cuenod et al. [82] used phosphorus MRS to study 24 patients with mild AD and 15 age-matched healthy volunteers. They found a significant increase in the phosphomonoester:total phosphorus (PME:P_{total}) ratio in AD patients. Use of a ratio above 11% yielded 83.3% sensitivity and 73.3% specificity. Other metabolite ratios (Pi, PD, PCr, nucleotide phosphates, to total P) were not significant. No metabolite ratio correlated with the score on MMSE. The results of an increase in the PME:P_{total} ratio in the prefrontal area in early AD patients confirmed some in vitro studies showing abnormalities of phospholipid turnover in AD. The authors suggest that conflicting results in in vivo studies may arise from differences in MRS techniques (e.g., location, sequence, and parameters) and/or patient characteristics (e.g., stage or type of disease and geographic origin).

Murphy et al. [83] studied brain slice phosphorus metabolism using proton MRS and glucose metabolism using positron emission tomography (PET) in 9 drug-free mild to moderately severe AD patients and 8 age- and sex-matched controls. Phosphorus metabolites examined included phosphocreatine, inorganic phosphate, phosphomonoesters, and phosphodiesters. While AD patients had significant brain glucose hypometabolism, there was no significant difference in any phosphorus metabolite concentration or ratio in the same volume of brain tissue. Within AD patients, there was no correlation between any phosphorus metabolite concentration or ratio and either severity or dementia or glucose metabolism. The authors conclude that altered high-energy phosphate levels in AD are not a consequence of reduced glucose metabolism and that they do not play a major role in the neuropathology of the disorder.

Moats et al. [84] performed quantitative 1H MRS in 10 AD patients and 7 normal elderly controls. They demonstrated a 50% increase in MI and a decrease in NA in occipital gray matter. Choline concentration increased with age, but was not elevated above normal in AD patients. Accounting for metabolite T_1 and T_2 effects using this quantitative method, the authors conclude that the MI concentration is even higher than first thought. They also suggest their results demonstrate the need for quantitative 1H MRS to substantiate metabolite ratios in future studies.

Brown et al. [85] used MRS to examine three groups: demented patients with multiple subcortical ischemic lesions ($n = 18$), nondemented, age-matched controls ($n = 21$), and 3 demented patients with neurodegenerative disease, probably of the Alzheimer type ($n = 19$). Demented patients with subcortical vascular lesions had an increase of phosphate energy charge in areas of the cerebral cortex (especially prominent in the frontal regions) superficial to and excluded from the subcortical lesions. They hypothesize that this increased energy charge might be caused by reduced metabolic activity or disconnected brain tissue or by astrocytic hypertrophy and hyperplasia that accompanies subtle ischemic, cortical alterations.

Smith et al. [86] examined phosphorus metabolites in gray and white matter in autopsy specimens of 9 subjects with late-stage AD, 3 with Pick's disease, and 7 age-matched controls using MRS. In the inferior parietal lobule gray and white matter, phosphomonoester and phosphodiester metabolites were greater than controls in both AD and Pick's disease. A significant correlation was found between phosphodiesters and neurofibrillary tangles in the parietal gray matter of AD patients. The authors suggest that since phosphorus metabolite alterations are present in two cortical degenerative diseases, they are not likely to be specific for AD.

Smith et al. [87] used P31 MRS to examine the frontal lobes of 17 patients with mild to moderate AD, 8 elderly controls, and 17 young controls. The phoshocreatine:inorganic phosphate ratio (PCr:Pi) was significantly lower in AD patients than in elderly controls and significantly higher in AD patients than in young controls. They did not find any differences between the groups on any other phosphate measure, including phosphomonoesters, phosphodiesters, and total nucleotide phosphates. The authors suggest that decreased energy-generating capacity may help explain their observation of decreased PCr/Pi in AD.

C. Other MRS Studies in AD

Besson et al. [88] performed in vitro spectrometric measures of T_1 and T_2 relaxation times of samples of gray and white matter of the brains of 15

AD patients, 5 patients with multi-infarct dementia, and 11 nondemented subjects. Relaxation times were significantly greater in the parietal and temporal white matter of AD patients compared with that of the other subjects. These greater relaxation times were associated with an increase in tissue water content.

Mohanakrishnan et al. [89] used in vitro high-resolution proton MRS to study concentrations of selected metabolites in the posterior temporoparietal cortex of 13 AD and 4 elderly control postmortem brains. Metabolites studied included acetate, alanine, aspartate, creatine, choline, glutamate, 4-aminobutyric acid (GABA), inositol, NAA, and N-acetyl glutamate. NAA was linearly correlated with creatine and with GABA. Severity of neurofibrillary tangles (using a three-level score of mild, moderate, or severe) was significantly correlated with NAA, creatine, glutamate, and GABA. These results support neuronal loss as a finding in the posterior temporoparietal cortices of AD brains. The authors suggest that proton MRS may offer a means to assess the severity and neuropathology of AD.

In a double-blind, placebo study by Pettegrew et al. [90], acetyl-L-carnitine was administered to 7 probable AD patients, who were then compared using P31 MRS to 5 placebo-treated probable AD patients and 21 age-matched controls over the course of one year. Acetyl-L-carnitine–treated patients showed significantly less deterioration in their MMSE and Alzheimer's Disease Assessment Scale [91] scores compared to AD patients on placebo. The decrease in phosphomonoester levels observed in both AD groups at entry was normalized in the acetyl-L-carnitine–treated but not in the placebo-treated patients. Similar normalization of high-enregy phosphate levels was observed in the acetyl-L-carnitine–treated but not in the placebo-treated patients. This important study is the first direct in vivo demonstration of a beneficial effect of a drug on both clinical and neurochemical parameters in AD.

D. Discussion

Magnetic resonance spectroscopic techniques may prove to be a useful adjunct in the early diagnosis of AD when used in combination with standard clinical and neuropsychological evaluations [92]. In addition, MRS may provide new insights into the pathogenesis of the disorder. However, we cannot recommend MRS for routine clinical use until further research is undertaken. Comparisons with autopsy-confirmed AD rather than with clinical diagnosis are required. Cross-validation and replication studies are needed, as are investigations of MRS in differentiating reversible and irreversible dementias, validity in varied populations, and longitudinal evaluation. Exciting, if preliminary, studies of MRS have emerged. We can expect future studies to further clarify findings and expand both clinical indications and research applications for MRS.

REFERENCES

1. P. C. Davis, L. Gray, M. Albert, W. Wilkinson, J. Hughes, A. Heyman, M. Gado, A. J. Kumar, S. Destian, C. Lee, E. Duvall, D. Kido, M. J. Nelson, J. Bello, S. Weathers, F. Jolesz, R. Kikinis, and M. Brooks, The Consortium to Establish a Registry for Alzheimer's Disease (CERAD). Part III. Reliability of a standardized MRI evaluation of Alzheimer's disease, *Neurology 42*:1676 (1992).
2. D. G. Murphy, C. D. DeCarli, E. Daly, J. A. Gillette, A. R. McIntosh, J. V. Haxby, D. Teichberg, M. B. Schapiro, S. I. Rapoport, and B. Horwitz, Volumetric magnetic resonance imaging in men with dementia of the Alzheimer type: Correlations with disease severity, *Biol. Psychiatry 34*:612 (1993).
3. T. L. Jernigan, D. P. Salmon, N. Butters, and J. R. Hesselink, Cerebral structure on NMR. Part II: Specific changes in Alzheimer's and Huntington's diseases, *Biol. Psychiatry 29*:68 (1991).
4. H. Rusinek, M. J. de Leon, A. E. George, L. A. Stylopoulos, R. Chandra, G. Smith, T. Rand, M. Mourino, and H. Kowalski, Alzheimer disease: Measuring loss of cerebral gray matter with magnetic resonance imaging, *Radiology 178*: 109 (1991).
5. O. Narkiewicz, M. J. de Leon, A. Convit, A. E. George, J. Wegiel, J. Morys, M. Bobinski, J. Golomb, and D. C. Miller, Dilatation of the lateral part of the transverse fissure of the brain in Alzheimer's disease, *Acta Neurobiol. Exp. 53*: 457 (1993).
6. J. P. Seab, W. J. Jagust, S. T. S. Wong, M. S. Roos, B. R. Reed, and T. F. Budinger, Quantitative NMR measurements of hippocampal atrophy in Alzheimer's disease, *Magn. Res. Med. 8*:200 (1988).
7. M. F. Folstein, S. E. Folstein, and P. R. McHugh, Mini-mental state, *J. Psychiatr. Res. 12*:189 (1975).
8. N. K. Tanna, M. I. Kohn, D. N. Horwich, P. R. Jolles, R. A. Zimmerman, W. M. Alves, and A. Alavi, Analysis of brain and cerebrospinal fluid volumes with MR imaging: Impact on PET data correction for atrophy. Part II. Aging and Alzheimer dementia, *Radiology 178*:123 (1991).
9. D. J. Meyerhoff, S. Mackay, J. M. Constans, D. Norman, C. van Dyke, G. Fein, and M. W. Weiner, Axonal injury and membrane alterations in Alzheimer's disease suggested by in vivo proton magnetic resonance spectrocopic imaging, *Ann. Neurol. 36*:40 (1994).
10. I. Slansky, K. Herholz, U. Pietrzyk, J. Kessler, M. Grond, R. Mielke, and W. D. Heiss, Cognitive impairment in Alzheimer's disease correlates with ventricular width and atrophy-corrected cortical glucose metabolism, *Neuroradiology 37*: 270 (1995).
11. P. V. Arriagada, T. H. Growdon, E. T. Hedley-Whyte, and B. T. Hyman,

Neurofibrillary tangles, but not senile plaques, parallel duration and severity of Alzheimer's disease, *Neurology 42*:631 (1992).

12. M. J. Ball, M. Fishman, V. Hachinski, W. Blume, A. Fox, V. A. Kral, A. J. Kirshen, H. Fox, and H. Merskey, A new definition of Alzheimer's disease: A hippocampal dementia. *Lancet 1 (8419)*:14 (1985).

13. M. C. Tierney, R. H. Fisher, A. J. Lewis, M. L. Zorzitto, W. G. Snow, D. W. Reid, and P. Nieuwstraten, The NINCS-ADRDA Work Group criteria for the clinical diagnosis of probable Alzheimer's disease: A clinicopathologic study of 57 cases, *Neurology 38*:359 (1988).

14. A. Convit, M. J. de Leon, J. Golomb, A. E. George, C. Y. Tarshish, M. Bobinski, W. Tsui, S. de Santi, J. Wegiel, and H. Wisniewski, Hippocampal atrophy in early Alzheimer's disease: Anatomic specificity and validation, *Psychiatr. O. 64*:371 (1993).

15. M. Ikeda, H. Tanabe, Y. Nakagawa, H. Kazui, H. Oi, H. Yamazaki, K. Harada, and T. Nishumura, MRI-based quantitative assessment of the hippocampal region in very mild to moderate Alzheimer's disease, *Neuroradiology 36*:7 (1994).

16. J. P. Kesslak, O. Nalcioglu, and C. W. Cotman, Quantification of magnetic resonance scans for hippocampal and parahippocampal atrophy in Alzheimer's disease, *Neurology 41*:51 (1991).

17. C. R. Jack Jr, R. C. Petersen, P. C. O'Brien, and E. G. Tangalos, MR-based hippocampal volumetry in the diagnosis of Alzheimer's disease, *Neurology 42*: 183 (1992).

18. P. H. Scheltens, D. Leys, F. Barkhof, D. Huglo, H. C. Weinstein, P. Vermersch, M. Kuiper, M. Steinling, E. C. Wolters, and J. Valk, Atrophy of medial temporal lobes on MRI in "probable" Alzheimer's disease and normal aging: Diagnostic value and neuropsychological correlates, *J. Neurol. Neurosurg. Psychiatry 55*:967 (1992).

19. J. T. O'Brien, P. Desmond, D. Ames, I. Schweitzer, V. Tuckwtell, and B. Tress, The differentiation of depression from dementia by temporal lobe magnetic resonance imaging, *Psychol. Med. 24*:633 (1994).

20. S. Lehericy, M. Baulac, J. Chiras, L. Pierot, N. Martin, B. Pillon, B. Deweer, B. Dubois, and C. Marsault, Amygdalohippocampal MR volume measurements in the early stages of Alzheimer's disease, *Am. J. Neuroradiol. 15*:929 (1994).

21. P. M. Desmond, J. T. O'Brien, B. M. Tress, D. J. Ames, J. G. Clement, P. Clement, I. Schweitzer, V. Tuckwell, and G. S. Robinson, Volumetric and visual assessment of the mesial temporal structures in Alzheimer's disease, *Aust. NZ J. Med. 24*:547 (1994).

22. C. A. Cuenod, A. Denys, J. L. Michot, P. Jehenson, F. Forette, D. Kaplan, A. Syrota, and F. Boller, Amygdala atrophy in Alzheimer's disease: an in vivo magnetic resonance imaging study, *Arch. Neurol. 50*:941 (1993).

23. T. Erkinjuntti, D. H. Lee, F. Gao, R. Steenhuis, M. Eliasziw, R. Fry, H. Merskey, and V. C. Hachinski, Temporal lobe atrophy on magnetic resonance imaging in the diagnosis of early Alzheimer's disease, *Arch. Neurol. 50*:305 (1993).

24. G. D. Pearlson, G. J. Harris, R. E. Powers, P. E. Barta, E. E. Camargo, G. A. Chase, J. T. Noga, and L. E. Tune, Quantitative changes in mesial temporal

volume, regional cerebral blood flow and cognition in Alzheimer's disease, *Arch. Gen. Psychiatry* 49:402 (1992).

25. R. J. Killiany, M. B. Moss, M. S. Albert, T. Sandor, J. Tieman, and F. Jolesz, Temporal lobe regions on magnetic resonance imaging identify patients with early Alzheimer's disease, *Arch. Neurol.* 50:949 (1993).
26. M. P. Laasko, H. Soininen, K. Partanen, E. -L. Helkala, P. Hartikainen, P. Vainio, M. Hallikainen, T. Hänninen, and P. J. Riekkinen Sr, Volumes of hippocampus, amygdala and frontal lobes in the MRI-based diagnosis of early Alzheimer's disease: correlation with memory functions, *J. Neural Transm. [P-D Sect]* 9:73 (1995).
27. T. Matsuzawa, T. Hishinuma, H. Matsui, K. Meguro, M. Ueda, S. Kinomura, and K. Yamada, Severe atrophy of amygdala and hippocampus in both Alzheimer's disease and multi-infarct dementia, *Sci. Rep. Res. Inst. Tohoko Univ.* 37:23 (1990).
28. B. Deweer, S. Lehiricy, B. Pillon, M. Baulac, J. Chiras, C. Marsault, Y. Agid, and B. Dubois, Memory disorders in probable Alzheimer's disease: The role of hippocampal atrophy as shown with MRI, *J. Neurol. Neurosurg. Psychiatry* 58:590 (1995).
29. P. C. Davis, M. Gearing, L. Gray, S. S. Mirra, J. C. Morris, S. D. Edland, T. Lin, and A. Heyman, Neuroimaging-neuropathology correlates of temporal lobe changes in Alzheimer's disease, *Neurology* 45:178 (1995).
30. C. T. Heusgen, P. C. Burger, B. J. Crain, and G. A. Johnson, In vitro MR microscopy of the hippocampus in Alzheimer's disease, *Neurology* 43:145 (1993).
31. S. W. Dahlbeck, K. W. McCluney, J. W. Yeakley, M. J. Fenstermacher, C. Bonmati, G. Van Horn, and J. Aldaq, The interuncal distance: a new magnetic resonance measurement for the hippocampal atrophy of Alzheimer's disease, *Am. J. Neuroradiol.* 12:931 (1991).
32. J. Howieson, J. A. Kaye, L. Holm, and D. Howieson, Interuncal distance: Marker of aging and Alzheimer disease, *Am. J. Neuroradiol.* 14:647 (1993).
33. M. Laasko, H. Soininen, K. Partanen, M. Hallikainen, M. Lehtovirta, T. Hänninen, P. Vainio, and P. J. Riekkinen Sr, The interuncal distance in Alzheimer disease and age-associated memory impairment, *Am. J. Neuroradiol.* 16:727 (1995).
34. B. Early, P. R. Escalona, O. B. Boyko, P. M. Doraiswamy, D. A. Axelson, L. Patterson, W. M. McDonald, and K. R. Krishnan, Interuncal distance measurements in healthy volunteers and in patients with Alzheimer disease, *Am. J. Neuroradiol.* 14:907 (1993).
35. P. Vermersch, P. Scheltens, F. Barkhof, M. Steinling, and D. Leys, Evidence for atrophy of the corpus callosum in Alzheimer's disease, *Eur. Neurol.* 34:83 (1994).
36. A. Biegon, J. Eberling, B. C. Richardson, M. S. Roos, S. T. S. Wong, B. R. Reed, and W. J. Jagust, Human corpus callosum in aging and Alzheimer's disease: A magnetic resonance imaging study, *Neurobiol. Aging* 15:393 (1994).
37. H. Yamauchi, H. Fukuyama, K. Harada, H. Nabatame, M. Ogawa, Y. Ouchi, J. Kimura, and J. Konoshi, Callosal atrophy parallels decreased cortical oxygen

metabolism and neuropsychological impairment in Alzheimer's disease, *Arch. Neurol. 50*:1070 (1993).

38. D. A. Wechsler, *Wechsler Adult Intelligence Scale*, Psychological Corp, New York, 1955.
39. M. Sasaki, S. Ehara, Y. Tamakawa, S. Takahashi, H. Tohgi, A. Sakai, and T. Mita, MR anatomy of the substantia innominata and findings in Alzheimer disease: a preliminary report, *Am. J. Neuroradiol. 16*:2001 (1995).
40. J. E. Goldman, N. Y. Calingasan, and G. E. Gibson, Aging and the brain, *Curr. Opin. Neurol. 7*:287 (1994).
41. M. Verny, C. Duyckaerts, L. Pierot, and J. J. Hauw, Leukoaraiosis, *Dev. Neurosci. 13*:245 (1991).
42. V. C. Hachniski, P. Potter, and H. Merskey, Leuko-araiosis, *Arch. Neurol. 44*: 21 (1987).
43. F. Fazekas, J. B. Chawluk, A. Alavi, H. Hurtig, and R. A. Zimmerman, Magnetic resonance signal abnormalities at 1.5 T in Alzheimer's dementia and normal aging, *Am. J. Neuroradiol. 8*:421 (1987).
44. P. H. Scheltens, F. Barkhof, D. Leys, J. P. Pruvo, J. J. P. Nauta, P. Vermersch, M. Steinling, and J. Valk, A semiquantative rating for the assessment of signal hyperintensities on magnetic resonance imaging, *J. Neurol. Sci. 114*:7 (1993).
45. D. A. Bennett, D. W. Gilley, R. S. Wilson, M. S. Huckman, and J. H. Fox, Clinical correlates of high signal lesions on magnetic resonance imaging in Alzheimer's disease, *J. Neurol. 239*:186 (1992).
46 K. Marder, M. Richards, J. Bello, K. Bell, M. Sano, L. Miller, M. Folstein, M. Albert, and Y. Stern, Clinical correlates of Alzheimer's disease with and without silent radiographic abnormalities, *Arch. Neurol. 52*:146 (1995).
47. G. Blessed, B. E. Tomlinson, and M. Roth, The association between quantitative measures of dementia and of senile changes in the cerebral grey matter of elderly subjects, *Br. J. Psychiatry 114*:797 (1968).
48. M. Brilliant, L. Hughes, D. Anderson, M. Ghobrial, and R. Elble, Rarefied white matter in patients with Alzheimer's disease, *Alz. Dis. Assoc. Disord. 9*: 39 (1995).
49. W. M. McDonald, K. R. Krishman, P. M. Doraiswamy, G. S. Figiel, M. M. Husian, O. B. Boyko, and A. Heyman, Magnetic resonance findings in patients with early-onset Alzheimer's disease, *Biol. Psychiatry 29*:799 (1991).
50. T. Erkinjuntti, F. Gao, D. H. Lee, M. Eliasziw, H. Merskey, and V. Hacfunski, Lack of difference in brain hyperintensies between patients with early Alzheimer's disease and control subjects, *Arch. Neurol. 51*:260 (1994).
51. A. Kumar, D. Yousem, E. Souder, D. Miller, G. Gottlieb, R. Gur, and A. Alavi, High-intensity signals in Alzheimer's disease without cerebrovascular risk factors: A magnetic resonance imaging evaluation, *Am. J. Psychiatry 149*:248 (1992).
52. G. Waldemar, P. Christainsen, H. B. Larsson, P. Hogh, H. Laursen, N. A. Lassen, and O. B. Paulson, White matter magnetic resonance hyperintensities in dementia of the Alzheimer type: Morphological and regional cerebral blood flow correlates, *J. Neurol. Neurosurg. Psychiatry 57*:1458 (1994).
53. P. H. Scheltens, F. Barkhof, J. Valk, P. R. Algra, R. G. van der Hoop, J.

Nauta, and E. C. Wolters, White matter lesions on magnetic resonance imaging in clinically diagnosed Alzheimer's disease: Evidence for heterogeneity, *Brain* *115*:735 (1992).

54. L. E. Harrell, E. Duvall, D. G. Folks, L. Duke, A. Bartolucci, T. Conboy, R. Callaway, and D. Kerns, The relationship of high-intensity signals on magnetic resonance images to cognitive and psychiatric state in Alzheimer's disease, *Arch. Neurol. 48*:1136 (1991).

55. D. Leys, G. Soetaert, H. Petit, A. Fauquette, J. -P. Pruvo, and M. Steinling, Periventricular and white matter magnetic resonance imaging hyperintensities do not differ between Alzheimer's disease and normal aging, *Arch. Neurol. 47*: 524 (1990).

56. P. Scheltens, F. Barkhof, D. Leys, E. C. Wolters, R. Ravid, and W. Kamphorst, Histopathologic correlates of white matter changes on MRI in Alzheimer's disease and normal aging, *Neurology 45*:883 (1995).

57. D. A. Bennett, D. W. Gilley, S. Lee, and E. J. Cochran, White matter changes: Neurobehavioral manifestations of Binswanger's disease and clinical correlates in Alzheimer's disease, *Dementia 5*:148 (1994).

58. L. O. Wahlund, H. Basun, O. Almkvist, G. Andersson-Lundman, P. Julin, and J. Saaf, White matter hyperintensities in dementia: Does it matter?, *Magn. Reson. Imaging 12*:87 (1994).

59. K. M. Reed, R. L. Rogers, and J. S. Meyer, Cerebral magnetic resonance imaging compared in Alzheimer's and multi-infarct dementia, *J. Neuropsychiatry Clin. Neurosci. 3*:51 (1991).

60. R. Schmidt, Comparison of magnetic resonance imaging in Alzheimer's disease, vascular dementia and normal aging, *Eur. Neurol. 32*:164 (1992).

61. D. Charletta, P. B. Gorelick, T. J. Dollear, S. Freels, and Y. Harris, CT and MRI findings among African-Americans with Alzheimer's disease, vascular dementia, and stroke without dementia, *Neurology 45*:1456 (1995).

62. H. Hanyu, S. Nakano, S. Abe, H. Arai, T. Iwamoto, and M. Takasaki, Differential diagnosis of Alzheimer-type dementia and vascular dementia based on neuroimaging study, *Brain Nerve 47*:665 (1995).

63. P. Julin, L- O. Wahlund, H. Basun, A. Persson, K. Måre, and U. Rudberg, Clinical diagnosis of frontal lobe dementia and AD: Relation to cerebral perfusion, brain atrophy and electroencephalography, *Dementia 6*:142 (1995).

64. S. J. Kirsch, R. W. Jacobs, L. L. Butcher, and J. Beatty, Prolongation of magnetic resonance t2 time in hippocampus of human patients marks the presence and severity of Alzheimer's disease, *Neurosci. Lett. 134*:187 (1992).

65. G. Bartzokis, D. Sultzer, J. Mintz, L. E. Holt, P. Marx, C. K. Phelan, and S. R. Marder, In vivo evaluation of brain iron in Alzheimer's disease and normal subjects using MRI, *Biol. Psychiatry 35*:480 (1994).

66. E. Howanitz, R. Bajulaiye, and M. Losonczy, Magnetic resonance imaging correlates of psychosis in Alzheimer's disease, *J. Nerv. Ment. Dis. 183*:548 (1995).

67. M. Lehtovirta, M. P. Laasko, H. Soininen, S. Helisalmi, A. Mannermaa, E. L. Helkala, K. Partanen, M. Ryynanen, P. Vainio, P. Hartikainen, and P. J. Riekkinen Sr, Volumes of hippocampus, amygdala and frontal lobe in Alzheimer

patients with different apolipoprotein E genotypes, *Neuroscience 67*:65 (1995).

68. W. J. Strittmatter, A. M. Saunders, D. Schmechel, M. Pericak-Vance, J. Enghild, G. S. Salvesen, and A. D. Roses, Apolipoprotein E: High avidity binding to beta-amyloid beta and increased frequency of type 4 allele in late-onset Alzheimer disease, *Proc. Natl. Acad. Sci. USA 90*:1977 (1993).

69. A. M. Saunders, W. J. Strittmatter, D. Schmechel, P. H. St. George-Hyslop, M. A. Pericak-Vance, S. H. Joo, B. L. Rosi, J. F. Gusella, D. R. Crapper-MacLachlan, M. J. Alberts, C. Hulette, B. Crain, D. Goldgaber, and A. D. Roses, Association of apolipoprotein E allele E4 with late-onset familial and sporadic Alzheimer's disease, *Neurology 43*:1467 (1993).

70. P. A. Locke, P. M. Conneally, R. E. Tanzi, J. F. Gusella, and J. L. Haines, Apolipoprotein E4 allele and Alzheimer disease: Examination of allelic association and effect on age at onset in both early- and late-onset cases, *Genetic Epidemiol. 12*:83 (1995).

71. E. H. Corder, A. M. Saunders, W. J. Strittmatter, D. E. Schmechel, P. C. Gaskell, G. W. Small, A. D. Roses, J. L. Haines, and M. A. Pericak-Vance, Gene dose of apolipoprotein E type 4 allele and the risk of Alzheimer's disease in late onset families, *Science 261*:921–923 (1993).

72. R. Longo, A. Giorgini, S. Magnaldi, L. Pascazio, and C. Ricci, Alzheimer's disease histologically proven studied by MRI and MRS; two cases, *Magn. Reson. Imaging 11*:1209 (1993).

73. T. K. Shonk, R. A. Moats, P. Gifford, T. Michaelis, J. C. Mandigo, J. Izumi, and B. D. Ross, Probable Alzheimer disease: diagnosis with proton MR spectroscopy, *Radiology 195*:65 (1995).

74. B. L. Miller, R. A. Moats, T. Shonk, T. Ernst, S. Wooley, and B. D. Ross, Alzheimer disease: Depiction of increased cerebral myo-inositol with proton MR spectroscopy, *Radiology 187*:433 (1993).

75. A. Shiino, M. Matsuda, S. Morikawa. T. Inubushi, I. Akiguchi, and J. Handa, Proton magnetic resonance spectroscopy with dementia, *Surg. Neurol. 39*:143 (1993).

76. W. E. Klunk, K. Panchalingam, J. Moossy, R. J. McClure, and J. W. Pettegrew, N-Acetyl-L-aspartate and other amino acid metabolites in Alzheimer's disease brain: A preliminary proton nuclear magnetic resonance study, *Neurology 42*: 1578 (1992).

77. P. F. Kwo-On-Yuen, R. D. Newmark, T. F. Budinger, J. A. Kaye, M. J. Ball, and W. J. Jagust, Brain N-acetyl-L-aspartic acid in Alzheimer's disease: A proton magnetic resonance spectroscopy study, *Brain Res. 667*:167 (1994).

78. P. Christiansen, A. Schlosser, and O. Henriksen, Reduced N-acetylaspartate content in the frontal part of the brain in patients with probable Alzheimer's disease, *Magn. Reson. Imaging 13*:457 (1995).

79. W. Block, F, Traber, C. K. Kuhl, M. Fric, E. Keller, R. Lamerichs, H. Rink, H. J. Moller, and H. H. Schild, 1H-MR-Spektroskopische Bildgebung bei Patienten mit klinischgesichertem Morbus Alzheimer, *Rofo Fortschr. Geb. Rontgenstr. Neuen Bildgeb. Verfahr 163*:230 (1995).

80. J. M. Constans, D. J. Meyerhoff, J. Gerson, S. MacKay, D. Norman, G. Fein, and M. W. Weiner, H-1 MR spectroscopic imaging of white matter signal hyper-

intensities: Alzheimer disease and ischemic vascular dementia, *Radiology 197*: 517 (1995).

81. P. A. Bottomley, J. P. Cousins, D. L. Pendrey, W. A. Wagle, C. J. Hardy, F. A. Eames, R. J. McCaffrey, and D. A. Thompson, Alzheimer dementia: quantification of energy metabolism and mobile phosphoesters with P-31 NMR spectroscopy, *Radiology 183*:695 (1992).

82. C. A. Cuenod, D. B. Kaplan, J. L. Michot, P. Jehenson, A. Leroy-Willig, F. Forette, A. Syrota, and F. Boller, Phospholipid abnormalities in early Alzheimer's disease. In vivo phosphorus 31 magnetic resonance spectroscopy, *Arch. Neurol. 52*:89 (1995).

83. D. G. Murphy, P. A. Bottomley, J. A. Salerno, C. deCarli, M. J. Mentis, C. L. Grady, D. Teichberg, K. R. Giacometti, J. M. Rosenberg, C. J. Hardy, M. B. Schapiro, S. I. Rapoport, J. R. Alger, and B. Horwitz, An in vivo study of phosphorus and glucose metabolism in Alzheimer's disease using magnetic resonance spectroscopy and PET, *Arch. Gen. Psychiatry 50*:341 (1993).

84. R. A. Moats, T. Ernst, T. K. Shonk, and B. D. Ross, Abnormal cerebral metabolite concentration in patients with probable Alzheimer disease, *Mag. Reson. Med. 32*:110 (1994).

85. G. G. Brown, J. H. Garcia, J. W. Gdowski, S. R. Levine, and J. A. Helpern, Altered brain energy metabolism in demented patients with multiple subcortical ischemic lesions. Working hypotheses, *Arch. Neurol. 50*:384 (1993).

86. C. D. Smith, L. G. Gallenstein, W. J. Layton, R. J. Kryscio, and W. R. Markesberry, 31P magnetic resonance spectroscopy in Alzheimer's and Pick's disease, *Neurobiol. Aging 14*:85 (1993).

87. C. D. Smith, L. C. Pettigrew, M. J. Avison, J. E. Kirsch, A. J. Tinkhtman, F. A. Schmidt, D. P. Wermeling, D. R. Wekstein, and W. R. Markesberry, Frontal lobe phosphorus metabolism and neuropsychological function in aging and in Alzheimer's disease, *Ann. Neurol. 38*:194 (1995).

88. J. A. Besson, P. V. Best, and E. R. Skinner, Post-mortem proton magnetic resonance spectrometric measures of brain regions in patients with a pathological diagnosis of Alzheimer's disease and multi-infarct dementia, *B. J. Psychiatry 160*:187 (1992).

89. P. Mohanakrishnan, A. H. Fowler, J. P. Vonsattel, M. M. Husain, P. R. Jolles, P. Liem, and R. A. Komoroski, An in vitro 1H nuclear magnetic resonance study of the temporoparietal cortex of Alzheimer brains, *Exp. Brain Res. 102*: 503 (1995).

90. J. W. Pettegrew, W. E. Klunk, K. Panchalingam, J. N. Kanfer, and R. J. McClure, Clinical and neurochemical effects of acetyl-L-carnitine in Alzheimer's disease, *Neurobiol. Aging 16*:1 (1995).

91. R. F. Zec, E. S. Landreth, S. K. Vicari, E. Feldman, J. Belman, A. Andrise, R. Robbs, V. Kumar, and R. Becker, Alzheimer disease assessment scale: Useful for both early detection and staging of dementia of the Alzheimer type, *Alzheimer Dis. Assoc. Disord. 6*:89 (1992).

92. S. M. Resnick and P. T. Costa, Comments on use of H-1 MR spectroscopy for diagnosis of probable Alzheimer disease, *Radiology 195*:14 (1995).

20

Positron Emission Tomography Studies in Dementia

John M. Hoffman
Emory University School of Medicine, Atlanta, Georgia

I. INTRODUCTION

Positron emission tomography (PET) is a functional imaging technique that allows for absolute quantitation of important variables such as blood flow (Fig. 1), glucose metabolism (Fig. 2), and receptor density as they relate to cerebral function [1–5]. Over the past decade, there have been tremendous

533

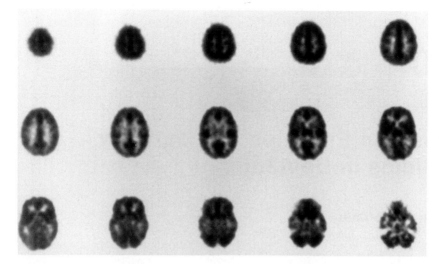

Fig. 1   Cerebral blood flow images of a 32-year-old, normal, healthy male obtained during the resting state—eyes open in a dimly lit, quiet room. The study is performed with approximately 50 mCi of O-15–labeled water. Image acquisition begins approximately 10 seconds after injection and a 90-second scan is obtained. Note the homogeneity of blood flow throughout the cortical and subcortical gray matter structures.

advancements in PET technology [6], with current tomographs now having resolution of approximately 4.0 mm. Development of various tracers, radioligands, and techniques have facilitated the use of PET in probing brain function including neurochemical and receptor systems [7–10]. Due to the improvement of the PET tomograph and refinement of techniques, there has been a tremendous increase in both temporal and spatial resolution [11]. PET methods have been applied to the study of normal physiology [12] and most neurological disorders [3,13,14], including dementia. Studies have explored human attention [15], cognition [16], intelligence [17], neuropsychological function [18], and memory function [19]. The initial fluorodeoxyglucose FDG–PET investigations of patients with various forms of dementia including Alzheimer's disease were performed at UCLA [20]. Alterations in regional and global glucose metabolism with preferential sparing of the primary motor sensory and visual cortex has been observed in those individuals with clinically diagnosed Alzheimer's disease [21,22] (Fig. 3). There appears to be an inverse correlation between the profoundness of Alzheimer's disease

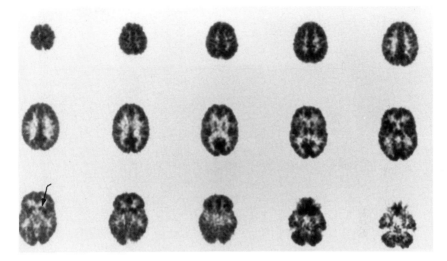

Fig. 2 FDG images of the same 32-year-old male shown in Fig. 1. The FDG images show homogeneous glucose uptake throughout the cortical and subcortical structures. The resolution of these scans is such that the internal capsule can be resolved (arrow). The typical FDG-PET study is performed in a dimly lit, quiet room. Approximately 45 minutes after tracer injection, the patient is imaged for approximately 20–30 minutes.

and the metabolic rate for glucose as determined with PET [23–29]. Since these initial studies, numerous investigations have been performed throughout the world examining FDG-PET in patients with dementia of various types [30–34]. Numerous studies have correlated clinical status, neuropsychological deficits [35–37] and other parameters such as glucose transport [38] with glucose metabolism. A common observation of the majority of these studies in subjects with probable Alzheimer's disease is decreased glucose metabolism in the temporal and parietal association cortex (Fig. 3). Many of the initial PET studies were performed prior to published NINCDS-ADRDA guidelines for the diagnosis of Alzheimer's disease [39]. Therefore, many of the initial studies describe discrepant and contradictory results. Several possible explanations for the discrepancies include ambient conditions in which the study was performed, psychological state of the subject, and numerous other variables known to alter glucose metabolism. Various laboratories use various ambient conditions, and this makes comparison between centers difficult. Also, in patients with various dementing illnesses, the pres-

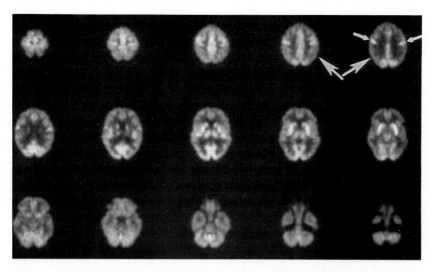

Fig. 3 Images of 58-year-old woman with a progressive dementing illness and questionable depression. The FDG-PET study was obtained to assist with differentiation of the dementia syndrome. The images at multiple levels reveal significant reduction in glucose metabolism in the temporal, parietal, and frontal areas. Note sparing of the motor sensory cortex (small arrows). The classic reduction in parietal association cortex metabolism is also present (large arrows).

ence of cerebral atrophy is important because it has known effects on the measured glucose metabolic rate, both globally and regionally [40–42]. PET methodology has been a valuable tool for neuropsychological and cognitive investigations in individuals with dementia and Alzheimer's disease [43]. PET techniques have found particular clinical usefulness in differentiating dementia syndromes [44–47] and in characterizing metabolic disturbances in the early stages of Alzheimer's disease [48–53]. This chapter reviews the contribution of PET imaging to our understanding of the normal aging process and differentiation and characterization of various dementing disorders.

Over the past 5 years, there has been tremendous interest in brain-activation and brain-mapping studies in normal [54–62] and dementia patients using PET [63–66]. During the study, the patient is engaged in a cognitive, sensory, motor, or other type of task. The radiolabeled water or sugar is injected during the particular activation paradigm, and a cross-sectional image of distribution of tracer is determined. The particular activation paradigm can then be compared (using subtraction techniques) to a baseline or control condition. The results of the distribution of subtracted activity localizes brain function, which would be secondary to the activation task itself. PET techniques are ideally suited for this particular type of approach since most studies are performed using the tracer H_2O, which has a short half-life of 2.0 minutes. This allows for repeated measurements and various tasks to be performed during one imaging session. This allows for powerful within-subject research designs as well as improved sensitivity and diminished variability of results [56,60].

II. NORMAL AGING

Prior to the study of patients with various neurological disorders, numerous studies were conducted to define normal glucose metabolism [12] (Fig. 2) and cerebral blood flow [2] (Fig. 1) and the effects of aging on these variables [67–75]. Age-related changes have been found [72]; however, there is discrepancy between results. In several studies, significant decreases in overall cerebral glucose metabolism as a function of age are reported [72], whereas in other studies no change is noted [41]. Methodological differences most likely account for these discrepancies. More recent studies have corrected for brain volume due to atrophic changes, which occur with aging [40–42]. In these particular studies, some age-related effects were noted [41], however, when the data were corrected for total brain volume and atrophy, no significant age-related decline in blood flow or metabolism was noted. Newer image-registration techniques [76–79] will allow for enhanced capability to correct for both global, as well as regional, atrophy. It should then be possible to better appreciate age-related changes, both structural and function [80]. More powerful statistical approaches [81,82] have been reported to examine brain function interrelationships in both health and disease [74,83].

III. DEMENTIA

Unlike structural imaging studies such as magnetic resonance imaging (MRI) and computed tomography (CT), PET provides a unique quantitative estimate of brain physiology [13], including cerebral blood flow, glucose metabolism, receptor binding kinetics, and neurotransmitter distribution. The majority of studies in dementia have been performed with FDG, a PET tracer used to determine glucose metabolism. The PET tomograph measures the cross-sectional tissue concentration of tracer, and when coupled with the plasma level of activity and a tracer kinetic model, absolute quantitation of glucose metabolism is possible. The majority of FDG-PET studies in dementia have been performed in the resting state with controlled ambient conditions. Various laboratories define this in different ways, but typically it involves the patient or subject being quiet with minimal stimulation in a quiet, dimly lit room. Since it takes approximately 45 minutes for the FDG to be incorporated prior to imaging, the ambient conditions are important, as various stimulations can alter the resting pattern.

Resting state FDG-PET studies have been correlated with various neuropsychological, cognitive, and intellectual variables. Studies conducted in healthy, normal individuals have failed to reveal significant relationships between resting state glucose metabolism and various cognitive test performance measures. In patients with dementia, however, regional metabolic rates do correlate with the severity of illness, type of dementia, the behavioral presentation, and various neuropsychological measures [21,22]. These particular findings allow studies of brain-behavior relationships, selective behavioral deficits, and the neurosubstrates for the specific disease process. PET is unique in that it allows for in vivo investigation of whole brain imaging and can be used to test whole brain and regional interrelationships [81,82] since multiple regional and brain systems can be probed using standard PET techniques. This particular rationale is the basis for brain-activation studies with PET.

IV. ALZHEIMER'S DISEASE

Numerous investigations using PET have been performed in individuals with Alzheimer's disease. It was hoped that an understanding of functional brain deficits determined with this methodology would be helpful in the early diagnosis of Alzheimer's disease [49] and differentiation of the various dementia syndromes [44]. Since Alzheimer's disease accounts for the vast majority of individuals with dementia in the United States [84–88], its impact is unquestioned. Recent investigations have supported a genetic predisposition [89–91]. Since the disease in its early stages can be quite insidious [85,86], it is often confused with the normal aging process. Isolated cognitive decline, particularly early in the illness, causes mild memory impairment, which is a common complaint in individuals in the early stages of Alzheimer's disease [85]. As the condition progresses, cognitive decline becomes more pervasive. Deficits in other aspects of cognition and behavior, including intelligence, orientation, visual-spatial abilities, language, and personality, are noted [92–101]. The clinical differentiation of the various dementia syndromes, including Alzheimer's disease, can be difficult [88,97]. Various diagnostic criteria have been used to assist clinicians in diagnosing Alzheimer's disease [102,103]. In 1984, NINCDS-ADRDA guidelines for the diagnosis of Alzheimer's disease were published [39]. In these particular criteria, clinicians can achieve approximately 80% reliability of diagnosis, particularly late in the disorder. Unfortunately, the majority of clinical studies suffer from a lack of definite pathological verification of disease [104,105]. PET studies which correlate certain metabolic findings and patterns with the diagnosis of probable Alzheimer's disease are somewhat compromised because of the lack of correlation with pathological verification [106–110]. The majority of FDG-PET studies in Alzheimer's patients have been performed in a standard resting state. A consistent finding among most studies is decreased brain glucose metabolism in individuals with moderate to severe Alzheimer's disease. The pattern of hypometabolism observed is typically localized to the parietal temporal regions and later in the disease, the frontal lobes [21,22] (Fig. 3). Numerous investigators have described heterogeneity in the metabolic patterns of AD [45]. Some asymmetry is common, with left temporal parietal hypometabolism more prominent than right parietal hypometabolism [33] (Fig. 4). Reduction in the frontal association cortices are typically correlated

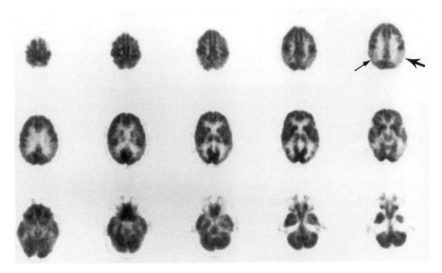

Fig. 4 Images of 55-year-old male with progressive dementia suspected to be Alzheimer's. However, the patient also had profound depression, and the possibility of pseudo-dementia was entertained. The FDG-PET images at multiple levels show reduction in the parietal and temporal FDG uptake. There is asymmetry of the uptake, with the left (large arrows) being more profoundly diminished than on the right (small arrows). In this particular individual, who had significant language disturbance, the metabolic asymmetry correlates with his predominant neuropsychological deficits of language.

with profound dementia. Primary visual cortex, the sensory motor area, cerebellum, and brainstem are typically least affected and usually show normal metabolism. Extensive neuropsychological correlative studies with FDG-PET suggest specific dysfunction of neocortex, both clinically and with metabolic determination with PET [35–37]. The findings with FDG-PET appear to correlate with the regional distribution of AD neuropathology [111–119]. Parietal cortical association cortex typically shows numerous plaques and tangles, and it is postulated that the alteration in metabolism may reflect areas of neuronal vulnerability or disconnection [120–129]. Since FDG-PET measures glucose metabolism of neurons, altered and reduced cortical metabolism may be due to decreased neuronal activity secondary to cell loss or abnormal cellular function in specific brain regions [109]. Recent studies have suggested that the reduced metabolism is primarily due to neuronal loss and gliosis. Other investigators have noted that cortical neurochemical changes [114] in AD may far exceed the actual neuronal cell loss in these areas, thus suggesting that hypometabolism observed with FDG-PET may reflect dysfunctional neurons as well as neuronal loss. It appears that FDG-PET is measuring the combined effects of neuronal cell loss, altered neuronal function in viable cells, and components of synaptic disconnection [130].

Reduction in cerebral metabolism in the temporal and parietal areas has become the hallmark finding in FDG-PET studies of Alzheimer's disease. This particular pattern can be noted very early in the disease and often precedes the appearance of significant cognitive, visual-spatial, or language symptoms [50–52]. The pattern appears relatively stable over time and with advancing dementia [131–133]. However, there can be progression of the metabolic asymmetries in frontal and other neocortical areas. Numerous studies have correlated FDG-PET metabolic abnormalities with cognitive and behavioral changes. Again, heterogeneity of results is noted, particularly in the AD group. This is partly due to the variable clinical presentation of Alzheimer's disease and variable progression and severity of disease. One major difficulty has been the heterogeneity of various patient groups studied by different investigators. In many studies, only individuals with very mild symptoms have been studied. In others, a more representative cross section of individuals with mild to severe disease has been studied. In some cases, individuals with more prominent visual-spatial or language difficulties have been investigated, thus giving asymmetrical metabolic results, as one would expect. In general, impairments in verbal abilities in AD subjects, such as naming and verbal learning, seem to correlate with reduced glucose metabolism in the left hemisphere. Visual-spatial deficits including apraxia and nonverbal intelligence seem to be associated with right temporal and parietal metabolic dysfunction. Several studies have hypothesized that FDG-PET changes may not be temporally related with observed symptoms, but rather predate clinical symptoms. Other investigators have explored PET as a diagnostic tool in predicting familial Alzheimer's disease [134].

V. VASCULAR DEMENTIA

The dementia of small vessel disease, typically termed vascular dementia or multi-infarct dementia, is becoming of increasing interest to both clinicians and researchers [135–144]. In these particular disorders, the observed dementia is believed to arise when a significant amount of cortical and/or subcortical brain tissue has been compromised by a series of vascular insults [136,140,142,145]. Investigators have determined that approximately half of the dementia seen in elderly individuals is secondary to Alzheimer's disease. It is estimated that between 12 and 20% are due to multi-infarct dementia or a vascular dementia syndrome and that an additional 16% may be secondary to combined Alzheimer's disease and vascular dementia [143].

Several recent investigations have attempted to better define vascular dementia [143]. Since vascular dementias compromise the second most common form of dementia in the elderly, it is becoming increasingly important to rule out this potentially treatable form of dementia [146]. These particular syndromes are difficult to characterize because of the heterogeneous and variable pathology. Vascular dementia can include infarction, demyelination secondary to small vessel disease, and various lesion sizes including lacunar infarcts versus large vessel occlusions [146,147]. Since lesions occur in various vascular distributions, a characteristic pattern of symptoms is difficult to define. Studies attempting to correlate neuropsychological deficits in vascular dementia syndromes [136] are complicated by pathological findings of AD in numerous individuals with vascular disease. Furthermore, plaques and tangles characteristic of Alzheimer's disease can be seen in neurologically normal elderly individuals and individuals with vascular dementia [116]. These particular findings have led many investigators to note that a discrete pathological profile of dementia—vascular or Alzheimer's disease—is difficult to define.

Differentiation of Alzheimer's disease and vascular dementia is important because the prognosis, treatment, and associated risk for further difficulty is quite different. Various expert panels have published criteria for the diagnosis and differentiation of vascular dementia and other cerebral vascular dementing conditions [137,138]. In vascular dementia, the patient's history often assists with the differential diagnosis. Certain clinical historical findings, particular evidence of previous stroke on CT or MRI [148,149], abrupt onset and stepwise deterioration in function, or focal neurological deficits on examination all make the possibility of a vascular etiology of dementia more likely. Individuals with vascular dementia often have a history of hypertension. Various clinical standards for differentiation of vascular dementia from AD are used in which a sensitivity and specificity of 70–80% can be achieved [138]. In individuals with overlap syndromes, such as AD and a vascular dementia, the standardized criteria have significantly reduced diagnostic accuracy.

Due to the difficulty of differentiating between Alzheimer's disease and vascular dementia, it is not surprising that techniques such as FDG-PET have failed to provide a specific metabolic pattern for vascular dementia [149] (Fig. 5). Typical findings in FDG-PET studies in multi-infarct dementia

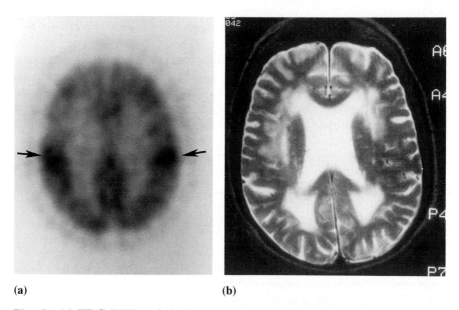

(a)   (b)

Fig. 5 (a) FDG-PET and (b) T_2 MRI images of a 67-year-old woman with stepwise progressive dementia. (a) FDG-PET study shows inhomogeneous FDG uptake throughout the frontal and parietal areas. In this particular individual, the frontal reduction is more profound than the parietal. However, both are abnormal, with significant reduction. Note sparing of the motor sensory strip (arrows). (b) T_2 MRI study of the same individual shows extensive white matter changes consistent with small vessel and vascular disease. In this particular individual, the clinical course was atypical for Alzheimer's disease because of steplike episodes of worsening. The FDG-PET study could be confused with that of Alzheimer's disease if the MRI study showing small vessel disease and clinical course was not known.

are focal, cortical metabolic defects [150,151] (Fig. 6). These defects are often asymmetrical and variable in their distribution. Regional hypometabolic changes may appear in sites distant from the area of known infarction, thus providing evidence of diaschisis [123,127,128]. An example may be reduced FDG uptake in the cerebral cortex secondary to ipsilateral thalamic infarction [152]. Similarly, the visual cortex has been shown to have significantly reduced metabolism in lesions involving the optic radiations [59]. Cerebellar cortex may be effected by contralateral parietal and frontal supratentorial lesions. These particular metabolic abnormalities are felt to reflect dysfunction in anatomically connected brain areas. Several studies have examined FDG-PET findings in demented individuals with multi-infarct dementia and patients with AD [150]. Investigators have failed to reveal a distinctive

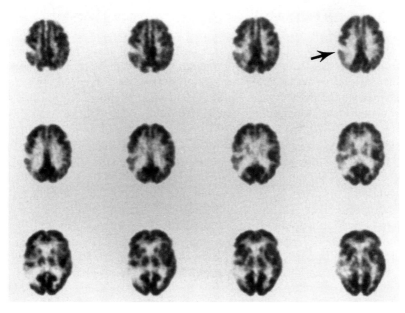

Fig. 6 FDG-PET images of a 72-year-old male with uncharacterized movement disorder and history of a remote right brain stroke. The FDG-PET images show normal distribution of tracer except in the right parietal area (arrow). This particular individual had a large right middle cerebral artery distribution stroke. The typical metabolic findings of markedly diminished FDG uptake in an area of stroke is noted throughout the right parietal and right superior temporal regions.

metabolic defect that would allow for differentiation of these disorders in patient groups. Duara et al. [149] described in 1989 a sensitivity of 92% for Alzheimer's disease and 87% for multi-infarct dementia. However, specificity in this study was only 54%. The overlap between the conditions can be difficult to discern on FDG-PET. When MRI studies are obtained at the same time as the FDG-PET, they can be extremely helpful in differentiating the cause of certain metabolic patterns. Although Alzheimer's disease cannot be completely excluded, a history of stepwise deterioration and an MRI study suggesting widespread vascular changes can assist with definitive diagnosis. In this particular instance, structural and functional brain imaging studies provide complementary information.

VI. SUBCORTICAL DEMENTIAS

Subcortical dementia represents the next most frequent group of disorders affecting individuals in middle to late life. This is not a specific disease process, rather a clinical syndrome characterized by certain neuropsychological impairments secondary to involvement of the brainstem, thalamus, basal ganglia, and frontal lobes [153,154]. These individuals typically present with bradyphrenia, depression, personality change, memory deficits, visual spatial deficits, attention deficits, and alteration in executive function. In rare individuals, language disturbance, apraxia, and visual agnosia can be present. Subcortical dementias include Huntington's disease [155,156]. Parkinson's disease [157–160], progressive supranuclear palsy [161–163], diffuse Lewy body disease [164–166], amyotrophic lateral sclerosis (167), Wilson's disease, spinal cerebellar degeneration syndromes, thalamic degeneration, multiple sclerosis [168], and AIDS dementia [169].

Huntington's disease is one of the most well understood of the subcortical dementing processes. This particular disorder is transmitted in an autosomal dominant fashion with a known defect on the distal end of the short arm of chromosome 4 [170]. Recently, the gene for Huntington's disease was isolated [171]. Huntington's disease affects approximately 5–10 per 100,000 individuals. This particular disorder is progressive and invariably fatal. Subtle changes in motor function [172,173], perception [174], neuropsychological function [175–177], language [178], and behavior are typical. In more advanced disease states, personality changes [179] and extrapyramidal abnormalities [180] including chorea are observed. Neurodegenerative changes in the caudate and putamen and their projection areas are noted [181]. Neuropathological studies note alteration in the caudate, putamen, lateral and medial globus pallidus, substantia nigra, frontal cortex, thalamus, and subthalamic nuclei. Structural imaging studies initially showed atrophy of the caudate and loss of definition between caudate and the adjacent ventricle.

More recent studies have shown cortical atrophy as the disease progresses, particularly in the frontal lobes. FDG-PET studies have been shown to be more sensitive than structural imaging studies in characterizing Huntington's disease. Striatal hypometabolism was noted in symptomatic individuals with Huntington's disease and in the very early, asymptomatic stages of the disorder [182,183] (Fig. 7). The typical FDG-PET finding is that of caudate hypometabolism. Mazziotta et al. studied, in depth, persons at risk for Huntington's disease with serial FDG-PET studies [184–186]. In these studies, at risk individuals with striatal hypometabolism eventually developed Huntington's disease, whereas individuals with normal metabolism remained disease free. The reduction of striatal glucose metabolism correlated extremely well with individuals with positive genetic markers for Huntington's disease. These results have been confirmed by others [187]. These results, again, suggest that PET is able to detect neuronal change prior to any morphological change observed on MRI or CT. Other investigators have not found such significant

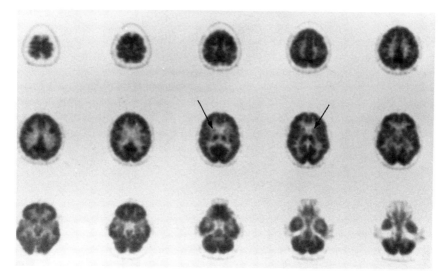

Fig. 7 FDG-PET images of a 55-year-old female with a progressive movement disorder suspected to be Huntington's disease. The patient has a family history of Huntington's disease. MRI was obtained showing no obvious abnormalities and no evidence of caudate atrophy. The FDG-PET images show diminished FDG uptake at several brain levels in the caudate bilaterally. (arrows). In this particular individual, no significant cortical metabolic abnormalities were noted.

results [188]. With the recent development of specific genetic testing, clinical applications of FDG-PET in Huntington's disease is less important. Although the technique is quite sensitive, specificity was not perfect. Striatal changes in FDG-PET are not specific to Huntington's disease. Reduced striatal glucose metabolism can be seen in other disorders affecting the basal ganglia, including benign hereditary chorea [189], Lesch-Nyhan syndrome, and Wilson's disease [3]. Diminished cortical metabolism has also been documented using PET in Huntington's disease [190,191].

Classic Parkinson's disease involves bradykinesia, tremor, and rigidity secondary to striatal-nigral dopaminergic cell loss. Neuropathologically, loss of pigmented cells within the substantia nigra and other brainstem nuclei is noted [157,159]. The dementia seen in Parkinson's disease is difficult to characterize and remains controversial [192]. Memory deficits and visual spatial difficulties can occur in approximately 60% of cases. However, stud-

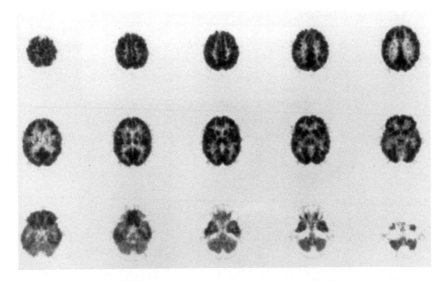

Fig. 8 Images of a 55-year-old female with Parkinson's disease. The patient was being evaluated for a pallidotomy procedure and FDG-PET images were obtained. In this particular individual, there is essentially normal FDG uptake throughout all cortical and subcortical structures. Somewhat increased metabolism in the striatum and thalamus is noted, which can be seen in patients with Parkinson's disease off medication. The FDG-PET studies are obtained in these patients to exclude cortical metabolic deficits as well as superimposed mild Alzheimer's disease.

ies have estimated incidences of 4–93%. This tremendous variability is most likely due to different clinical criteria applied to the dementia of Parkinson's disease. It is now recognized that Parkinson's disease can occur in isolation, in combination with Alzheimer's disease, or with diffuse Lewy body disease [193]. Differentiation and characterization of these disorders is further compromised by the fact that dementia is the hallmark of both Alzheimer's disease and diffuse Lewy body disease [194]. Parkinson's dementia may be secondary to cortical and subcortical changes [195] associated with these diseases rather than nigral striatal changes of Parkinson's disease. Some preliminary evidence suggests that brain behavior alterations associated with Parkinson's disease are neuropsychologically and neuropathologically distinct from those of Alzheimer's disease [196]. FDG-PET studies have shown different patterns of glucose metabolism in patients with Alzheimer's disease, striatonigral degeneration [197] compared with Parkinson's disease [198–204]. Often individuals with Parkinson's disease show diffusely diminished metabolism throughout the cerebral cortex and in the frontal lobes.

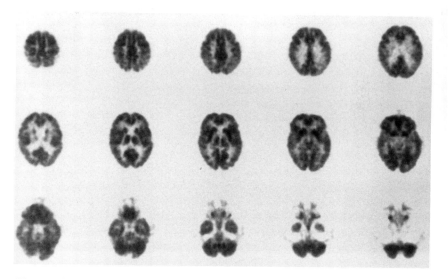

Fig. 9 Images of a 66-year-old male with progressive Parkinson's disease. This particular individual was a pallidotomy candidate. The FDG-PET shows markedly increased FDG uptake in the striatum and thalamus. This particular finding has been observed previously (see text) and may be a potential reliable finding in patients with idiopathic Parkinson's disease. This particular individual was studied off Parkinson's medications.

Interestingly, individuals with Parkinson's disease do not show striatal hypo-metabolic changes as are seen in Huntington's disease. The majority of stud-ies have not shown significant alterations in striatal metabolism compared to control individuals (Fig. 8). Some investigators have noted increased puta-men metabolism in individuals after withdrawal of anti-Parkinsonian medica-tions [201,205] (Fig. 9). In individuals with severe Parkinson's disease and dementia, the FDG-PET abnormalities may be indistinguishable from those seen in Alzheimer's disease (namely temporal parietal hypometabolism) [206] (Fig. 10). It should be noted that the FDG-PET changes in metabolism noted with PET are not absolute in defining Parkinson's disease. The future role of PET imaging in Parkinson's disease will most likely be the study of presynaptic dopaminergic ligands such as F-DOPA [207–213] labeled with positron-emitting radionuclides. These particular studies would allow quanti-tation of presynaptic dopaminergic function [209,213]. Initial studies with fluorodopa have shown and correlated reduction in FDOPA uptake with neuronal cell loss in Parkinson's disease [214] (Fig. 11).

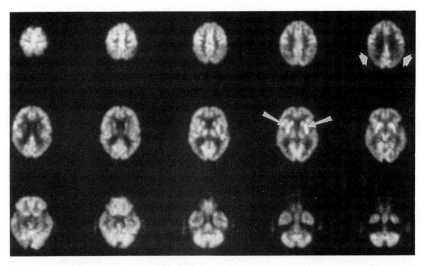

Fig. 10 Images of a 74-year-old male with a progressive dementing illness and classic Parkinson's disease. This particular individual shows increased putamenal uptake bilaterally (small arrows) and parietal and temporal corti-cal reduction in FDG uptake (large arrows). Increased putamenal activity can be seen in idiopathic Parkinson's disease. The diminished cortical FDG uptake is consistent with a mixed disorder of Parkinson's disease and Alzhei-mer's disease.

Progressive supranuclear palsy (PSP), also known as Steele-Richardson-Olszewski syndrome [163], is a neurological disorder that can be difficult to clinically differentiate from Parkinson's disease [215]. PSP is a chronic progressive condition with extrapyramidal motor involvement and dementia. The illness includes certain unique features, notably supranuclear gaze palsy, pseudobulbar palsy, and motor axial involvement including dystonia [163,215]. Pathologically, the illness appears to have many Parkinsonian features. There is neuronal degeneration in brainstem nuclei, subthalamic nuclei, the pallidum, and tegmentum [163]. The cerebral and cerebellar cortex is typically spared. Structural imaging studies have been used to confirm expected atrophy in midbrain structures, calliculi, the pons, and neocortex [216]. Unfortunately, these studies have not been of significant value, particularly early in the disease process. Several FDG-PET investigations have

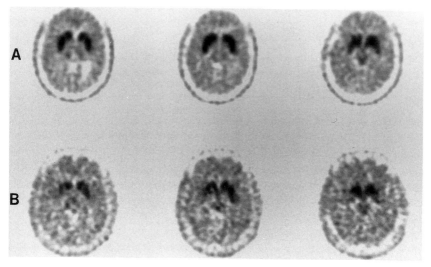

Fig. 11 F-dopa images at three different levels of (A) a normal and (B) a Parkinson's patient. These parametric images are obtained by knowing the plasma activity of the tracer, metabolite quantities, and the rate of F-dopa uptake into the striatum. Note the significantly higher uptake rate in the normal compared to the Parkinsonian patient. This particular finding has been used to assist with the early diagnosis of Parkinson's disease. Other studies have correlated striatal nigral cell loss with F-dopa uptake and showed a significant correlation.

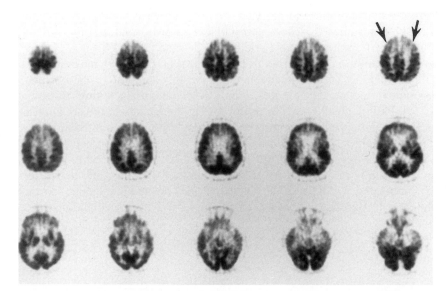

Fig. 12 Images of a 67-year-old male with a 1½ history of progressive dementia. The FDG-PET study shows marked reduction in FDG uptake in the frontal lobes (arrow). These particular findings and the patient's eventual clinical course were consistent with progressive supranuclear palsy.

been performed in patients with PSP. Prominent frontal hypometabolism has been noted in several investigations [217–220] (Fig. 12). The profound involvement of the frontal lobe in PSP is in contradistinction to metabolic patterns observed in Parkinson's disease. It has been postulated that these observations may allow FDG-PET studies to help in distinguishing Parkinson's disease from PSP.

VII. MISCELLANEOUS DISORDERS

Pick's disease is a progressive cortical dementing illness that can often be difficult to distinguish from Alzheimer's disease [221,222]. However, dramatic changes in personality, judgment, and impulse control are typically seen in Pick's disease compared to Alzheimer's disease. In certain cases, isolated language deficits have been observed [223]. Pick's disease typically has an earlier age of onset than Alzheimer's disease [222], and variable memory impairment is present. Due to the overlap and similarity between Alzheimer's disease and Pick's disease, the diagnosis can only be made definitively with biopsy or autopsy. The classic neuropathological change in Pick's disease is that of lobar atrophy in the frontal and temporal regions. Swollen neurons and neurons containing the classic Pick inclusion bodies are noted in these cortical areas. Several FDG-PET studies in individuals with Pick's disease have been performed. Typical FDG-PET findings are focal hypometabolism in frontal and anterior temporal cortical regions [224–226]. Although there is tremendous clinical overlap in AD and Pick's disease, the hypometabolism seen in Pick's disease is typically localized to the frontal and temporal areas and not the temporal parietal areas. Representative images of an individual with biopsy-proven Pick's disease are shown in Fig. 13. Other conditions with frontal degeneration, such as PSP, can be difficult to differentiate with FDG-PET. However, the clinical presentation and clinical course can be quite different.

Creutzfeldt-Jakob disease (CJD) is a rare dementing disorder [227,228] which is transmitted via a prion [229,230]. The disease is typically differen-

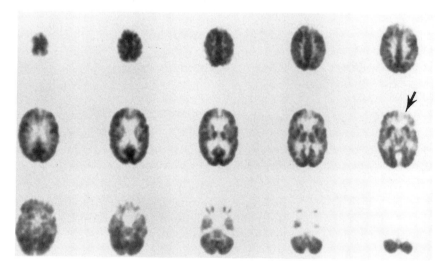

Fig. 13 FDG-PET images of a 57-year-old male with a history of chronic alcohol abuse and prominent personality changes. An MRI showed prominent frontal atrophy. The patient had progressive memory problems and significant cognitive dysfunction. FDG-PET images show diminished FDG uptake in the frontal lobes (left greater than right) (arrow). This particular patient eventually had a biopsy performed in the left frontal lobe, which showed the classic neuropathological changes of Pick's disease.

tiated from Alzheimer's disease and other dementias by its rapid progression with death occurring typically within 3 years of diagnosis. Several biological similarities between AD and CJD and the co-occurrence of the conditions in certain family members purport a genetic contribution to both conditions [231]. A few studies of FDG-PET in CJD have been described [232–234]. In several instances, a pattern of FDG uptake similar to Alzheimer's disease is noted with involvement of temporal, parietal, and frontal association cortex (Fig. 14).

Cortico-basal ganglionic degeneration (CBGD) is an unusual movement disorder characterized by extrapyramidal symptoms, progressive unilateral

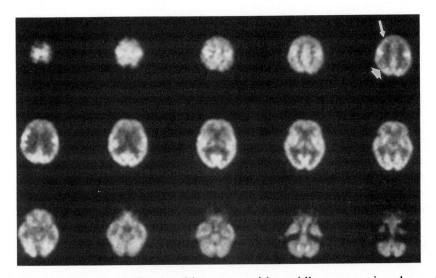

Fig. 14 Images of 65-year-old woman with rapidly progressive dementia and ataxia. A FDG-PET study was performed to assist in the diagnostic differentiation of the patient's clinical syndrome. The FDG-PET images show marked cortical hypometabolism, particularly in the frontal (small arrows) and parietal (large arrows) lobes in the more superior aspects of the brain. Asymmetry between the left and right is also noted. Because of the patient's progressive and rapid decline, a brain biopsy was performed, which showed evidence of Jakob-Creutzfeld disease. Note in this particular individual that the FDG-PET study could be interpreted as Alzheimer's disease. However, the rapid and uncharacteristic clinical course makes the FDG-PET diagnosis of Alzheimer's disease much less likely. This again emphasizes the importance of correlating metabolic and clinical information when evaluating the patient with metabolic imaging.

rigidity, and lateralized cortical signs, including apraxia and involuntary movements [235]. This syndrome can also involve sensory impairment, myoclonus, and alien limb syndrome. In rare instances, clinical signs, such as supranuclear gaze palsy, action tremor, and gait disturbance have been noted. These typically develop dementia late in the clinical course. This unusual disorder is typically refractory to standard parkinsonian drug therapy. Structural imaging studies may show slight asymmetry and atrophy. However, this is not always present. In the early course of the illness, it may be difficult to differentiate from other extrapyramidal disorders, such as PSP and Parkinson's disease. PET studies have revealed metabolic asymmetries in CBGD, particularly involving parietal cortex and thalamus [235] (Fig. 15). The typical metabolic disturbance is contralateral to the side of motor involvement; however, bilateral FDG-PET abnormalities have been described. The neuropathology for CBGD is pale, swollen neurons with ec-

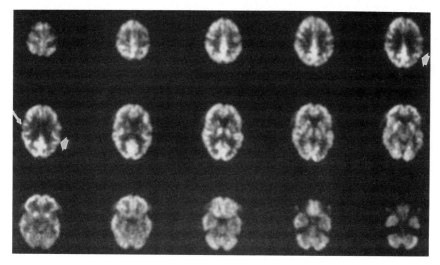

Fig. 15 FDG-PET images of a 50-year-male with a progressive neurological syndrome characterized by profound apraxia, the right extremities more involved than the left. The patient was also beginning to experience mild cognitive impairment. The FDG-PET images show profound metabolic abnormalities, particularly on the left (large arrow), but also on the right in the frontal and parietal areas adjacent to the motor sensory strip (small arrow). This asymmetrical pattern, which shows cortical dysfunction in a brain area felt to be responsible for apraxia, is consistent with the patient's clinical diagnosis of cortical basal ganglionic degeneration.

centric nuclei in cortical areas of involvement. Achromasia is typically seen in the neurons in the substantia nigra and caudate. The substantia nigra also shows significant neuronal loss and gliosis.

Over the past 10 years, there has been increasing evidence of progressive focal cerebral degenerative syndromes which early in their course are extremely difficult to differentiate from other disorders [236]. These syndromes include progressive aphasia, frontal lobe dementia [237], parietal degeneration, and aphasia without dementia. These particular disorders are often confused with asymmetrical presentation of Alzheimer's disease, Pick's disease, and CJD. Over time, however, the patients continue to progress and begin having focal cognitive dysfunction and eventually dementia. Pathological studies are rare; however, they can show mild cortical changes, including nonspecific changes, achromasia, neuronal loss, and mild gliosis. Many of these pathological findings can be seen in other degenerative disorders such as CJD and Pick's disease. Often there is evidence of bilateral involvement late in the course of the illness. Both single photon emission computed tomography (SPECT) and PET studies have been performed in these particular syndromes. Structural imaging studies such as MRI have shown focal asymmetrical atrophy with corresponding dilatation of the ventricular system. SPECT and PET studies have shown metabolic and perfusion defects in the areas that correspond to the primary neurological dysfunction [238,239]. However, the metabolic and perfusion abnormalities are often more extensive than would be predicted from the atrophy and asymmetry on the MRI study. Again, there is no specific metabolic pattern that allows differentiation of this particular syndrome from the early and asymmetrical presentations of Alzheimer's disease, Pick's disease, or CJD.

VIII. FUTURE ROLE OF PET IN DEMENTIA SYNDROMES

This chapter provides an overview of the various metabolic abnormalities noted in various dementia syndromes. It would be ideal if the patterns of altered glucose metabolism observed with PET in various diseases were unique and specific for each disease. Unfortunately, there is tremendous overlap in the metabolic patterns seen with the various diseases. Numerous studies have shown that FDG-PET is very sensitive in determining Alzheimer's disease; however, specificity is lacking [149,240]. Various disorders, including vascular dementia, Parkinson's disease, and Creutzfeldt-Jakob disease, can have the same metabolic abnormalities. The problem of FDG-PET specificity in dementia has been described and discussed in detail by Duara and colleagues [149]. In a manner similar to the clinical overlap of symptoms, FDG-PET results can also overlap. Reliance upon FDG-PET imaging as a diagnostic marker for AD is not possible at this time due to a lack of specificity [149,240]. Furthermore, overlap of both clinical and neuropathological findings makes it difficult to clearly define the sensitivity and specificity of FDG-PET. In spite of these limitations, however, PET continues to be a valuable tool in both research and clinical studies. It provides important information about brain function [3] with a degree of sensitivity not possible with other imaging modalities. FDG-PET may allow us to better understand the mechanisms of behavior in both health and disease. With continued advances in imaging technology, increased diagnostic accuracy may be possible in the evaluation of the dementia patient [241–243]. Combined data, including neuropsychological variables [243] and FDG-PET results, may be helpful in statistical modeling procedures that can predict disease [242]. Initial studies using these techniques have shown a 87% ability to correctly classify mild and moderate demented patients with AD from normal elderly controls [49]. Clinically useful diagnostic algorithms [244] might be constructed using certain FDG-PET variables [242] and quantitative measures of neuropsychological functioning. Furthermore, MRI volumetric measures may provide additional statistical power and thus enhance diagnostic accuracy. At the present time, reliance on FDG-PET imaging alone as a standard diagnostic marker [245–247] is not possible. In certain cases, however, the appropriate use of FDG-PET imaging and clinical history will allow for the differentiation of dementia syndromes. FDG-PET may be particularly helpful in diagnostically difficult cases. A relevant example would be an individual with an unusual clinical history, a nonfocal neurological examination, a normal CT or MRI study, and an FDG-PET which showed bilateral temporal-parietal hypometabolism. In this particular instance, the information would be supportive of the diagnostic impression of Alzheimer's disease. Conversely, a scan unlike that typically seen in Alzheimer's disease may help the clinician in considering other disorders in the differential diagnosis.

In the future, using the techniques of brain mapping and brain activation, it will be possible to explore dementia and Alzheimer's disease and better understand the differences associated with disease by directly challenging involved systems. Furthermore, by designing studies to assess cognition, language, and memory, important information regarding the functional organization of the nervous system will be accumulated. The basic premise of these types of studies would be the fact that, when stimulated, certain brain regions in individuals with dementia do not respond in a manner typically seen in normal individuals. Initial studies in Alzheimer's disease were performed by various investigators using FDG. These particular studies involved a double injection of the tracer with imaging during a cognitive or neuropsychological task. Unfortunately, use of a long half-life isotope such as FDG has the disadvantage of the study being long and difficult for individuals with dementia. These studies, however, have shown interesting changes occurring in dementia and point out how certain capacities remain preserved even when stressed with certain cognitive demands. Investigators have shown that the patterns of brain activation in certain visual, verbal, and memory tasks are similar in AD patients and age-matched controls [64–66]. In these particular individuals, there may hypometabolic abnormalities in the resting state, but it is possible for these involved brain regions to activate in a manner similar to those of normal individuals. Numerous investigative groups are beginning to explore sophisticated behavioral activation paradigms based on cognitive psychological theories. In all brain-activation studies it is critical that the control or baseline task be appropriately designed. For example, if a certain cognitive task is performed that requires visual input as well as verbal output, then the control baseline task should be devised to include visual input and verbal output. The variable of choice would be the specific cognitive task. Since the images are subtracted, it is critical that the baseline or control task be carefully designed so that only the variable of interest is localized.

REFERENCES

1. M. E. Phelps, J. C. Mazziotta, and S. C. Huang, Study of cerebral function with positron computed tomography, *J. Cereb. Blood Flow Metab.* 2:113 (1982).
2. R. S. J. Frackowiak, G. L. Lenzi, T. Jones, and J. D. Heather, Quantitative measurement of regional cerebral blood flow and oxygen metabolism in man using ^{15}O and positron emission tomography: Theory, procedure, and normal values, *J. Comput. Assist. Tomog.* 4:727 (1980).
3. J. Mazziotta and M. Phelps, Positron emission tomography studies of the brain, *Positron Emission Tomography and Autoradiography: Principles and Applications for the Brain and Heart* (M. Phelps, J. Mazziotta, and H. R. Schelbert, eds.), Raven Press, New York, 1986, p. 493.
4. M. E. Raichle, Quantitative in vivo autoradiography with positron emission tomography, *Brain Res. Rev.* 1:47 (1979).
5. M. E. Phelps, S. C. Huang, E. J. Hoffman, et al., Tomographic measurement of local cerebral metabolic rate in humans with (F-18) 2-fluoro-2-deoxy-D-glucose: Validation of method, *Ann. Neurol.* 6:371 (1979).
6. Workshop Panel, National Cancer Institute workshop statement: Advances in clinical imaging using positron emission tomography, *Arch. Intern. Med. 150*: 735 (1990).
7. R. F. Dannals, Synthesis of radiotracers, *J. Neuropsychiatry Clin. Neurosci. (Suppl) 1*:S14 (1989).
8. J. H. Greenberg, M. Reivich, A. Alavi, P. Hand, A. Rosenquist, W. Rintelmann, A. Stein, R. Tusa, R. Dann, D. Christman, J. Fowler, B. MacGregor, and A. Wolf, Metabolic mapping of functional activity in human subjects with the [18F]fluorodeoxyglucose technique, *Science 212*:678 (1981).

9. L. Sokoloff, L. Reivich M., C. Kennedy, M. H. Des Rosiers, C. S. Patlak, K. D. Pettigrew, O. Sakurada, and M. Shinohara, The [^{14}C]deoxyglucose method for the measurement of local cerebral glucose utilization: Theory, procedure, and normal values in the conscious and anesthetized albino rat, *J. Neurochem.* 28:897 (1977).

10. L. Sokoloff, Localization of functional activity in the central nervous system by measurement of glucose utilization with radioactive deoxyglucose, *J. Cereb. Blood Flow Metab.* 1:7 (1981).

11 J. M. Links, Data acquisition, display, and quantification, *J. Neuropsychiatry Clin. Neurosci. (Suppl) 1*:S7 (1989).

12. J. C. Mazziotta, M. E. Phelps, J. Miller, and D. E. Kuhl, Tomographic mapping of human cerebral metabolism: Normal unstimulated state, *Neurology 31*:503 (1981).

13. J. M. Hoffman, M. W. Hanson, and R. E. Coleman, Clinical positron emission tomography imaging, *Radiol. Clin. North Am.* 31:935 (1993).

14. P. R. Jolles, P. R. Chapman, and A. Alavi, PET, CT, and MRI in the evaluation of neuropsychiatric disorders: Current applications, *J. Nucl. Med. 30*:1589 (1989).

15. M. I. Posner and S. E. Petersen, The attention system of the human brain, *Ann. Rev. Neurosci. 13*:2542 (1989).

16. R. W. Parks, D. A. Loewenstein, and J. Y. Chang, Brain imaging: Positron emission tomography and cognitive functioning, *Cognitive Approaches to Neuropsychology* (J. M. Williams and C. J. Long, eds.), Plenum Press, New York, 1988, p. 189.

17. T. N. Chase, P. Fedio, N. L. Foster, R. Brooks, G. Di Chiro, and L. Mansi, Wechsler Adult Intelligence Scale Performance: Cortical localization by fluorodeoxyglucose F 18-positron emission tomography, *Arch. Neurol. 41*:1244 (1984).

18. G. Pawlik and W. D. Heiss, Positron emission tomography and neuropsychological function, *Neuropsychological Function and Brain Imaging* (E. D. Bigler, R. A. Yeo, and E. Turkheimer, eds.), New York, Plenum Press, 1989, p. 65.

19. F. Fazio, D. Perani, M. C. Gilardi, F. Colombo, S. F. Cappa, G. Vallar, V. Bettinardi, E. Paulesu, M. Alberoni, S. Bressi, M. Franceschi, and G. L. Lenzi, Metabolic impairment in human amnesia: A PET study of memory networks, *J. Cereb. Blood Flow Metab. 12*:353 (1992).

20. D. F. Benson, D. E. Kuhl, R. A. Hawkins, M. E. Phelps, J. L. Cummings, and S. Y. Tsai, The fluorodeoxyglucose 18F scan in Alzheimer's disease and multi-infarct dementia, *Arch. Neurol. 40*:711 (1983).

21. J. M. Hoffman, B. H. Guze, L. R. Baxter, J. C. Mazziotta, and M. E. Phelps, [18F]-Fluorodeoxyglucose (FDG) and positron emission tomography (PET) in aging and dementia: A decade of studies, *Eur. Neurol. 29* (Suppl 3):16 (1989).

22. S. I. Rapoport, Positron emission tomography in Alzheimer's disease in relation to disease pathogenesis: A critical review, *Cerebrovasc. Brain Metab. Rev. 3*:297 (1991).

23. N. L. Foster, T. N. Chase, L. Mansi, R. Brooks, P. Fedio, N. J. Patronas, and G. DiChiro, Cortical abnormalities in Alzheimer's disease, *Ann. Neurol. 16*:649 (1984).

24. K. J. Friston and R. S. J. Frackowiak, Cerebral function in aging and Alzheimer's disease: the role of PET, *Electroencephalogr. Clin. Neurophysiol. 42*: 355 (1991).

25. R. Duara, C. Grady, J. Haxby, M. Sundaram, N. R. Cutler, L. Heston, A. Moore, N. Schlageter, S. Larson, and S. I. Rapoport, Positron emission tomography in Alzheimer's disease, *Neurology 36*:879 (1986).

26. N. L. Foster, T. N. Chase, P. Fedio, et al., Alzheimer's disease: Focal changes shown by positron emission tomography, *Neurology 33*:961 (1983).

27. T. N. Chase, N. L. Foster, P. Fedio, R. Brooks, L. Mansi, and G. Di Chiro, Regional cortical dysfunction in Alzheimer's disease as determined by positron emission tomography, *Ann. Neurol. 15* (Suppl):S170 (1984).

28. R. P. Friedland, T. F. Budinger, E. Ganz, Y. Yano, C. A. Mathid, E. Koss, B. A. Ober, R. H. Huesman, and S. E. Derenzo, Regional cerebral metabolic alterations in dementia of the Alzheimer type: Positron emission tomography with [18F]-fluoro-deoxyglucose, *J. Comput. Assist. Tomogr. 7*:590 (1983).

29. B. H. Guze, J. M. Hoffman, L. R. Baxter Jr., J. C. Mazziota, and M. E. Phelps, Functional brain imaging in Alzheimer-type dementia, *Alzheimer Dis. Assoc. Disord. 5*:215 (1991).

30. W. J. Jagust and J. L. Eberling, MRI, CT, SPECT, PET: Their use in diagnosing dementia, *Geriatrics 46*:28 (1991).

31. R. P. Friedland, Positron emission tomography in dementia, *Semin. Neurol. 150*:735 (1989).

32. R. S. J. Frackowiak, C. Pozzili, N. N. J. Legg, G. H. Du Boula, J. Marshall, G. L. Lenzi, and T. Jones, Regional cerebral oxygen supply and utilization in dementia: A clinical and physiological study with oxygen-15 and positron emission tomography, *Brain 104*:753 (1981).

33. D. A. Loewenstein, W. W. Barker, J. Y. Chang, A. Apicella, F. Yoshii, P. Kothari, B. Levin, and R. Duara, Predominant left hemisphere metabolic dysfunction in dementia, *Arch. Neurol. 46*:146 (1989).

34. T. N. Chase, H. Burrows, and E. Mohr, Cortical glucose utilization patterns in primary degenerative dementias of the anterior and posterior type, *Arch. Gerontol. Geriatr. 6*:289 (1987).

35. J. V. Haxby, R. Duara, C. L. Grady, N. R. Cutler, and S. I. Rapoport, Relations between neuropsychological and cerebral metabolism asymmetries in early Alzheimer's disease, *J. Cereb. Blood Flow Metab. 5*:193 (1985).

36. K. A. Welsh, J. M. Hoffman, N. L. Earl, and M. W. Hanson, Neural correlates of dementia: Regional brain metabolism and the CERAD neuropsychological battery, *Arch. Clin. Neuropsychol. 9*(5):395 (1994).

37. K. A. Welsh, J. M. Hoffman, W. M. McDonald, N. L. Earl, and J. C. S. Breitner, Concordant but different: Cognitive function, cerebral anatomy, and metabolism in monozygotic twins with Alzheimer's disease, *Neuropsychology 7*:158 (1993).

38. W. J. Jagust, J. P. Seab, R. H. Huesman, P. E. Valk, C. A. Mathis, B. R. Reed, P. G. Coxson, and T. F. Budinger, Diminished glucose transport in Alzheimer's disease: Dynamic PET studies, *J. Cereb. Blood Flow Metab.* *11*(2):323 (1991).

39. G. McKhann, D. Drachman, M. Folstein, R. Katzman, D. Price, and E. M. Stadlan, Clinical diagnosis of Alzheimer's disease: Report of the NINCDS-ADRDA Work Group under the auspices of the Department of Health and Human Services Task Force on Alzheimer's Disease, *Neurology 34*:939 (1984).

40. J. B. Chawluk, R. Dann, A. Alavi, H. I. Hurtig, R. E. Gur, S. Resnick, R. A. Zimmersman, and M. Reivick, The effect of focal cerebral atrophy in positron Emission tomography studies of aging and dementia, *Nucl. Med. Biol. 17*:797 (1990).

41. F. Yoshii, W. W. Barker, J. Y. Chang, D. Loewenstein, A. Apicella, D. Smith, T. Boothe, M. D. Ginsberg, S. Pascal, and R. Duara, Sensitivity of glucose metabolism to age, gender, brain volume, brain atrophy, and cerebrovascular risk factors, *J. Cereb. Blood Flow Metab. 8*:654 (1988).

42. N. L. Schlageter, B. Horwitz B, H. Creasey, R. Carson, R. Duara, G. W. Berg, and S. I. Rapoport, Relation of measured brain glucose utilization and cerebral atrophy in man, *J. Neurol. Neurosurg. Psychiatry 50*:779 (1987).

43. W. H. Riege and E. J. Metter, Cognitive and brain imaging measures of Alzheimer's disease: Review, *Neurobiol. Aging 9*:69 (1988).

44. E. Salmon, B. Sadzot, P. Maquet, C. Degueldre, C. Lemaire, P. Rigo, D. Comar, and G. Franck, Differential diagnosis of Alzheimer's disease with PET, *J. Nucl. Med. 35*:391 (1994).

45. J. V. Haxby, C. L. Grady, E. Koss, B. Horowitz, M. Schapiro, R. P. Friedland, and S. I. Rapoport, Heterogenous anterior-posterior metabolic patterns in dementia of the Alzheimer type, *Neurology 38*:1853 (1988).

46. C. L. Grady, J. V. Haxby, M. B. Schapiro, A. Gonzalez-Aviles, A. Kumar, M. J. Ball, L. Heston, and S. I. Rapoport, Subgroups in dementia of the Alzheimer type identified using positron emission tomography, *J. Neuropsychiatry Clin. Neurosci. 2*:373 (1990).

47. K. Herholz, D. Perani, E. Salmon, G. Franck, F. Fazio, W.-D. Heiss and D. Comar, Comparability of FDG PET studies in probable Alzheimer's disease, *J. Nucl. Med. 34*:1460 (1993).

48. E. Koss, R. P. Friedland, B. A. Ober, and W. J. Jagust, Differences in lateral hemispheric assymmetries of glucose utilization between early and late onset Alzheimer-type dementia, *Am. J. Psychiatry 142*:638 (1985).

49. N. P. Azari, K. D. Pettigrew, M. B. Schapiro, J. V. Haxby, C. L. Grady, P. Pietrini, J. A. Salerno, L. L. Heston, S. I. Rapoport, and B. Horwitz, Early detection of Alzheimer's disease: A statistical approach using positron emission tomographic data, *J. Cereb. Blood Flow Metab. 13*:438 (1993).

50. D. E. Kuhl, G. W. Small, W. H. Riege, D. G. Fujikawa, E. J. Metter, D. F. Benson, J. W. Ashford, J. C. Mazziotta, A. Maltese, and D. A. Dorsey, Cerebral metabolic patterns before the diagnosis of probable Alzheimer's disease, *J. Cereb. Blood Flow Metab. 7*:S406 (1987).

51. J. V. Haxby, C. L. Grady, R. Duara, N. Schlageter, G. Berg, and S. I. Rapoport, Neocortical metabolic abnormalities precede nonmemory cognitive deficits in early Alzheimer's type dementia, *Arch. Neurol.* *43*:882 (1986).

52. J. M. Hoffman, K. A. Welsh, M. W. Hanson, N. Earl, and R. E. Coleman, FDG-PET is useful in early detection and confirmation of Alzheimer's disease (AD), *Neurology 42* (Suppl. 3):315 (1992).

53. W. Ammann, R. Harrop, J. Rogers, T. Ruth, C. Sayre, and B. D. Pate, Positron emission tomography in the early diagnosis of Alzheimer's disease, *Neurology 36*:888 (1986).

54. P. T. Fox, F. M. Miezin, J. M. Allman, D. C. Van Essen, and M. E. Raichle, Retinotopic organization of the human visual cortex mapped with positron emission tomography, *J. Neurosci. 7*:913 (1987).

55. P. T. Fox, M. A. Mintun, M. E. Raichle, R. M. Miezin, J. M. Allman, and D. C. Van Essen, Mapping human visual cortex with positron emission tomography, *Nature 323*:806 (1986).

56. P. T. Fox, M. A. Mintun, E. M. Reiman, and M. E. Raichle, Enhanced detection of focal brain responses using intersubject averaging and change-distribution analysis of subtracted PET images, *J. Cereb. Blood Flow Metab. 8*:642 (1988).

57. R. C. Gur, R. E. Gur, A. D. Rosen, S. Warach, A. Alavi, J. Greenberg, and M. Reivich, A cognitive-motor network demonstrated by positron emission tomography, *Neuropsychologia 21*:601 (1983).

58. J. V. Haxby, C. L. Grady, L. G. Ungerleider, and B. Horwitz, Mapping the functional neuroanatomy of the intact human brain with brain work imaging, *Neuropsychologia 29*:539 (1991).

59. W. D. Heiss, K. Vyska, G. Klcster, H. Traupe, C. Freundlieb, A. Hoeck, L. E. Feinendegen, and G. Stoecklin, Demonstration of decreased functional activity of visual cortex by ^{11}C-methylglucose and positron emission tomography, *Neuroradiology 23*:4547 (1982).

60. J. C. Mazziotta, S. C. Huang, M. E. Phelps, R. E. Carson, N. S. MacDonald, and K. Mahoney, A noninvasive positron computed tomography technique using oxygen-15-labeled water for the evaluation of neurobehavioral task batteries, *J. Cereb. Blood Flow Metab. 5*:70 (1985).

61. J. C. Mazziotta, M. E. Phelps, and R. E. Carson, Topographic mapping of human cerebral metabolism: Sensory deprivation, *Ann. Neurol. 12*:435 (1982).

62. M. E. Raichle, Positron emission tomography, *New Perspectives in Cerebral Localization* (R. A. Thompson and J. R. Green, eds.), Raven Press, New York, 1982, pp. 145–156.

63. R. Duara, D. A. Loewenstein, and W. W. Barker, Utilization of behavioral activation paradigms for positron emission tomography studies in normal young and elderly subjects and in dementia, *Positron Emission Tomography in Dementia. Frontiers of Clinical Neuroscience.* Vol. 10 (R. Duara, ed.), Wiley-Liss, New York, 1990, p. 131.

64. R. Duara, W. W. Barker, J. Chang, F. Yoshii, D. A. Loewenstein, and S. Pascal, Viability of neocortical function shown in behavioral activation state

PET studies in Alzheimer's disease, *J. Cereb. Blood Flow Metab.* *12*:927 (1992).

65. J. D. Miller, M. J. de Leon, S. H. Ferris, A. Kluger, A. E. George, B. Reisberg, H. J. Sachs, and A. P. Wolf, Abnormal temporal lobe response in Alzheimer's disease during cognitive processing as measured by ^{11}C-2-deoxy-d-glucose and PET, *J. Cereb. Blood Flow Metab.* *7*:248 (1987).

66. J. Kessle, K. Herholz, M. Grond, and W.-D. Heiss. Impaired metabolic activation in Alzheimer's disease: A PET study during continuous visual recognition, *Neuropsychologia 29*:229 (1991).

67. M. J. de Leon, S. H. Ferris, A. E. George, B. Reisberg, D. R. Christman, I. Kricheff, and A. P. Wolf, Computed tomography and positron emission transaxial tomography evaluations of normal aging and Alzheimer's disease, *J. Cereb. Blood Flow Metab.* *3*:391 (1983).

68. M. J. de Leon, A. E. George, S. H. Ferris, D. R. Christman, J. S. Fowler, C. I. Gentes, J. Brodie, B. Reisberg, and A. P. WoH, Positron emission tomography and computed tomography assessments of the aging human brain, *J. Comput. Assist. Tomogr. 8*:88 (1984).

69. R. Duara, C. Grady, J. Haxby, D. Ingvar, L. Sokoloff, R. Margolin, R. G. Manning, N. R. Cutler, and S. I. Rapoport, Human brain glucose utilization and cognitive function in relation to age, *Ann. Neurol. 16*:702 (1984).

70. R. Duara, R. A. Margolin, E. A. Roberson-Tchabo, E. D. London, M. Schwartz, J. W. Renfrew, B. J. Koziarz, M. Sundaram, C. Grady, A. M. Moore, D. H. Ingvar, L. Sokoloff, H. Weingartner, R. M. Kessler, R. G. Manning, M. A. Channing, N. R. Cutler, and S. I. Rapoport, Cerebral glucose utilization as measured with positron emission tomography in 21 resting healthy men between the ages of 21 and 83 years, *Brain 106*:761 (1983).

71. J. V. Haxby, C. L. Grady, R. Duara, E. A. Robertson-Tchabo, B. Koziarz, N. R. Cutler, and S. I. Rapoport, Relations among age, visual memory, and resting cerebral metabolism in 40 healthy men, *Brain Cognition 5*:412 (1986).

72. D. E. Kuhl, E. J. Metter, W. H. Riege, and M. E. Phelps, Effects of human aging on patterns of local cerebral glucose utilization determined by (^{18}F) fluorodeoxyglucose method, *J. Cereb. Blood Flow Metab. 2*:163 (1982).

73. E. J. Metter, W. H. Riege, D. E. Kuhl, and M. E. Phelps, Differences in regional glucose metabolic intercorrelations with aging, *J. Cereb. Blood Flow Metab. 4*:500 (1983).

74. B. Horwitz, R. Duara, and S. I. Rapoport, Age differences in intercorrelations between regional cerebral metabolic rates for glucose, *Ann. Neurol. 19*:60 (1986).

75. A. Loessner, A. Alavi, K.-U. Lewandrowski, D. Mozley, E. Souder, and R. E. Gur, Regional cerebral function determined by FDG-PET in healthy volunteers: Normal patterns and changes with age, *J. Nucl. Med. 36*:1141 (1995).

76. S. Minoshima, R. A. Koeppe, K. A. Frey, and D. E. Kuhl, Anatomic standardization: Linear scaling and nonlinear warping of functional brain images, *J. Nucl. Med. 35*(9):1528 (1994).

77. C. A. Pelizzari, G. T. Chen, D. R. Spelbring, R. R. Weischselbaum, and C. T. Chen, Accurate three-dimensional registration of CT, PET, and/or MRI images of the brain, *J. Comput. Assist. Tomogr.* *13*:20 (1989).

78. R. P. Wood, S. R. Cherr, and J. C. Mazziotti, Rapid automated Algorithm for aligning and reslicing PET images, *J. Comput. Assist. Tomogr.* *16*(4):620 (1992).

79. R. P. Woods, J. C. Mazziotta, and S. R. Cherry, MRI-PET registration with automated algorithm, *J. Comput. Assist. Tomogr.* *17*(4):536 (1993).

80. M. C. Mazziotta and S. H. Koslow, Assessment of goals and obstacles in data acquisition and analysis from emission tomography: Report of a series of international workshops, *J. Cereb. Blood Flow Metab.* *7*(Suppl 1):S1 (1987).

81. J. R. Moeller and S. C. Strother, A regional covariance approach to the analysis of functional patterns in positron emission tomographic data, *J. Cereb. Blood Flow Metab.* *11*:A121 (1991).

82. C. King and R. Cohen, Alternative statistical models for the examination of clinical positron emission tomography fluorodeoxyglucose data, *J. Cereb. Blood Flow Metab.* *5*:142 (1985).

83. S. Minoshima, K. A. Frey, R. A. Koeppe, N. L. Foster, and D. E. Kuhl, A diagnostic approach in Alzheimer's disease using three-dimensional stereotactic surface projections of fluorine-18-FDG PET, *J. Nucl. Med.* *36*(7):1238 (1995).

84. D. A. Evans, H. H. Funkenstein, M. S. Albert, P. A. Scherr, N. R. Cook, M. J. Chown, L. E. Hebert, C. H. Hennekens, and J. O. Taylor, Prevalence of Alzheimer's disease in a community sample of older persons: Higher than previously reported, *J. Am. Med. Assoc.* *262*:2251 (1989).

85. D. R. Crapper-McLachlan, A. J. Dalton, H. Galin, G. Schlotterer, and E. Daicar, Alzheimer's disease: Clinical course and cognitive disturbances, *Acta Neurol. Scand.* *99*:83 (1984).

86. R. Katzman, Alzheimer's disease, *N. Engl. J. Med.* *314*:217 (1986).

87. M. B. Moss and M. S. Albert, Alzheimer's disease and other dementing disorders, *Geriatric Neuropsychology* (M. S. Albert and M. B. Moss, eds.), Guilford Press, New York, 1988, p. 145.

88. R. Katzman, M. Aronson, P. A. Fuld, C. Kawas, T. Brown, H. Morgenstern, W. Frishman, L. Gidez, H. Eder, and W. L. Ooi, Development of dementing illness in an 80 year old volunteer cohor, *Ann. Neurol.* *25*:317 (1989).

89. G. D. Schellenberg, T. D. Bird, E. M. Wijsman, H. T. Orr, L. Anderson, E. Nemens, J. A. White, L. Bonnycastel, J. L. Weber, M. E. Alonso, H. Potter, L. L. Heston, and G. M. Martin, Genetic linkage evidence for a familial Alzheimer's disease locus on chromosome 14, *Science* *258*:668 (1992).

90. G. St. George-Hyslop, R. Tanzi, R. Polinsky, J. L. Haines, L. Nee, P. C. Watkins, R. H. Myers, R. G. Feldman, A. Pilleri, D. Drachman, J. Growdon, A. Bruni, J. F. Foncin, D. Salvion, P. Frannelt, L. Amaducci, S. Sorbi, S. Piacentino, G. D. Steward, W. Hobbs, P. M. Conneally, and J. F. Gusella, The genetic defect causing familial Alzheimer's disease maps on chromosome 21, *Science* *235*:885 (1987).

91. W. J. Strittmatter, A. M. Saunders, D. Schmechel, M. Pericak-Vance, J. Enghild, G. S. Salvesen, and A. D. Roses, Apolipoprotein E: high affinity binding to beta amyloid and increased frequency of type 4 allele in late onset familial Alzheimer's, *Proc. Natl. Acad. Sci. 90*:1977 (1993).

92. P. A. Fuld, D. M. Masur, A. D. Bla, H. Crystal, and M. K. Aronson, Object-memory evaluation for prospective detection of dementia in normal functioning elderly: Predictive and normative data, *J. Clin. Exp. Neuropsychol. 12*:539 (1990).

93. D. S. Knopman and S. Ryberg, A verbal memory test with high predictive accuracy for dementia of the Alzheimer type, *Arch. Neurol. 46*:141 (1989).

94. D. M. Masur, P. A. Fuld, A. D. Blau, H. Crystal, and M. K. Aronson, Predicting development of dementia in the elderly with the selective reminding test, *J. Clin. Exp. Neuropsychol. 12*:529 (1990).

95. K. A. Welsh, N. Butters, J. Hughes, R. C. Mohs, and A. Heyman, Detection and staging of dementia in Alzheimer's disease: Use of the neuropsychological measures developed for the Consortium to Establish a Registry for Alzheimer's disease, *Arch. Neurol. 49P*:448 (1992).

96. M. Storandt, R. J. Botwinick, W. L. Danziger, L. Berg, and C. P. Hughes, Psychometric differentiation of mild senile dementia of the Alzheimer type, *Arch. Neurol. 41*:497 (1984).

97. A. Martin, P. Brouwers, F. Lalonde, C. Cox, P. Teleska, P. Fedio, N. L. Foster, and T. N. Chase, Towards a behavioral typology of Alzheimer's disease, *J. Clin. Exp. Neuropsychol. 8*:594 (1986).

98. K. A. Welsh, N. Butters, J. Hughes, R. C. Mohs, and A. Heyman, Detection of abnormal memory decline in mild cases of Alzheimer's disease using CERAD neuropsychological measures, *Arch. Neurol. 48*:278 (1991).

99. G. Rebok, J. Brandt, and M. Folstein, Longitudinal cognitive decline in patients with Alzheimer's disease, *J. Geriat. Psychiatry Neurol. 3*:91 (1990).

100. I. C. Siegler, K. A. Welsh, D. V. Dawson, G. G. Fillenbaum, N. L. Earl, E. B. Kaplan, and C. M. Clark, Ratings of personality change in patients being evaluated for memory disorders, *Alzheimer's Dis. Assoc. Disord. 3*:240 (1991).

101. Z. S. Khachaturian, Diagnosis of Alzheimer's disease, *Arch. Neurol. 42*:1097 (1985).

102. W. A. Kukull, E. B. Larson, B. V. Reifler, et al., The validity of three clinical diagnostic criteria for Alzheimer's disease, *Neurology 40*:1364 (1990).

103. D. P. Salmon, P. R. Kwo-on Yuen, W. C. Heindel, N. Butters, and L. J. Thal, Differentiation of Alzheimer's disease and Huntington's disease with the dementia rating scale, *Arch. Neurol. 46*:1204 (1989).

104. C. L. Joachim, J. H. Morris, and D. J. Selkoe, Clinically diagnosed Alzheimer's disease: Autopsy results in 150 cases, *Ann. Neurol. 24*:50 (1988).

105. M. C. Tierney, R. H. Fisher, A. J. Lewis, M. L. Zorzitto, W. G. Snow, D. W. Reid, and P. Nieuwstraten, The NINCDS-ADRDA Work group criteria for the clinical diagnosis of probable AD: A clinicopathologic study of 57 cases, *Neurology 38*:359 (1988).

106. J. M. Hoffman, K. A. Welsh, M. W. Hanson, B. Crain, and N. Earl, FDG-

PET imaging in pathologically verified dementia, *Neurology 45* (Suppl 4):A324 (1995).

107. P. L. McGeer, H. Kamo, R. Harop, D. K. B. Li, H. Tuokko, E. G. McGeer, M. J. Adam, W. Ammann, B. L. Beattie, D. B. Calne, W. R. W. Martin, B. D. Pate, J. G. Rogers, T. J. Ruth, C. I. Sayre, and A. J. Stoessl, Positron emission tomography in patients with clinically diagnosed Alzheimer's disease, *Can. Med. Assoc. J. 134*:597 (1986).

108. P. L. McGeer, H. Kamo, R. Harop, E. G. McGeer, W. R. W. Martin, B. D. Pate, and D. K. B. Li, Comparison of PET, MRI and CT with pathology in a proven case of Alzheimer's disease, *Neurology 36*:1569 (1986).

109. E. G. McGeer, P. L. McGeer, R. Harrop, H. Akiyama, and H. Kamo, Correlations with regional postmortem enzyme activities with premortem local glucose metabolic rates in Alzheimer's disease, *J. Neurosc. Res. 27*:612 (1990).

110. E. G. McGeer, R. P. Peppard, P. L. McGeer, H. Tuokko, C. Crockett, R. Parks, H. Akiyama, D. B. Calne, B. L. Beattie, and R. Harop, [18]Fluorodeoxyglucose positron emission tomography studies in presumed Alzheimer's cases, including 13 serial scans, *Can. J. Neurol. Sci. 17*:1 (1990).

111. S. E. Arnold, B. T. Hyman, J. Flory, A. R. Damasio, and G. W. Van Hoesen, The topographical and neuroanatomical distribution of neurofibrillary tangles and neuritic plaques in the cerebral cortex of patients with Alzheimer's disease, *Cereb. Cortex 1*:103 (1991).

112. P. V. Arriagada, K. Marzloff, and B. T. Hyman, Distribution of Alzheimer-type pathologic changes in nondemented elderly individuals matches the pattern in Alzheimer's disease, *Neurology 42*:1681 (1992).

113. D. G. Blessed, B. E. Tomlinson, and M. Roth, The association between quantitative measures of dementia and of senile change in the cerebral gray matter of elderly subjects, *Br. J. Psychiatry 114*:797 (1968).

114. L. A. Hansen, R. DeTeresa, P. Davies, and R. D. Terry, Neocortical morphometry, lesion counts, and choline acetyltransferase levels in the age spectrum of Alzheimer's disease, *Neurology 38*:48 (1988).

115. E. M. Martin, R. S. Wilson, R. D. Penn, J. H. Fos, R. A. Clasen, and S. M. Jaroy, Cortical biopsy results in Alzheimer's disease: Correlation with cognitive deficits, *Neurology 37*:1201 (1987).

116. S. S. Mirra, M. N. Hart, and R. D. Terry, Making the diagnosis of Alzheimer's disease: A primer for practicing pathologists, *Arch. Pathol. Lab. Med. 117*: 132 (1993).

117. R. C. A. Pearson, M. M. Esiri, R. W. Hjorns, G. K. Wilcock, and T. P. S. Powell, Anatomical correlates of the distribution of pathological changes in the neocortex in Alzheimer's disease, *Proc. Natl. Acad. Sci. 82*:4531 (1985).

118. B. E. Tomlinson, G. Blessed, and M. Roth, Observations on the brains of nondemented old people, *J. Neurol. Sci. 7*:331 (1968).

119. B. E. Tomlinson and G. Henderson, Some quantitative cerebral findings in normal and demented old people, *Neurobiology of Aging* (R. D. Terry and S. Gershon, ed.), Raven Press, New York, 1976, p. 183.

120. B. T. Hyman, G. W. Van Hoesen, A. R. Damasio, and C. L. Barnes, Alzhei-

mer's disease: Cell-specific pathology isolates the hippocampal formation, *Science 225*:1168 (1984).

121. J. R. Absher and D. F. Benson, Disconnection syndromes: An overview of Geschwind's contributions, *Neurology 43*:862 (1993).

122. H. Akiyama, R. Harrop, P. L. McGeer, R. Peppard, and E. G. McGeer, Crossed cerebellar and uncrossed basal ganglia and thalamic diaschisis in Alzheimer's disease, *Neurology 39*:541 (1989).

123. J. C. Baron, M. G. Bousser D. Comar, et al., Crossed-cerebellar diaschesis: A remote functional depression secondary to supra-tentorial infarction in man, *J. Cereb. Blood Flow Metab.* (Suppl 1):S500 (1981).

124. J. C. Baron, R. D'Antona, P. Pantano, M. Serdaru, Y. Samson, and M. G. Bousser, Effects of thalamic stroke on energy metabolism of the cerebral cortex: A positron emission tomography study in man, *Brain 109*:1243 (1986).

125. N. Geschwind, Disconnection syndromes in animals and man, Parts I and II, *Brain 88*:237, 585 (1965).

126. A. F. Leuchter, T. F. Newton, I. A. Cook, D. O. Walter, S. Rosenberg-Thompson, and P. A. Lachenbruch, Changes in brain functional connectivity in Alzheimer type and multi-infarct dementia, *Brain 115*:1543 (1992).

127. P. Pantano, J. C. Baron, Y. Samson, M. G. Bousser, C. Derouesne, and D. Comar, Crossed cerebellar diaschisis: Further studies, *Brain 109*:677 (1986).

128. M. Kushner, A. Alavi, M. Reivich, et al. Contralateral cerebellar hypometabolism following cerebral insult: A positron emission tomographic study, *Ann. Neurol. 15*:425 (1984).

129. P. Satz, Brain reserve capacity on symptom onset after brain injury: A formulation and review of evidence for threshold theory, *NeuroPsychology 7*:273 (1993).

130. G. S. Smith, M. J. de Leon, A. E. George, A. Kluger, N. D. Volkow, T. McGrae, J. Golomb, S. H. Ferris, B. Reisberg, J. Ciaravino, and M. E. La Regina, Topography of cross-sectional and longitudinal glucose metabolic deficits in Alzheimer's disease: Pathophysiologic implications, *Arch. Neurol. 49*: 1142 (1992).

131. J. V. Haxby, C. L. Grady, E. Koss, B. Horowitz, L. Heston, M. Schapiro, R. P. Friedland, and S. I. Rapoport, Longitudinal study of cerebral metabolic asymmetries and associated neuropsychological patterns in early dementia of the Alzheimer type, *Arch. Neurol. 47*:753 (1990).

132. C. L. Grady, J. V. Haxby, B. Horwitz, M. Sundaram, G. Berg, M. Schapiro, R. P. Friedland, and S. I. Rapoport, Longitudinal study of the early neuropsychological and cerebral metabolic changes in dementia of the Alzheimer type, *J. Clin. Exp. Neuropsychol. 10*:579 (1988).

133. N. R. Cutler, J. V. Haxby, R. Duara, C. L. Grady, A. M. Moore, J. E. Parisi, J. White, L. Heston, R. M. Margolin, and S. I. Rapoport. Brain metabolism as measured with positron emission tomography: Serial assessment in a patient with familial Alzheimer's disease, *Neurology 35*:1556 (1985).

134. P. Pietrini, C. L. Grady, J. V. Haxby, L. Heston, J. A. Salerno, A. Gonzales-Aviles, and M. B. Shapiro, Resting cerebral glucose metabolism (CMRglc)

does not identify subjects "at risk" for familial Alzheimer disease, *Ann. Neurol. 30*:287 (1991).

135. D. A. Bennett, R. S. Wilson, D. W. Gilley, and J. H. Fox, Clinical diagnosis of Binswanger's disease, *J. Neurol. Neurosurg. Psychiatry 53*:961 (1990).

136. K. B. Boone, B. L. Miller, I. M. Lesser, M. Mehringer, E. Hill-Gutierrez, M. A. Goldberg, and N. G. Berman, Neuropsychological correlates of white-matter lesions in healthy elderly subjects: A threshold effect, *Arch. Neurol. 49*: 549 (1992).

137. G. C. Roman, T. K. Tatemichi, T. Erkinjuntti, J. L. Cummings, J. C. Masdeu, J. H. Garcia, L. Amaducci, J. M. Orgogozo, A. Brun, A. Hofman, D. M. Moody, M. D. Obrien, T. Yamaguchi, J. Grafman, B. P. Drayer, D. A. Bennett, M. Fisher, J. Ogata, E., Kokmen, F. Bermego, P. A. Wolf, P. B. Gorelick, K. L. Bick, A. D. Pajeau, M. A. Bell, C. DeCarli, A. Culebras, A. D. Korczyn, J. Bogousslavsky, A. Hartmann, and P. Scheinberg, Vascular dementia: Diagnostic criteria for research studies. Report of the NINDS-AIREN International Workshop, *Neurology 43*:250 (1993).

138. H. C. Chui, J. I. Victoroff, D. Margolin, W. Jagust, R. Shankle, and R. Katzman, Criteria for the diagnosis of ischemic vascular dementia proposed by the State of California Alzheimer's Disease Diagnostic and Treatment Centers, *Neurology 42*:473 (1992).

139. P. Fischer, K. Jellinger, G. Gatterbi, and G. Danielcyzk, Prospective neuropathological validation of Hachinski's ischaemic score in dementias, *J. Neurol. Neurosurg. Psychiatry 54*:580 (1991).

140. V. C. Hachinski, N. A. Lassen, and J. Marshall, Multi-infarct dementia. A cause of mental deterioration in the elderly, *Lancet 2*:207 (1974).

141. W. B. Kannel, T. R. Dawber, P. Sorlie, and P. A. Wolf, Component blood pressure and risk of atherothrombotic brain infarct: The Framingham Study, *Stroke 7*:327 (1976).

142. C. A. Kooistra and K. M. Heilman, Memory loss from a subcortical white matter infarct, *J. Neurol. Neurosurg. Psychiatry 51*:866 (1988).

143. D. B. Larson, J. S. Lyons, J. C. Bareta, B. J. Burns, D. G. Blazer, and I. D. Goldstrom, The construct validity of the ischemic score of Hachinski for the detection of dementias, *J. Neuropsychiatry 1*:181 (1988).

144. G. C. Roman, The epidemiology of vascular dementia, *Cerebral Ischemia and Dementia* (A. Hartmann, W. Kuschinsky, and S. Hoyer, eds.), Springer-Verlag, Berlin, 1991, p. 9.

145. W. G. Rosen, R. D. Terry, P. A. Fuld, R. Katzman, and A. Peck, Pathological verification of ischemic score in differentiation of dementias, *Ann. Neurol. 7*: 486 (1980).

146. P. Scheinberg, Dementia due to vascular disease—a multifactorial disorder, *Stroke 19*:1291 (1988).

147. T. K. Tatemichi, How acute brain failure becomes chronic: A view of the mechanisms of dementia related to stroke, *Neurology 40*:1652 (1990).

148. S. Pappata, S. Tran Dinh, J. C. Baron, H. Cambon, and A. Syrota, Remote metabolic effects of cerebrovascular lesions: Magnetic resonance and positron tomography imaging, *Neuroradiology 29*:1 (1987).

149. R. Duara, W. Barker, D. Loewenstein, S. Pascal, and B. Bowen, Sensitivity and specificity of positron emission tomography and magnetic resonance imaging studies in Alzheimer's disease and multi-infarct dementia, *Eur. Neurol.* *29*:9 (1989).

150. D. E. Kuhl, E. J. Metter, and W. H. Riege, Patterns of cerebral glucose utilization in depression, multiple infarct dementia, and Alzheimer's disease, *Brain Imaging and Brain Function, Vol.* 63 (L. Sokoloff, ed.), Raven Press, New York, 1985, p. 211.

151. D. E. Kuhl, M. E. Phelps, A. P. Kowell, E. J. Metter, C. Selin, and J. Winter, Effect of stroke on local cerebral metabolism and perfusion: Mapping by emission computed tomography of ^{18}FDG and ^{13}NH$_3$, *Ann. Neurol. 8*:47 (1980).

152. E. C. Laterre, A. G. De Volder, and A. M. Goffinet, Brain glucose metabolism in thalamic syndrome, *J. Neurol. Neursurg. Psychiatry 51*:427 (1988).

153. J. L. Cummings, *Subcortical Dementia*, New York, Oxford University Press, 1990.

154. M. Freedman, Parkinson's disease, *Subcortical Dementia* (J. Cummings, ed.), Oxford University Press, New York, 1990, p. 108.

155. S. E. Folstein, J. Brandt, and M. R. Folstein, Huntington's disease, *Subcortical Dementia* (J. Cummings, ed.), Oxford University Press, New York, 1990, p. 87.

156. J. B. Martin and J. F. Gusella, Huntington's disease: Pathogenesis and management (review), *N. Engl. J. Med. 315*(20):1267 (1986).

157. H. Bernheimer, W. Birkmeyer, O. Hornykiewicz, K. Mellinger, and F. Seitelberger, Brain dopamine and the syndromes of Parkinson and Huntington, *J. Neurol. Sci. 20*:415 (1973).

158. I. Kessler, Parkinson's disease in epidemiological perspective, *Advances in Neurology, Vol.* 19 (B. S. Schoenberg, ed.), Raven Press, New York, 1978, p. 355.

159. J. B. Penney and A. B. Young, Huntington's disease, *Parkinson's Disease and Movement Disorders* (J. Jankovio and E. Toloso, eds.), Urban & Schwarzenberg Press, Baltimore, 1988, p. 167.

160. A. M. Hakim and G. Mathieson, Dementia in Parkinson's disease: a neuropathologic study, *Neurology 29*:1209 (1979).

161. P. H. Davis, C. Bergeron, and D. R. McLachlan, Atypical presentation of progressive supranuclear palsy, *Ann. Neurol. 17*:373 (1985).

162. K. Jellinger, P. Riederer, and M. Tomonga, Progressive supranuclear palsy: Clinicopathological and biochemical studies, *J. Neural Trans. Suppl. 16*:111 (1980).

163. J. C. Richardson, J. Steele, and J. Olszewski, Supranuclear ophthalmoplegia, pseudobulbar palsy, nuchal dystonia and dementia: A clinical report on eight cases of "heterogenous system degeneration." *Trans. Am. Neurol. Assoc. 88*: 25 (1963).

164. K. Kosaka, M. Yoshimira, K. Ikeda, and H. Budka, Diffuse type of Lewy body disease: progressive dementia with abundant cortical Lewy bodies and senile changes of varying degree: A new disease?, *Clin. Neuropathol. 3*:185 (1984).

165. W. I. Rosenblum and N. R. Ghatak, Lewy bodies in the presence of Alzheimer's disease, *Arch. Neurol. 36*:170 (1979).

166. W. R. G. Gibb, Idiopathic parkinsons disease and the Lewy body disorders, *Neuropathol. Appl. Neurobiol. 12*:223 (1986).

167. A. J. Hudson, Amyotrophic lateral sclerosis and its association with dementia, parkinsonism, and other neurological disorders: A review, *Brain 104*:217 (1981).

168. S. M. Rao, Multiple sclerosis, *Subcortical Dementia* (J. Cummings, ed.), Oxford University Press, New York, 1990, p. 164.

169. B. A. Navia, The AIDS dementia complex, *Subcortical Dementia* (J. Cummings, ed.), Oxford University Press, New York, 1990, p. 181.

170. J. F. Gusella, N. S. Wexler, P. M. Conneally, S. L. Nayler, M. A. Anderson, R. E. Tanki, P. C. Watkins, K. Ottina, M. R. Wallace, A. Y. Sakaguchi, A. B. Young, I. Shoulson, E. Bonilla, and J. B. Martin, A polymorphic DNA marker genetically linked to Huntington's disease, *Nature 306*:234 (1983).

171. Huntington's Disease Collaborative Research Group, A novel gene containing a trinucleotide repeat that is expanded and unstable on Huntington's disease chromosomes, *Cell 72*:971 (1993).

172. J. L. Bradshaw, J. G. Phillips, C. Dennis, J. B. Mattingley, D. Andrewes, E. Chiu, J. M. Pierson, and J. A. Bradshaw, Initiation and execution of movement sequences in those suffering from and at risk of developing Huntington's disease, *J. Clin. Exp. Neuropsychol. 14*:179 (1992).

173. J. Hefter, V. Homberg, H. W. Lange, and H. J. Freud, Impairment of rapid movement in Huntington's disease, *Brain 110*:585 (1987).

174. P. Brouwers, C. Cox, A. Martin, T. Chase, and P. Fedio, Differential perceptual-spatial impairment in Huntington's and Alzheimer's dementias, *Arch. Neurol. 41*:1073 (1984).

175. N. Butters, D. Sax, K. Montgomery, and S. Tarlow, Comparison of the neuropsychological deficits associated with early and advanced Huntington's disease, *Arch. Neurol. 35*:585 (1978).

176. R. C. Josiassen, L. M. Curry, and E. L. Mancall, Development of neuropsychological deficits in Huntington's disease, *Arch. Neurol. 40*:791 (1983).

177. N. Butters, J. WoHe, M. Martone, E. Granholm, and L. S. Cermak, Memory disorders associated with Huntington's disease: Verbal recall, verbal recognition, and procedural memory, *Neuropsychologia 23*:729 (1985).

178. K. Podoll, P. Caspary, H. W. Lange, and J. Noth, Language functions in Huntington's disease, *Brain 111*:1475 (1988).

179. S. E. Folstein, M. H. Abbott, G. A. Chase, B. A. Jensen, and M. F. Folstein, The association of affective disorder with Huntington's disease in a case series and in families, *Psvchol. Med. 13*:537 (1983).

180. P. D. Thompson, A. Berardelli, J. C. Rothwell, B. L. Day, J. P. R. Dick, R. Benecke, and C. D. Marsden, The coexistence of bradykinesia and chorea in Huntington's disease and its implications for theories of basal ganglia control of movement, *Brain 111*:223 (1988).

181. J. P. Von Sattel, R. H. Myers, T. J. Stevens, R. J. Ferrante, E. D. Bird, and

E. P. Richardson, Neuropathological classification of Huntington's disease, *J. Neuropathol. Exp. Neurol. 44*:559 (1985).

182. D. E. Kuhl, E. J. Metter, W. H. Riege, and C. H. Markham, Patterns of cerebral glucose utilization in Parkinson's disease and Huntington's disease, *Ann. Neurol. 15* (Suppl):S119 (1984).
183. E. S. Garnett, G. Firnau, C. Nahmias, R. Carbotte, and G. Bartolucci, Reduced striatal glucose consumption and prolonged reaction time are early features in Huntington's disease, *J. Neurol. Sci. 65*:231 (1984).
184. J. C. Mazziotta, M. E. Phelps, J. J. Pahl, S. C. Huang, L. R. Baxter, W. H. Riege, J. M. Hoffman, D. E. Kuhl, A. B. Lanto, J. A. Wapenski, and C. H. Markham, Reduced cerebral glucose metabolism in asymptomatic subjects at risk for Huntington's disease, *N. Engl. J. Med. 316*:357 (1987).
185. S. T. Grafton, J. C. Mazziotta, J. J. Pahl, P. St. George-Hyslop, J. L. Haines, J. Gusella, J. M. Hoffman, L. R. Baxter, and M. E. Phelps. A comparison of neurological, metabolic, structural, and genetic evaluations in persons at risk for Huntington's disease, *Ann. Neurol. 28*:614 (1990).
186. S. T. Grafton, J. C. Mazziotta, J. J. Pahl, P. St. George-Hyslop, J. L. Haines, J. Gusella, J. M. Hoffman, L. R. Baxter, and M. E. Phelps, Serial changes of cerebral glucose metabolism and caudate size in persons at risk for Huntington's disease, *Arch. Neurol. 49*:1161 (1992).
187. M. R. Hayden, J. Hewitt, A. J. Stoessl, C. Clark, W. Ammann, and W. R. W. Martin, The combined use of positron emission tomography and DNA polymorphisms for preclinical detection of Huntington's disease, *Neurol. 37*: 1441 (1987).
188. A. B. Young, J. B. Penney, S. Starosta-Rubinstein, D. Markel, S. Berent, J. Rothley, A. Betley, and R. Hichwa, Normal caudate glucose metabolism in persons at risk for Huntington's disease, *Arch. Neurol. 44*:254 (1987).
189. O. Suchowersky, M. R. Hayden, M. R. W. Marti, A. J. Stoessl, A. M. Hildebrand, and B. D. Pate, Cerebral metabolism of glucose in benign hereditary chorea, *Movement Disord. 1*:3346 (1986).
190. W. R. W. Martin, C. Clark, W. Ammann, A. J. Stoessl, W. Shtybel, and M. R. Hayden, Cortical glucose metabolism in Huntington's disease, *Neurology 42*:223 (1992).
191. T. Kuwert, H. W. Lange, K. -J. Langen, H. Herzog, A. Aulick, and L. E. Feinendegen, Cortical and subcortical glucose consumption measured by PET in patients with Huntington's disease, *Brain 113*:1405 (1990).
192. J. O. Rinne, J. Rummukainen, L. Paljarvi, and U. K. Rinne, Dementia in Parkinson's disease is related to neuronal loss in the medial substantia nigra, *Ann. Neurol. 26*:47 (1989).
193. M. E. Mahler and J. L. Cummings, Alzheimer disease and the dementia of Parkinson disease: Comparative investigations, *Alzheimer Dis. Assoc. Disord. 14*:133 (1990).
194. M. Yoshimura, Cortical changes in the parkinsonian brain: A contribution to the delineation of "diffuse Lewy body disease," *J. Neurol. 229*:17 (1983).
195. J. H. Xuereb, B. E. Tomlinson, D. Irving, R. H. Perry, G. Blessed, and E.

K. Perry, Cortical and subcortical pathology in Parkinson's disease: Relationship to Parkinsonian dementia, *Advances in Neurology*, Vol. 53: *Parkinson's Disease: Anatomy, Pathology, and Therapy* (M. B. Streifler, A. D. Korczn, E. Melamed, and M. B. H. Youdin, eds.), Raven Press, New York, 1990, p. 35.

196. M. F. Mendez, N. L. Adams, and S. K. Lewandowski, Neurobehavioral changes associated with caudate lesions, *Neurology* 39:349 (1989).

197. D. Eidelberg, S. Takikawa, J. R. Moeller, V. Dhawan, K. Redington, T. Chaly, W. Robeson, J. R. Dahl, D. Margouleff, E. Fazzini, S. Przedborski, and S. Fahn, Striatal hypometabolism distinguishes striatonigral degeneration from Parkinson's disease, *Ann. Neurol.* 33:518 (1993).

198. D. Eidelberg, J. R. Moeller, V. Dhawan, J. J. Sidtis, J. Z. Ginos, S. C. Strother, J. Cedarbaum, P. Greene, S. Fahn, and D. A. Rottenberg, The metabolic anatomy of Parkinson's disease: Complementary [^{18}F]fluorodeoxyglucose and [^{18}F]fluorodopa positron emission tomographic studies, *Movement Disord.* 5(3):203 (1990).

199. D. Eidelberg, J. R. Moeller, V. Dhawan, P. Spetsieris, S. Takikawa, T. Ishikawa, T. Chaly, W. Robeson, D. Margouleff, S. Przedborski, and S. Fahn, The metabolic topography of parkinsonism, *J. Cereb. Blood Flow Metab.* 14: 783 (1994).

200. D. Eidelberg, J. R. Moeller, T. Ishikawa, V. Dhawan, P. Spetsieris, T. Chaly, A. Belakhlef, F. Mandel, S. Przedborski, and S. Fahn, Early differential diagnosis of Parkinson's disease with ^{18}F-fluorodeoxyglucose and positron emission tomography, *Neurology* 45:1995 (1995).

201. D. Eidelberg, J. R. Moeller, T. Ishikawa, V. Dhawan, P. Spetsieris, T. Chaly, W. Robeson, J. R. Dahl, and D. Margouleff, Assessment of disease severity in parkinsonism with fluorine-18-fluorodeoxyglucose and PET, *J. Nucl. Med.* 36:378 (1995).

202. W. R. W. Martin, J. H. Beckman, D. B. Calne, M. J. Adam, R. Harrop, J. G. Rogers, T. J. Ruth, C. I. Sayre, and B. D. Pate, Cerebral glucose metabolism in Parkinson's disease, *Can. J. Neurol. Sci.* 11:169 (1984).

203. J. S. Perlmutter, New insights into the pathophysiology of Parkinson's disease: The challenge of positron emission tomography, *Trends Neurosci.* 11:203 (1988).

204. E. J. Metter, D. E. Kuhl, and W. H. Riege, Brain glucose metabolism in Parkinson's disease, *Advances in Neurology*, Vol. 53: *Anatomy, Pathology, and Therapy* (M. B. Streifler, A. D. Korczyn, E. Melamed and M. B. H. Youdim, eds.), Raven Press, New York, 1990, p. 135.

205. D. Rougemont, J. C. Baron, P. Collard, P. Bustany, D. Comar, and Y. Agid, Local cerebral glucose utilization in treated and untreated patients with Parkinson's disease. *J. Neurol. Neurosurg. Psychiatry* 47:824 (1984).

206. R. F. Peppard, W. R. W. Martin, G. D. Carr, E. Grochowski, M. Schulzer, M. Guttman, P. L. McGeer, A. G. Phillips, J. K. C. Tsui, and D. B. Calne, Cerebral glucose metabolism in Parkinson's disease with and without dementia, *Arch. Neurol.* 49:1262 (1992).

207. D. J. Brooks, E. D. Playford, V. Ibanez, G. V. Sawle, P. D. Thompson, L. J. Findley, and C. D. Marsden, Isolated tremor and disruption of the nigrostriatal dopaminergic system: An 18F-dopa PET study, *Neurology 42*:1554 (1992).

208. D. J. Brooks, V. Ibanez, G. V. Sawle, N. Quinn, A. J. Lees, C. J. Mathias, R. Bannister, C. D. Marsden, and R. S. J. Frackowiak, Differing patterns of striatal ^{18}F-dopa uptake in Parkinson's disease, multiple system atrophy, and progressive supranuclear palsy, *Ann. Neurol. 28*:547 (1990).

209. A. Gjedde, J. Reith, S. Dyve, G. Leger, M. Guttman, M. Diksic, A. Evans, and H. Kuwabara, Dopa decarboxylase activity of the living human brain, *Proc. Natl. Acad. Sci. USA 88*:2721 (1991).

210. D. J. Brooks, PET studies on the early and differential diagnosis of Parkinson's disease, *Neurology 43* (Suppl 6):S6 (1993).

211. K. L. Leenders, A. J. Palmer, N. Quinn, J. C. Clark, G. Firnau, E. S. Garnett, C. Nahmias, T. Jones, and C. D. Marsden, Brain dopamine metabolism in patients with Parkinson's disease measured with positron emission tomography, *J. Neurol. Neurosurg. Psychiatry 49*:853 (1986).

212. G. V. Sawle, E. D. Playford, D. J. Burn, V. J. Cunningham, and D. J. Brooks, Separating Parkinson's disease from normality, *Arch. Neurol. 51*:237 (1994).

213. H. Kuwabara, P. Cumming, Y. Yasuhara, G. C. Leger, M. Guttman, M. Diksic, A. C. Evans, and A. Gjedde, Regional striatal DOPA transport and decarboxylase activity in Parkinson's disease, *J. Nucl. Med. 36*(7):1226 (1995).

214. B. J. Snow, I. Tooyama, E. G. McGeer, T. Yamada, D. B. Calne, H. Takahashi, and H. Kimura, Human positron emission tomographic [18F]fluorodopa studies correlate with dopamine cell counts and levels, *Ann. Neurol. 34*:324 (1993).

215. R. C. Duvoisin, L. I. Golbe, and F. E. Lepore, Progressive supranuclear palsy, *Can. J. Neurol. Sci. 14*:547 (1987).

216. S. M. Schonfeld, L. I. Golbe, J. I. Sage, J. N. Safer, and R. C. Duvoisin, Computed tomographic findings in progressive supranuclear palsy: Correlation with clinical grade, *Movement Disord. 2*:263 (1987).

217. M. H. Bhatt, B. J. Snow, W. R. W. Martin, R. Peppard, and D. B. Calne, Positron emission tomography in progressive supranuclear palsy, *Arch. Neurol. 48*:389 (1991).

218. R. D'Antona, J. C. Baron, Y. Samson, M. Serdaru, F. Viader, Y. Agid, and J. Cambier, Subcortical dementia. Frontal cortex hypometabolism detected by positron emission tomography in patients with progressive supranuclear palsy, *Brain 108*:785 (1985).

219. N. L. Foster, S. Gilman, S. Berent, E. M. Morin, M. B. Brown, and R. A. Koeppe, Cerebral hypometabolism in progressive supranuclear palsy studied with positron emission tomography, *Ann. Neurol. 24*:399 (1988).

220. A. M. Goffinet, A. G. De Volder, C. Gullain, D. Rectem, A. Bol, C. Michel, M. Cogneau, D. Labar, and C. Laterre, Positron tomography demonstrates frontal lobe hypometabolism in progressive supranuclear palsy, *Ann. Neurol. 25*:131 (1989).

221. N. R. Graff-Radford, A. R. Damasio, B. T. Hyman, M. N. Hart, D. Tranel,

H. Damasio, G. W. Van Hoesen, and K. Rezai, Progressive aphasia in a patient with Pick's disease: A neuropsychological, radiologic, and anatomic study, *Neurology 40*:620 (1990).

222. L. L. Heston and A. R. Mastri, Age at onset of Pick's and Alzheimer's dementia: Implications for diagnosis and research, *J. Gerontol. 4*:422 (1982).

223. A. J. Holland, D. H. McBurney, J. Moossy, and O. M. Reinmuth, The dissolution of language in Pick's disease with neurofibrillary tangles: A case study, *Brain Lang. 24*:36 (1985).

224. H. Kamo, P. L. McGeer, R. Harrop, E. G. McGeer, D. B. Calne, W. R. W. Martin, and B. D. Pate, Positron emission tomography and histopathology in Picks disease, *Neurology 37*:439 (1987).

225. E. Salmon and G. Franck, Positron emission tomographic study in Alzheimer's disease and Picks disease, *Arch. Gerontol. Geriatr. 1* (Suppl):241 (1989).

226. D. S. Knopman, K. J. Christensen, L. J. Schut, R. E. Harbaugh, T. Reeder, T. Ngo, and W. Frey, The spectrum of imaging and neuropsychological findings in Picks disease, *Neurology 39*:362 (1989).

227. C. L. Masters and E. P. Richardson, Subacute spongiform encephalopathy (Creutzfeldt-Jakob disease), *Brain 101*:333 (1978).

228. R. Roos, D. C. Gajdusek, and C. J. Gibbs, The clinical characteristics of transmissible Creutzfeldt-Jakob disease, *Brain 96*:1 (1973).

229. S. B. Prusiner, Novel proteinaceous infectious particles cause scrapie, *Science 216*:136 (1982).

230. P. J. Harrison and G. W. Roberts, "Life Jim, but not as we know it?" Transmissible dementias and the prion protein, *Br. J. Psychiatry 158*:457 (1991).

231. P. Brown, L. G. Goldfarb, W. R. McCombie, A. Nieto, D. Squillacote, W. Sheremata, B. W. Little, M. S. Godec, C. J. Gibbs, and D. C. Gajdusek, Atypical Creutzfeldt-Jakob disease in an American family with an insert mutation in the PRNP amyloid precursor gene, *Neurology 42*:422 (1992).

232. R. P. Friedland, S. B. Pruisner, W. J. Jagust, T. F. Budinger, and R. L. Davis, Bitemporal hypometabolism in Creutzfeldt-Jakob disease measured by positron emission tomography with [18F]-2Fluorodeoxyglucose, *J. Comput. Assist. Tomogr. 8*:978 (1984).

233. V. A. Holthoff, J. Sandmann, F. Pawlik, R. Schroder, and W. D. Heiss, Positron emission tomography in Creutzfeldt-Jakob disease, *Arch. Neurol. 47*:1035 (1990).

234. S. Horowitz, D. F. Benson, D. E. Kuhl, and J. L. Cummings, FDG scan to confirm Creutzfeldt-Jakob diagnosis (abstract), *Neurology 32*:A167 (1982).

235. D. Eidelberg, V. Dhawan, J. R. Moeller, J. J. Sidtis, J. Z. Ginos, S. C. Strother, J. Cederbaum, P. Greene, S. Fahn, J. M. Powers, and D. A. Rottenberg, The metabolic landscape of cortico-basal ganglionic degeneration: regional asymmetries studied with positron emission tomography, *J. Neurol. Neurosurg. Psychiatry 54*:856 (1991).

236. R. J. Caselli, C. R. Jack, Jr., R. C. Petersen, H. W. Wahner, and T. Yanagihara, Asymmetric cortical degenerative syndromes: Clinical and radiologic correlations, *Neurology 42*:1462 (1992).

237. D. Neary, J. S. Snowden, B. Northen, and P. Goulding, Dementia of the frontal lobe type, *J. Neurol. Neurosurg. Psychiatry 51*:353 (1988).
238. J. B. Chawluk, M. M. Mesulam, H. Hurtig, M. Kushner, S. Weintraub, A. Saykin, N. Rubin, A. Alavi, and M. Reivich, Slowly progressive aphasia without generalized dementia: Studies with positron emission tomography, *Ann. Neurol. 19*:68 (1986).
239. N. L. Foster, T. N. Chas, N. J. Patronas, M. M. Gillespie, and P. Fedio. Cerebral mapping of apraxia in Alzheimer's disease by positron emission tomography, *Ann. Neurol. 19*:139 (1986).
240. W. J. Powers, J. S. Perlmutter, T. O. Videen, P. Herscovitch, L. K. Griffeth, H. D. Royal, B. A. Siegel, J. C. Morris, and L. Berg, Blinded clinical evaluation of positron emission tomography for diagnosis of probable Alzheimer's disease, *Neurology 42*:765 (1992).
241. J. M. Hoffman, M. W. Hanson, K. A. Welsh, N. Earl, S. Paine, R. E. Coleman, Interpretation variability of ^{18}F-fluoro-2-deoxyglucose (FDG) positron emission tomography (PET) in dementia, *Invest. Radiol. 31(6)*:316 (1996).
242. S. J. McCrory and I. Ford, Multivariate analysis of SPECT images with illustrations in Alzheimer's disease, *Stat. Med. 10*:1711 (1991).
243. R. J. Naugle and E. D. Bigler, Brain imaging and neuropsychological identification of dementia of the Alzheimer's type, *Neuropsychological Function and Brain Imaging* (E. D. Bigler, R. A. Yeo, and E. Turkheimer, eds.), Plenum Press, New York, 1989, p. 185.
244. W. E. Reichman and J. L. Cummings, Diagnosis of rare dementia syndromes: An algorithmic approach, *J. Geriatr. Psychiatry Neurol. 3*:73 (1990).
245. B. J. Carroll, M. Feinberg, J. F. Greden, J. Tarika, A. A. Albala, R. F. Haskett, N. Mcl. James, Z. Kronfol, N. Lohr, M. Steiner, J. P. deVigne, and E. Young, A specific laboratory test for the diagnosis of melancholia: Standardization, validation, and clinical utility, *Arch. Gen. Psychiatry 38*:15 (1981).
246. N. Cutler, Utility of biological markers in the evaluation and diagnosis of Alzheimer's disease, *Brain Dysfunction 1*:12 (1988).
247. A. A. Nierenberg and A. R. Feinstein, How to evaluate a diagnostic marker test: Lessons from the rise and fall of the dexamethaxone suppression test, *J. Am. Med. Assoc. 259*:1699 (1988).

21

Application of Positron Emission Tomography to Age-Related Cognitive Changes

David J. Madden
Duke University Medical Center, Durham, North Carolina

John M. Hoffman
Emory University School of Medicine, Atlanta, Georgia

I. INTRODUCTION

Behavioral and neuropsychological research has documented a complex mosaic of changes in cognitive function during human aging [1–3]. Although the quality of decision making can improve as the result of older adults' increased experience [4], other abilities, especially those relying on the speed of perceptual processing, exhibit significant age-related decline, even for relatively healthy individuals. The specific changes in the central nervous system that are responsible for the age-related pattern of cognitive performance have been difficult to identify. The postmortem examination of brain tissue has revealed significant age-related changes in the structure of the brain, including decrease in total brain mass, gyral atrophy, widening of sulci, enlargement of the lateral ventricles, and neural cell loss [5–7]. Although studies vary with regard to the regional specificity of age-related neuronal loss, Kemper [7] noted that losses appeared to be greatest in the frontal and temporal lobes, with association cortex being more affected than primary sensory/motor cortex. Terry et al. [8], however, proposed that the predominant effect of aging is a decrease in neuronal size rather than a reduction in the number of cells.

A major advantage of neuroimaging methods such as computed tomography (CT) and magnetic resonance imaging (MRI) is that structural neuroanatomical changes can be observed in vivo [9]. The age-related changes observed with these neuroimaging methods are in general consistent with the results of postmortem studies [10–12]. Raz et al. [13], for example, found that the observable differentiation between gray and white matter in the medial temporal lobes decreased as a function of adult age. Using MRI-based estimates of cortical volume, Raz et al. [14] reported that an age-related decline was present in association cortex but not in primary sensory cortex. Using MRI volumetric measures, Coffey et al. [15] found a significant age-related reduction in both total and regional cerebral volume, particularly of the frontal lobes, in 76 healthy adults between 30 and 91 years of age. In the Coffey et al. [15] study, there was a concomitant increase with age both in ventricular volume and in the presence of subcortical hyperintensities in the MRI images. The age-related volumetric decrease in subcortical gray matter structures, such as the caudate and lenticular nuclei, may be even greater than the decrease in cortical gray matter [16]. Coffey et al. [15] noted that many older subjects exhibited no structural neuroanatomical changes and emphasized that the typical changes were not clinically significant.

The limitation of conventional CT and MRI scans is that the data reflect brain structure, and inferences regarding function are necessarily correlational. An important challenge for neuroimaging methodology is the development of techniques for identifying the age-related changes in neural function that accompany the structural changes. One possible approach is functional MRI, which maps the changes in the MR signal corresponding to areas of increased cerebral blood flow (CBF) [17–19]. Functional MRI, however, typically requires high-strength magnets and other specialized technologies not widely available, although advances are being made in the extraction of functional data from conventional MRI scanners [20,21]. A second and more frequently used approach is positron emission tomography (PET), which was developed specifically as an imaging modality for brain metabolic activity and CBF [22–25]. Research using PET has provided a wealth of information regarding the functional organization of the neural systems mediating human cognitive performance [26–30]. An important aspect of the PET methodology is that measures of CBF and cerebral metabolic activity can be obtained during the performance of a cognitive task, thus providing information on the pattern of regional activity associated with cognitive performance. Investigations using PET, however, have been primarily concerned with young adults' performance. Although a number of reports of age-related changes in PET measures have also been published, the studies of adult age differences in PET have not been guided by current theories of cognitive performance to the degree that PET studies of young adults have.

In this chapter, we review current models of the neural systems underlying cognitive function based on PET studies of young adults, focusing on studies of word identification, attention, and memory. We examine current findings from behavioral studies on adult age differences in these abilities, as well as the PET studies that have included adult age as a variable. Our goal is to suggest ways in which PET methodology can be used to obtain relevant information regarding the functional neuroanatomy of age-related cognitive changes. We focus on the age-related changes that occur in healthy individuals. Research on clinically significant cognitive deficits (e.g., Alzheimer's disease) using PET measures has been reviewed by Hoffman et al. [31], Duara et al. [32], Goldstein and Reivich [33] and Parasuraman and Haxby [34].

II. PET METHODOLOGY

The basis of PET methodology is the hypothesis proposed by Roy and Sherrington [35] that the blood supply within a neural region varies in relation to the chemical changes underlying the functional activity of that region. Kety and Schmidt [36] made an important advance by devising a method for measuring whole-brain blood flow, which involved measuring arteriovenous differences in the level of an inert gas (nitrous oxide) following inhalation. Since the introduction of the Kety-Schmidt technique, several functional neuroimaging methodologies have been developed for measuring cerebral metabolic activity and CBF within specific neural regions as well as in the brain as a whole [37–39]. These methodologies rely on the assumption that neural activity, energy metabolism, and blood flow are tightly coupled, that is, increased blood flow supports the oxygen consumption and glucose utilization of nerve impulse activity [40,41]. This assumption holds under most conditions [42,43], although in certain situations (e.g., intense sensory stimulation) CBF and metabolic responses become uncoupled [44].

In PET, cerebral metabolic activity and CBF are measured from the tissue clearance of radionuclides that are either injected or inhaled. Radioisotopes of several elements with short half-lives, such as ^{15}O (oxygen) and ^{18}F (flourine), produce positrons. These and other radioisotopes are incorporated into radionuclides, such as $H_2^{15}O$ (i.e., ^{15}O-labeled water) and $[^{18}F]$flurorodeoxyglucose (i.e., ^{18}F-labeled deoxyglucose). Following radionuclide administration, the interaction of a positron with an electron in tissue leads to the emergence of two annihilation photons. External radiation detectors, arranged in a series of rings around the head, record the level of radioactivity in tissue along lines of coincidence between pairs of detectors.

The most frequently measured indices of metabolic activity are regional cerebral blood flow (rCBF) and the regional cerebral metabolic rates for oxygen ($rCMRO_2$) and glucose (rCMRglc). In the majority of studies relevant to cognitive function, changes in rCMRglc are measured following injection of ^{18}F-labeled deoxyglucose; changes in rCBF are measured following either the injection of ^{15}O-labeled water or the inhalation of ^{15}O-labeled carbon dioxide ($C^{15}O_2$). The technique for measuring $rCMRO_2$ involves the sequential administration of three ^{15}O-labeled tracers and the combined assessment of rCBF, regional cerebral blood volume, and the regional oxygen extraction ratio, obtained in separate scans. Because the utilization of glucose and oxygen are metabolic activities of nerve cells, rCMRglc and $rCMRO_2$ are direct measures of cerebral metabolism, whereas rCBF, representing the transport of oxygen and glucose to nerve cells, is an indirect measure. Studies of cognitive function have most frequently measured rCBF, however, because the radionuclides incorporating ^{15}O are cleared from the body within 15 minutes, allowing repeated task-specific scans, whereas ^{18}F[fluorodeoxyglucose] does not clear the body for 9 hours, precluding a repeated scan on the same day. The measurement of $rCMRO_2$ has not been widely used in studies of cognitive function because of its operational complexity and the possibility of $rCMRO_2$ becoming uncoupled from rCBF and rCMRglc under some task conditions [44]. The acquisition of radioactivity counts occurs over a 1-minute integration period for ^{15}O-labeled radionuclides and over a 45-minutes integration period for ^{18}F[fluorodeoxyglucose]. Each PET image consequently represents all of the neural events occurring during the integration period. To obtain quantitative values for rCMRglc and rCBF (e.g., in units of ml/100 g of tissue/min), the local radioactivity counts must be combined mathematically with the time-activity curve obtained from sampling of arterial blood during radionuclide administration.

In many instances, PET measures of metabolic activity or CBF are obtained while subjects are in a resting state, without an assigned cognitive task (e.g., Ref. 45). In the analysis of cognitive performance, however, a more informative approach is to examine the pattern of increased neural activity that occurs while a subject is actually performing a particular cognitive task. The pattern of metabolic or CBF values obtained during performance of a control task can be subtracted from the values obtained during performance of an activation task, yielding a pattern of task-specific change [46,47]. In addition, the radioactivity counts for CBF are a nearly linear function of blood flow in the tissue, so that when the measure of interest is the difference between scans (i.e., a subtraction), quantitative estimates of rCBF can be obtained without sampling arterial blood [48]. This subtraction methodology has been applied extensively to the interpretation of rCBF changes in PET activation studies of word identification, attention, and memory [29,49–52]. The subtraction approach, however, does require assumptions (e.g., that two tasks differ only in a prespecified cognitive operation) that are not always valid, and the pattern of activation yielded by the subtraction depends on the cognitive processes associated with the control task [53,54]. In the context of a PET experiment, it may consequently be informative to perform subtractions among different activation task conditions, as well as between activation and control conditions, to obtain converging evidence regarding the cognitive processes leading to a particular pattern of rCBF activation.

The analysis of PET data can focus either on specific brain regions that are expected to exhibit functional change or on the pattern of changes across the whole brain. Frackowiak and Friston [55] noted that these different analytical approaches represent different (but related) interpretations of the change in rCBF between task conditions: the change may be best explained either in terms of functional localization alone or in terms of distributed patterns of neural activity in networks of functionally specialized cortical regions. Although both approaches can be hypothesis-driven, somewhat different analytic procedures are employed. The first approach leads to univariate or multivariate analysis of variance designs in which regions of interest (ROIs) are considered as levels of an independent variable and function measures such as rCBF are dependent variables [56]. The second approach uses the data from the complete PET image without specifying ROIs in advance. For example, in statistical parametric mapping (SPM) [57–59], a map is formed that represents, for each pixel in the PET image, the difference between an activation condition and a baseline condition, using global CBF as a covariate. The set of *t*-statistic values, one for each pixel, representing the significance of change in that pixel, constitutes the statistical parametric map. The *t*-values are corrected for the effects of multiple comparisons, transformed to the unit normal distribution, and thresholded at a specified probability level. Unlikely regional excursions within the map are interpreted as regionally specific effects. The resulting foci of rCBF activation are characterized in terms of the spatial extent and peak height of their local maxima. The locations of the local maxima within a standard stereotaxic space [60] are also identified. The analysis of distributed activity, especially SPM analyses, is used widely in the investigation of cognitive performance, because it is difficult to specify a priori all of the ROIs that may be relevant for a particular cognitive task. The analysis of distributed activity has also led to the development of correlational methods for characterizing the functional connectivity among brain regions [61,62].

Advances in the precision of PET measurements have been accompanied by increased awareness of the many limitations to the quantitative interpretation of PET data and the complexity of the statistical issues involved [56,59,63,64]. For example, there is typically substantial variability between subjects at several levels: the shape of the brain and gyral pattern, the functional localization of elementary cognitive operations, and the pattern of metabolic activation associated with complex task performance. In addition, the magnitude of task-dependent activation is often only 2–5% above that of the control task, and it is difficult to separate this signal from background noise.

The effects of intersubject variability can be taken into account statistically in analyses that average PET images across subjects and localize activation in a standard stereotaxic space [46,58]. On the data-acquisition side, the signal-to-noise ratio of subtraction images can be increased by the use of three-dimensional imaging in which the interplane septa of the tomograph are removed and the system is reconfigured to accept coincidences between all combinations of detector rings [65–67]. With three-dimensional imaging, radioactivity counts equivalent to those of conventional two-dimensional PET imaging can be obtained with one quarter of the radionuclide dosage used in two-dimensional studies. As a result, several additional scans can be performed within a subject for a given cumulative dose limit. The increased sensitivity may permit the detection of statistically significant activation effects within a single subject.

III. WORD IDENTIFICATION

Behavioral research on word identification has proceeded from the assumption that the definitions of individual words are represented in long-term memory independently of lower-level features such as letters and phonemes.

Comprehension of an individual word involves access to the mental lexicon through an analysis of the word's perceptual features and (perhaps in parallel) the available semantic context [68,69]. A basic distinction in this research area is between access to semantic information that occurs automatically (as the result of stimulus presentation) and the access that occurs as the result of subject-initiated retrieval [70,71]. A substantial number of PET studies of young adult subjects have focused on the processes involved in word identification and lexical access, and these studies have been reviewed by Wise et al. [72], Petersen and Fiez [29], Liotti et al. [73], Démonet et al. [74], and Démonet [75]. The PET data have in general indicated that the component processes of feature extraction and the retrieval of word meaning are represented in specific neural regions and that word identification involves the coordination of activity from different regions. In addition, the pattern of rCBF activation associated specifically with word meaning appears to vary as a function of the degree of self-directed retrieval of semantic information that is required.

The separation of feature-level and semantic processing by PET was first reported by Petersen et al. [76,77]. These authors used a PET activation paradigm that included a fixation-point-only baseline condition, plus activation conditions involving passive presentation of words, repeating presented words aloud, and generating uses for presented words. Petersen et al. [76,77] found that passive presentation of words led to increased rCBF in separate cortical areas for visual and auditory presentation, relative to a fixation point baseline condition. In the former instance, striate and extrastriate regions were active; in the latter instance, primary auditory cortex (temporal) and tempoparietal areas were active. These activations were bilateral but more pronounced in the left hemisphere. During word repetition, other areas, near the sylvian fissure bilaterally, were active, and these areas did not vary as a function of word presentation modality. Two areas exhibited increased rCBF, relative to the passive presentation condition, during the "generate uses" (i.e., semantic association) task. These were the left dorsolateral prefrontal cortex and the anterior cingulate gyrus, which were active regardless of presentation modality.

Petersen et al. [78] followed up these findings by visually presenting words, pronounceable nonwords, consonant strings, and letterlike forms (false fonts) in separate activation scans. Each scan was a "passive-viewing" condition in which no response to the stimuli was required. Relative to a fixation-point condition, all of the stimuli produced lateral extrastriate activation, but only the words and pronounceable nonwords led to increased rCBF in left medial extrastriate cortex. When the false font condition was used as a control condition in the subtraction analysis, left inferior prefrontal cortex exhibited increased rCBF for words, but not for nonwords. This area was located near the one reported by Petersen et al. [76,77] to be active during the semantic association (generate uses) task. During the identification of visually presented words, there consequently appear to be separate areas for visual feature extraction (lateral extrastriate), word-form analysis (left medial extrastriate), and semantic analysis (left frontal).

Wise et al. [79] and Frith et al. [61] reported data that confirm the role of left frontal cortex in semantic retrieval, but also indicate a contribution of posterior temporal cortex. In the Wise et al. study, the activation conditions included the tasks of listening to nonwords, detecting category superordinate-exemplar word pairs, and silently generating verbs that were appropriate for presented nouns. Relative to a resting state control condition, all three activation conditions led to increased rCBF in superior temporal cortex bilaterally. The verb-generation task was in addition associated with activation in left posterior frontal areas and the supplementary motor area bilaterally. During the verb generation task, only Wernicke's area (left posterior superior temporal gyrus) exhibited activation with a reduced rate of stimulus presentation. Wise et al. [79] suggested that whereas word comprehension activates only temporal lobe structures, the retrieval of specific word meaning involves interrelated activity in Wernicke's area, left dorsolateral prefrontal cortex, and the supplementary motor area. The authors discussed several methodological differences between their design and that of Petersen et al. [76,77] that may have led to the different patterns of rCBF activation between the studies.

Frith et al. [61] used tasks that were similar to those of Wise et al. [79]; the activation conditions contrasted verbal fluency tasks (e.g., naming as many jobs as possible) with the discrimination of auditorily presented words and nonwords (i.e., lexical decision). Vocal counting was used as a control condition. Relative to lexical decision and counting, verbal fluency was associated with activation in left dorsolateral prefrontal cortex and left parahippocampal gyrus; significant rCBF decreases were observed in superior temporal regions bilaterally. In the lexical decision condition, in contrast, there was bilateral activation in the superior temporal regions and decreased rCBF in the posterior cingulate bilaterally. Frith et al. proposed that words are represented in a distributed neural network in the superior temporal cortex of both cerebral hemispheres. Comprehension of extrinsically presented words, as in the lexical decision condition, can be completed within the network, whereas the intrinsic generation of specific words, as in the verbal fluency condition, requires a selective and inhibitory control process originating in left dorsolateral prefrontal cortex. Friston et al. [80] confirmed this model in an independent comparison of rCBF activations in extrinsic and intrinsic word retrieval tasks.

Démonet and colleagues [53,81] also emphasized the contribution of distributed neural networks to processing different components of word identification. They [81] used a nonverbal auditory task (monitoring for pure tones) as a reference task for two PET activation tasks (sequential phoneme monitoring and semantic categorization) representing different aspects of word processing. Subtracting the control task from each of the activation tasks yielded separate patterns of rCBF activation for phonemic and semantic processing. Subsequent analyses [53], in which the phoneme monitoring and semantic categorization tasks were subtracted from each other, indicated that rCBF in a common set of neural regions was activated, to varying degrees, in both tasks. One region, including the left inferior supramarginal gyrus, was more active during phoneme monitoring than during semantic categorization, whereas the converse was true for foci distributed among left inferior temporal, left superior frontal, and bilateral inferior parietal regions. Démonet [75] concluded that it is more useful to view the results of these rCBF subtractions as graded differences in distributed neural systems than as all-or-none localizations of specific processing components.

It is also important to note that task design variables such as subjects' level of practice and the duration and presentation rate of the stimuli may influence rCBF activation during cognitive performance in ways that are not currently understood. Raichle et al. [82], for example, proposed that two neural pathways mediate verbal response selection and that these pathways contribute differentially according to subjects' degree of familiarity with the task. These authors examined rCBF activation in a verb-generation task similar to the semantic association task used by Petersen et al. [76,77]. During subjects' first (unpracticed) performance of this task, the PET data indicated the presence of rCBF activation, relative to word repetition, in several areas constituting one pathway: left prefrontal cortex, left posterior temporal cortex, anterior cingulate, and right cerebellar hemisphere. Following 10–15 minutes of practice with the verb-generation task, another PET scan of the same subjects revealed an rCBF decrease in these cortical areas, with a concomitant rCBF increase in a second pathway: bilateral sylvian-insular cortex and left medial extrastriate cortex. Price et al. [83] reported several changes in rCBF activation during visual word identification as a function of stimulus duration. These authors found that increasing stimulus duration from 150 to 1000 ms in a lexical decision task with vocal responses led to increased rCBF bilaterally in the posterior fusiform gyri; other areas, such as dorsolateral prefrontal cortex, tended to exhibit greater activation at the briefer duration. Increased presentation rate of visual stimuli has been observed to lead to increased activation of visual cortical areas, as measured by both PET [84] and functional MRI [85].

IV. SELECTIVE AND DIVIDED ATTENTION

Investigations of attentional processes using PET methodology have also suggested that component operations are localized within specific neural regions. Tasks that require the use of selective attention define relevant and irrelevant sources of information for task performance, allowing attention to be focused selectively on the relevant information; in divided attention tasks, multiple sources of information must be attended simultaneously [86]. Corbetta et al. [49,50] investigated the functional neuroanatomy of selective and divided attention. These authors measured rCBF during subjects' performance of a visual attention task—the same/different discrimination of two sequentially presented displays of small bars. In the selective attention condition, the single stimulus dimension (shape, color, or velocity) relevant for the same/different judgment was specified in advance of each trial block and remained constant within a block. In the divided attention condition, the two displays of bars could differ in any of the three dimensions. Control conditions included passive viewing of the stimuli without responding and passive viewing of a fixation point.

Corbetta et al. [49,50] obtained different patterns of rCBF activation for the selective and divided attention tasks. Using the passive task as a control, the subtraction images for the three selective attention conditions exhibited both commonality and regional specificity as a function of the relevant stimulus dimension. All three selective attention conditions led to rCBF activation in primary visual cortex and the left globus pallidus. Selective attention for both shape and color were associated with specific activation in the left collateral sulcus. There were additional responses to shape bilaterally in fusiform and parahippocampal gyri. Right-sided activation also occurred for the shape dimension at the intersection between the calcarine and parieto-occipital sulci and in the superior temporal cortex. Activations for attending to speed, relative to the passive task, were localized on the lateral surface of the occipital gyri and in the inferior parietal lobule.

The divided attention condition activated fewer regions than the selective attention conditions, but there was activation for divided attention (relative to the passive task) in the locations associated with attending to color (left collateral sulcus) and speed (left lateral occipital gyrus). Unlike the selective attention condition, however, the divided attention condition was also associated with specific activations in the medial frontal region (anterior cingulate) and right prefrontal cortex.

Corbetta et al. [49,50] suggested that the specific rCBF activations associated with selective attention to shape and color are consistent with a distinction between ventral occipitotemporal and dorsal occipitoparietal cortical visual pathways introduced by Ungerleider and Mishkin [87]. The ventral pathway is hypothesized to be relatively more critical for visual object identification processes, whereas the dorsal pathway is hypothesized to be relatively more critical for spatial localization processes. The posterior attention system, by involving the maintenance of a set for a particular visual feature, would be linked to the ventral occipitotemporal pathway. According to Corbetta et al. [50], the adoption of a selective set could depend on a circuit connecting lateral orbitofrontal cortex and basal ganglia. The set would be implemented in the extrastriate regions (where the display matching operations are performed) through the thalamus, which would route the activation to the appropriate extrastriate region (see Ref. 88). Performance in the divided-attention condition, in contrast, requires greater memory demands during the interdisplay interval and the coordination of several sources of feature information. The system mediating divided-attention performance is thus not as dependent on extrastriate functioning, but is instead implemented by an anterior attentional system involving lateral prefrontal cortex and the anterior cingulate.

Corbetta et al. [89] demonstrated that the posterior attention system is particularly important for shifting attention across spatial location. During the rCBF measurement, subjects responded manually to each of a series of appearances of a visually presented target (an asterisk) along a probabilistically determined path. Subjects' responses were faster when the target occurred in a predicted (i.e., validly cued) location than in a nonpredicted (i.e., invalidly cued) location, indicating that subjects were shifting attention on the basis of the spatial cue. The rCBF activation that occurred during the validly cued trials (relative to target detection at a central location) varied as a function of the visual field in which the target was located. Shifting attention to the left visual field primarily activated right superior parietal cortex; shifting attention to the right visual field led to activation in superior parietal cortex of both the left and right hemispheres. Thus, the right superior parietal cortex may contain the neural system for directing spatial shifts of attention both contralaterally and ipsilaterally. This system for attending to spatial location is part of the posterior attention system but is distinct anatomically from the extrastriate regions mediating selective attention to other dimensions such as shape, color, and speed [49,50].

Whereas the association of the posterior attention system with selective attention process is supported relatively consistently by the PET data, the anterior attention system is more difficult to characterize functionally. Posner and Petersen [90] noted that because in a divided-attention search task an increase in the number of relevant display locations does not lead to a performance decrement unless a target is detected [91], the defining characteristic of the anterior attention system may be target detection. Results of several investigations, however, are difficult to reconcile with a target-detection interpretation of the anterior attention system. Pardo et al. [92] and Bench et al. [93] measured rCBF activation in the Stroop color-naming paradigm. They found that when subjects attempted to name the color of incongruent words (e.g., the word "red" printed in green), there was increased activation in anterior cingulate cortex, relative to a condition in which the word and its printed color were congruent. The target detection demands of the Stroop task would appear to be comparable across conditions; the difference is in whether a highly practiced response (i.e., pronouncing the actual word presented) must be inhibited. Frith et al. [94] found that when subjects were required to select the response (i.e., to determine which finger to move or which series of words to pronounce), there was rCBF activation in dorsolateral prefrontal cortex. Pardo et al. [95] reported that vigilance for a somatosensory stimulus (i.e., sustained attention) was associated with rCBF activation in prefrontal and superior parietal regions in the right hemisphere. When a semantic association task has not been practiced extensively, verbal response selection appears to involve the anterior attention system [82].

It may thus be premature to use a single performance characteristic (e.g., target detection or response inhibition) to define the anterior attention system. At the present time, it appears that a broader characterization, such as the monitoring of multiple sources of task-relevant information and selection of potential responses, is more accurate. The characterization must also be sufficiently broad to incorporate the fact that the anterior attention system appears to contribute significantly to performance in memory tasks.

V. MEMORY

A. Declarative and Nondeclarative Memory

An important distinction in behavioral studies of memory is between declarative memory, which involves the conscious intention to remember, and nondeclarative memory, which involves the effects of past experience as expressed without the intention to remember [96,97]. Performance on the widely used laboratory tests of recall and recognition represents declarative memory processes, whereas nondeclarative memory abilities are expressed in tasks such as perceptual identification, fragment completion, repetition priming, and skill learning.

Squire et al. [98] found that declarative and nondeclarative memory tasks led to different patterns of rCBF activation. Participants in this study memorized a list of words prior to each PET scan; rCBF was measured during two activation conditions. Each of the activation conditions involved the presentation of 20 three-letter stems, 10 of which could be completed with one of the recently studied words. One of the activation conditions (priming) required subjects to complete a series of three-letter stems with the first word that came to mind. In the other activation condition (memory), subjects were instructed to use the stems as cues to recall the recently studied words.

A baseline condition involved completing stems that could not form words in the study list. In the subtraction image for both of the activation conditions, relative to the baseline, there was increased rCBF in the right posterior medial temporal lobe in the area occupied by the hippocampus and parahippocampal gyrus. The magnitude of the rCBF increase, however, was greater for the memory task than for the priming task. In addition, priming was associated with a decrease in rCBF, relative to the baseline, in right occipital cortex. The memory task was associated with an activation in right prefrontal cortex.

Squire et al. [98] suggested that the rCBF decrease in occipital cortex associated with priming reflects the decreased visual processing demands of stimulus repetition, a form of nondeclarative memory. The hippocampal activation occurring in the performance of the memory task, in contrast, appears to represent the retrieval demands of cued recall from declarative memory. The prefrontal activation indicates in addition that these retrieval processes involve the anterior attention system [90]. Subsequent experiments by Buckner et al. [99] demonstrated that the right prefrontal activation reported by Squire et al. [98] was replicable under conditions in which the to-be-remembered items and recall cues were presented in different formats (e.g., auditory presentation of the study list and visual presentation of the cues), whereas the medial temporal activation did not occur in these conditions.

A related finding is that of Grafton et al. [100]. These authors found that the rCBF changes associated with learning in a pursuit rotor task (a form of nondeclarative memory) were located in the left primary motor cortex, left supplementary motor area, and left thalamus. These areas were a subset of the more widely distributed network that exhibited rCBF activation during motor execution. Thus, in both the Squire et al. [98] and Grafton et al. [100] studies, nondeclarative memory performance was mediated primarily by the same sensory/motor areas that were responsible for the initial registration of the stimuli in the task. In the Squire et al. experiment, however, the effects of nondeclarative memory were expressed as a decrease in rCBF, whereas in the Grafton et al. experiment the corresponding effects occurred as rCBF increases.

B. Episodic Memory

A theoretical distinction is frequently made between two forms of declarative memory: episodic memory, in which remembered events have a specific context (e.g., the most recent list of words or pictures presented), and semantic memory, in which remembered events are context-independent (e.g., the definitions of individual words) [101]. From this perspective, the PET studies discussed in Section III can be viewed as investigations of semantic memory, whereas the cued recall task used by Squire et al. [98] and Buckner et al. [99] would represent the episodic component of declarative memory. Episodic memory processes form a continuum ranging from the conscious manipulation of a limited number of recently presented items (i.e., working memory) [102] to the long-term memory processes responsible for the retention of information over many years [103].

The PET studies of working memory processes have suggested that these processes depend on the functioning of specific areas in frontal cortex. Petrides et al. [104] found that either vocally generating a random sequence of the numbers 1 to 10 or monitoring an auditorily presented sequence of these numbers for the omission of a single item led to bilateral activation of middorsolateral frontal cortex. Jonides et al. [105] used a spatial task in which subjects decided whether one of three dots was surrounded by a circle. Delaying the onset of the circle for 3 seconds after the offset of the dots led to rCBF activation (relative to simultaneous presentation) in several areas of the right hemisphere: prefrontal cortex, posterior parietal cortex, and premotor cortex. Petrides et al. [106] also used spatial stimuli (abstract designs) in a task that relied on working memory. When subjects were required to point to a sequence of eight designs without repeating any (the self-ordered task), there was rCBF activation (relative to a condition in which the same design could be selected repeatedly) in middorsolateral frontal cortex bilaterally, but predominantly in the right hemisphere.

Other working memory tasks, however, appear to activate more posterior cortical regions. Grasby et al. [107] presented a series of nine five-word lists auditorily, and subjects recalled each list following presentation (i.e., a subspan task). Compared to a resting condition, rCBF during recall exhibited activation in the superior temporal gyrus and thalamus bilaterally, the right parahippocampal gyrus and cerebellum, and left anterior cingulate. Without a control task involving the repetition of spoken words, however, it is difficult to conclude that the activation represents memory processes specifically. Paulesu et al. [108] examined the activation associated with a recognition memory task that required subjects to decide whether a visually presented probe letter was a member of a previously displayed set of six consonants. Relative to a control task involving rhyming judgments regarding consonants, there was rCBF activation in the left supramarginal gyrus, which the authors suggest may represent storage of phonological information. When the data for the memory and rhyming task were combined and compared to data from similar tasks using abstract forms and visual similarity judgments, rCBF activation was evident bilaterally (but more pronounced in the left hemisphere) for frontal, superior temporal, and supramarginal gyri, as well as the insulae and cerebellum. Paulesu et al. proposed that these areas represent an articulatory loop involved in subvocal rehearsal.

Smith et al. [109] proposed that different forms of working memory processing could be differentiated in terms of the ventral (feature identification) and dorsal (spatial localization) visual processing pathways described by Ungerleider and Mishkin [87]. Smith et al. [109] investigated the changes in rCBF activation associated with the identification and spatial localization of unfamiliar geometric shapes (polygons) over a brief (3-s) delay. These authors found that when the task involved object identification (i.e., same/different comparison regarding the identity of successively presented items), two areas in the occipitotemporal pathway of the left hemisphere exhibited rCBF activation. When the working memory task required spatial localization (i.e., same/different comparison of item location), however, there was rCBF activation in several regions that were located predominantly in the right hemisphere. These included occipitoparietal cortex, but also inferior and dorsolateral prefrontal cortex, and anterior cingulate. In a separate behavioral experiment with subjects who had not undergone the PET testing, Smith et al. [109] demonstrated that, for the object memory task, performance was affected by the featural similarity of the display items but not by their location, whereas performance in the spatial memory task was influenced by the spatial proximity of the items and not by their featural similarity.

Processes involved in the encoding and retrieval of information beyond the limits of working memory (i.e., long-term episodic memory) appear to have a neural representation that is distinct from working memory. Subjects in the Petrides et al. [106] study learned a prespecified pairing of eight colors and eight abstract designs. In the conditional task, subjects pointed to the design associated with each color. When the rCBF activation associated with working memory (the self-ordered task discussed previously in this section) was subtracted from the conditional task, there was activation in the posterior cingulate bilaterally and in the superior frontal sulcus and insula of the left hemisphere. Similarly, Grasby et al. [107] included a supraspan task (recall of three previously presented 15-word lists) that relied on long-term episodic memory. These authors subtracted the activation associated with working memory (the subspan task discussed previously in this section) from the activation associated with the supraspan task. The result was a pattern of increased rCBF in the middle and superior frontal gyri bilaterally, combined with decreased rCBF in the middle and superior temporal gyri, and in the insular and lower part of the postcentral gyrus. This pattern resembled the Frith et al. [61] findings (see Sec. III), in which the retrieval of long-term semantic memory information was associated with decreased rCBF in superior temporal cortex, perhaps as the result of an inhibitory control process.

These studies of long-term episodic memory did not include conditions that allow the effects of encoding and retrieval processes to be distinguished. Mazziotta and Metter [110] reported changes in rCMRglc as a function of preparing to remember (i.e., encoding) in an episodic memory task. Listening to an auditorily presented story led, relative to a resting state baseline, to a diffuse left-sided increase in rCMRglc, with regional activations in left frontal and temporo-occipital areas. Only when subjects were instructed to remember the story, however, was activation evident in bilateral medial temporal areas, including hippocampus and parahippocampus. Shallice et al. [111] separated encoding and retrieval processes in a between-subjects design. Participants in the encoding study listened to 15 paired associates for later recall; those in the retrieval study vocally recalled lists of 15 paired associates that had been presented previously. Subtraction images of control conditions indicated that encoding was associated with increased rCBF in left dorsolateral prefrontal and retrosplenial cortex. Retrieval led to activation in right prefrontal cortex and the precuneus bilaterally. Kapur et al. [112] obtained related findings in a within-subjects comparison of different encoding conditions. During the PET scan, subjects performed either a shallow (checking for the letter a) or a deeper (living/nonliving categorization) processing task with visually presented words. Later recognition memory was better for the more deeply processed words, and subtracting the rCBF image for the shallow encoding task from the image for the deeper encoding task yielded a focus of activation in the left inferior prefrontal cortex. Tulving et al. [113] focused on retrieval by subtracting the rCBF images associated with listening to unfamiliar sentences from those associated with listening to previously learned sentences. Activation was evident in the frontal lobes, especially in right dorsolateral prefrontal cortex and in areas of the parietal lobe bilaterally.

Tulving et al. [52] summarized PET studies of memory in terms of a hemispheric encoding/retrieval asymmetry (HERA) model of episodic memory. In the HERA model, the left and right prefrontal lobes are part of an extensive neural network that mediates memory performance. Prefrontal regions in the left cerebral cortex are differentially active during the encoding of novel episodic information and the retrieval of semantic information. Prefrontal regions in the right cerebral cortex are differentially active during the retrieval of episodic information.

VI. ADULT AGE DIFFERENCES IN PET

Research using nontomographic methods indicated that a decrease in CBF and cerebral metabolic activity occurs during aging. Kety [114] reviewed the data on age-related changes based on studies that had used the nitrous oxide method for measuring CBF for the whole brain [36]. Kety noted that there was a monotonic decrease as a function of adult age for both CBF and cerebral oxygen consumption. The rate of this decrease paralleled closely the age-related decrease in cortical density as measured by cell count. Kety viewed the age-related decrease in metabolic rate as a consequence of neuronal loss. More recent studies using other nontomographic methods such as [133]Xe (xenon) inhalation have reported, consistent with Kety [114] an age-related decline in rCBF, even in the absence of risk factors for stroke [115]. The ^{133}Xe inhalation studies also suggest, however, that the pattern of rCBF activation during cognitive performance may be relatively constant as a function of age [116,117].

The PET studies that have compared healthy adults of varying ages are summarized in Table 1. These studies have yielded mixed results, but it is evident from the table that when age differences are obtained, they are in the direction of decline in CBF and metabolic activity as a function of age. The trend of the data obtained from PET is thus consistent with the results of nontomographic studies. The regional pattern of age-related change, however, is difficult to determine. Age-related changes in frontal lobe functioning have emerged in several studies. Kuhl et al. [118] and Loessner et al. [119] reported age-related declines in rCMRglc for frontal cortex. Kuhl et al. [118] and de Leon et al. [120] found that the ratio of frontal to parietal values for rCMRglc exhibited disproportionate age-related decline. This pattern was replicated by de Leon et al. [120] when the data were combined with those of a previous study [121]. Hoffman et al. [122] found that age-related decline in rCMRglc was restricted to relatively few frontal and subcortical regions.

Other investigators have reported more diverse age-related changes. Leenders et al. [123] found that rCMRO$_2$ declined significantly as a function of age in 7 of 14 ROIs, whereas the age-related decline in rCBF was significant only for frontal and insular cortices. Martin et al. [124] obtained significant age-related declines in rCBF for the cingulate, parahippocampal, superior temporal, medial frontal, and posterior parietal cortices bilaterally, and for the left insular and left posterior prefrontal cortices. The changes in the parietal cortex, however, were located in several scattered foci and were less reliable statistically than the other changes. Horwitz et al. [125] found that in a sample of male subjects, mean rCMRglc did not vary significantly as a function of age, but there were age differences in the pattern of intercorrelations of rCMRglc values. Specifically, when the matrix of all possible correlations among 59 ROIs was examined, there were fewer significant correlations for the older men than for the young men, especially for pairs of ROIs in the frontal and parietal lobes. Azari et al. [126] obtained a similar pattern of results using a higher resolution scanner and women subjects.

All of these aforementioned studies of age differences used resting state measures in which subjects did not perform any specific task during the PET scan, and, as is evident in Table 1, few studies have investigated age differences in PET activation paradigms. Tempel and Perlmutter [127] found

Table 1 PET Studies of Age-Related Changes

Authors	Ref.	n	Gender; age range (yr)	Scan conditions	Metabolic measure	Changes with increasing age
Frackowiak et al.	160	14	M,F; 26–74	Resting	rCBF; rCMRO$_2$	Decrease in both rCBF and rCMRO$_2$
Lenzi et al.	161	27	NR; NR	Resting	rCBF; rCMRO$_2$	Decrease in both rCBF and rCMRO$_2$
Kuhl et al.	118 162	40	M,F; 18–78	Resting	rCMRglc	Decrease in ratio of metabolic rates; frontal and parietal ROIs
de Leon et al.	163 121	37	NR; 26–67	Resting	rCMRglc	Cortical atrophy, but no change in rCMRglc
Duara et al.	164	21	M; 21–83	Resting	rCMRglc	None
Hawkins et al.	165	8	M,F; 18–68	Resting	rCMRglc	No change in either FDG rate constant or rCMRglc
Duara et al.	166	40	M; 21–83	Resting	rCMRglc	None
Pantano et al.	167	27	M,F; 19–76	Resting	rCBF; rCMRO$_2$	Decrease in both rCBF and rCMRO$_2$, multiple ROIs
Riege et al.	168	23	M,F; 27–78	Resting	rCMRglc	Decrease, Broca's region
Haxby et al.	169	40	M; 21–83	Resting	rCMRglc	None; no relation of visual memory to rCMRglc
Herscovitch et al.	132	18	NR; 22–84	Resting	rCBF; rCMRO$_2$	Cortical atrophy, but no change in either rCBF or rCMRO$_2$
Horwitz et al.	125	30	M; 20–83	Resting	rCMRglc	Decrease in correlations among metabolic rates for ROIs, frontal and parietal
Yamaguchi et al.	170	22	M,F; 26–64	Resting	rCBF; rCMRO$_2$,	Decrease in rCMRO$_2$, multiple ROIs; none in rCBF
de Leon et al.	120	53	NR; 30–69	Resting	rCMRglc	None, except for hypofrontality in combined sample
Kushner et al.	171	30	NR; 18–73	Resting	rCMRglc	None, for either global or cerebellar values

Table 1 *(Continued)*

Authors	Ref.	*n*	Gender; age range (yr)	Scan conditions	Metabolic measure	Changes with increasing age
Schlageter et al.	172	49	M; 21–83	Resting	rCMRglc	None
Hoffman et al.	122	36	M,F; 21–74	Resting	rCMRglc	Decrease; frontal and subcortical ROIs
Yoshii et al.	137	76	M,F; 21–84	Resting	rCMRglc	None, when adjusted for brain volume and atrophy
Duara et al.	32	22	NR; 42–63	Activation with reading/memory and verbal fluency tasks	rCMRglc	Decrease bilaterally; orbitofrontal and premotor
Itoh et al.	173	28	M,F; 50–85	Resting	rCBF; rCMRO$_2$	Cortical atrophy, but no change in either rCBF or rCMRO$_2$
Leenders et al.	123	34	M,F; 22–82	Resting	rCBF; rCMRO$_2$	Decrease in rCMRO$_2$ multiple ROIs; decrease in rCBF, two ROIs
Martin et al.	124	30	M,F; 30–85	Resting	rCBF	Decrease, multiple ROIs
Azari et al.	126	32	F; 21–90	Resting	rCMRglc	Decrease in correlations among metabolic rates for ROIs, frontal and parietal
Burns and Tyrrell	174	14	M,F; 51–85	Resting	rCMRO$_2$	Decrease; parietal
Grady et al.	128	20	M; 27–72	Activation with face-matching and dot location–matching tasks	rCBF	Difference in pattern of activation across across ROIs
Marchal et al.	175	25	M,F; 20–68	Resting	rCBF; rCMRO$_2$	rCMRO$_2$ (corrected for atrophy) decrease; rCBF decrease, multiple ROIs
Takada et al.	176	32	M,F; 27–67	Resting	rCBF; rCMRO$_2$	rCMRO$_2$ decrease, multiple ROIs; rCBF decrease, left temporal
Tempel and Perlmutter	127	26	M,F; 20–72	Activation with vibrotactile stimulation	rCBF	None

(continued)

Table 1   (*Continued*)

Authors	Ref.	*n*	Gender; age range (yr)	Scan conditions	Metabolic measure	Changes with increasing age
Grady et al.	129	50	M; 26–67	Activation with face matching and spatial localization	rCBF	Difference in SPM pattern of activation
Grady et al.	131	20	M,F; 25–69	Activation with visual encoding and recognition memory tasks	rCBF	Difference in SPM pattern of activation
Loessner et al.	119	120	M,F; 19–79	Resting	rCMRglc	Decrease, frontal ROI
Madden et al.	130	20	M; 18–75	Activation with visual word identification	rCBF	Difference in SPM pattern of activation

For studies including patient groups (e.g., dementia), only healthy subjects are considered; *n* refers to total number of healthy subjects. M = males; F = females; NR = not reported; rCBF = regional cerebral blood flow; rCMRglc = regional cerebral metabolic rate for glucose; rCMRO$_2$ = regional cerebral metabolic rate for oxygen; ROI = region of interest; SPM = Statistical Parametric Mapping.

that the change in rCBF associated with vibrotactile stimulation did not vary significantly as a function of adult age, which is consistent with the results of nontomographic studies [116,117]. Other results, however, suggest that with a more cognition-dependent activation paradigm, age-related changes may be evident. Grady et al. [128] found that rCBF activation during two visual tasks exhibited a pattern in which occipitotemporal cortex was relatively more active during a face-matching task and superior parietal cortex was relatively more active during dot location matching. This differential pattern of activation was more clearly evident in the young adults' data than in the older adults' data.

Grady et al. [129] followed up on their initial findings in two experiments, the first of which was a replication and reanalysis of the Grady et al. [128] face-matching and dot-location tasks, using additional subjects and more anatomically precise image subtraction analyses. The second experiment included the same types of tasks, but the complexity of the location task stimuli was increased so that it more closely approximated the complexity of the face stimuli. For each task, passive viewing of the stimuli was used as a control condition. Grady et al. [129] replicated the general pattern of the results of their earlier study. Relative to the control condition, both young and older adults exhibited occipitotemporal activation during face matching and occipitoparietal activation during location matching, with less functional differentiation between the tasks being evident for older adults than for young adults. During both tasks, there was more activation in ventral and medial occipital (prestriate) cortex for young adults than for older adults, whereas the older adults exhibited relatively more activation in occipitotemporal cortex. For the location-matching tasks, the older adults exhibited greater activation than the young adults in several areas of prefrontal cortex, bilateral inferior parietal cortex, and in left medial parietal cortex. Grady et al. [129] proposed that the efficiency of visual processing in occipital cortex was greater for young adults than for older adults; as a result, the older adults relied more heavily on cortical areas outside these pathways, such as the frontal and parietal regions. In addition, the authors suggested that the more widespread prefrontal activation exhibited by the older adults, during location matching, may indicate that spatial vision is more vulnerable than object vision to the effects of aging.

The Grady et al. [128,129] studies examined visual processing for nonverbal stimuli (faces and noise patterns). Madden et al. [130] investigated age-related changes in rCBF during visual processing of verbal stimuli. These authors used a word/nonword discrimination (lexical decision) task as the activation task. The individual words and nonwords were presented either intact or degraded (by asterisks located between adjacent letters). Control conditions involved passive viewing of either the words and nonwords or a series of fixation points. Task condition subtractions indicated that rCBF activation in regions of the inferior aspect of the left occipital and temporal lobes was significantly greater for young adults than for older adults. These data complement those of Grady et al. [128,129] by demonstrating that age-related change in the functioning of the ventral occipitotemporal pathway is not limited to activation tasks involving nonverbal stimuli. The Madden et al. [130] data also suggest that the retrieval of semantic information sufficient to identify individual words can be mediated by the ventral occipitotemporal pathway, without the involvement of left frontal cortex [76–78].

Two PET activation studies have focused specifically on age-related changes in memory functioning. Duara et al. [32] measured rCMRglc during two tasks, one of which involved reading and recalling a series of verbal passages, the other which involved recalling as many words as possible beginning with a specific letter (i.e., verbal fluency). Relative to a resting state baseline, older adults exhibited less rCMRglc activation, bilaterally, than young adults, in the orbitofrontal regions during the reading/recalling task. An age-related decline in rCMRglc activation was evident for the premotor region, bilaterally, during the verbal fluency task.

The second memory study, that of Grady et al. [131], separated the effects of encoding and recognition for visually presented faces. During separate scans, subjects viewed faces to be remembered (i.e., encoding), performed a face-matching control task and completed a recognition memory test for the previously viewed items. Behavioral data indicated that the older adults' recognition memory performance was worse than that of the young adults. The rCBF date suggested that, for young adults, memory processes are mediated by dissociable systems for encoding (left prefrontal cortex) and recognition (right prefrontal cortex), as proposed by the HERA model of Tulving et al. [52] (discussed in Sect. V). An age-related decline was evident in the rCBF activation associated with both encoding and recognition, but was particularly pronounced during encoding, leading Grady et al. [131] to conclude that the age-related decline in memory performance for this type of task is due, at least in part, to the neural processes occurring at encoding.

The trend from PET studies of age differences in cognitive activation is an age-related decline in the magnitude of the regionally specific activations associated with task performance. An important issue in the interpretation of these age-related changes is cerebral atrophy. This issue does not affect nontomographic measurements of whole brain CBF (e.g., as obtained by the Kety-Schmidt nitrous oxide inhalation technique) because these measures record data only per unit of extant tissue. The data obtained from regional tomographic measures such as PET, however, represent activity per unit volume of intracranial contents. As a result of age-related cortical atrophic changes [6], a volume of space of constant size is more likely to contain metabolically inactive elements (e.g., ventricular and sulcal spaces) for older adults than for young adults. The age-related decline in CBF and cerebral metabolic rate obtained from PET may consequently reflect these atrophic changes rather than metabolic or CBF changes per se [37].

Several methods have developed for correcting PET data for the effects of cerebral atrophy [132–134]. These methods involve combining estimates of actual neural tissue volume, from CT or MRI scans, with the PET data. The application of these types of methods has indicated that age- and dementia-related changes in global CBF and metabolic rate are reduced by the use of atrophy-corrected values [135–137], although the effect of these corrections on rCBF activation measures has not been investigated. Current methods of analyzing rCBF activation, such as SPM [58], use each subject's global flow as a covariate, and Grady et al. [129] found that, in an SPM analysis of rCBF activation, age was associated with both increases and decreases in regional activation, as a function of task condition. Madden et al. [130] found that an age-related decrease in rCBF activation was evident in the absence of age differences in the volume of cortical gray matter as estimated from MRI. Thus, it will be important to consider the potential effects of cerebral atrophy; indeed, as Kety [114] noted, neuronal loss may be an important physiologic mechanism underlying age-related functional change. It is unlikely that age differences in rCBF activation, however, can be attributed entirely to cortical atrophy.

VII. DIRECTIONS FOR RESEARCH ON AGE DIFFERENCES IN PET

The PET methodology provides a unique opportunity to identify the age-related changes in neural functioning that mediate adult age differences in cognitive performance. From the studies listed in Table 1, however, it is evident that, with the exception of Duara et al. [32], Tempel and Perlmutter [127], Grady et al. [128,129,131], and Madden et al. [130], age has not been included as a variable in PET activation paradigms. We believe that the most important direction for further PET research on aging is the use of $H_2^{15}O$ activation paradigms in which the changes in rCBF in response to specific task components can be measured. Although an overall reduction in the rate of neural metabolic activity may occur as a function of age, the more informative measure is the pattern of regional activation, relative to an appropriate baseline, associated with a particular cognitive activity. In addition, the PET activation studies that have been conducted with young adult subjects [29,49,50,98] have investigated aspects of cognitive performance in which adult age differences have been documented in behavioral research [2]. It will consequently be useful to take into account, in the design of PET activation studies, the pattern of age-related cognitive changes obtained from behavioral measures. We mention here three areas of investigation: word identification, attention, and memory, for which extensive behavioral data are available.

A. Word Identification

Verbal knowledge, in terms of vocabulary size and the pattern of associations produced to a stimulus word, appears to remain stable as a function of age [138]. There is an age-related decline in performance on word-identification tasks that is related to the efficiency of feature extraction. The effect of degrading the stimulus quality of visually presented words, for example, is often greater for older adults than for young adults [139–141], and older adults require a relatively longer segment of an auditorily presented word to achieve identification [142]. In contrast, the activation and use of semantic information during word identification appear to be relatively resistant to age-related decline. The degree to which the identification of a visually presented target word is influenced by a preceding word or sentence context (i.e., semantic priming) is typically comparable for young and older adults [138,143]. When stimulus quality is degraded, older adults may even rely on semantic context to a greater degree than young adults [140,142,144]. This relative preservation of semantic activation processes, however, is observed under conditions that Frith et al. [61] described as extrinsic generation: when the target stimulus is presented externally. Under conditions of intrinsic generation, when subjects must initiate a memory search for a specific word, age-related decline has been observed. Bowles and Poon [145] reported that young and older adults exhibited comparable semantic priming on a lexical decision task, but that older adults were less successful than young adults in accessing the specific word fitting a given definition. Burke et al. [146] found that retrieval failures in everyday word-retrieval tasks (tip-of-the-tongue phenomena) increased as a function of age.

This pattern of age-related changes in word-identification performance leads to the prediction that under extrinsic generation conditions, age differences in PET measures of rCBF activation would be associated primarily with the neural systems mediating feature extraction processes. Thus, for visual and auditory presentation, respectively, there may be an age-related decrease in activation for the medial occipital cortex and the middle superior temporal cortex. The pattern of age-related change in rCBF for visual word identification reported by Madden et al. [130] is consistent with this interpretation. When words are intrinsically generated, however, as in the semantic association and verbal fluency tasks of Frith et al. [61], Petersen et al. [76–78], and Wise et al. [79], the activation of left prefrontal cortex, anterior cingulate, and Wernicke's area reported by these authors is likely to exhibit age-related change.

B. Attention

The vast majority of behavioral studies of age-related changes in attention have investigated visual information processing [147,148]. Adult age differences in visual search performance have been often observed when the task relies primarily on divided-attention processes. The prototypical finding is that as the number of required comparisons increases, in terms of either the number of items in the target set or the visual display, the magnitude of the age difference in reaction time also increases [149]. Similarly, under some conditions the ability to ignore irrelevant information appears to undergo age-related decline [150]. Selective attention processes, however, appear to be more resistant to the effects of aging. For example, comparable patterns of task performance have been reported for young and older adults when a visual cue (e.g., a bar marker) specifying the potential spatial location of the target is presented prior to display onset [151].

Hartley [152] and Madden and Plude [148] noted that the PET studies of attentional processes in young adults lead to the prediction that the anterior and posterior attentional systems [90] exhibit differential age-related change. If age-related performance decrements are greater for divided attention processes than for selective attention processes, then the degree of rCBF activation in the anterior attention system during divided-attention tasks should be lower (or more regionally diffuse) for older adults than for young adults. In the visual discrimination task used by Corbetta et al. [49,50], for example, the divided-attention condition (in which subjects were not given advance information regarding the stimulus dimension that would differ between displays) would be expected to elicit greater rCBF activation in the medial frontal region (e.g., anterior cingulate cortex) for young adults than for older adults. Conversely, the rCBF activation in the extrastriate areas (i.e., posterior attention system), which Corbetta et al. [49,50,89] reported was associated with selective attention to a specific stimulus dimension, would be expected to remain relatively constant as a function of adult age.

C. Memory

Behavioral studies of memory have indicated that the episodic component of declarative memory is particularly vulnerable to age-related decline [153]. When, for example, following presentation of a word list (without instructions to remember), subjects are given a cued recall test (i.e., an assessment of episodic memory), performance is typically higher for young adults than for older adults. When the same cues are given as a fragment completion test, however, without reference to the original list (i.e., priming of nondeclarative memory), the proportion of completed fragments matching the original list is often comparable for young and older adults [154]. In addition, significant age-related decline has been observed in the performance of working memory tasks [150,155,156]. These findings suggest that self-directed encoding, maintenance, and retrieval processes are an important aspect of age-related decline in episodic memory function. The retrieval component appears to be particularly vulnerable; evidence for age differences in encoding processes is variable [157], whereas there is a consistent relation between the degree of retrieval support and age differences in episodic memory performance. As retrieval support is decreased (e.g., in recall tasks relative to recognition tasks), the age-related decline is magnified [158].

If, as the results of Squire et al. [98] and Grafton et al. [100] suggest, the neural systems mediating declarative and nondeclarative memory can be distinguished by PET, a corresponding distinction should be evident in age-related changes in rCBF activation. The magnitude of decrease in rCBF for right occipital cortex during repetition priming [98] and increase in rCBF in the regions mediating motor learning [100], for example, should be comparable for young and older adults, in view of the similarity of the two age groups' performance on tests of nondeclarative memory [153]. Tasks that rely on the episodic component of declarative memory, in contrast, should exhibit significant age-related change in rCBF. Given the age-related decline in working memory [150,155], the rCBF activation of prefrontal (predominantly dorsolateral) cortex associated with working memory performance [104–106] would be expected to be lower in magnitude for older adults than for young adults. A similar age effect would be predicted for the cortical regions mediating the articulatory loop described by Paulesu et al. [108]. Tasks that involve self-directed retrieval from long-term episodic memory (e.g., Ref. 111) would be particularly likely to yield age-related changes in rCBF. The HERA model of Tulving et al. [52] suggests that age differences in episodic retrieval processes would be evident in the pattern of rCBF activation in the right prefrontal cortex. Age differences in rCBF generally consistent with the HERA model have been reported by Grady et al. [131] (see Sec. VI), although these authors found that encoding processes were more important than retrieval processes in determining age effects.

Moscovitch and Winocur [159] developed a theoretical model of the age-related changes in neural functioning associated with changes in memory performance. In this framework, the age-related decline frequently observed in tests of declarative memory represent decrements in associative and consolidation processes mediated by the hippocampus and in the implementation of encoding and retrieval strategies mediated by frontal regions. The authors viewed the relative preservation of older adults' performance on nondeclarative memory tests as a result of the fact that the cortical and subcortical areas involved in the initial registration of perceptual events can mediate nondeclarative memory for those events. Moscovitch and Winocur used the similarity between the effects of aging and the effects of hippocampal/frontal lesions on memory performance as evidence for their theory. The PET investigations of nondeclarative memory in young adults [98,100] support the theory, as does the Grady et al. [131] report of an age-related decline in rCBF activation of left prefrontal cortex during memory encoding. An additional aspect of the Grady et al. [131] data, relevant to the Moscovitch and Winocur theory, is the finding that, during the encoding task, young adults exhibited a significant correlation between the rCBF values of the right hippocampus and those of a left frontal region (anterior cingulate). This correlation, which suggests a neural system mediating the consolidation of encoded events, was not significant in the older adults' data.

VIII. CONCLUSION

Measures of CBF and metabolic activity obtained from PET have led to the development of detailed models of the functional neuroanatomy of cognitive performance in young adults (e.g., Refs. 29, 30, 49–51). Behavioral investigations of adult age differences in cognitive performance have revealed a pattern of age-related change and constancy in the types of tasks that have been used in PET studies of young adults. Extensive research has been conducted on age differences in selective attention, visual word identification, and memory functioning [2]. Theoretical distinctions applied in PET research, such as selective versus divided attention, intrinsic versus extrinsic semantic activation, and declarative versus nondeclarative memory, have also been used to guide behavioral studies of age-related changes in cognitive function. As a result, clear predictions are possible regarding age differences in the pattern of rCBF activation during PET. Although substantial research using PET has been conducted on age-related changes in resting state CBF cerebral metabolic activity (Table 1), few empirical studies of age differences in PET activation paradigms have been conducted, and such studies are important both theoretically and practically. This kind of data would provide a new and fundamental source of evidence regarding the age-related changes in neural functioning that mediate the changes in cognitive performance. The data would also be relevant to the neuropsychological theories of cognitive functioning (e.g., Ref 159) developed based on lesion studies and animal models. The practical implication of such data would be an improvement in both the ability to detect cognitive impairments such as dementia [34] and the ability to distinguish the effects of aging from those of disease.

ACKNOWLEDGMENT

This work was supported by Research Grant R01 AG11622 from the National Institute on Aging.

REFERENCES

1. J. Cerella, J. Rybash, W. Hoyer, and M. L. Commons (eds.), *Adult Information Processing: Limits on Loss*, Academic Press, San Diego, 1993.
2. F. I. M. Craik and T. A. Salthouse (eds.), *The Handbook of Aging and Cognition*, Erlbaum, Hillsdale, NJ, 1992.
3. D. H. Kausler, *Experimental Psychology, Cognition, and Human Aging*, Springer-Verlag, New York, 1991.
4. D. A. Walsh and D. A. Hershey, Mental models and the maintenance of complex problem solving-skills in old age, *Adult Information Processing: Limits on Loss* (J. Cerella, J. Rybash, W. Hoyer, and M. L. Commons, eds.), Academic Press, San Diego, 1993, p. 553.
5. P. D. Coleman and D. G. Flood, Neuron numbers and dendritic extent in normal aging and Alzheimer's disease, *Neurobiol. Aging 8*:521 (1987).

6. H. Creasey and S. I. Rapoport, The aging human brain, *Ann. Neurol. 17*:2 (1985).
7. T. Kemper, Neuroanatomical and neuropathological changes in normal aging and in dementia, *Clinical Neurology of Aging* (M. L. Albert, ed.), Oxford University Press, New York, 1984, p. 9.
8. R. D. Terry, R. DeTeresa, and L. A. Hansen, Neocortical cell counts in normal human adult aging, *Ann. Neurol. 21*:530 (1987).
9. W. W. Orrison, Jr. and J. A. Sanders, Clinical brain imaging: computerized axial tomography and magnetic resonance imaging, *Functional Brain Imaging* (W. W. Orrison, Jr., J. D. Lewine, J. A. Sanders, and M. F. Hartshorne, eds.), Mosby, St. Louis 1995, p. 97.
10. F. Fazekas, J. B. Chawluk, A. Alavi, H. I. Hurtig, and R. A. Zimmerman, MR signal abnormalities at 1.5 T in Alzheimer's dementia and normal aging, *Am. J. Neuroradiol. 8*:421 (1987).
11. K. R. R. Krishnan, Neuroanatomic substrates of depression in the elderly, *J. Geriatr. Psychiatry Neurol. 6*:39 (1993).
12. M. Schwartz, H. Creasey, C. L. Grady, J. M. DeLeo, H. A. Frederickson, N. R. Cutler, and S. I. Rapoport, Computed tomographic analysis of brain morphometrics in 30 healthy men, aged 21 to 81 years, *Ann. Neurol. 17*:146 (1985).
13. N. Raz, D. Millman, and G. Sarpel, Cerebral correlates of cognitive aging: Gray-white matter differentiation in the medial temporal lobes, and fluid versus crystallized abilities, *Psychobiology 18*:475 (1990).
14. N. Raz, I. J. Torres, W. D. Spencer, and J. D. Acker, Pathoclysis in aging human cerebral cortex: Evidence from in vivo MRI morphometry, *Psychobiology 21*:151 (1993).
15. C. E. Coffey, W. E. Wilkinson, I. A. Parashos, S. A. R. Soady, R. J. Sullivan, L. J. Patterson, G. S. Figiel, M. C. Webb, C. E. Spritzer, and W. T. Djang, Quantitative cerebral anatomy of the aging human brain: A cross-sectional study using magnetic resonance imaging, *Neurology 42*:527 (1992).
16. D. G. M. Murphy, C. DeCarli, M. B. Schapiro, S. I. Rapoport, and B. Horwitz, Age-related differences in volumes of subcortical nuclei, brain matter, and cerebrospinal fluid in healthy men as measured with magnetic resonance imaging, *Arch. Neurol. 49*:839 (1992).
17. K. K. Kwong, J. W. Belliveau, D. A. Chesler, I. E. Goldberg, R. M. Weisskoff, B. P. Poncelet, D. N. Kennedy, B. E. Hoppel, M. S. Cohen, R. Turner, H. M. Cheng, T. J. Brady, and B. R. Rosen, Dynamic magnetic resonance imaging of human brain activity during primary sensory stimulation, *Proc. Natl. Acad. Sci. USA 89*:5675 (1992).
18. J. W. Prichard and B. R. Rosen, Functional study of the brain by NMR, *J. Cereb. Blood Flow Metab. 14*:365 (1994).
19. J. A. Sanders and W. W. Orrison, Jr., Functional magnetic resonance imaging, *Functional Brain Imaging* (W. W. Orrison, Jr., J. D. Lewine, J. A. Sanders, and M. F. Hartshorne, eds.), Mosby, St. Louis 1995, p. 239.
20. J. D. Cohen, D. C. Noll, and W. Schneider, Functional magnetic resonance

imaging: Overview and methods for psychological research, *Behav. Res. Meth. Inst. Comp. 25*:101 (1993).

21. T. Constable, G. McCarthy, T. Allison, A. W. Anderson, and J. C. Gore, Functional brain imaging at 1.5 T using conventional gradient echo MR imaging techniques, *Magn. Reson. Imaging 11*:451 (1993).

22. M. F. Hartshorne, Positron emission tomography, *Functional Brain Imaging* (W. W. Orrison, Jr., J. D. Lewine, J. A. Sanders and M. F. Hartshorne, eds.), Mosby, St. Louis 1995, p. 187.

23. J. C. Mazziotta, M. E. Phelps, D. Plummer, R. Schwab, and E. Halgren, Optimization and standardization of anatomical data in neurobehavioral investigations using positron computed tomography, *J. Cereb. Blood Flow Metab. 3*:S266 (1983).

24. M. E. Raichle, W. R. W. Martin, P. Herscovitch, M. A. Mintun, and J. Markham, Brain blood flow measured with intravenous $H_2^{15}O$. II. Implementation and validation, *J. Nucl. Med. 24*:790 (1983).

25. M. Reivich, D. Kuhl, A. Wolf, J. Greenberg, M. Phelps, T. Ido, V. Casella, J. Fowler, E. Hoffman, A. Alavi, P. Som, and L. Sokoloff, The ^{18}F fluorodeoxyglucose method for the measurement of local cerebral glucose utilization in man, *Circ. Res. 44*:127 (1979).

26. D. J. Chadwick and J. E. Whelan (eds.), *Exploring Brain Functional Anatomy with Positron Tomography*, Wiley, Chichester, UK, 1991.

27. J. V. Haxby, C. L. Grady, L. G. Ungerleider, and B. Horowitz, Mapping the functional neuroanatomy of the intact human brain with brain work imaging, *Neuropsychologia 29*:539 (1991).

28. J. C. Mazziotta, Brain metabolism: Measurement and correlates with neuropsychological performance, *Handbook of Neuropsychology*, Vol. 10 (F. Boller and J. Grafman, eds.), Elsevier, Amsterdam, 1995, p. 331.

29. S. E. Petersen and J. A. Fiez, The processing of single words studied with positron emission tomography, *Ann. Rev. Neurosci. 16*:509 (1993).

30. M. E. Raichle, Images of the mind: Studies with modern imaging techniques, *Ann. Rev. Psychol. 45*:333 (1994).

31. J. M. Hoffman, B. H. Guze, L. R. Baxter, J. C. Mazziotta, and M. E. Phelps, ^{18}F-Fluorodeoxyglucose (FDG) and positron emission tomography (PET) in aging and dementia: A decade of studies, *Eur. Neurol. 29*:16 (1989).

32. R. Duara, D. A. Loewenstein, and W. W. Barker, Utilization of behavioral activation paradigms for positron emission tomography studies in normal young and elderly subjects and in dementia, *Positron Emission Tomography in Dementia* (R. Duara, ed.), Wiley-Liss, New York, 1990, p. 131.

33. S. Goldstein and M. Reivich, Cerebral blood flow and metabolism in aging and dementia. *Clin. Neuropharmacol. 14*:S1 (1991).

34. R. Parasuraman and J. V. Haxby, Attention and brain function in Alzheimer's disease: A review, *Neuropsychology 7*:242 (1993).

35. C. S. Roy and C. S. Sherrington, On the regulation of the blood supply of the brain, *J. Physiol. (Lond). 11*:85 (1890).

36. S. S. Kety and C. F. Schmidt, The nitrous oxide method for the quantitative

determination of cerebral blood flow in man: Theory, procedure, and normal values, *J. Clin. Invest.* *27*:476 (1948).

37. M. E. Raichle, Circulatory and metabolic correlates of brain function in normal humans, *Handbook of Physiology: Section 1. The Nervous System*, Vol. 5 (F. Plum, ed.), American Physiological Society, Bethesda, MD, 1987, p. 643.

38. J. C. Mazziotta and S. Gilman, *Clinical Brain Imaging: Principles and Applications*, F. A. Davis, Philadelphia, 1992.

39. W. W. Orrison, Jr., J. D. Lewine, J. A. Sanders, and M. F. Hartshorne (eds.), *Functional Brain Imaging*, Mosby, St. Louis, 1995.

40. P. Horowicz and M. G. Larrabee, Clucose consumption and lactate production in a mammalian sympathetic ganglion at rest and in activity, *J. Neurochem.* *2*:102 (1958).

41. P. Horowicz and M. G. Larrabee, Oxidation of glucose in a mammalian sympathetic ganglion at rest and in activity, *J. Neurochem.* *9*:1 (1962).

42. J. C. Baron, P. Lebrun-Grandie, P. Collard, C. Crouzel, G. Mestelan, and M. G. Bousser, Noninvasive measurement of blood flow, oxygen consumption, and glucose utilization in the same brain regions in man by positron emission tomography: Concise communication, *J. Nucl. Med.* *23*:391 (1982).

43. M. E. Raichle, R. L. Grubb, Jr., M. L. Gado, J. O. Eichling, and M. M. Ter-Pogossian, Correlation between regional cerebral blood flow and oxidative metabolism, *Arch. Neurol.* *33*:523 (1976).

44. P. T. Fox and M. E. Raichle, Focal physiological uncoupling of cerebral blood flow and oxidative metabolism during somatosensory stimulation in normal subjects, *Proc. Natl. Acad. Sci. USA 83*:1140 (1986).

45. J. C. Mazziotta, M. E. Phelps, R. E. Carson, and D. E. Kuhl, Tomographic mapping of human cerebral metabolism: Sensory deprivation, *Ann. Neurol.* *12*:435 (1982).

46. P. T. Fox, M. A. Mintun, E. M. Reiman, and M. E. Raichle, Enhanced detection of focal brain responses using intersubject averaging and change-distribution analysis of subtracted PET images, *J. Cereb. Blood Flow Metab.* *8*:642 (1988).

47. J. C. Mazziotta, S. C. Huang, M. E. Phelps, R. E. Carson, N. S. MacDonald, and K. Mahoney, A non-invasive positron computed tomography technique using oxygen-15-labeled water for the evaluation of the neurobehavioral task batteries, *J. Cereb. Blood Flow Metab.* *5*:70 (1985).

48. P. T. Fox, M. A. Mintun, M. E. Raichle, and P. Herscovitch, A noninvasive approach to quantitative functional mapping of $H_2^{15}O$ and positron emission tomography, *J. Cereb. Blood Flow Metab.* *4*:329 (1984).

49. M. Corbetta, F. M. Miezin, S. Dobmeyer, G. L. Shulman, and S. E. Petersen, Attentional modulation of neural processing of shape, color, and velocity in humans, *Science 248*:1556 (1990).

50. M. Corbetta, F. M. Miezin, S. Dobmeyer, G. L. Shulman, and S. E. Petersen, Selective and divided attention during visual discriminations of shape, color, and speed: Functional anatomy by positron emission tomography, *J. Neurosci.* *11*:2383 (1991).

51. R. L. Buckner and E. Tulving, Neuroimaging studies of memory: Theory and recent PET results, *Handbook of Neuropsychology*, Vol. 10 (F. Boller and J. Grafman, eds.), Elsevier, Amsterdam, 1995, p. 439.

52. E. Tulving, S. Kapur, F. I. M. Craik, M. Moscovitch, and S. Houle, Hemispheric encoding/retrieval asymmetry in episodic memory: Positron emission tomography findings, *Proc. Natl. Acad. Sci. USA 91*:2016 (1994).

53. J.-F. Démonet, C. Price, R. Wise, and R. S. J. Frackowiak, Differential activation of right and left posterior sylvian regions by semantic and phonological tasks: A positron-emission tomography study in normal human subjects, *Neurosci. Lett. 182*:25 (1994).

54. J. Sergent, E. Zuck, M. Levesque, and B. MacDonald, Positron emission tomography study of letter and object processing: Empirical findings and methodological considerations, *Cereb. Cortex 2*:68 (1992).

55. R. S. J. Frackowiak and K. J. Friston, Methodology of activation paradigms, *Handbook of Neuropsychology*, Vol. 10 (F. Boller and J. Grafman, eds.), Elsevier, Amsterdam, 1995, p. 369.

56. J. C. Mazziotta, C. C. Pelizzari, G. T. Chen, F. L. Bookstein, and D. Valentino, Region of interest issues: The relationship between structure and function in the brain, *J. Cereb. Blood Flow Metab. 11*:A51 (1991).

57. K. J. Friston, C. D. Frith, P. F. Liddle, R. J. Dolan, A. A. Lammertsma, and R. S. J. Frackowiak, The relationship between global and local changes in PET scans, *J. Cereb. Blood Flow Metab. 10*:458 (1990).

58. K. J. Friston, A. P. Holmes, K. J. Worsley, J. P. Poline, C. D. Frith, and R. S. J. Frackowiak, Statistical parametric mapping in functional imaging: A general linear approach, *Hum. Brain Mapp. 2*:189 (1995).

59. K. J. Friston, C. D. Frith, P. F. Liddle, and R. S. J. Frackowiak, Comparing functional (PET) images: The assessment of significant change, *J. Cereb. Blood Flow Metab. 11*:690 (1991).

60. J. Talairach and P. Tournoux, *Co-Planar Stereotaxic Atlas of the Human Brain*, Thieme, Stuttgart, 1988.

61. C. D. Frith, K. J. Friston, P. F. Liddle, and R. S. J. Frackowiak, A PET study of word finding, *Neuropsychologia 29*:1137 (1991).

62. B. Horwitz, C. L. Grady, J. V. Haxby, L. G. Ungerleider, M. B. Schapiro, M. Mishkin, and S. I. Rapoport, Functional associations among human posterior extrastriate brain regions during object and spatial vision, *J. Cog. Neurosci. 4*:311 (1992).

63. I. Ford, J. H. McColl, A. G. McCormack, and S. J. McCrory, Statistical issues in the analysis of neuroimages, *J. Cereb. Blood Flow Metab. 11*:A89 (1991).

64. H. Steinmetz and R. J. Seitz, Functional anatomy of language processing: Neuroimaging and the problem of individual variability, *Neuropsychologia 29*: 1149 (1991).

65. S. R. Cherry, R. P. Woods, E. J. Hoffman, and J. C. Mazziotta, Improved detection of focal cerebral blood flow changes using three-dimensional positron emission tomography, *J. Cereb. Blood Flow Metab. 13*:630 (1993).

66. D. W. Townsend, Optimization of signal in positron emission tomography

scans: Present and future developments, *Exploring Brain Functional Anatomy with Positron Tomography* (D. J. Chadwick and J. Whelan eds.), Wiley, Chichester, UK, 1991, p. 57.

67. D. A. Silbersweig, E. Stern, C. D. Frith, C. Cahill, L. Schnorr, S. Grootoonk, T. Spinks, J. Clark, R. Frackowiak, and T. Jones, Detection of thirty-second cognitive activations in single subjects with positron emission tomography: A new low-dose $H_2^{15}O$ regional cerebral blood flow three-dimensional imaging technique, *J. Cereb. Blood Flow Metab. 13*:617 (1993).

68. D. Besner and J. C. Johnston, Reading and the mental lexicon: On the uptake of visual information, *Lexical Representation and Process* (W. Marslen-Wilson, ed.), MIT Press, Cambridge, MA, 1989, p. 291.

69. U. H. Frauenfelder and L. K. Tyler, The process of spoken word recognition: An introduction, *Cognition 25*:1 (1987).

70. J. H. Neely, Semantic priming effects in visual word recognition: A selective review of current findings and theories, *Basic Processes in Reading: Visual Word Recognition* (D. Besner and G. W. Humphreys, eds.), Erlbaum, Hillsdale, NJ, 1991, p. 264.

71. M. I. Posner and C. R. R. Snyder, Attention and cognitive control, *Information Processing and Cognition: The Loyola Symposium* (R. L. Solso, ed.), Erlbaum, Hillsdale, NJ, 1975, p. 55.

72. R. J. Wise, U. Hadar, D. Howard, and K. Patterson, Language activation studies with positron emission tomography, *Exploring Brain Functional Anatomy with Positron Tomography* (D. J. Chadwick and J. Whelan, eds.), Wiley, Chichester, UK, 1991, p. 218.

73. M. Liotti, C. T. Gay, and P. T. Fox, Functional imaging and language: Evidence from positron emission tomography, *J. Clin. Neurophysiol. 11*:175 (1994).

74. J.-F. Démonet, R. Wise, and R. S. J. Frackowiak, Language functions explored in normal subjects by positron emission tomography: A critical review, *Hum. Brain Mapp. 1*:39 (1993).

75. J.-F. Démonet, Studies of language processing using positron emission tomography, *Handbook of Neuropsychology*, Vol. 10 (F. Boller and J. Grafman, eds.), Elsevier, Amsterdam, 1995, p. 423.

76. S. E. Petersen, P. T. Fox, M. I. Posner, M. Mintun, and M. E. Raichle, Positron emission tomographic studies of the cortical anatomy of single-word processing, *Nature 331*:585 (1988).

77. S. E. Petersen, P. T. Fox, M. I. Posner, M. Mintun, and M. E. Raichle, Positron emission tomographic studies of the processing of single words, *J. Cog. Neurosci. 1*:153 (1989).

78. S. E. Petersen, P. T. Fox, A. Z. Snyder, and M. E. Raichle, Activation of extrastriate and frontal cortical areas by visual words and word-like stimuli, *Science 249*:1041 (1990).

79. R. Wise, F. Chollet, U. Hadar, K. Friston, E. Hoffner, and R. Frackowiak, Distribution of cortical neural networks involved in word comprehension and word retrieval, *Brain 114*:1803 (1991).

80. K. J. Friston, C. D. Frith, P. F. Liddle, and R. S. J. Frackowiak, Investigating a network model of word generation with positron emission tomography, *Proc. R. Soc. London Ser. B 244*:101 (1991).

81. J.-F. Démonet, F. Chollet, S. Ramsay, D. Cardebat, J.-L. Nespoulous, R. Wise, A. Rascol, and R. S. J. Frackowiak, The anatomy of phonological and semantic processing in normal subjects, *Brain 115*:1753 (1992).

82. M. E. Raichle, J. A. Fiez, T. O. Videen, A. K. MacLeod, J. V. Pardo, P. T. Fox, and S. E. Petersen, Practice-related changes in human brain functional anatomy during nonmotor learning, *Cereb. Cortex 4*:8 (1994).

83. C. J. Price, R. J. S. Wise, J. D. G. Watson, K. Patterson, D. Howard, D., and R. S. J. Frackowiak, Brain activity during reading: The effects of exposure duration and task, *Brain 117*:255 (1994).

84. P. T. Fox and M. E. Raichle, Stimulus rate determines regional brain blood flow in striate cortex, *Ann. Neurol. 17*:303 (1985).

85. W. Schneider, B. J. Casey, and D. Noll, Functional MRI mapping of stimulus rate effects across visual processing stages, *Hum. Brain Mapp. 1*:117 (1994).

86. R. M. Shiffrin, Attention, *Stevens' Handbook of Experimental Psychology*, Vol. 2 (R. C. Atkinson, R. J. Herrnstein, G. Lindzey, and R. D. Luce, eds.), Wiley, New York, 1988, p. 739.

87. L. G. Ungerleider and M. Mishkin, Two cortical visual systems, *Analysis of Visual Behavior* (D. J. Ingle, M. A. Goodale, and R. J. W. Mansfield, eds.), MIT Press, Cambridge, MA, 1982, p. 549.

88. D. LaBerge, Thalamic and cortical mechanisms of attention suggested by recent positron emission tomographic experiments, *J. Cog. Neurosci. 2*:358 (1990).

89. M. Corbetta, F. M. Miezin, G. L. Shulman, and S. E. Petersen, A PET study of visuospatial attention. *J. Neurosci. 13*:1202 (1993).

90. M. I. Posner and S. E. Petersen, The attention system of the human brain, *Ann. Rev. Neurosci. 13*:25 (1990).

91. J. Duncan, The locus of interference in the perception of simultaneous stimuli, *Psychol. Rev. 87*:272 (1980).

92. J. V. Pardo, P. J. Pardo, K. E. Janer, and M. E. Raichle, The anterior cingulate cortex mediates processing selection in the Stroop attentional conflict paradigm, *Proc. Natl. Acad. Sci. USA 87*:256 (1990).

93. C. J. Bench, C. D. Frith, P. M. Grasby, K. J. Friston, E. Paulesu, R. S. J. Frackowiak, and R. J. Dolan, Investigations of the functional anatomy of attention using the Stroop test, *Neuropsychologia 31*:907 (1993).

94. C. D. Frith, K. Friston, P. F. Liddle, and R. S. J. Frackowiak, Willed action and the prefrontal cortex in man: A study with PET, *Proc. R. Soc. London Ser. B 244*:241 (1991).

95. J. V. Pardo, P. T. Fox, and M. E. Raichle, Localization of a human system for sustained attention by positron emission tomography, *Nature 349*:61 (1991).

96. P. Graf and M. E. J. Masson (eds.), *Implicit Memory: New Directions in Cognition, Development, and Neuropsychology*, Erlbaum, Hillsdale, NJ, 1993.

97. L. R. Squire, S. Zola-Morgan, C. B. Cave, F. Haist, G. Musen, and W. A.

Suzuki, Memory: Organization of brain systems and cognition, *Attention and Performance XIV: Synergies in Experimental Psychology, Artificial Intelligence, and Cognitive Neuroscience* (D. E. Meyer and S. Kornblum, eds.), MIT Press, Cambridge, MA, 1993, p. 393.

98. L. R. Squire, J. G. Ojemann, F. M. Miezin, S. E. Petersen, T. O. Videen, and M. E. Raichle, Activation of the hippocampus in normal humans: A functional anatomical study of memory, *Proc. Natl. Acad. Sci. USA 89*:1837 (1992).

99. R. L. Buckner, S. E. Petersen, J. G. Ojemann, F. M. Miezin, L. R. Squire, and M. E. Raichle, Functional anatomical studies of explicit and implicit memory retrieval tasks, *J. Neurosci. 15*:12 (1995).

100. S. Grafton, J. C. Mazziotta, S. Presty, K. J. Friston, R. S. J. Frackowiak, and M. E. Phelps, Functional anatomy of human procedural learning determined with regional cerebral blood flow and PET, *J. Neurosci. 12*:2542 (1992).

101. E. Tulving, *Elements of Episodic Memory*, Oxford University Press, New York, 1983.

102. A. D. Baddeley, *Working Memory*, Oxford University Press, London, 1986.

103. H. P. Bahrick, P. O. Bahrick, and R. P. Wittlinger, Fifty years of memory for names and faces: A cross-sectional approach, *J. Exp. Psychol. [Gen.] 104*:54 (1975).

104. M. Petrides, B. Alivisatos, E. Meyer, and A. C. Evans, Functional activation of the human frontal cortex during the performance of verbal working memory tasks, *Proc. Natl. Acad. Sci. USA 90*:878 (1993).

105. J. Jonides, E. E. Smith, R. A. Koeppe, E. Awh, S. Minoshima, and M. A. Mintun, Spatial working memory in humans as revealed by PET, *Nature 363*:623 (1993).

106. M. Petrides, B. Alivisatos, A. C. Evans, and E. Meyer, Dissociation of human mid-dorsolateral from posterior dorsolateral frontal cortex in memory processing, *Proc. Natl. Acad. Sci. USA 90*:873 (1993).

107. P. M. Grasby, C. D. Frith, K. J. Friston, C. Bench, R. S. J. Frackowiak, and R. J. Dolan, Functional mapping of brain areas implicated in auditory-verbal memory function. *Brain 116*:1 (1993).

108. E. Paulesu, C. D. Frith, and R. S. J. Frackowiak, The neural correlates of the verbal component of working memory, *Nature 362*:342 (1993).

109. E. E. Smith, J. Jonides, R. A. Koeppe, E. Awh, E. H. Schumacher, and S. Minoshima, Spatial versus object working memory: PET investigations, *J. Cog. Neurosci. 7*:337 (1995).

110. J. C. Mazziotta and E. J. Metter, Brain cerebral metabolic mapping of normal and abnormal language and its acquisition during development, *Language, Communication, and the Brain* (F. Plum, ed.), Raven Press, New York, 1988, p. 245.

111. T. Shallice, P. Fletcher, C. D. Frith, P. Grasby, R. S. J. Frackowiak, and R. J. Dolan, Brain regions associated with acquisition and retrieval of verbal episodic memory, *Nature 368*:633 (1994).

112. S. Kapur, F. I. M. Craik, E. Tulving, A. A. Wilson, S. Houle, and G. M. Brown, Neuroanatomical correlates of encoding in episodic memory: Levels of processing effect, *Proc. Natl. Acad. Sci. USA 91*:2008 (1994).

113. E. Tulving, S. Kapur, H. J. Markowitsch, F. I. M. Craik, R. Habib, and S. Houle, Neuroanatomical correlates of retrieval in episodic memory: Auditory sentence recognition, *Proc. Natl. Acad. Sci. USA 91*:2012 (1994).

114. S. S. Kety, Human cerebral blood flow and oxygen consumption as related to aging, *J. Chronic Dis. 3*:478 (1956).

115. J. S. Meyer, Y. Terayama, and S. Takashima, Cerebral circulation in the elderly, *Cerebrovasc. Brain Metab. Rev. 5*:122 (1993).

116. J. R. Ewing, G. C. Brown, J. W. Gdowski, R. Simkins, S. R. Levine, and K. M. A. Welch, Stroke risk and age do not predict behavioral activation of brain blood flow, *Ann. Neurol. 25*:571 (1989).

117. R. C. Gur, R. E. Gur, W. D. Obrist, B. E. Skolnik, and M. Reivich, Age and regional cerebral blood flow at rest and during cognitive activity, *Arch. Gen. Psychiatry 44*:617 (1987).

118. D. E. Kuhl, E. J. Metter, W. H. Riege, and M. E. Phelps, Effects of human aging on patterns of local cerebral glucose utilization determined by the ^{18}F fluorodeoxyglucose method, *J. Cereb. Blood Flow Metab. 2*:163 (1982).

119. A. Loessner, A. Alavi, K.-U. Lewandrowski, D. Mozley, E. Souder, and R. E. Gur, Regional cerebral function determined by FDG-PET in healthy volunteers: Normal patterns and changes with age, *J. Nucl. Med. 36*:1141 (1995).

120. M. J. de Leon, A. E. George, J. Tomanelli, D. Christman, A. Kluger, J. Miller, S. H. Ferris, J. Fowler, J. D. Brodie, P. van Gelder, A. Klinger, and A. P. Wolf, Positron emission tomography studies of normal aging: A replication of PET III and 18-FDG using PET VI and 11-CDG, *Neurobiol. Aging 8*:319 (1987).

121. M. J. de Leon, A. E. George, S. H. Ferris, D. R. Christman, J. S. Fowler, C. I. Gentes, J. Brodie, B. Reisberg, and A. P. Wolf, Positron emission tomography and computed tomography assessments of the aging human brain, *J. Comput. Assist. Tomogr. 8*:88 (1984).

122. J. M. Hoffman, B. H. Guze, T. C. Hawk, J. P. Pahl, R. Sumida, L. R. Baxter, J. C. Mazziotta, and M. E. Phelps, Cerebral glucose metabolism in normal individuals: Effects of aging, sex, and handedness, *Neurology 38*(Suppl. 1): 371 (1988).

123. K. L. Leenders, D. Perani, A. A. Lammertsma, J. D. Heather, P. Buckingham, M. J. R. Healy, J. M. Gibbs, R. J. S. Wise, J. Hatazawa, S. Herold, R. P. Beaney, D. J. Brooks, T. Spinks, C. Rhodes, R. S. J. Frackowiak, and T. Jones, Cerebral blood flow, blood volume and oxygen utilization: Normal values and effect of age, *Brain 113*:27 (1990).

124. A. J. Martin, K. J. Friston, J. G. Colebatch, and R. S. J. Frackowiak, Decreases in regional cerebral blood flow with normal aging, *J. Cereb. Blood Flow Metab. 11*:648 (1991).

125. B. Horwitz, R. Duara, and S. I. Rapoport, Age differences in intercorrelations between regional cerebral metabolic rates for glucose, *Ann. Neurol. 19*:60 (1986).

126. N. P. Azari, S. I. Rapoport, J. A. Salerno, C. L. Grady, A. Gonzalez-Aviles, M. B. Schapiro, and B. Horwitz, Interregional correlations of resting cerebral glucose metabolism in old and young women, *Brain Res. 589*:279 (1992).

127. L. W. Tempel and J. S. Perlmutter, Vibration-induced regional cerebral blood flow responses in normal aging, *J. Cereb. Blood Flow Metab. 12*:554 (1992).
128. C. L. Grady, J. V. Haxby, B. Horwitz, M. B. Schapiro, S. I. Rapoport, L. G. Ungerleider, M. Mishkin, R. E. Carson, and P. Herscovitch, Dissociation of object and spatial vision in human extrastriate cortex: Age-related changes in activation of regional cerebral blood flow measured with ^{15}O water and positron emission tomography, *J. Cog. Neurosci. 4*:23 (1992).
129. C. L. Grady, J. Ma. Maisog, B. Horwitz, L. G. Ungerleider, M. J. Mentis, J. A. Salerno, P. Pietrini, E. Wagner, and J. V. Haxby, Age-related changes in cortical blood flow activation during visual processing of faces and location, *J. Neurosci. 14*:1450 (1994).
130. D. J. Madden, T. G. Turkington, R. E. Coleman, J. M. Provenzale, T. R. DeGrado, and J. M. Hoffman, Adult age differences in regional cerebral blood flow during visual word identification: Evidence from H$_2$^{15}O PET, *NeuroImage 3*:127 (1996).
131. C. L. Grady, A. R. McIntosh, B. Horwitz, J. Ma. Maisog, L. G. Ungerleider, M. J. Mentis, P. Pietrini, M. B. Schapiro, and J. V. Haxby, Age-related reductions in human recognition memory due to impaired encoding, *Science 269*: 218 (1995).
132. P. Herscovitch, A. Auchus, M. Gado, D. Chi, and M. Raichle, Correction of positron emission tomography data for cerebral atrophy, *J. Cereb. Blood Flow Metab. 6*:120 (1986).
133. H. W. Muller-Gartner, J. M. Links, J. L. Prince, R. N. Bryan, E. McVeigh, J. P. Leal, C. Davatzikos, and J. J. Frost, Measurement of radiotracer concentration in brain gray matter using positron emission tomography: MRI-based correction for partial volume effects, *J. Cereb. Blood Flow Metab. 12*:571 (1992).
134. T. O. Videen, J. S. Perlmutter, M. A. Mintun, and M. E. Raichle, Regional correction of positron emission tomography data for the effects of cerebral atrophy, *J. Cereb. Blood Flow Metab. 8*:662 (1988).
135. A. Alavi, A. B. Newberg, E. Souder, and J. A. Berlin, Quantitative analysis of PET and MRI data in normal aging and Alzheimer's disease: Atrophy weighted total brain metabolism and absolute whole brain metabolism as reliable discriminators, *J. Nucl. Med. 34*:1681 (1993).
136. J. B. Chawluk, A. Alavi, R. Dann, H. Hurtig, S. Bais, M. J. Kushner, R. A. Zimmerman, and M. Reivich, Positron emission tomography in aging and dementia: Effect of cerebral atrophy, *J. Nucl. Med. 28*:431 (1987).
137. F. Yoshii, W. W. Barker, J. Y. Chang, D. Loewenstein, A. Apicella, D. Smith, T. Boothe, M. D. Ginsberg, S. Pascal, and R. Duara, Sensitivity of cerebral glucose metabolism to age, gender, brain volume, brain atrophy, and cerebrovascular risk factors, *J. Cereb. Blood Flow Metab. 8*:654 (1988).
138. L. L. Light, The organization of memory in old age, *The Handbook of Aging and Cognition* (F. I. M. Craik and T. A. Salthouse, eds.), Erlbaum, Hillsdale, NJ, 1992, p. 111.
139. P. A. Allen, D. J. Madden, T. A. Weber, and K. E. Groth, Influence of age and processing stage on visual word recognition, *Psychol. Aging 8*:274 (1993).

140. D. J. Madden, Adult age differences in the effects of sentence context and stimulus degradation during visual word recognition, *Psychol. Aging 3*:167 (1988).

141. D. J. Madden, Four to ten milliseconds per year: Age-related slowing of visual word identification, *J. Gerontol. [Psychol. Sci.] 47*:P59 (1992).

142. E. A. L. Stine and A. Wingfield, Older adults can inhibit high-probability competitors in speech recognition, *Aging Cognit. 1*:152 (1994).

143. J. M. Duchek and D. A. Balota, Sparing activation processes in older adults, *Adult Information Processing: Limits on Loss* (J. Cerella, J. Rybash, W. Hoyer, and M. L. Commons, eds.), Academic Press, San Diego, 1993, p. 384.

144. A. Wingfield, L. W. Poon, L. Lombardi, and D. Lowe, Speed of processing in normal aging: Effects of speech rate, linguistic structure, and processing time, *J. Gerontol. 40*:579 (1985).

145. N. L. Bowles and L. W. Poon, Aging and retrieval of words in semantic memory, *J. Gerontol. 40*:71 (1985).

146. D. M. Burke, D. G. MacKay, J. S. Worthley, and E. Wade, On the tip of the tongue: What causes word finding failures in young and older adults? *J. Mem. Lang. 30*:542 (1991).

147. A. A. Hartley, Attention, *The Handbook of Aging and Cognition* (F. I. M. Craik and T. A. Salthouse, eds.), Erlbaum, Hillsdale, NJ, 1992, p. 3.

148. D. J. Madden and D. J. Plude, Selective preservation of selective attention, *Adult Information Processing: Limits on Loss* (J. Cerella, J. Rybash, W. Hoyer, and M. L. Commons, eds.), Academic Press, San Diego, 1993, p. 273.

149. P. Rabbitt, Age and discrimination between complex stimuli, *Behavior, Aging, and the Nervous System* (A. T. Welford and J. E. Birren, eds.), Charles C. Thomas, Springfield, IL, 1965, p. 35.

150. L. Hasher and R. T. Zacks, Working memory, comprehension, and aging: A review and a new review, *The Psychology of Learning and Motivation*, Vol. 22 (G. H. Bower, ed.), Academic Press, Orlando, FL, 1988.

151. D. J. Plude and W. J. Hoyer, Age and the selectivity of visual information processing, *Psychol. Aging 1*:4 (1986).

152. A. A. Hartley, Evidence for the selective preservation of spatial selective attention in old age, *Psychol. Aging 8*:371 (1993).

153. L. L. Light and D. La Voie, Direct and indirect measures of memory in old age, *Implicit Memory: New Directions in Cognition, Development, and Neuropsychology* (P. Graf and M. E. J. Masson, eds.), Erlbaum, Hillsdale, NJ, 1993, p. 207.

154. L. L. Light and A. Singh, Implicit and explicit memory in young and older adults, *J. Exp. Psychol. [Learn. Mem. Cognit.] 13*:531 (1987).

155. T. A. Salthouse, Working-memory mediation of adult age differences in integrative reasoning, *Mem. Cognit. 20*:413 (1992).

156. T. A. Salthouse, D. R. D. Mitchell, E. Skovronek, and R. L. Babcock, Effects of adult age and working memory on reasoning and spatial abilities, *J. Exp. Psychol. [Learn. Mem. Cognit.] 15*:507 (1989).

157. F. I. M. Craik and J. M. Jennings, Human memory, *The Handbook of Aging*

and Cognition (F. I. M. Craik and T. A. Salthouse, eds.), Erlbaum, Hillsdale, NJ, 1992 p. 51.

158. D. M. Burke and L. L. Light, Memory and aging: The role of retrieval processes, *Psychol. Bull. 90*:513 (1981).

159. M. Moscovitch and G. Winocur, The neuropsychology of memory and aging, *The Handbook of Aging and Cognition* (F. I. M. Craik and T. A. Salthouse, eds.), Erlbaum, Hillsdale, NJ, 1992, p. 315.

160. R. S. J. Frackowiak, G. L. Leniz, T. Jones, and J. D. Heather, Quantitative measurement of regional cerebral blood flow and oxygen metabolism in man using ^{15}O and positron emission tomography: Theory, procedure, and normal values, *J. Comput. Assist. Tomogr. 4*:727 (1980).

161. G. L. Lenzi, R. S. J. Frackowiak, T. Jones, J. D. Heather, A. A. Lammertsma, C. G. Rhodes, and C. Pozzilli, $CMRO_2$ and CBF by the oxygen-15 inhalation technique, *Eur. Neurol. 20*:285 (1981).

162. D. E. Kuhl, E. J. Metter, W. H. Riege, and R. A. Hawkins, The effect of normal aging on patterns of local cerebral glucose utilization, *Ann. Neurol. 15*:S133 (1984).

163. M. J. de Leon, S. H. Ferris, A. E. George, D. R. Christman, J. S. Fowler, C. Gentes, B. Reisberg, B. Gee, M. Emmerich, Y. Yonekura, J. Brodie, I. I. Kricheff, and A. P. Wolf, Positron emission tomography (PET) studies of aging and Alzheimer's disease, *Am. J. Neurorad. 4*:568 (1983).

164. R. Duara, R. A. Margolin, E. A. Robertson-Tchabo, E. D. London, M. Schwartz, J. W. Renfrew, B. J. Koziarz, M. Sundaram, C. Grady, A. M. Moore, D. H. Ingvar, L. Sokoloff, H. Weingartner, R. M. Kessler, R. G. Manning, M. A. Channing, N. R. Cutler, and S. I. Rapoport, Cerebral glucose utilization as measured with positron emission tomography in 21 resting healthy men between the ages of 21 and 83 years, *Brain 106*:761 (1983).

165. R. A. Hawkins, J. C. Mazziotta, M. E. Phelps, S. C. Huang, D. E. Kuhl, R. E. Carson, E. J. Metter, and W. H. Riege, Cerebral glucose metabolism as a function of age in man: Influence of the rate constants in the fluorodeoxyglucose method, *J. Cereb. Blood Flow Metab. 3*:250 (1983).

166. R. Duara, C. Grady, J. Haxby, D. Ingvar, L. Sokoloff, R. A. Margolin, R. G. Manning, N. R. Cutler, and S. I. Rapoport, Human brain glucose utilization and cognitive function in relation to age, *Ann. Neurol. 16*:702 (1984).

167. P. Pantano, J.-C. Baron, P. Lebrun-Grandie, N. Duquesnoy, M. G. Bousser, and D. Comar, Regional cerebral blood flow and oxygen consumption in human aging, *Stroke 15*:635 (1984).

168. W. H. Riege, E. J. Metter, W. E. Kuhl, and M. E. Phelps, Brain glucose metabolism and memory functions: Age decrease in factor scores, *J. Gerontol. 40*:459 (1985).

169. J. V. Haxby, C. L. Grady, R. Duara, E. A. Robertson-Tchabo, B. Koziarz, N. R. Cutler, and S. I. Rapoport, Relations among age, visual memory, and resting cerebral metabolism in 40 healthy men, *Brain Cognit. 5*:412 (1986).

170. T. Yamaguchi, I. Kanno, K. Uemura, F. Shishido, A. Inugami, T. Ogawa, M. Murakami, and K. Suzuki, Reduction in regional cerebral metabolic rate of oxygen during human aging, *Stroke 17*:1220 (1986).

171. M. Kushner, M. Tobin, A. Alavi, J. Chawluk, M. Rosen, F. Fazekas, J. Alavi, and M. Reivich, Cerebellar glucose consumption in normal and pathologic states using fluorine-FDG and PET, *J. Nucl. Med. 28*:1667 (1987).

172. N. L. Schlageter, B. Horwitz, H. Creasey, R. Carson, R. Duara, G. W. Berg, and S. I. Rapoport, Relation of measured brain glucose utilisation and cerebral atrophy in man, *J. Neurol. Neurosurg. Psychiatry 50*:779 (1987).

173. M. Itoh, J. Hatazawa, H. Miyazawa, H. Matsui, K. Meguro, K. Yanai, K. Kubota, S. Watanuki, T. Ido, and T. Matsuzawa, Stability of cerebral blood flow and oxygen metabolism during normal aging, *Gerontology 36*:43 (1990).

174. A. Burns and P. Tyrrell, Association of age with regional cerebral oxygen utilization: A positron emission tomography study, *Age Ageing 21*:316 (1992).

175. G. Marchal, P. Rioux, M. C. Petit-Taboue, G. Sette, J. M. Travere, C. Le Poec, P. Courtheoux, J. M. Derlon, and J. C. Baron, Regional cerebral oxygen consumption, blood flow, and blood volume in healthy human aging, *Arch. Neurol. 49*:1013 (1992).

176. H. Takada, K. Nagata, Y. Hirata, Y. Satoh, Y. Watahiki, J. Sugawara, E. Yokoyama, Y. Kondoh, F. Shishido, A. Inugami, H. Fujita, T. Ogawa, M. Murakami, H. Iida, and I. Kanno, Age-related decline of cerebral oxygen metabolism in normal population detected with positron emission tomography, *Neurol. Res. 14*:S128 (1992).

22

Neuroimaging of HIV Infection

Christopher E. Byrum
Duke University Medical Center, Durham, North Carolina

Jill E. Thompson
University of North Carolina Hospitals, Chapel Hill, North Carolina

615

I. INTRODUCTION

Acquired immunodeficiency syndrome (AIDS), caused by the retrovirus designated the human immunodeficiency virus (HIV), is a rapidly growing health problem in the United States and worldwide. It is estimated that more than 22 million people have been infected by the HIV virus. Since the recognition of AIDS in 1981, it has become a global epidemic afflicting more than 6 million people worldwide. In the United States, AIDS has become the leading cause of death in young men and the fourth leading cause of death in young women, with increasing frequency of heterosexual transmission [1].

The HIV virus is neurotropic and can involve both the peripheral and central nervous system. A number of infectious and noninfectious complications of immunodeficiency that herald the onset of AIDS in HIV-infected patients can involve the central nervous system (CNS). Based on autopsy findings, 75% of AIDS patients have CNS involvement, with 30% having multiple CNS lesions [2]. The HIV virus itself is responsible for the majority of CNS infections in AIDS patients, followed by *Toxoplasma gondii* and *Cryptococcus neoformans* [3].

HIV-infected patients can manifest a variety of psychiatric syndromes, ranging from adjustment disorders, to affective and anxiety disorders, to delirium and psychosis [4,5]. In as many as 20% of HIV-infected individuals, neurological or neuropsychiatric symptoms may be the presenting features [6,7]. Most initially present for brain imaging with altered mental status, which occurs in 50–75% of HIV patients [5]. Typically, these mental status changes are characterized by confusion or other signs of delirium. Delirium, or acute confusional state, is relatively common throughout the course of HIV disease, with up to 43% of hospitalized HIV-infected patients sustaining a delirium at some point during hospitalization [5].

In addition, an important new disease entity has been recognized manifesting as progressive cognitive impairment, representing the clinical manifestations of subacute HIV encephalitis. This has been termed AIDS dementia complex (ADC), or HIV dementia, and comprises motor, cognitive, and behavioral abnormalities. This complex, increasingly recognized as a sequela of HIV infection, is characterized by the insidious onset of psychomotor retardation, especially slowing of thought processes (bradyphrenia), speech, and movement. Other salient features include memory loss, impaired concentration, apathy, lethargy, and social withdrawal. Incoordination, tremor, and gait disturbances are also seen [8–13].

Recently Grant and Atkinson [4] proposed a revised terminology, suggesting that the term *dementia* implied exclusion of milder cognitive disorders associated with HIV infection. They recommended that the neurocognitive complications be classed as two syndromes differing in level of severity: HIV-associated dementia (HAD) and HIV-associated mild neurocognitive disorder (HIV-MND) [4].

The prevalence of mild neurocognitive disorder increases with disease progression. For example, approximately 50% of patients diagnosed with AIDS have neuropsychological deficit [4]. The rate of MND among asymptomatic or early symptomatic HIV patients has not been clearly determined. Grant and Atkinson concluded that subtle cognitive changes occur in 20–30% of patients in the early and middle phases of disease [4].

HIV-associated dementia occurs more commonly in advanced AIDS. Estimates of incidence vary from 7 to 38% of AIDS patients, with up to 66% of advanced cases of AIDS exhibiting dementia [8–13]. It is not clear whether mild neurocognitive disorder progresses inevitably to dementia. Some studies indicate that among patients followed for 2 years after AIDS onset, the annual incidence of dementia is 7–14% [4]. There have been reports of dementia as the presenting feature of AIDS, although this is uncommon [14,15].

Neurological complications of HIV infection can be classified as *primary* or *secondary*. Primary complications comprise HIV encephalopathy or leukoencephalopathy and are believed to be a direct result of the HIV virus in the CNS. Other primary complications include myelopathy and peripheral neuropathy. Secondary complications are those arising as a consequence of the immunodeficiency state. These include opportunistic infections and neoplasms, which can present as focal, multifocal, or diffuse lesions in the CNS. Infections and neoplasms can also indirectly compromise CNS functioning due to systemic dysfunction, such as respiratory or cardiovascular compromise.

Neuroimaging has become essential to neurologists and psychiatrists in the initial diagnosis and evaluation of disease progression. The most important use of neuroimaging in these patients is to determine whether a CNS lesion is present and its diagnostic and therapeutic significance. Most mass lesions are well visualized by both magnetic resonance imaging (MRI) and computed tomography (CT). However, for other types of lesions, specifically those that are diffuse in nature as in encephalopathy or encephalitis, the superior tissue contrast and resolution provided by MRI is desirable.

II. PRIMARY NEUROLOGICAL COMPLICATIONS OF HIV INFECTION

The primary complications of HIV infection appear as an encephalopathy, which is due to direct toxic effects of the virus on brain tissue. HIV encephalopathy is a progressive subcortical dementia that is a form of subacute encephalitis [3]. The eventual development of encephalopathy occurs in approximately 60% of patients with AIDS and can be demonstrated in the brain within 2 weeks of infection [7,16,17].

The pathological changes of HIV encephalopathy are better seen on MRI than on CT [8,9,18,19]. The most common MR findings in HIV-infected patients who present for imaging include mild to severe cortical atrophy, marked by sulcal and ventricular enlargement, and periventricular white matter abnormalities without edema [8,9,18–23] (Fig. 1). The white matter lesions are usually bilateral but asymmetrical, with the frontal lobes most frequently involved. Meningeal fibrosis can occasionally be seen. Gray matter is typically spared. In nondemented HIV-positive patients, T2-weighted MR images may show only a few scattered, nonspecific white matter foci of hyperintensity. This finding may or may not be accompanied by cortical atrophy.

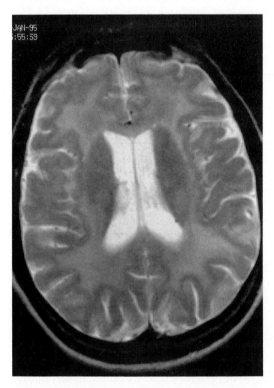

Fig. 1 T$_2$-weighted axial image demonstrates high signal intensity (HSI) throughout the periventricular white matter in HIV-positive male with encephalopathy. Note associated mild central and cortical atrophy.

Notably, while severe atrophy has been demonstrated in demented patients, atrophy has also been demonstrated in nondemented but symptomatic HIV patients [20,23–28]. The presence of brain atrophy in asymptomatic HIV patients is more controversial [22,25–27,29,30]. However, a number of studies have demonstrated a relationship between neuropsychological impairment and atrophy in HIV-seropositive patients [24,31–36].

White matter abnormalities, without mass effect or contrast enhancement, have been noted in the periventricular and subcortical regions, internal capsule, corpus callosum, and fornix [9,23,26,37,38]. The white matter lesions are typically bilateral but asymmetrical, with the frontal lobes most frequently involved.

The prevalence of focal white matter lesions has been found to be no higher in the asymptomatic HIV patients than in appropriate seronegative controls [26,29,39]. The incidence of high-signal intensity lesions reportedly is slightly higher in symptomatic, nondemented AIDS patients [39]. However, the development of the AIDS dementia complex has been reported to have a significant association with the occurrence of MRI white matter lesions [25,26]. Diffuse, widespread involvement of a large area of white matter appears to correlate well with dementia [20,23,26,38,40]. Thus the presence of white matter abnormalities is not specific for dementia, but they are more prevalent and show greater severity in patients with HIV dementia. Longitudinal studies by Post and colleagues indicate that severity of white matter abnormalities correlates with clinically detectable neurological disease and that progression of abnormalities correlates with neurological deterioration [35].

The development of dementia in HIV encephalopathy appears to correlate most closely with basal ganglia atrophy. Aylward et al. [22] reported that smaller basal ganglia volumes, after corrections for intracranial volume, distinguished demented HIV patients from nondemented HIV patients and uninfected controls. The authors concluded that HIV infection causes generalized brain atrophy, but that the clinical features of HIV dementia develop with selective basal ganglia atrophy, consistent with the characterization of HIV dementia as subcortical. Dal-Pan et al. [21] used standardized planimetry on MR images to measure the ventricular-brain ratio (VBR) and the bifrontal (BFR) and bicaudate (BCR) ratios, three measures of cerebral atrophy. They found significant correlations between HIV dementia and both the VBR (a general measure of overall cerebral atrophy) and the BCR (a measure of atrophy in the region of the caudate nucleus). The association was stronger for BCR enlargement than for VBR enlargement, suggesting that selective caudate region atrophy is associated with HIV dementia. Hestad et al. [32] similarly found that the BCR was most closely associated with poor performance on specific neuropsychological tests.

A. Neuropathology of HIV Encephalitis and Encephalopathy

On pathological examination of the HIV-infected brain, the most characteristic finding is that of microglial nodules in the cortex, white matter, and basal ganglia [42]. The microglial nodules are composed of HIV-infected multinucleated glial cells [8,10,16,18,43]. The multinucleated glial cells are also found scattered individually throughout the white matter early in the disease progression. Additionally, atrophy, loss of neurons, and gliosis are present, accompanied by periventricular and central white matter pallor [9].

Budka in 1991 proposed that HIV-specific CNS pathology shows two patterns: HIV encephalitis, which is multifocal and inflammatory, and HIV leukoencephalopathy, which is diffuse, noninflammatory, and degenerative in nature. Microglial nodules are found in both patterns [43]. HIV encephalitis involves primarily cerebral white matter, basal ganglia, and brainstem. HIV leukoencephalopathy is characterized by diffuse and progressive damage to cerebral white matter. Pathological findings in leukoencephalopathy include myelin pallor and reactive astrogliosis in the absence of inflammation, multinucleated giant cells, or brain atrophy [43,44]. It is clear that these findings overlap and two distinct and unique patterns are not definable. For the purposes of description and definition in our chapter, we will refer to the following: HIV encephalitis is characterized as the aforementioned pathological entity, namely, that of microglial nodules in the cortex, white matter, and basal ganglia. On structural imaging examinations this presents as atrophy with diffuse and asymmetrical white matter abnormalities that neither cause mass effect nor enhance with contrast. HIV encephalopathy is the clinical and functional entity that results from direct HIV infection of the CNS. The associated structural imaging findings overlap those seen in HIV encephalitis, which likely antedates the emergence of encephalopathy. Encephalopathy may be associated with a greater degree of atrophy, marking the sequelae of the encephalitis. We use the term "HIV leukoencephalopathy" to refer to clinical findings specifically associated with white matter abnormalities. Once again, the structural imaging findings may be similar to that seen in HIV encephalitis and HIV encephalopathy.

B. Functional Imaging

Based on clinical-radiological-pathological studies, it is believed that HIV encephalitis usually antedates the convincing radiological diagnosis of infection [40,45]. For this reason positron emission tomography (PET) and single photon emission computed tomography (SPECT) have been performed in an attempt to detect metabolic and perfusion abnormalities in the early stages of HIV infection. HIV encephalopathy is characterized by hypometabolic areas in the white matter and subcortical gray matter on PET [5,46–49] and

SPECT [50–54]. The frontal lobes were most significantly affected in many cases. The functional imaging pattern is similar to that seen in progressive supranuclear palsy [55]. Several studies have reported alterations in relative regional metabolism in the basal ganglia [5,48,53,56]. Regional or diffuse hypometabolism may precede the appearance of abnormalities on MR scans or the obvious cognitive impairment [5,47,49]. These results suggest that PET may be more sensitive than traditional neuropsychological evaluation to subtle central nervous system changes in association with AIDS.

Magnetic resonance spectroscopy (MRS) allows investigators to measure the biochemical and physiological state of tissue, demonstrating subtle changes before the process has progressed to cause significant structural damage. Proton spectroscopy has recently revealed reductions in cerebral N-acetyl aspartate (NAA), often without abnormal MR findings [57–64]. NAA is a neuronal marker, with decreased levels indicating neuronal damage in early stages of HIV infection. In a recent study, Jarvik et al. [1993] found 87% of HIV-positive patients had significantly abnormal spectroscopy features as compared with normal subjects [37]. Reductions of NAA ratios were greater in patients with dementia [57,59–61,64]. [^{31}P] phosphorus spectroscopy shows reduced ATP and phosphocreatine in HIV encephalopathy, indicating significant impairment in brain cellular oxidative metabolism [65,66]. MR spectroscopic imaging may demonstrate the detectable metabolic changes of HIV encephalopathy and may be more sensitive than conventional MR imaging in the demonstration of CNS involvement.

III. SECONDARY NEUROLOGICAL COMPLICATIONS OF HIV INFECTION

Secondary neurological complications of HIV, including infection and neoplasia, generally present as delirium, ranging from clouding of consciousness, confusion, and disorientation to visual or auditory hallucinations or paranoid delusions. However, other psychiatric syndromes can result, including depression, mania, anxiety, and schizophreniform psychoses [4,5]. These opportunistic infections or neoplasms probably precipitate altered mental status by mass effect or edema. As such, they are little different from other primary or secondary space-occupying lesions in the CNS. Psychiatric symptoms associated with space-occupying lesions of any etiology are referable to direct or indirect disruption of neural pathways by compression or edema. Specific neurological or psychiatric symptoms or syndromes reflect the brain structures and systems involved. However, the phenomenon of diaschisis may produce cerebral dysfunction that does not appear to correspond to extent of the lesion. Diaschisis refers to dysfunction of brain structures or

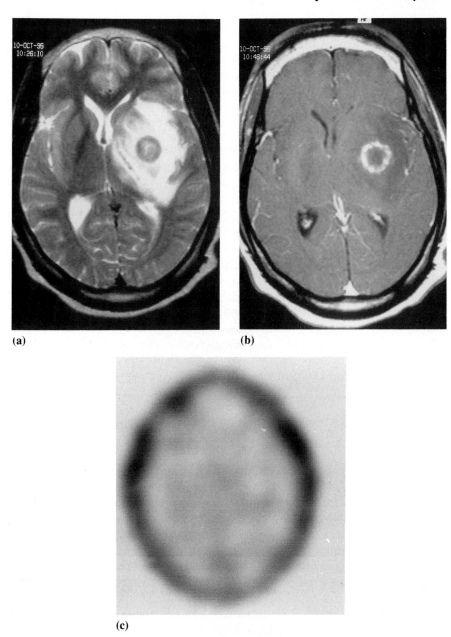

(a)   (b)

(c)

Fig. 2 Toxoplasmosis. (a) T$_2$-weighted axial image demonstrates a hypointense ring with a moderate amount of surrounding edema located in the left
basal ganglia. (b) Corresponding T$_1$-weighted image demonstrates a solitary,

systems remote from the site of the lesion and reflects the disruption of excitatory or inhibitory afferent inputs to the remote systems [67].

A. *Toxoplasma gondii* Infection

Toxoplasmosis is caused by an obligate intracellular protozoan. In the immunocompetent adult, acquired infection typically has a benign and self-limiting course. The incidence of seropositivity in the United States is approximately 20–70% [42]. *Toxoplasma gondii* infection is the most common opportunistic CNS infection in the AIDS population. The infection may cause fulminant and necrotizing encephalitis in the immunocompromised individual. In neonates with congenitally acquired infection, severe brain destruction is apparent.

Pathologically, toxoplasmosis lesions are characterized by three distinct zones: a central zone with coagulative necrosis and few organisms; an intermediate zone with engorged blood vessels, numerous inflammatory cells and tachyzoites, and few areas of necrosis; and a peripheral zone with many encysted organisms (bradyzoites), few vessels, and infrequent necrosis [3,42]. The lesions are usually surrounded by edema. There are no capsules surrounding the toxoplasma lesions. The most common sites of involvement are the basal ganglia and cerebral hemispheres near the corticomedullary junctions.

Contrast-enhanced computed tomography (CECT) reveals solitary or multiple ring-enhancing lesions in the basal ganglia or at gray-white junctions with significant surrounding edema and mass effect. In the immunocompromised patient, the possibility of lymphoma should be included in the differential diagnosis with the aforementioned imaging findings. MR is more sensitive for the detection of new or additional lesions. On T_2-weighted images (T2WI), the lesions have variable intensity but are surrounded by hyperintense edema (Fig. 2a). T_1-weighted images (T1W1) after contrast demonstrate focal nodular or rim enhancement patterns similar to that seen with CECT (Fig. 2b). Treated lesions usually become at least partially calcified, which is easily detected with non-enhanced computed tomography (NECT) scans. On MR these lesions appear hypointense on both long and short TR sequences. A small percentage of toxoplasma lesions will hemorrhage, which MR is more sensitive in detecting than CT.

Due to the overlapping of structural imaging findings between toxoplasmosis and lymphoma, PET and SPECT imaging have recently been advo-

---

nodular enhancing lesion. **(c)** Thallium SPECT axial image at the same level reveals **no** evidence of increased perfusion, suggesting infectious rather than neoplastic entity. This lesion responded to toxoplasmosis therapy.

cated. CNS lymphoma has been shown to accumulate [^{18}F]-fluoro-2-deoxy-glucose (FDG) on PET studies [68] with similar findings seen on SPECT studies. *Toxoplasma gondii* lesions do not demonstrate increased perfusion or hypermetabolism (Fig. 2c).

B. *Cryptococcus neoformans* Infection

Cryptococcosis is caused by a ubiquitous fungus that enters via the respiratory tract and then involves the CNS by hematogenous spread. It is the third most common opportunistic CNS infection in the AIDS population, with approximately 5% of patients eventually developing cryptococcal infection [3]. Disseminated infection is more common in AIDS patients versus meningitis, which is usually seen in immunocompetent patients.

Early in the disease, nonspecific or no imaging abnormalities will be present. Dilated perivascular spaces, focal cryptococcomas, atrophy, and communicating hydrocephalus may be present. Characteristic lesions consist of inflammatory cells, organisms, gelatinous masses, and dilated perivascular spaces [3,17]. The meninges and brainstem are also frequently involved.

CT findings, as mentioned earlier, are commonly nonspecific, and for this reason MR is preferred for imaging patients with suspected cryptococcal infection. T2WI reveal multifocal hyperintensities in the basal ganglia and brainstem (Fig. 3) [69]. These findings represent gelatinous pseudocysts and dilated perivascular spaces [3]. On postcontrast images there is variable enhancement, although cerebral cortical microabscesses have been reported [42]. MR allows us to differentiate cryptococcal lesions from toxoplasma lesions by the less widely distributed foci and less edema in the latter.

C. Progressive Multifocal Leukoencephalopathy

Progressive multifocal leukoencephalopathy (PML), caused by the papovavirus, is a progressive demyelinating disease of the CNS seen almost exclusively in the immunocompromised host. Approximately 1–4% of the AIDS population will develop PML [3]. The virus attacks the oligodendrocytes and primarily involves the subcortical white matter, the cerebellum, and brainstem. The most commonly affected areas are the occipital and parietal lobes. The most important pathological finding is that of intranuclear inclusions found within edematous oligodendroglial nuclei [17].

Patients frequently present with a progressive dementia, cerebellar or brainstem signs, and hemiparesis. The neuropsychiatric symptoms are simi-

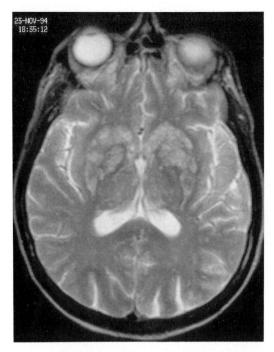

Fig. 3 Cryptococcus: T_2-weighted image at level of basal ganglia demonstrates clusters of HSI lesions most prominently located around perivascular spaces.

lar to those of other demyelinating diseases, such as multiple sclerosis. Occasionally, patients will present with seizures and/or spinal cord symptoms. Due to the progressive nature of the disease, rapid deterioration leading to death in a few months is the usual clinical course.

Imaging findings include subcortical white matter involvement, manifest by low attenuation on CT (Fig. 4a) and high signal on T_2-weighted MR images (Fig. 4b, c) located bilaterally and asymmetrically in the parieto-occipital lobes [17]. On postcontrast images no enhancement is present (Fig. 4d). Eventually the involvement progresses and all or most cerebral white matter becomes involved with occasional involvement of the gray matter of the thalamus and basal ganglia.

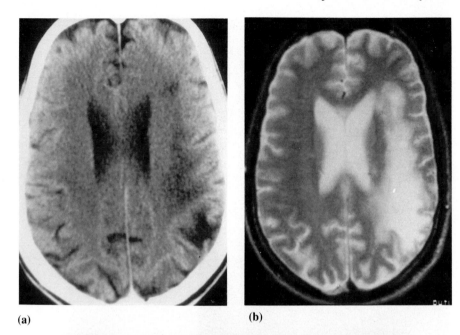

(a)   (b)

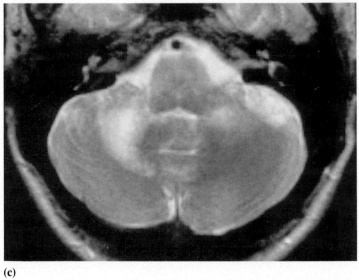

(c)

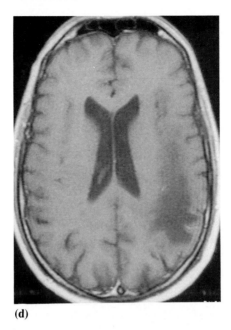

(d)

Fig. 4 Progressive multifocal leukoencephalopathy. **(a)** Nonenhanced computed tomography image demonstrates low attenuation in the periventricular and subcortical white matter of the left parietal-occipital lobe. Note lack of symmetry and mass effect. **(b)** T2WI at same level reveals HSI corresponding to lesion seen on CT. **(c)** T2WI demonstrates an additional lesion located in the dentate nuclei of the cerebellum. **(d)** T1WI postenhancement image from the same patient reveals asymmetrical white matter lesion with no evidence of contrast enhancement.

IV. OTHER LESS COMMON CNS INFECTIONS IN HIV PATIENTS

Mycobacterium infection usually results in meningitis in the AIDS population, however abscesses, tuberculomas, and encephalitis can also occur [17]. Tuberculous abscesses present as large, focal masses with edema and ring enhancement, commonly located at the gray-white junction (Fig. 5). Additionally, MR may demonstrate a hypointense T2WI ring with marked postcontrast enhancement. Basilar meningitis with thick enhancement of the me-

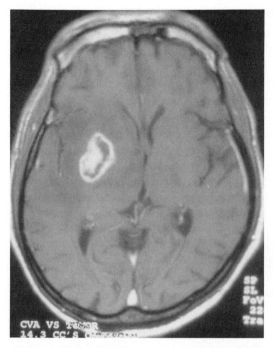

Fig. 5 Tuberculous abscess: T1WI postenhancement image demonstrates a nodular and irregular ring-enhancing lesion located in the region of the external capsule. Note associated edema and mass effect with compression of the right frontal and occipital horns and third ventricle.

ninges, which may be associated with hydrocephalus, is seen in tuberculous meningitis. Biopsy and CSF studies are needed for definitive diagnoses.

Neurosyphilis, caused by *Treponema pallidum*, occurs in up to 1.5% of HIV-infected individuals [17]. Infection can result in meningoencephalitis or vasculitis with resultant ischemia and infarction. Focal and well-circumscribed lesions (gummas) may present as masses that are adherent to the dura overlying the cerebral convexities.

Cytomegalovirus (CMV) is an opportunistic virus frequently seen in association with HIV. Infection may represent reactivation of previously silent infection [3]. It involves both the peripheral and central nervous system and is well known for causing retinitis. Other organ systems may also be infected. CMV may result in subacute encephalitis with radiographic studies that are nonspecific. The most common finding is that of atrophy. Low-attenuation white matter lesions and subependymal enhancement may be seen on CT [17]. MR also demonstrates diffuse and regular subependymal enhancement.

Other infections of the CNS seen in the AIDS population include *Candida albicans*, *Nocardia asteroides*, *Aspergillus fumigatus* (Fig. 6a&b), *Histoplasma capsulatum*, *Coccidioides immitis*, cysticercosis, and herpes simplex virus (HSV) (Fig. 7a&b).

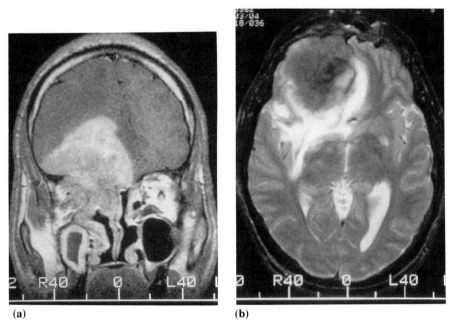

(a)   (b)

Fig. 6 Aspergillus. (a) T1WI coronal postenhancement image reveals a large, heterogeneously enhancing lesion arising from the right paranasal sinuses and invading the right frontal lobe. Associated edema and mass effect are present. (b) Corresponding T2WI demonstrates low signal intensity (LSI) lesion with HSI surrounding edema involving the right frontal lobe. Subfalcial herniation, ipsilateral ventricular compression, and contralateral hydrocephalus are present.

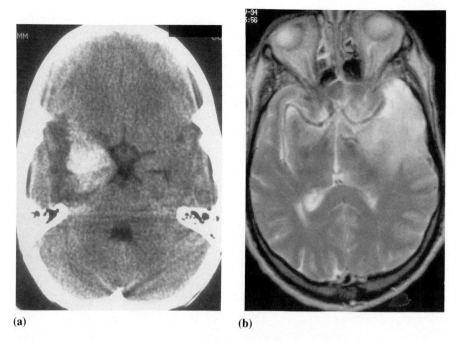

(a)   (b)

Fig. 7   Herpes simplex virus. **(a)** NECT image shows a hemorrhagic lesion in the right medial temporal lobe. **(b)** T2WI in a different patient reveals HSI in the left temporal lobe with mild mass effect and edema. These were both proven to represent HSV.

Fig. 8   Cerebral lymphoma. **(a)** T1WI postenhancement coronal image demonstrates homogeneously enhancing lesions involving and crossing the corpus callosum (CC) and causing mass effect. **(b)** T2WI in the same patient once again demonstrates crossing of the CC with surrounding edema. **(c)** Contrast enhanced CT in a different patient demonstrates a ring-enhancing lesion in the right frontal lobe with surrounding low attenuation edema. **(d)** Corresponding thallium SPECT image at the same level reveals increased uptake (perfusion) in the lesion. These were both biopsy-proven lymphomas.

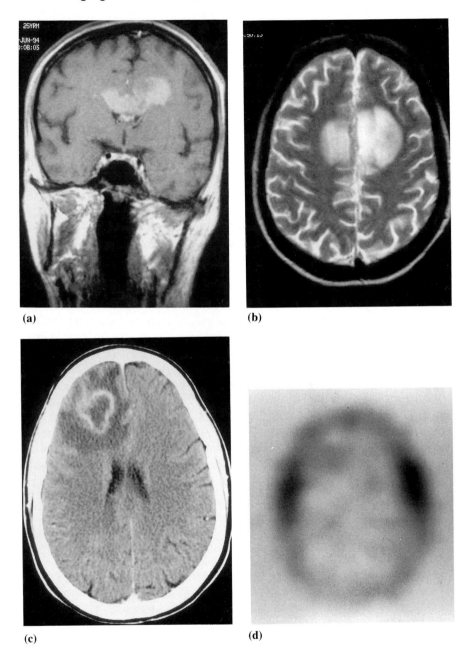

(a)

(b)

(c)

(d)

V. CEREBRAL LYMPHOMA

Primary CNS lymphoma ultimately develops in approximately 2.0% of AIDS patients, a figure that is rapidly increasing [70]. The tumors are of B-cell origin and result in both large-cell immunoblastic and small noncleaved lymphomas. Most patients present with impaired cognitive function and focal neurological deficits [17]. Cerebral lymphoma typically presents as solitary or multiple discrete focal masses in the brain parenchyma. They are more frequently necrotic in the AIDS population. The tumors are often responsive to radiation therapy, although death usually ensues within a year. Imaging findings demonstrate focal lesions with ring, solid, or inhomogeneous enhancement (Fig. 8a). Associated edema and and mass effect are frequently present (Fig. 8b). The most common sites of involvement include the corpus callosum, subependymal-periventricular region, basal ganglia, and vermis. As previously mentioned, lymphoma can be radiologically indistinguishable from toxoplasma infection and functional imaging may be helpful (Fig. 8c, d).

VI. CONCLUSION

By the year 2000, it is projected that 40 million men, women, and children will be infected with the HIV virus [1]. Brain-imaging techniques will be invaluable to the psychiatrist, neurologist, and internist in the diagnostic evaluation and follow-up of HIV infection of the CNS. Structural brain imaging will remain the mainstay of diagnostic and therapeutic imaging in most infectious and neoplastic complications of HIV disease. However, it is apparent that functional imaging, including PET, SPECT, functional MR, and magnetoencephalography will emerge as primary imaging modalities in the evaluation of HIV dementia. Functional imaging will also expand our knowledge of brain systems or structures involved in the specific neuropsychiatric symptoms.

REFERENCES

1. T. C. Quinn, The epidemiology of the acquired immunodeficiency syndrome in the 1990s, *Emerg. Med. Clin. North Am. 13*:1 (1995).
2. F. Gray, R. Gherardi, and F. Scaravilli, The neuropathology of the acquired immune deficiency syndrome (AIDS), *Brain 111*:245 (1988).
3. A. G. Osborne, Infections of the brain and its linings, *Diagnostic Neuroradiology* (A. G. Osborne, ed.), Mosby, St. Louis, 1994, p. 673.
4. I. Grant and J. H. Atkinson, Psychiatric aspects of acquired immune deficiency syndrome, *Comprehensive Textbook of Psychiatry/VI* (H. I. Kaplan and B. J. Sadock, eds.), Williams and Wilkins, Baltimore, 1995, pp. 1644–1669.

5. C. H. Hinkin, W. G. van Gorp, and P. Satz, Neuropsychological and neuropsychiatric aspects of HIV infection in adults, *Comprehensive Textbook of Psychiatry/VI* (H. I. Kaplan and B. J. Sadock, eds.), Williams and Wilkins, Baltimore, 1995, pp. 1669–1680.
6. J. R. Berger, B. Kaszowitz, G. Dickinson, et al., Progressive multifocal leukoencephalopathy associated with human immunodeficiency virus infection: A review of the literature and report of 16 cases, *Ann. Intern. Med.* *107*:78 (1987).
7. C. H. Flowers, M. F. Mafee, R. Crowell R, et al., Encephalopathy in AIDS patients: Evaluation with MR imaging, *AJNR 11:*1235 (1990).
8. B. A. Navia, B. D. Jordan, and R. W. Price, The AIDS dementia complex: I. Clinical features, *Ann. Neurol.* *19*:517 (1986).
9. B. A. Navia, E.-S. Cho, C. K. Petito, et al., The AIDS dementia complex: II. Neuropathology, *Ann. Neurol.* *19*:525 (1986).
10. C. K. Petito, E. -S. Cho, W. Lemann, et al., Neuropathology of acquired immunodeficiency syndrome (AIDS): An autopsy review, *J. Neuropathol. Exp. Neurol.* *45*:635 (1986).
11. R. S. Janssen, O. C. Nwanyanwu, R. M. Selik, et al., Epidemiology of human immunodeficiency virus encephalopathy in the United States, *Neurology 42*: 1472 (1992).
12. J. C. McArthur, D. R. Hoover, H. Bacellar, et al., Dementia in AIDS patients: Incidence and risk factors. Multicenter AIDS Cohort Study, *Neuroloy 43*:2245 (1993).
13. F. Gray, L. Belec, C. Keohane, et al., Zidovudine therapy and HIV encephalitis: A 10-year neuropathological survey, *AIDS 8*:489 (1994).
14. B. A. Navia and R. W. Price, The acquired immunodeficiency syndrome dementia complex as the presenting or sole manifestation of human immunodeficiency virus infection, *Arch. Neurol. 44*:65 (1987).
15. R. M. Levy, R. S. Janssen, T. J. Bush, et al. Neuroepidemiology of acquired immune deficiency syndrome, *AIDS and the Nervous System* (M. L. Rosenblum, R. M. Levy, and D. E. Bredesen, eds.), Raven Press, New York, 1988, p. 13.
16. R. W. Price, B. Brew, J. Sidtis, et al., The brain in AIDS: Central nervous system HIV-1 infection and AIDS dementia complex, *Science 239*:586 (1988).
17. J. R. Berger, M. J. Post, and R. M. Levy, The acquired immunodeficiency syndrome, *Neuroimaging* (J. O. Greenberg, ed.), McGraw-Hill, New York, 1995, p. 413.
18. M. J. Post, L. G. Tate, B. M. Quencer, et al., CT, MR, and pathology in HIV encephalitis and meningitis, *AJR 151*:373 (1988).
19. H. S. Chrysikopoulos, G. A. Press, M. R. Grafe, et al., Encephalitis caused by human immunodeficiency virus: CT and MR imaging manifestations with clinical and pathologic correlation, *Radiology 175*:185 (1990).
20. A. Sönnerborg, J. Sääf, B. Alexius, et al., Quantitative detection of brain aberrations in human immunodeficiency virus type 1-infected individuals by magnetic resonance imaging, *J. Infect. Disc. 162*:1245 (1990).
21. G. J. Dal-Pan, J. H. McArthur, E. Aylward, et al., Patterns of cerebral atrophy

in HIV-1-infected individuals: Results of a quantitative MRI analysis, *Neurology 42*:2125 (1992).

22. E. H. Aylward, J. D. Henderer, J. C. McArthur, et al., Reduced basal ganglia volume in HIV-1-associated dementia: Results from quantitative neuroimaging, *Neurology 43*:2099 (1993).

23. D. F. Broderick, F. J. Wippold, D. B. Clifford, et al., White matter lesions and cerebral atrophy on MR images in patients with and without AIDS dementia complex, *AJR 161*:177 (1993).

24. I. Grant, J. H. Atkinson, J. R. Hesselink, et al., Evidence for early central nervous system involvement in the acquired immunodeficiency syndrome (AIDS) and other human immunodeficiency virus (HIV) infections. Studies with neuropsychologic testing and magnetic resonance imaging, *Ann. Intern. Med. 107*:828 (1987).

25. C. Pedersen, C. Thomsen, S. P. Arlien, et al., Central nervous system involvement in human immunodeficiency virus disease. A prospective study including neurological examination, computerized tomography, and magnetic resonance imaging, *Dan. Med. Bull. 38*:379 (1991).

26. R. Raininko, I. Elovaara, A. Virta, et al., Radiological study of the brain at various stages of human immunodeficiency virus infection: Early development of brain atrophy, *Neuroradiology 34*:190 (1992).

27. T. L. Jernigan, S. Archibald, J. R. Hesselink, et al., Magnetic resonance imaging morphometric analysis of cerebral volume loss in human immunodeficiency virus infection. The HNRC Group, *Arch. Neurol. 50*:250 (1993).

28. S. Oster, P. Christoffersen, H. J. Gundersen, et al., Cerebral atrophy in AIDS: A stereological study, *Acta Neuropathol. Berl. 85*:617 (1993).

29. H. Manji, S. Connolly, R. McAllister, et al., Serial MRI of the brain in asymptomatic patients infected with HIV: Results from the UCMSM/Medical Research Council neurology cohort, *J. Neurol. Neurosurg. Psychiatry 57*:144 (1994).

30. M. N. Paley, W. K. Chong, I. D. Wilkinson, et al., Cerebrospinal fluid-intracranial volume ratio measurements in patients with HIV infection: CLASS image analysis technique, *Radiology 190*:879 (1994).

31. I. Elovaara, E. Poutiainen, R. Raininko, et al., Mild brain atrophy in early HIV infection: the lack of association with cognitive deficits and HIV-specific intrathecal immune response, *J. Neurol. Sci. 99*:121 (1990).

32. K. Hestad, J. H. McArthur, G. J. Dal Pan, et al., Regional brain atrophy in HIV-1 infection: association with specific neuropsychological test performance, *Acta Neurol. Scand. 88*:112 (1993).

33. J. Jakobsen, C. Gyldensted, B. Brun, et al., Cerebral ventricular enlargement relates to neuropsychological measures in unselected AIDS patients, *Acta Neurol. Scand. 79*:59 (1989).

34. H. S. Levin, D. H. Williams, M. J. Borucki, et al., Magnetic resonance imaging and neuropsychological findings in human immunodeficiency virus infection, *JAIDS 3*:757 (1990).

35. M. J. Post, J. R. Berger, R. Duncan, et al., Asymptomatic and neurologically

symptomatic HIV-seropositive subjects: Results of long-term MR imaging and clinical follow-up, *Radiology 188*:727 (1993).

36. E. Poutiainen, I. Elovaara, R. Raininko, et al., Cognitive performance in HIV-1 infection: Relationship to severity of disease and brain atrophy, *Acta Neurol. Scand. 87*:88 (1993).

37. J. G. Jarvik, J. R. Hesselink, C. Kennedy, et al., Acquired immunodeficiency syndrome. Magnetic resonance patterns of brain involvement with pathologic correlation, *Arch. Neurol. 45*:731 (1988).

38. K. D. Kieburtz, L. Ketonen, A. E. Zettelmaier, et al., Magnetic resonance imaging findings in HIV cognitive impairment, *Arch. Neurol. 47*:643 (1990).

39. R. A. Bornstein, D. Chakeres, M. Brogan, et al., Magnetic resonance imaging of white matter lesions in HIV infection, *J. Neuropsych. Clin. Neurosci. 4*:174 (1992).

40. W. L. Olsen, F. M. Longo, C. M. Mills, et al., White matter disease in AIDS: Findings at MR imaging, *Radiology 169*:445 (1988).

41. C. P. Hawkins, J. E. McLaughlin, B. E. Kendall, et al., Pathological findings correlated with MRI in HIV infection, *Neuroradiology 35*:264 (1993).

42. B. C. Bowen and M. J. Post, Intracranial infection, *Magnetic Resonance Imaging of the Brain and Spine* (S. W. Atlas, ed.), Raven Press, New York, 1991, p. 501.

43. H. Budka, Neuropathology of human immunodeficiency virus infection, *Brain Pathol. 1*:163 (1991).

44. J. C. McArthur, B. A. Cohen, O. A. Selnes, et al., Low prevalence of neurological and neuropsychological abnormalities in otherwise healthy HIV-1-infected individuals: results from the multicenter AIDS Cohort Study, *Ann. Neurol. 26*:601 (1989).

45. M. J. D. Post, Neuroimaging in various stages of human immunodeficiency virus infections, *Curr. Opin. Radiol. 2*:73 (1990).

46. D. A. Rottenberg, J. R. Moeller, S. C. Strother, et al., The metabolic pathology of the AIDS dementia complex, *Ann. Neurol. 22*:700 (1987).

47. S. Pascal, L. Resnick, W. W. Barker, et al., Metabolic asymmetries in asymptomatic HIV-1 seropositive subjects: Relationship to disease onset and MRI findings. *J. Nucl. Med. 32*:1725 (1991).

48. W. G. van Gorp, M. A. Mandelkern, M. Gee, et al., Cerebral metabolic dysfunction in AIDS: findings in a sample with and without dementia, *J. Neuropsych. Clin. Neurosci. 4*:280 (1992).

49. G. J. Harris, G. D. Pearlson, J. C. McArthur, et al., Altered cortical blood flow in HIV-seropositive individuals with and without dementia: A single photon emission computed tomography study, *AIDS 8*:495 (1994).

50. Y. R. Tran Dinh, H. Mamo, J. Cervoni, et al., Disturbances in the cerebral perfusion of human immune deficiency virus-1 seropositive asymptomatic subjects: A quantitative tomography study of 18 cases, *J. Nucl. Med. 31*:1601 (1990).

51. A. Ajmani, E. Habte-Gabr, M. Zarr, et al., Cerebral blood flow SPECT with Tc-

99m exametazine correlates in AIDS dementia complex stages. A preliminary report, *Clin. Nucl. Med. 16*:656 (1991).

52. J. C. Masdeu, A. Yudd, H. R. L. Van, et al., Single-photon emission computed tomography in human immunodeficiency virus encephalopathy: A preliminary report, *J. Nucl. Med. 32*:1471 (1991).

53. B. L. Holman, B. Garada, K. A. Johnson, et al., A comparison of brain perfusion SPECT in cocaine abuse and AIDS dementia complex, *J. Nucl. Med. 33*: 1312 (1992).

54. M. A. Rosci, F. Pigorini, A. Bernabei, et al., Methods for detecting early signs of AIDS dementia complex in asymptomatic HIV-1-infected subjects, *AIDS 6*: 1309 (1992).

55. W. W. Orrison, *Functional Brain Imaging*, Mosby, St. Louis, 1995.

56. C. C. Kuni, F. S. Rhame, M. J. Meier, et al., Quantitiative I-123-IMP brain SPECT and neuropsychological testing in AIDS dementia, *Clin. Nucl. Med. 16*:174 (1991).

57. D. K. Menon, J. G. Ainsworth, I. J. Cox, et al., Proton MR spectroscopy of the brain in AIDS dementia complex, *J. Comput. Assist. Tomogr. 16*:538 (1992).

58. W. K. Chong, B. Sweeney, I. D. Wilkinson, et al., Proton spectroscopy of the brain in HIV infection: Correlation with clinical, immunologic, and MR imaging findings, *Radiology 188*:119 (1993).

59. W. K. Chong, M. Paley, I. D. Wilkinson, et al., Localized cerebral proton MR spectroscopy in HIV infection and AIDS, *AJNR 15*:21 (1994).

60. D. J. Meyerhoff, S. MacKay, L. Bachman, et al., Reduced brain N-acetylaspartate suggests neuronal loss in cognitively impaired human immunodeficiency virus-seropositive individuals: In vivo 1H magnetic resonance spectroscopic imaging, *Neurology 43*:509 (1993).

61. J. R. McConnell, S. Swindells, C. S. Ong, et al., Prospective utility of cerebral proton magnetic resonance spectroscopy in monitoring HIV infection and its associated neurological impairment, *AIDS Res. Hum. Retroviruses 10*:977 (1994).

62. I. D. Wilkinson, M. Paley, W. K. Chong, et al., Proton spectroscopy in HIV infection: Relaxation times of cerebral metabolites, *Magn. Reson. Imaging 12*: 951 (1994).

63. J. Vion-Dury, G. S. Confort, F. Nicoli, et al., Localized brain proton MRS metabolic patterns in HIV-related encephalopathies, *CR Acad. Sci. III 317*:833 (1994).

64. P. B. Barker, R. R. Lee, and J. C. McArthur, AIDS dementia complex: Evaluation with proton MR spectroscopic imaging, *Radiology 195*:58 (1995).

65. P. A. Bottomley, C. J. Hardy, J. P. Cousins, et al., AIDS dementia complex: Brain high-energy phosphate metabolite deficits, *Radiology 176*:407 (1990).

66. R. F. Deicken, B. Hubesch, P. C. Jensen, et al., Alterations in brain phosphate metabolite concentrations in patients with human immunodeficiency virus infection, *Arch. Neurol. 48*:203 (1991).

67. D. M. Feeney, and J. -C. Baron, Diaschisis, *Stroke 17*:817 (1986).

68. J. M. Hoffman, H. A. Waskin, T. Schifter, et al., FDG-PET in differentiating

lymphoma from nonmalignant central nervous system lesions in patients with AIDS, *J. Nucl. Med. 34*:567 (1993).

69. J. Balakrishnan, P. S. Becker, A. J. Kumar, et al., Acquired immunodeficiency syndrome: Correlation of radiologic and pathologic findings in the brain, *Radiographics 10*:201 (1990).

70. A. G. Osborne, Brain tumors and tumorlike masses: Classification and differential diagnosis, *Diagnostic Neuroradiology* (A. G. Osborne, ed.), Mosby, St. Louis, 1994, p. 673.

23

Brain Imaging in Chronic Fatigue Syndrome

Jennifer Cousins and Michael Gonzalez
Duke University Medical Center, Durham, North Carolina

I. INTRODUCTION

Chronic fatigue syndrome (CFS) is a debilitating disorder characterized by sustained easy fatigability with a cluster of neurological, immunological, affective, and cognitive symptoms not attributable to other medical conditions [1]. The illness usually presents with a sudden onset of flulike symptoms followed by a chronic state of fatigue with other somatic signs and symptoms including fevers, myalgia, sore throat, headaches, arthralgia, muscle weakness, enlarged lymph nodes, as well as affective and neuropsychological complaints. Depression, memory impairment, difficulty concentrating, word searching, and disturbances in abstract thinking are common neurocognitive findings and implicate the central nervous system in the CFS disease process [2].

II. CASE DEFINITION

The syndrome of chronic fatigue has been described in medical literature since the early seventeenth century and has been referred to by terms including neuromyasthenia, myalgic encephalopathy, chronic Epstein-Barr virus (EBV) syndrome, postviral fatigue syndrome, as well as chronic fatigue syndrome. Due to the similarities of clinical presentation of this syndrome and variability of nomenclature applied by clinicians, the Centers for Disease Control (CDC) proposed a research case definition for CFS in 1988 [1]. According to the case definition, diagnosis of CFS requires the patient to meet two defined "major criteria" and eight or more "minor criteria." The major criteria include abrupt onset of persistent or relapsing fatigue or a state of easy fatigability that does not resolve with bedrest, is severe enough to impair average daily activity below 50% of premorbid level, and lasts for a period of 6 months or more. Exclusion of other potentially causative clinical conditions is also required. The minor criteria are subdivided into 11 "symptom criteria" and 3 "physical criteria." The symptom criteria include sore throat, muscle weakness, and myalgias, and the three physical criteria are low-grade fever, nonexudative pharyngitis, and palpable lymph nodes [1,3].

A. Etiology Hypotheses

Although chronic fatigue syndrome has been described clinically by various names throughout the world and has been defined according to the CDC's "uniform" case definition, the origin and pathophysiology of CFS remains unclear. Several hypotheses exist regarding the etiology of CFS [4]. One theory focuses on the syndrome as an immunological dysfunction. Viral infection has been proposed as the possible source of the immune dysfunction, either by causing a persistent immune activation or by inefficient destruction of virus-infected cells. Immunological laboratory findings support the theory of a low-grade immune system activation. Another hypothesis emphasizes the neuropsychological abnormalities of CFS, attributing symptoms to a primary affective disorder, specifically depression. Due to the presence of biological as well as behavioral findings in a large portion of CFS patients, it has recently been theorized that CFS may be a result of endocrine dysfunction of the hypothalamic-pituitary-adrenal axis (HPA) [4]. The occurrence of immunological, neuroendocrine, neurological, affective, as well as cognitive abnormalities suggests that the CNS plays a role in the pathophysiology of CFS. Researchers, therefore, have begun to utilize brain imaging and cerebral blood flow techniques to investigate potential neuroanatomical and neu-robiological abnormalities.

Due to the lack of conclusive evidence regarding the etiology and patho-physiology of CFS, controversy exists in the medical field. Many have ar-gued that CFS is a heterogeneous disorder with multiple origins. A high lifetime prevalence of depression and dysthymia in the CFS patient popula-tion begs the question of what role affective disorders play. Some clinicians quickly dismiss CFS as being solely an atypical depression. Recent research has utilized disorders with similar presentations, such as depression, multiple sclerosis (MS), or AIDS dementia complex (ADS), as control groups. Subse-quently, differences between these groups have been illuminated, fueling the debate. Given the affective findings in the CFS patient population, neuroim-aging abnormalities that have been demonstrated thus far, and the current controversy within the medical community, further review of neuroimaging abnormalities is warranted.

B. Magnetic Resonance Imaging

Several recent studies using magnetic resonance imaging (MRI) have all dem-onstrated brain abnormalities in patients with CFS [3,5–9]. The abnormalities most frequently found by MRI are T_2-weighted signal hyperintensities in white matter regions. Daugherty et al. [3] found that 15 out of 20 CFS patients showed punctate foci of increased T_2-weighted signal intensity in the upper centrum semiovale and bilaterally in the upper parasagital convolutional white matter tracts. Less commonly seen in this study were nonperiventricu-lar deep frontal and peripheral white matter patchy areas of increased signal intensity [3]. Similarly, Buchwald et al. [5] reported that 113 of 144 (78%) patients with CFS showed MRI abnormalities, most commonly foci of T2 signal hyperintensities in subcortical white matter regions compared to 10 of 47 (21%) matched healthy controls. Strayer et al. [6] also found that 40% of 89 CFS patients showed MRI abnormalities as judged by three different readers. These abnormalities also typically involved white matter regions. Another study, in which two blinded neuroradiologists rated MRI scans, found that 14 of 52 CFS patients' scans were rated as abnormal compared to 1 of 52 matched controls who had received clinical MRI scans due to history of head trauma or headache [7]. Abnormalities included signal hyper-intensities and ventricular and sulcal enlargement. Schwartz et al. [8] also reported that 8 of 16 (50%) CFS subjects demonstrated T2 punctate signal hyperintensities in the centrum semiovale, corona radiata, internal capsule, periventricular region, or subcortical white matter compared to 3 of 15 (20%) age-matched controls. On average, patients demonstrated 2.06 foci of signal hyperintensity, while controls had an average of 0.80 of these abnormal foci.

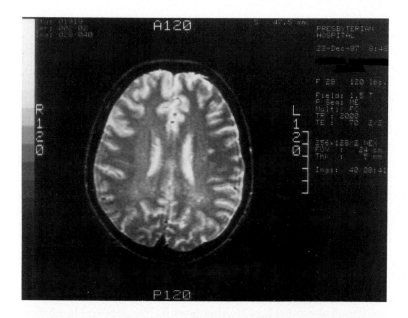

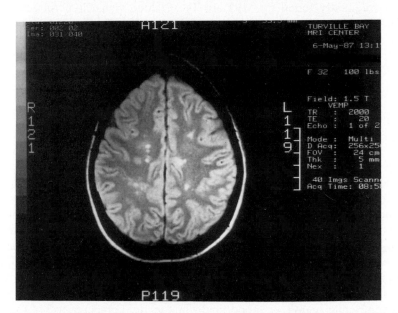

Fig. 1 Typical T_2-weighted white matter signal hyperintensities found in CFS patients on axial MRI. (Images courtesy of Paul R. Cheney, M.D., Ph.D., of The Cheney Clinic, Charlotte, NC.)

When MRI and single-photon emission computed tomography (SPECT) scans were compared in these same patients, SPECT revealed more abnormalities. Regional coorelation between abnormalities was not found when the two neuroimaging techniques were compared. Follow-up (10 weeks to 4 years) MRI scans in 4 of these patients did not reveal any changes over time in the pattern of MRI abnormalities, suggesting that the changes may be irreversible. Figure 1 illustrates T_2-weighted white matter signal hyperintensities in a CFS patient on axial MRI.

C. Single-Photon Emission Computed Tomography

In addition to MRI, recent SPECT studies have also shown brain abnormalities in CFS patients [6,8,10]. Ishise et al. [10] demonstrated that 48 of 60 (80%) CFS subjects showed significantly diminished ratios of regional cerebral blood flow versus 14 normal control subjects. The major brain regions with diminished blood flow were 63% in the frontal lobe, 35% in the temporal lobe, 53% in the parietal lobe, 38% in the occipital lobe, and 40% in the basal ganglia [10]. Schwartz et al. [8] also found SPECT evidence for impaired regional cerebral blood flow (rCBF) in CFS. This study showed that 13 of 16 CFS patients had significantly more defects throughout the cerebral cortex compared to 3 of 14 normal subjects. Four patients had follow-up SPECT studies within a 6-month period. Three of these patients improved clinically, and, in these subjects a decrease in the number of perfusion deficits appeared to correlate with clinical improvement [8]. Additionally, Schwartz et al. [9] conducted a study in which 45 CFS patients were compared to 27 AIDS dementia complex patients, 14 unipolar depression patients, and 38 healthy controls. The CFS, ADS, and depression groups all tended to have perfusion defects in the frontal and temperal lobes. It is speculated that these regionally similar defects may explain the similar cognitive and affective symptoms associated with these disorders. Of the four groups, the ADS patients showed the highest number of perfusion defects, while the CFS and depressed patients demonstrated a similar number of defects, and the normal controls had the fewest number of defects. SPECT also revealed that CFS and ADS patients had significantly lower indices of midcerebral uptake than depressed patients and controls. A negative correlation was found between defect number and midcerebral uptake index for CFS and ADS patients. This correlation was not found in depressed patients or controls [8].

III. CONCLUSION

Clinical presentation as well as evidence from imaging research indicate that the CNS plays a role in the pathophysiology of CFS. The MRI and SPECT studies to date collectively suggest an organic basis for the neurocognitive and affective symptoms found in CFS. Specifically, neuroimaging indicates that the pathophysiology of CFS involves brain white matter and subcortical regions and may be analogous to other chronic inflammatory viral disorders, such as AIDS dementia.

As CFS becomes better characterized and aspects of this controversial disorder become more clearly delineated, the relationship between affective findings and CFS will also become better understood. In the meantime, the debate regarding etiology and pathophysiology will likely continue. More research is necessary to further illuminate the neurobiology of this syndrome as well as the potential neuroanatomical correlates of clinical symptoms such as depression and cognitive impairment. As further imaging studies are undertaken and newer imaging techniques, such as magnetic resonance spectroscopy, are applied to CFS, greater understanding will be attained.

REFERENCES

1. G. P. Holmes, J. E. Kaplan, N. M. Gnatz, A. L. Komaroff, L. B. Shonberger, S. E. Straus, J. F. Jones, R. E. Bubois, C. Cunningham-Rundles, S. Pahwa, G. Tosato, L. S. Zegans, D. T. Purtilo, N. Brown, R. T. Schooley, and I. Brus, Chronic fatigue syndrome: A working case definition, *Ann. Intern. Med. 108*: 387 (1988).
2. A. L. Komaroff and D. Buchwald, Symptoms and signs of chronic fatigue syndrome, *Rev. Infect. Dis. 13* (Suppl 1):S8 (1991).
3. S. A. Daugherty, B. E. Henry, D. L. Peterson, R. L. Swarts, S. Bastien, and R. S. Thomas, Chronic fatigue syndrome in northern Nevada, *Rev. Infect. Dis. 13* (Suppl 1):S39 (1991).
4. C. M. A. Swanink, J. H. M. M. Vercoulen, G. Bleijenberg, J. F. M. Fennis, J. M. D. Galama, and J. W. M. Van der Meer, Chronic fatigue syndrome: A clinical and laboratory study with a well matched control group, *J. Int. Med. 237*:499 (1995).
5. D. Buchwald, P. Cheney, D. Peterson, H. Berch, S. Wormsley, A. Geiger, D. Ablashi, Z. Salahuddin, C. Saxinger, R. Biddle, R. Kikinis, F. Jolesz, T. Folks, N. Balachandran, J. Perter, R. Gallo, and A. Komaroff, A chronic illness characterized by fatigue, neurologic and immunologic disorders, and active human herpesvirus type 6 infection, *Ann. Intern. Med. 116* (2):103 (1992).
6. D. R. Strayer, W. A. Carter, I. Brodsky, P. Cheney, D. Peterson, P. Salvato, C. Thompson, M. Loveless, D. E. Shapiro, W. Elsasser, and D. H. Gillespie, A controlled clinical trial with a specifically configures RNA drug, Poly(I)-Poly(C12U), in chronic fatigue syndrome, *Clin. Infect. Dis. 18* (Suppl 1):S88 (1994).
7. B. H. Natelson, J. M. Cohen, I. Brassloff, and H. J. Lee, A controlled study of brain magnetic resonance imaging in patients with the chronic fatigue syndrome, *J. Neurol. Sci. 120* (2):213 (1993).
8. R. Schwartz, B. Garada, A. Komaroff, H. Tice, M. Gleit, F. Jolesz, and B. L.

Holman, Detection of intracranial abnormalities in patients with chronic fatigue syndrome: Comparison of MR imaging and SPECT, *Am. J. Roentgenol. 162* (4):935 (1994).

9. R. Schwartz, A. Komaroff, B. Garada, M. Gleit, T. Doolittle, D. Bates, R. Vasile, and B. L. Holman, SPECT imaging of the brain: Comparison of findings in patients with chronic fatigue syndrome, AIDS dementia complex, and major unipolar depression, *Am. J. Roentgenol. 162* (4):943 (1994).
10. M. Ishise, I. E. Salit, S. E. Abbey, D. G. Chung, B. Gray, J. C. Kirsh, and M. Freedman, Assessment of regional cerebral perfusion by 99T cm-HMPAO SPECT in chronic fatigue syndrome, *Nuclear Med. Commun. 13* (10):767 (1992).

Index

About the Editors

K. RANGA RAMA KRISHNAN is a Professor of Psychiatry, the Head of the Division of Biological Psychiatry, and the Director of the Affective Disorders Program, Duke University Medical Center, Durham, North Carolina. The coeditor of a book and author or coauthor of nearly 200 book chapters and journal publications, he is a member of the American Psychiatric Association, the Society of Biological Psychiatry, and the International Society of Psychoneuroendocrinology, among others. Dr. Krishnan received the M.B.B.S. degree (1978) from the University of Madras, India.

P. MURALI DORAISWAMY is an Assistant Professor of Biological Psychiatry, the Director of Clinical Trials in the Department of Psychiatry, and a Senior Fellow at the Center for the Study of Aging and Human Development, Duke University Medical Center, Durham, North Carolina. The author or coauthor of over 70 book chapters and journal publications, he is also the recipient of the Paul Beeson Faculty Physician Scholars in Aging Research Award from the American Federation for Aging Research. Dr. Doraiswamy received the M.B.B.S. degree (1987) from the University of Madras, India.